TRENDS IN EPIDEMIOLOGY

Publication Number 836

AMERICAN LECTURE SERIES®

A Monograph in

The BANNERSTONE DIVISION *of*
AMERICAN LECTURES IN EPIDEMIOLOGY

Edited by

GORDON T. STEWART, M.D.
Henry Mechan Professor of Public Health
University of Glasgow
Glasgow, Scotland

TRENDS IN EPIDEMIOLOGY

Application to Health Service Research and Training

Edited by

GORDON T. STEWART, M.D.
Henry Mechan Professor of Public Health
University of Glasgow
Glasgow, Scotland

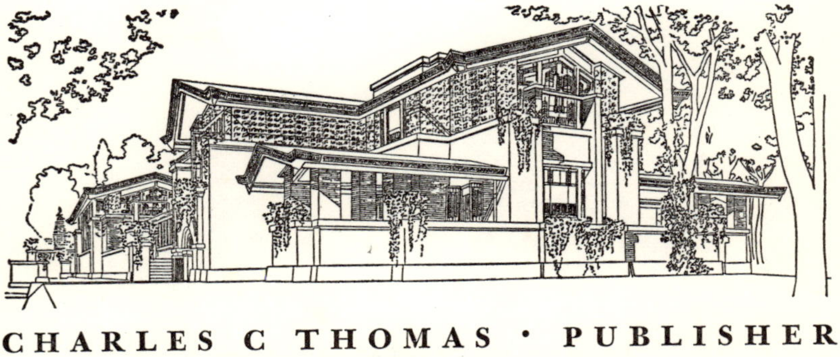

CHARLES C THOMAS · PUBLISHER
Springfield · Illinois · U.S.A.

Published and Distributed Throughout the World by

CHARLES C THOMAS • PUBLISHER

BANNERSTONE HOUSE

301-327 East Lawrence Avenue, Springfield, Illinois, U.S.A.

ISBN 0-398-02422-7

Library of Congress Catalog Card Number 71-175089

With THOMAS BOOKS *careful attention is given to all details of manufacturing and design. It is the Publisher's desire to present books that are satisfactory as to their physical qualities and artistic possibilities and appropriate for their particular use.* THOMAS BOOKS *will be true to those laws of quality that assure a good name and good will.*

Printed in the United States of America

N-1

CONTRIBUTORS

Henry Blackburn, M.D.: Professor of Physiological Hygiene, University of Minnesota, Minneapolis, Minnesota 55455, and Visiting Professor, Institute of Social and Preventive Medicine, University of Geneva, Geneva 1205, Switzerland.

Frederick H. Epstein, M.D.: Professor of Epidemiology, School of Public Health, and Director, Center for Research in Diseases of the Heart, Circulation, and Related Disorders, University of Michigan, Ann Arbor, Michigan 48108.

Oscar Felsenfeld, M.D., M.Sc., D.T.M. & H., F.A.C.P., F.R.S.H., Col. (Ret.) M.C.: Chief, Division of Communicable Diseases, Tulane University Delta Primate Research Center, Covington, Louisiana 70433; Professor, Tulane University School of Public Health and Tropical Medicine; Consultant, World Health Organization; and Temporary Advisor, International Atomic Energy Agency.

George R. Gay, M.D., F.A.C.A.: Chief, Heroin Section and Director, Haight-Ashbury Free Medical Clinic Detoxification, Rehabilitation and Aftercare Project, San Francisco, California 94117; Lecturer in Toxicology (Pharmacology), University of California Medical Center, San Francisco; and Public Health Officer, City and County of San Francisco.

Tavia Gordon: Supervisory Statistician, Biometrics Research Branch, National Heart and Lung Institute, U.S. Public Health Service, Bethesda, Maryland 20014.

C. David Jenkins, Ph.D.: Professor of Epidemiology, The School of Public Health, and Clinical Associate Professor, Department of Psychiatry, The University of North Carolina at Chapel Hill 27514.

KENNETH G. JOHNSON, M.D.: Chairman and Professor, Department of Community Medicine, Dartmouth Medical School, Hanover, New Hampshire 03755; former Professor of Community Medicine, Department of Public Health, Cornell University Medical College, New York, New York 10021.

WILLIAM B. KANNEL, M.D., F.A.C.P., F.A.C.C.: Heart Disease Epidemiology Study, Framingham, Massachusetts.

THEODORE D. LAMPTON, B.S., M.D.: Assistant Professor, Department of Medicine, and Instructor, Department of Preventive Medicine, University of Mississippi School of Medicine, Jackson, Mississippi 39216; Coordinator and Director, Mississippi Regional Medical Program, Jackson, Mississippi 39216.

JEANNE MAGAGNA, R.N., M.A.: Research Associate in Epidemiology, Department of Public Health, Cornell University Medical College, New York, New York 10021.

EDMOND A. MURPHY, M.D., Sc.D.: Associate Professor of Medicine and Biostatistics, Division of Medical Genetics, Department of Medicine, Johns Hopkins University School of Medicine, Baltimore, Maryland 21205.

MICHAEL A. MUSTILLE: Medical student, Cornell University Medical College, New York, New York 10021.

PETER B. PEACOCK, M.D., D.P.H., D.I.H.: Professor and Chairman, Department of Public Health and Epidemiology, University of Alabama in Birmingham 35233, and Visiting Professor of Epidemiology, University of Pennsylvania.

SHERMAN C. RAFFEL, Ph.D.: Associate Professor, Department of Psychiatry, Department of Public Health and Epidemiology, University of Alabama in Birmingham 35233.

CHARLES P. RILEY, M.D.: Fellow in Division of Cardiology, Department of Medicine, University of Alabama.

PHILIP E. SARTWELL, M.D., M.P.H.: Professor of Epidemiology, School of Hygiene and Public Health, The Johns Hopkins University, Baltimore, Maryland 21205.

DAVID SCHOTTENFELD, M.D., F.A.C.P., F.A.C.P.M.: Chief, Clinical Epidemiology and Statistics, Memorial Hospital for Cancer and Allied Diseases, and Associate Professor of Public Health, Cornell University Medical College, New York, New York 10021.

RYAN S. SEARLE: Medical student, Cornell University Medical College, New York, New York 10021.

ROGER SIMON, M.D.: Intern, Department of Medicine, New York Hospital, Cornell Medical Center, New York, New York 10021.

GORDON T. STEWART, M.D., D.T.M. & H., F.R.C. Path.: Henry Mechan Professor of Public Health and Head of the Department of Epidemiology and Social Medicine, University of Glasgow, Glasgow, Scotland; and Consultant Physician, Western Regional Hospital Board, Scotland. Visiting Professor of Epidemiology (1970-71), Cornell University Medical College, New York, New York.

MERVYN SUSSER, M.B., B.Ch., F.R.C.P. (Ed.), D.P.H.: Professor and Head, Division of Epidemiology, School of Public Health and Administrative Medicine, Columbia University, New York, New York 10032.

JOHN S. WALKER, D. Juris.: Assistant Professor, University of Alabama in Birmingham 35233.

KATSUHIKO YANO, M.D.: Assistant Professor of Epidemiology, Department of Public Health, Cornell University Medical College, New York, New York 10021.

PREFACE

TRENDS IN ACADEMIC DISCIPLINES, as in other styles of life, are governed by forces of drift as well as of drive. Epidemiology has drifted from its traditional engagement with infectious disease toward a more diversified involvement in chronic disabilities and diseases. In so doing, it has raised its sight from parasites to hosts, from germs to people, and from people to persons; it has begun to look through demography to society, and through groups to individuals. This drift is part of a movement of academe into the problems of contemporary society and symbolizes increasing awareness in the health sciences generally of the societal and behavioral forces which affect community and personal health, whether or not other etiologic agents are medically identifiable. To extend its competence in these fields, epidemiology has sought and acquired assistance from other disciplines and has converted its drift into a drive of enquiry into practically all aspects of human health and ecology.

This book is intended to present examples of the epidemiological drive into new problems along with renewals of its traditional exploration of older problems, and the Editor is very fortunate indeed in having the cordial cooperation of several well-known experts for the purpose. The first two chapters, by Sartwell and Susser, present historical, philosophical, social and methodological considerations of the subject, as it is presently taught and practiced. Chapters Three (Murphy) and Four (Jenkins) describe the application of two external disciplines, genetics and psychology, which have contributed fresh energy to the new drive. In Chapters Five (Epstein), Six (Gordon and Kannel) and Seven (Blackburn) the numerous etiologic facets of coronary and atherosclerotic disease are reviewed in ways which, collectively, illustrate epidemiological design, prospective study, prediction and multifactor control. Stroke as a major problem of rehabilitation as well as of prevalence is described by Peacock *et al.* in Chapter Eight and communicable disease, as a resurgent threat in developed and underdeveloped communities is examined in Chapter Nine. Cancer in its diversity is discussed by Schottenfeld in Chapter Ten. Following this are three chapters on subjects which are less familiar but potentially very relevant to epidemiology: Chapter Eleven, by Felsenfeld, describing a technical advance which could extend the scope and sensitivity of serochemical surveillance; Chapter Twelve, by Gay, depicting the new epidemic of youth, drug dependence; and Chapter Thirteen, in which students and faculty at Cornell University Medical College together explore health problems and community needs simultaneously in an area of urban decay a few miles away from the golden strip of Manhattan. In the final chapter, an attempt is made to relate the lessons and implications of these trends in epidemiology to service and academic improvement.

The book therefore includes some traditional problems posing new questions about infectious diseases; the new leading causes of chronic morbidity and death—heart, cancer and stroke; the new epidemics, like drug abuse and venereal disease; and, in less detail, the gross national by-products of our civilization—pollution and social upheavals. But the price of selectivity is loss of comprehensiveness and the present volume lacks separate chapters on mental disorders, accidents, arthritis, metabolic and pulmonary disease, each of which deserves attention epidemiologically even if new trends are in these subjects less striking. With these exceptions, the advances handled by the expert authors all have immediate applications to various health services and to the basic role of epidemiology in the health sciences.

The book was compiled by the Editor during a year spent at Cornell University Medical College as Visiting Professor of Epidemiology, and he is indebted to many colleagues and students there for stimulating discussions, especially to Professors Walsh McDermott, Kenneth G. Johnson, Walter Lynn and Thomas Hodgson. Opportunities to view and enter the health arena in New York City were freely provided by Doctor Mary McLaughlin, Commissioner of Health, and Doctor Lawrence Bergner, Assistant Commissioner. Acknowledgment is made gratefully also to Professor John Cassel and his colleagues at the University of North Carolina in Chapel Hill, North Carolina, for instructive years spent in one of the first interdisciplinary departments of epidemiology; and to many students, at all levels and in different disciplines, at the University of North Carolina, at Tulane University, at Cornell University Medical College and at Colleges participating in the Health Research Training Program of New York, for sharing their experiences in community health projects.

This is the first volume of the American Lecture Series on Community Health. It is appropriate therefore that the various authors are contributing their chapters from some of the great Schools of Medicine and Public Health in the United States. To these authors, who are the book, acknowledgment is made most gratefully for their time and cooperativeness no less than for the quality of their chapters. The Editor's preparation for his editorship is largely due to experience gained in the United States, so it behooves him also to acknowledge help in the form of generous research and training grants during the past eight years from the National Science Foundation, the National Institutes of Health and the National Center for Health Service Research and Development. He is indebted also to Miss Berniece Hess and Miss Caroline Sdano for careful editorial assistance, indexing and typing of the manuscripts.

GORDON T. STEWART

CONTENTS

TRENDS IN EPIDEMIOLOGY

Chapter 1

TRENDS IN EPIDEMIOLOGY

PHILIP E. SARTWELL

THE INVITATION which I received to address this group was a very flattering one. It was suggested that my broad experience and years be put to use in giving you a broad view of epidemiology from my vantage point. Naturally, a person who can claim at least the years probably is likely to feel that he can claim the breadth of view as well. And so I rashly accepted the invitation; the qualms came later. I hope that you will bear with me while I make some rather philosophical general comments about trends in epidemiology as I see them.

There is a popular phrase having to do with some of the current ills of mankind which speaks of a crisis of identity. Now I do not know just what a crisis of identity is, but I understand it to refer to uncertainties that now plague people about what their position is in society and, fundamentally, what kind of people they are. I see no evidence that epidemiology as a profession is afflicted, at the present time, with any crisis of identity. I do think, however, a case might be made for such a situation, in a mild way, at about the time when I entered the public health field, in the 1930's. At that time, epidemiology was a little-understood field—perhaps even by its practitioners, who were quite a small number, at least compared with today's. There were a few very competent epidemiologists in the universities, the federal government, and some of the state governments, and that was about it. To be sure, quite a few other people were officially labeled as epidemiologists because in various health departments there were needed young recruits who could be taken on in a training capacity to do various odd jobs, and a convenient label for such apprentices was epidemiologist.

Note: This paper is based on a lecture delivered to the Society for Epidemiologic Research, Minneapolis, Minnesota, on June 26, 1970.

It was about this time that there appeared a series of articles and editorials—some serious, some humorous—dealing with the question, What is an epidemiologist? The definition which I have always liked best was attributed to a former colleague of mine, Doctor Alexander Gilliam. It went this way: "Epidemiology is what an epidemiologist does." Doctor Gilliam denied the authorship of this aphorism, but his name has stuck to it. I am suggesting that the search for a definition of epidemiology which would be acceptable to anybody besides the author of it was symptomatic of a crisis of identity. Since we had some other crises to deal with, including a depression and a world war, we did not react to this one as vigorously as young people react to crises in 1970.

Today the role of epidemiology is much clearer, its definition is less widely divergent among different people, and I think we have a pretty good idea of where we are going. There is perhaps a little danger in this situation, for we may have been more productive when we were on our mettle than we are now that we think we have arrived. I certainly do not intend either to pose a new definition or to suggest a new route. Rather, I should like to examine the question of who speaks most broadly and authoritatively for medicine in these days of fragmentation of medical services and specialties.

In the nineteenth century, when epidemiology made its most dramatic achievements—one thinks of Jenner, Snow, Budd, Panum, and the rest of the great figures of that day—there was no particular specialization in medicine and these people whom I have cited were general practitioners of medicine. It is particularly evident in the work of John Snow that he drew on all of the relevant information from the fields of clinical medicine and pathology in arriving at his hypothesis regarding the transmissibility of cholera, which he tested by epidemiological means when the opportunity arose. As medical specialties began to develop in the latter part of the century, it became evident that the field which had the most to offer at that time in the way of synthesis of ideas and development of unified concepts of disease was pathology. The term pathology really embraced all of the laboratory elements of medicine, including the bacteriology of the day. The pathologist did not treat patients and hence could stand off and take an objective look at sickness. He was the ultimate authority on diagnosis of disease and has tended to be looked upon as the scientific arbiter of medicine since the time of Virchow, or earlier.

I believe a gradual change has been occurring in this respect, and that this change began perhaps in the 1920's or 1930's. It is a change which has placed the epidemiologist in a more central position, in my opinion, than that of practitioners in most other fields of medicine, although this is a position which he certainly must still share with the pathologist and with some other groups, such as internists. The change came about through the recognition that the distribution of disease in a population is a tremendously important facet of disease: that its interpretation goes to the roots of the causation of disease, and that if one hopes to really understand disease, he must understand its epidemiology and must try to integrate the epidemiologic findings with the other known findings, such as the pathological, immunological, biochemical, and clinical findings—in fact, the entire description and natural history of disease. Also, the epidemiologist finds himself in the position of helping to define disease. To classify disease entities is an activity which is not entirely clinical and to which the epidemiologist is able to bring to bear a special set of skills.

Another phenomenon that has come into play is the advent of team research. You are all familiar with this trend; one simple illustration of it that I would like to mention this morning concerns the number of coauthors on scientific papers. For this purpose I chose two periods in the evolution of the *American Journal of Epidemiology,* which was formerly known as the *American Journal of Hygiene*. The distribution of numbers of coauthors of papers published in the first three volumes of the *Journal,* back in the period 1921-23 inclusive, has been tabulated along with the number of authors of papers published in the most recent complete volume to which I had access (Fig. 1.1). There has been a dramatic shift from predominance of single-author papers to ones with several authors. In the earlier period, 59 percent of papers had a single author; in the second period, forty-six years later, the mode was at three authors, only 7 percent having a

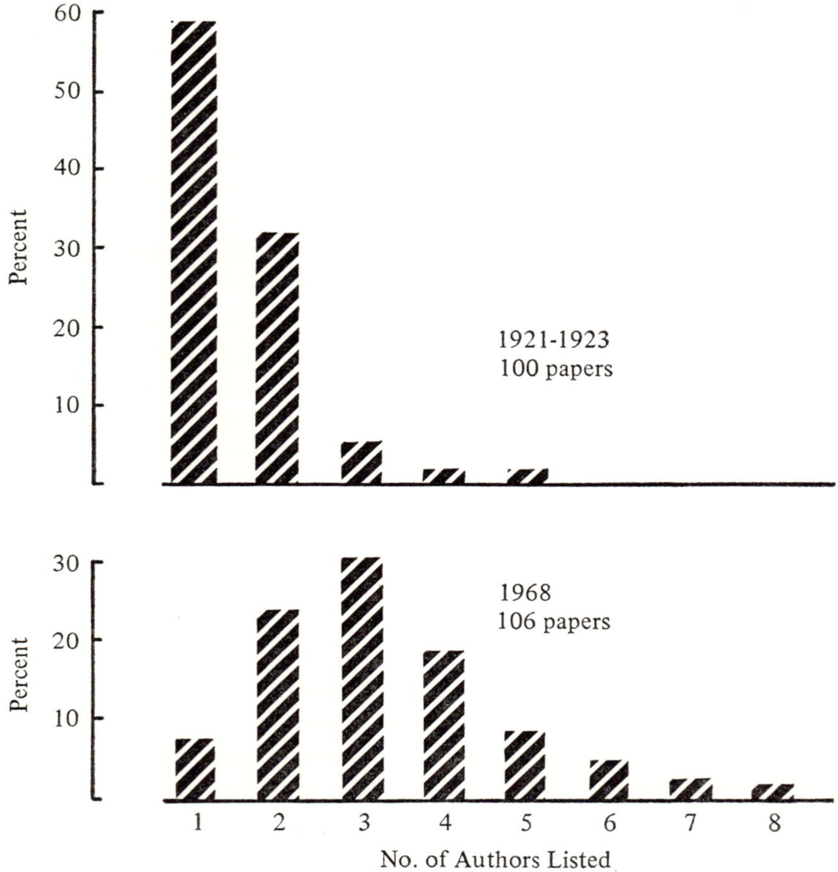

Figure 1.1 Percent distribution of papers published in *American Journal of Hygiene (Epidemiology)* according to number of authors, in two periods.

single author, the maximum number being eight. What this means is that epidemiologists have tended increasingly to seek out collaborators in other fields. They have had to do this because their studies have been interdisciplinary in a great many cases. The explosion of scientific knowledge has made it impossible for such studies to be undertaken by a single individual and so we find epidemiologists collaborating with internists, pediatricians, microbiologists, biochemists, pathologists, and statisticians, to name but a few of the many groups involved. In these research endeavors the epidemiologist frequently takes a prominent position. He may be the individual who puts the findings of the group together and develops and defends the hypothesis of the study. It is in this sense that I suggest that epidemiology has somewhat supplanted the laboratory sciences and particularly pathology as an integrating element in medical science.

We applaud this interdisciplinary approach to problems. It is well illustrated, for instance, when speakers on chemical carcinogenesis bring the results of experimental pathology, industrial medicine, biochemistry, and molecular biology into consideration. It is essential that epidemiologists get into a corner at times, but equally essential that they keep in touch with the extraordinary advances in other fields.

A corollary to the burgeoning number of collaborators is the pace at which research proceeds. One might expect it to have accelerated because of the added manpower available, but a case can be made for the opposite having occurred with respect to individual projects. Let me illustrate and, following in the footsteps of far more illustrious people, use as my illustration John Snow.[1] The first edition of his monograph on the mode of communication of cholera was published in 1849. With the revisit of cholera to London in 1854 he was presented with another chance to study it, and having a prepared mind he made the most of his chance. Let me remind you of the chronology of events in that hectic summer of 1854. The Broad Street epidemic began on August 31 of that year. His investigation of the epidemic in the south districts of London evidently took place in July and August, some data becoming available only late in the year. As he states, "The inquiry was necessarily attended with a good deal of trouble," trouble which he goes on to describe and then to explain the means used to circumvent it. He did employ one assistant for a part of the study. He made his own chemical analyses of the water, paid his own visits to the affected houses, made his own arrangements with the Registrar General, and submitted the manuscript on December 11, 1854, three months after the Golden Square episode and less than that after the subsidence of the epidemic south of the Thames. It may be supposed that during this period he had to pay some attention to his medical practice as well.

One may reflect on how such an investigation might be conducted in, let us say, 1970 in the United States. I am sure the principal investigator, an epidemiologist, would feel it necessary to have a clinician, a biostatistician, and a sanitary engineer on his team at a minimum. After recruiting this group, a study plan and a budget would need to be developed. Next would come submission of the project to a granting agency, probably the federal government. In the course of time a site visit would follow. At this point my discussion becomes unrealistic, for I will assume the project would be approved and funded on its first submission, which probably would not happen in this year of federal economy. The time assigned to these successive steps is anyone's guess, but unless the Epidemic Intelligence Service made the investigation, it would take a long time. Nor is this all. A modern investigator would no doubt want to put his data on a computer. Now my experience with computers is unenlightened. I find that by the time you have located and instructed a programmer, have had a program written and debugged, and then have obtained machine time and secured printouts of the data analyses, you have spent several times as long as would be required to secure the same analyses by old-fashioned methods. This view of computer science is a penalty you have to pay for listening to an aging epidemiologist, but I can document it.

Seriously, my example is intended to point up a distressing characteristic of contemporary epidemiology, especially in chronic disease. This is the slow pace of research. The biochemist, as it seems to an outsider, gets a clue from his last experiment; he sets up a fresh experiment in his laboratory to test his new hypothesis and he gets an answer and the whole process can sometimes take less than a week. Contrast this to the pace of a prospective study of a chronic disease. There may be some useful side products along the way, but it is likely to take five years before there is any payoff in terms of the hypothesis. It is hard for the scientist so to steel himself and curb his impatience as to be satisfied with this way of life, and many of us cannot be happy with it. Also, it does not enhance our reputations and our bibliographies very fast, to put the matter in perhaps too cynical a way.

The development of interdisciplinary interest has gone on in parallel with the increasing breadth of application of epidemiology, from a field which was almost exclusively concerned with infectious disease to one which rather ambitiously declares itself as being concerned with all disease and abnormalities of physiological state, as well as trauma. I think that a cohort analysis of the interests of epidemiologists would be of interest. Among the most senior group there are few who did not first have an interest in infectious disease. One of the most distinguished of our epidemiologic leaders has unfortunately just left the scene; I am thinking of Dr. Thomas Francis, Jr. In his early days, Dr. Francis was a clinical and laboratory investigator whose interest centered on influenza. From this he broadened out to encompass a great many interests, including a vital role in broadening the investigations conducted by the Atomic Bomb Casualty Commission. Among the members of this audience, on the other hand, I imagine the majority have not had a primary preoccupation with infectious disease even at the outset of their careers. Viewing epidemiology as the application of a special method, I cannot see why we should worry about making any distinctions between infectious disease and chronic disease epidemiology. The methods of approach have been different in the past, but this has been by historical accident and I think that the distinction is unimportant.

I have traced what has seemed to me to be a common bond of epidemiology and pathology, namely, that they have both attempted the task of integrating medical findings. This is borne out by the fact that pathologists sometimes refer to the field of "geographic pathology," which is pretty close to what we mean by epidemiology, and by the fact that August Hirsch,[2] a German worker of the latter part of the nineteenth century, gave a definition of the field that he was treating in his comprehensive three-volume work which I think would serve admirably as a definition of epidemiology today, ninety years after it was written. Most of you, I hope, are familiar with this definition, but I will quote it again:

> In these considerations lie the germs of a science which in an ideally complete form would furnish a medical history of mankind but which treated more narrowly and so as to embrace only the pathological side of human life will give firstly, a picture of the occurrence, distribution and the types of the diseases of mankind, in distinct epochs of time and at various points of the earth's surface; and secondly, will render an account of the relations of those diseases to the external conditions surrounding the individual and determining his manner of life. And this science I have named from the dominating point of view the science of Geographical and Historical Pathology.

My suggestion is that were Hirsch writing this paragraph today, he would change the words hardly at all, except that he might change the name of the science to epidemiology.

Among the many diseases to which epidemiology has contributed heavily, I would like to use as an example one which still is in a pretty unsatisfactory state but much better understood than formerly. This is chronic nonspecific respiratory disease, or, if you will, chronic bronchitis. I can well remember being told while in medical school that the latter term was just a cover-up for ignorance, that no such thing as a primary chronic bronchitis existed and the term should never be used. This kind of denial is one way of dealing with an uncomfortable problem but is not to be recommended. This was pretty much the state of affairs for a good many years. The main reasons were that we had no diagnostic tools such as x-ray, culture, or blood test by which a case could be confirmed, the lesions were not accessible to pathological examination, and few persons died as a direct consequence of the disease.

The main advances in understanding chronic respiratory disease have been made by British workers, which should not surprise us, for its prevalence appears higher in Britain than elsewhere. A notable advance was the development of a standardized questionnaire, as distinguished from a clinical history. This evolved into the now widely known MRC questionnaire, which has recently been translated into Japanese and independently translated back into English to see if any change in meaning had been introduced. In the hands of properly trained interviewers this questionnaire is a reasonably precise tool for judging the presence and degree of severity of any chosen combination of respiratory symptoms. Combined with simple ventilatory function tests, it has made possible for the first time the conducting of meaningful international comparative surveys and has permitted the firm documentation of the quantitative role of cigarette smoking and atmospheric pollution in this disease. The point I wish to emphasize is that epidemiology has contributed largely to the clinical definition of this disease and has also established some of the important and avoidable etiologic agents. I can see no other way in which these goals could have been reached.

This example points up well two of the characteristics of the so-called "epidemiologic method," a favored term which people seldom bother to define and which most of us probably could not define without considerable pause. These two characteristics are, firstly, employing standardized, meaningful tests of known accuracy or, if this is impossible, at least known and hopefully high precision, and making these tests as quantitative in nature as is feasible, and secondly, basing the investigation on the whole population and not merely on the hospitalized ill segment of the population. There are situations in which studies must be limited to hospitalized patients and appropriate controls, always remembering their relation to the population, but with a ubiquitous condition like bronchitis, for which medical care may never be sought, it is imperative to study the whole population, or—a less satisfactory substitute—a group such as industrial workers, who may be considered reasonably representative.

An equally good example of the importance of both these elements in the epidemiologic method is seen in the development of knowledge about tuberculosis through use of the tuberculin test. Here, quantitation of dosage and reaction size in relation to exposure and geography and application of the test to whole populations produced a reversal of several strongly held beliefs which were hampering progress.

At this point, I should like to raise for consideration the questions of what some of the directions are in which epidemiology should and will go, and what some of the problems are that it should attempt to solve in the future. I do not refer to the distant future, for this would be too hazardous, but to the immediate future. Our field has come of age; it is now recognized widely as being useful to medicine. I do not mean to imply that clinicians now call upon epidemiological personnel, concepts, and methods as often as they should, but many of them are moving in that direction. Teaching of this subject in medical schools is improving.

One valuable undertaking is to put epidemiology more effectively to work in aiding the clinician to identify disease syndromes and find their causes. This is the same task described earlier for chronic respiratory disease. It should be directed especially toward the diseases seen by those medical specialists who have not been especially aware of the epidemiologic approach in the past. An interest in ophthalmological problems has involved some of my associates, for example, in studies of certain lesions of the uveal tract and this group, led by a clinical ophthalmologist, has now shown convincingly that certain chorioretinal scars are closely related to histoplasmin sensitivity and presumably have *H. capsulatum* as their etiologic agent.[3]

The process of differentiation of syndromes and diseases has come a long way from the days of "fever hospitals." Doubtless there are many further differentiations that need to be made, but I also wonder if we do not have some distinctions without a difference. Just as the essential unity of streptococcal infection and scarlet fever was long ago shown, and as the probable identity of Hashimoto's disease with chronic thyroiditis was more recently demonstrated, other such identities remain to be discovered. Another aspect of this topic is the interrelationship of distinct diseases when they coexist in the same patient. Often the attempt to study one condition when others are highly prevalent in the population will lead to conflicting or erroneous findings unless the patient's whole burden of diseases is considered. For an elementary example, serological tests for a particular disease may be greatly influenced in either direction by other common infections which the patient may have or have had.

I shall only mention three very important areas, simply because their importance requires no documentation. They are cancer, mental illness, and cardiovascular disease. All are susceptible to advances through intensified epidemiologic study.

Another broad field for investigation is, at the moment, and will continue to be, the effects of the environment on health. While this general problem seems to have come to public attention recently, it has of course been of concern to our profession ever since Potts commented on scrotal cancer of chimney sweeps and Baker showed that lead poisoning was the cause of Devonshire colic—both in the eighteenth century. In fact, it is the central problem of epidemiology.

There is a tendency to regard environmental degradation of all sorts, and especially that which is esthetically offensive, as necessarily harmful to health. One example is pollution of swimming areas; another, the railroad's practice of dumping human wastes on the tracks. It has not been proven that sewage pollution of beaches which is not too severe to be esthetically tolerated is dangerous to health; and Dr. Maxcy, at a time when the railroads were carrying many more passengers than they do now, was unable to find evidence that the waste disposal practice produced typhoid or other enteric diseases. The difficulty of showing whether atmospheric pollution, pollution of water supplies with certain industrial chemical wastes, and wide use of herbicides, insecticides, and food additives are harmful is well known. We should not assume that theoretical hazards are of actual importance, although in many cases it is wisest to act as though they were until we can find out. These are all gigantic tasks which the microbiologist and toxicologist cannot solve without epidemiological assistance.

Finally, I wish to stress one very important area which comes under the general heading of environment but is a special problem, namely, iatrogenic disease. I apologize to the few in this audience who have already heard this part of my remarks.

There have been many forms of iatrogenic disease. I do not mean disease resulting from deliberate quackery but from standard medical practice. The most common of course is drug reactions. Recent studies have for the first time given us an insight into how common these are and how much they contribute to the burden of morbidity and prolongation of hospital stay. This problem is going to grow in importance with the proliferation of new drugs and the unstemmed tendency to administer many drugs in the course of a patient's illness. Some adverse drug reactions are fatal and some do not occur in any close temporal relationship to the administration of the drug. The relation of Chloramphenicol® to aplastic anemia is an example. It is likely that there are others, still unrecognized.

But we should not think that drug reactions are the only form of iatrogenic disease. For two examples of other types, we may turn back again to the nineteenth century. It was before the middle of that century that Semmelweis, Holmes, and other workers concluded that puerperal sepsis was frequently communicated by the medical attendant from patient to patient. Evidence of an epidemiological nature supported by statistical tests of significance was followed by what should have been convincing experimental evidence. Yet it was not until 1878, over a quarter of a century later, that conviction was generally provided by the demonstration of visible microscopic agents of disease and death. Furthermore, the earlier assertions drew fire and vituperation from leaders of the profession.

The case of serum hepatitis is equally curious. In the early 1880's, at least two German physicians reported episodes of jaundice somehow connected with smallpox vaccination using human vaccinia lymph. Yet it was not until the late 1930's that suspicion took shape regarding the capacity of human serum to produce jaundice, and not until 1942 that the matter was established, by epidemiological methods, of course, since these were the only kind of methods available. Over half a century had passed, and while blood transfusion did not enjoy popularity over much of that period, there must have been many cases of serum hepatitis resulting from injections of plasma or serum as well as whole blood. By contrast, the discovery of the bad effects of administration of high concentrations of oxygen to premature infants came about within relatively few years of the first appearance, as a recognized entity, of retrolental fibroplasia.

The facility with which such relationships are recognized depends on the immediacy of the adverse response; reactions coming on a day following use of a drug are easily related to it, while the reason for the delay in understanding serum hepatitis was the interval usually of several months that elapsed between exposure and onset, which obscured the relationship. Another factor, of course, is the incidence of the adverse reaction; another, the frequency of the same or an indistinguishable condition occurring spontaneously in the population; and still another is the frequency of use of the drug or agent in the population. Finally, what has been termed the "biological reasonableness" of the phenomenon must be invoked to explain the refusal to accept such things as the contagiousness of puerperal sepsis. The medical profession was not prepared on the basis of mid-nineteenth century knowledge, understanding, and philosophy to accept the theory of contagion except as applied to a few diseases.

A recent instance that illustrates these points and, in fact, may serve as a prototype is the case of birth-control pills and thromboembolism. Assuming, although not all would agree with this, that oral contraceptives have been shown to be related to thromboembolism, we may see that the difficulty in showing a relationship, despite the extremely large number of women who took the pill, was due to the fact that the disease did not usually come on at once but might be delayed until the pill had been used for months or even years, that it did occur spontaneously with considerable frequency, and that the increase in frequency under the influence of female sex hormones was not of great magnitude.

The usual sequence of events leading to the recognition of an iatrogenic condition has been, first, the publication of case reports, with speculation as to their meaning, next, the accumulation of such reports and publication of summary reviews of the situation, and then, the attempt at an orderly system of complete reporting. At this point, if not before, it becomes evident to all that strong and convincing evidence of etiology cannot be anticipated from such data in a case like the oral contraceptive-thromboembolism one. There are several reasons for this. Until there exists a suspicion of causation, one cannot expect any case reports to be made, while afterward, there is likely to be overreporting of the association from some quarters and underreporting from others, particularly if there is any reason to fear medico-legal complications. And the situation at this point can be summed up in one or both of the epidemiological expressions, "no denominator" or "no controls." Case reporting cannot be expected to be complete and unbiased, and even if it were, that would not be enough. In short, except where the risk is very great, systems of individual "adverse reaction reports" solicited from hospitals or practicing physicians will not suffice for the identification of risks and certainly not for their quantification.

Assuming that animal experiments cannot provide an answer, the next step needs to be a specifically epidemiological study, of one of two types: population-based or case-control. I shall return to these contrasting methods and their respective advantages a little later.

Another area where collaborative epidemiologic research is urgently needed is the possible carcinogenicity of oral contraceptives. I mention this not because I think there is any substantial evidence to worry about this problem, but because with so many women using these products it is imperative that surveillance be maintained.

There are, of course, other potential hazards with which modern technology has presented us which are not iatrogenic but which might yield to similar methods. The cases of acute myocardial failure attributed to consumption of large quantities of beer containing trace amounts of cobalt have attracted attention recently. The risk of cancer from ingestion of cyclamates was decided on the basis of animal experiments which do not seem entirely relevant to human experience. The number of substances classified as GRAS (generally regarded as safe) and added for various technical reasons to foods and beverages is very large and new additives are being developed almost daily. There is need for long-term study of persons occupationally heavily exposed to various chemicals, such as insecticides and herbicides, which in much smaller doses have been feared as potentially injurious. But the medical profession has a special obligation to maintain surveillance over the possible risks that may some day be laid at its own door.

The recognition of iatrogenic disease is technically the type of problem for which epidemiologic methods are well suited. As with the common-vehicle epidemic of typhoid of yesteryear—and the hepatitis epidemic of 1970, for this type of hazard has not disappeared, though it appears in new guises—it is satisfying to get back to the single-etiology situation, where one seeks to identify a specific cause or vehicle of disease, the effects of which may be modified by host and environment factors but which is still essentially unitary.

Attitudes toward the retrospective type of study have changed in the past two decades, at least among epidemiologists and statisticians. Any discussion of this topic nowadays demands a definition of the term at the outset, as its usage varies, especially in clinical circles, and this has led to much confusion. The terms "retrospective" and "prospective," often used to denote two contrasting types of study, should really be abandoned because of this confusion. I have for some years employed the terms "case-control" (or "case-history") for the type of investigation which begins by identifying a series of already diagnosed cases of a disease or condition to be studied, selects a control group, who may be either well persons or cases of other (often a variety of) diseases, and obtains information as to pertinent attributes of both groups for comparative purposes. The most widely known of these studies were the many which with impressive regularity found that cases of lung cancer gave histories of smoking cigarettes much more frequently and heavily than did controls.

By contrast, a prospective, population-based, or cohort type of study identifies groups of people who are well or who at any rate do not at present have the disease under investigation, characterizes them as to the attribute of interest, and follows them over time to observe the incidence of one or more diseases or conditions. Thus, a cigarette-smoking contingent and as comparable a control group of nonsmokers as could be found might be followed to observe the incidence of lung cancer—and coronary artery disease, too, if desired. Such a study generally begins with the identification of persons who are *presently* free from disease, but this is not necessary. For example, Seltser and I[4] undertook in the 1950's to examine the mortality experience of radiologists and other medical specialist groups from the date of joining specialty societies. We went back to 1920 to identify these individuals and carried the observations up to 1958. Was this a prospective or retrospective study? The events examined were in the past, hence the study in the most familiar sense of the word was a retrospective one. But in fact, according to the definition provided above, it was a typical population-based, or cohort, study. This illustrates the confusion over the terms and supports the abandonment of the term "retrospective."

Suspicion of case-control studies, in the past, has been on the basis of unavoidable and undetectable biases that were thought to exist in the selection of cases. A second factor was the difficulty of selecting controls representative of whatever population one felt they should represent. But the bias was the more important question. Two studies in particular may have contributed to this fear. One was a comparison of all autopsied patients at a hospital who died of cancer with all autopsied patients who did not have cancer. The issue of interest was the frequency with which active tuberculous lesions were found at autopsy in the two groups. A marked dissociation of cancer and tuberculosis was claimed, but this was soon found to be erroneous. Later, Berkson[5] showed that it was readily possible for biases to produce a spurious association of diseases among hospital patients. However, the use of this type of study for testing associations between a disease and an attribute (not another disease) seems to be less subject to these concerns. Most statisticians have been guarded in their acceptance of the case-control method; Dorn[6] made a thoughtful appraisal of it.

Yet this method has great appeal. It is the natural way in which clinicians confronted with patients get their initial hypotheses of etiologic factors in disease. Their "controls" are generally only vaguely formulated impressions of the usual frequency of the attributes in other patients they have seen. While many such hypotheses turn out to be wrong, they are a main wellspring of new ideas in epidemiology and must not be disregarded.

One type of bias is common to case-and-control studies which rely upon historical information given by the patient. This is the tendency of patients or their families to give affirmative answers to questions more often than controls would do. It may be expected to operate when the patient is aware of the suspicion that the factor is connected with the disease and when the disease is a very serious one that has led the patient, or the patient's mother, to reflect at length on the past history. A remedy for this kind of bias lies in verification from an independent source of the historical information in question, when this is possible.

The list of diseases in which the case-control method has been effective in pointing to important associations, later confirmed by other and supposedly more reputable methods, is a long one. On the other side of the coin, there are not many instances in which a conclusion reached by this method has been invalidated. This pragmatic observation should convince the skeptic that the method has great utility. There are kinds of studies in which the population-based approach has obvious advantages: for example, the trial of an immunizing agent against a frequent disease like influenza. In rare diseases, on the other hand, one either does a case-control study or no study at all, for the prospective method is impossibly difficult to carry out within a reasonable time span.

Apart from the frequency of the disease, a main issue which will determine which type of study to do is whether a hypothesis already exists that can be explored by the case-control method or whether one is primarily concerned with an attribute which might have a variety of health consequences. Thus, employees in an industry with exposure to a possibly toxic chemical would best be studied by the population-based method, since this if done in appropriate detail will reveal any major medical outcome of the exposures, rather than just those already suspected.

Perhaps the most important advantage of the population-based approach is its ability to provide comparative incidence figures. The case-control method allows the estimation of relative risks, but a fivefold excess risk of a rare condition is of different consequence from a similar excess risk in a common (and equally serious) condition. Often, however, it is possible to estimate disease frequencies from independent sources without relying on a population-based study.

One reason for the popularity of the population-based method may be that it is confused in some people's minds with the experimental method, in which deliberate random allocation to alternate groups is carried out. No one doubts the greater power of experimental as contrasted with observational methods, but experimental methods can seldom be used in human epidemiology. The population-based studies under discussion are observational in character. Therefore we cannot be sure, in this kind of study any more than in the other kind, that associations between an attribute and a disease are not due to some other, hidden covariable.

Optimal methods for case-control studies have not yet been attained, by any means. The central problems concern the control group. If the patient series is derived from one or more hospitals, should the controls, too, be hospital patients or should they be a sample of the local population? No general answer to this question can yet be given, and indeed the answer must probably depend on how completely the selected hospitals provide service to a definable population. If patients are chosen as controls, what conditions are best to select? Any disease or injury chosen will of course have its own epidemiologic features. Another problem is how to select controls on the basis of such characteristics as will make them more nearly like the cases of the disease under investigation. Clearly, their sex and age distribution must somewhat resemble those of the cases, but there exists a problem of "overmatching" that I have discussed elsewhere.[7] Many workers prefer to do only minimal or no matching because they fear the occurrence of unwanted and unrecognized forms of selectivity from close matching. The alternative to matching is, of course, some form of adjustment for influential factors. One of the strongest arguments in favor of matching arises when ascertainment of characteristics of controls is difficult or expensive (as when a home interview must be conducted or an elaborate biochemical determination done). In this situation available funds, if limited, may permit inclusion of only a limited number of controls. Rather close matching is then more efficient in providing a directly comparable control group of adequate size.

Along with the wider use of the case-control method has come an increase in the exploitation of human communities for epidemiologic purposes. It has been demonstrated that the opportunities for population-based studies are multiplied when single communities are selected for intensive study. Examples in this country which come to mind are the diabetes studies in Oxford, Massachusetts,[8] and other places, the investigations of tuberculosis and, secondarily, of several other diseases in Williamson County, Tennessee, and, later, Muscogee County, Georgia,[9] the heart disease studies in Framingham, Massachusetts, and the wide-ranging studies now going on in Tecumseh, Michigan, and Washington County, Maryland. All these have relied on one or both of two principles: finding out everything that is feasible to learn of the attributes of the inhabitants, by special censuses, and concentrating on the study of incidence or prevalence of selected diseases.

What has been said has been largely colored by the situation in highly developed countries, where most infectious diseases are on the wane. Exceptions are venereal disease (sadly neglected by epidemiologists), influenza and other respiratory infections, viral hepatitis, and a few other problems. But in many developing countries virtually nothing is known about infectious disease incidence outside the largest cities. Here is an area of urgent need for intensive studies, not of one disease at a time but of all diseases and environmental conditions in a few villages selected as representative of geographic, hygienic, or social conditions, as Buck[10] has done. One reason for this different approach is that disease interactions need to be understood before a community's health problems can be most intelligently approached, and multiple infections are the rule in many such places. Another is that, once having put a team in a remote community, it is a waste not to find out all one can about the health of that community. We now possess an impressive armamentarium of serological and biochemical tests, skin tests, bacteriological and parasitological tests, x-rays, clinical procedures, and standardized medical history taking, all adaptable for field use. It is obvious that both for the sake of the residents in these communities and to take advantage of the opportunity to learn more about "exotic" diseases, the present state of ignorance of their problems should no longer be countenanced.

These, then, are some of the directions that seem most fruitful for epidemiologic research in the immediate future. We may be sure of one thing: the needs are for increased exploitation of this method in the period ahead of us. The implications for training and funding in this field are clear.

REFERENCES

1. Snow, J. On the mode of communication of cholera. In *Snow on Cholera: A Reprint of Two Papers.* New York, Commonwealth Fund, 1936.
2. Hirsch, A. *Handbook of Geographical and Historical Pathology.* Trans. from 2nd German ed. London, The New Sydenham Society, 1883, Vols. I-III.
3. Smith, R.E., and Ganley, J.P. An epidemiologic study of presumed ocular histoplasmosis. *Trans. Amer. Acad. Ophthal. Otolaryng.,* in press.
4. Seltser, R., and Sartwell, P.E. The influence of occupational exposure to radiation on the mortality of American radiologists and other medical specialists. *Amer. J. Epidem., 81*:2-22, 1963.
5. Berkson, J. Limitations of the application of fourfold table analysis to hospital data. *Bio. Bull., 2*:47-53, 1946.
6. Dorn, H.F. Philosophy of inferences from retrospective studies. *Amer. J. Public Health, 43*:677-83, 1953.
7. Sartwell, P.E. Oral contraceptives and thromboembolism: a further report. *Amer. J. Epidem., 94*:192-201, 1971.
8. Wilkerson, H.L.C., and Krall, L.P. Diabetes in a New England town. *J.A.M.A., 135*:209-216, 1947.
9. Comstock, G.W. Community research in tuberculosis, Muscogee County, Georgia. *Public Health Rep., 79*:1045-1056, 1964.
10. Buck, A.A., Sasake, T.T., and Anderson, R.I. *Health and Disease in Four Peruvian Villages: Contrasts in Epidemiology.* Baltimore, Johns Hopkins Press, 1968.

Chapter 2

PROCEDURES FOR ESTABLISHING CAUSAL ASSOCIATIONS

MERVYN SUSSER

VEXATION AND CONTROVERSY have surrounded efforts to establish causal factors in disease. It is essential, in this central concern of epidemiologists, to clarify ideas and sharpen the tools that are used. This chapter had its origin in an effort to conceptualize causation in a manner that would help to free epidemiological thinking from outmoded concepts. The most serviceable concepts involve multiple causality,[1,1a] and from this point of view the text of MacMahon *et al.*[2] has provided a useful statement. For the purposes of the present chapter, that statement is accepted as a starting point, and I have not included here my own attempts to develop it further. Given the conceptual framework of sequences and networks of multiple causes, I have aimed to provide a systematic framework for thinking about the procedures by which causation can be established.

The chapter reviews various types of association that have been recognized under the general classifications of symmetrical, asymmetrical, and reciprocal relationships. These relationships present problems of logical inference. The distinctions between them are not self-evident. Associations often appear to be what they are not, and concealed factors give rise to false appearances. A number of strategies for dispelling false inferences are considered in turn. Some are considered more fully than others, according to my own competence and the needs I perceive. Thus research design and statistical approaches are discussed briefly; the search for extraneous sources of variation that can produce

---

Note: The material in this chapter has been expanded by the author in a book *Causal Thinking in the Health Sciences,* to be published by Oxford University Press.

observed associations between variables, the elaboration of the analysis of associated variables, and criteria of judgment are treated at greater length.

The gallimaufry of ill-defined terms that overlap with each other, and their promiscuous use in the literature, make choices among them difficult. For lack of time and resources I have not made a systematic search of the literature. Instead, I have tried to define my own terminology with care, and to indicate clearly the meaning I have either selected for each term, or assigned to it. Sometimes, in the absence of any existing term known to me, an idiosyncratic usage could not be avoided.

One fundamental condition of cause-and-effect relationships is that they are asymmetrical. Another fundamental condition of cause-and-effect relationships is the time sequence of the variables: a causal variable must precede its effects. The determination of a time sequence is not sufficient in itself to demonstrate causality. One variable may precede another in time with absolute regularity, but it is causal only if it produces an effect and the relationship is asymmetrical. Night follows day, and in duration varies inversely with it. But day follows night, and neither causes the other; their relationship is symmetrical.

The search for causes and effects being a central concern of epidemiology, epidemiologists must learn and develop a language of causality. This is not to say that the symmetrical mathematical equation is not useful. For instance, epidemiology has only begun to exploit the full potential of the simple and basic equation $P_t = ID$: the prevalence of a manifestation (P: the ratio of the number existing at a point in time to the defined population at that time) equals the product of the two elements, incidence of the manifestation (I: the rate at which it occurs in a defined population over a defined period of time) and its duration. If two of these three elements are known, the third can be derived.[2] Thus the equation has been used to argue that such conditions as psychoneurosis, psychopathy, schizophrenia, and drug addiction need not be permanent afflictions.[2a]

Now we turn to elaborate types of symmetrical and asymmetrical relationships in more detail.[3]

Symmetrical Relationships

Fortuitous relationships. These occur by chance and need no further explanation.

Functional interdependence. $F = MA$, $P_t = ID$, and the relationship between night and day are of this kind. In such a relationship one variable cannot exist without the other.

Common complex. Many variables commonly occur together without being either interdependent or necessary to each other. An example of a common complex would be the combination in the "culture of poverty" of poor nutrition with crowding, weekly wages, and an orientation toward the present, or the combination of air pollution with crowding, poor housing, and the use of coal for domestic fuel.

Alternative indicators of the same entity. Alternative indicators are often put to use in the research strategies of epidemiology. For instance, exposure to an infectious disease like rubella might be inferred both from immune bodies in the serum and from a history of the disease.

The effects of a common cause. In causal analysis this type of symmetrical relationship is one of greatest concern. For example, low birth weight in the ghettoes of American cities is regularly associated with failure of the mother to obtain prenatal care. A part of this association is explained by the fact that premature labor gives rise both to low birth weight and to the inability of women to attend for prenatal care late in gestation. A premature labor prevents the late attender from signing up and entering the statistics of prenatal clinics late in pregnancy. Insofar as the association can be explained by the third variable, prematurity, the inference of a causal association may be "spurious."

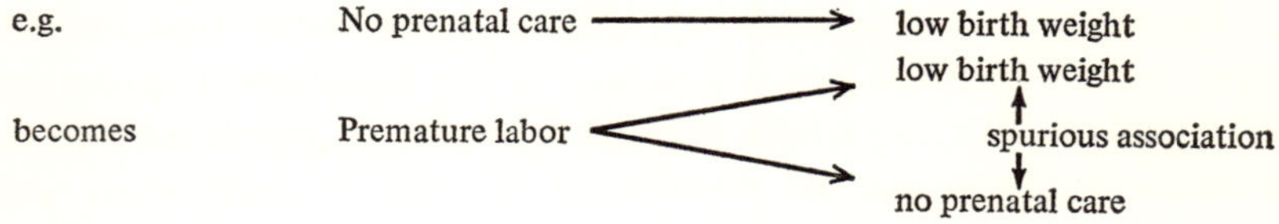

Asymmetrical Relationships

Where there is an asymmetrical connection between variables, then one variable can be said to determine the other. Not everyone would label every form of determination a cause, but for the purpose of this analysis the words are interchangeable. Some of the types of asymmetrical relationship can be described as follows.

Stimulus/response. Exposure to a stimulus, an agent, or an experience produces a response, or host reaction. This type of asymmetrical relationship would be accepted as "cause and effect" by almost all.

Host characteristics. A persisting property, attribute, or characteristic of persons may give rise either to a particular mode of response or to a predisposition to that mode. In epidemiology, characteristics regularly used as descriptive variables are sex, race, age, and place of residence. They can be viewed as determinants when they are associated with a higher risk than average of some manifestation.

Predispositions. A predisposition may precede and determine a particular host response. Persons or populations may have a latent potential to respond in a certain way; this latent predisposition can be activated by the proper circumstances. Predisposition is a special case of a high-risk attribute. Examples of such predispositions are allergies; the tendency of individuals with glucose-6-phosphate-dehydrogenase deficiency to react to drugs like sulphonamides and the malaria prophylactic primaquine, or to the favus bean; the constitution and immune state of the host; or values, attitudes, and beliefs, all of which may predispose to particular responses.

Preconditions. In some obvious cases there could be no outcome without certain preconditions. Motor vehicles are necessary to motor vehicle accidents; male sex is necessary to prostatic disease.

Immanence and heritability. These states imply that an outcome is built into the general nature of the situation, population, or organism. The capacities to walk upright, to speak, and to reproduce humans are all immanent in the human fetus and emerge with development. Freud argued that oedipal responses were immanent in the structure of the nuclear family. In a living organism, of course, much that is immanent is also heritable and genetic.

All these various types of asymmetrical relationships can be subsumed in the concept of multiple causality.

Reciprocal Relationships

Reciprocal relationships exhibit an alternating asymmetry. A first factor influences a second, which in turn influences the first in an alternating cycle. Action is followed by reaction, which feeds back into the situation. A common everyday example of such alternation is the thermostatic device for the control of household temperature. In physiology there are many examples of thermostatic mechanisms, and reciprocal interaction is characteristic of psychological and social relationships. A model for this reaction would be as follows:

$$X_{t0} \text{———} Y_{t1} \text{———} X_{t2} \text{———} Y_{t3} \text{———} X_{t4} \text{———} \ldots \text{etc.}$$

where X and Y are reciprocal variables, and $t0$, $t1$, $t2$. . .etc. represent successive points in time.

ASSOCIATIONS AND LOGICAL INFERENCE

The nub of epidemiology is a concern to establish causes and effects in relation to health disorders. Epidemiologists proceed to their answers by inference from the facts they know and from the facts brought to light in their studies. The empirical philosophers, however, have interposed an awkward objection to the procedure. To *infer* cause from the results of the most solid research is only to represent reality and to give an idealized model of it.

The empiricists argue, first, that perfect demonstration of a cause demands replicability and predictability. Change occurs as time passes, and therefore no event can exactly be repeated. To some degree any replication is an approximation. They add that knowledge is based on experience and ultimately derived through the senses. Knowledge is subjective and not objective.

The gaps between actual properties of the material world, on the one hand, and the measures devised to represent these properties, on the other, are filled by subjective assumptions. Eddington, a physicist of the first half of this century, argued that it was "only a pious opinion" that mass as a property is equivalent to mass inferred from readings of a pointer on a balance. The problem is made obvious when the property of heart function is derived from the variable electric tracing of cardiac impulses read by eye or from the shadow the heart casts on a radiograph.

How do we tolerate this uncertainty in epidemiology? Like public health and medicine generally, epidemiology is an action-oriented discipline. The orientation towards action grows from the charge placed upon the health professional to cut back the afflictions of disease. Uncertainty can sap the will to action. The dominant philosophical adaptation of epidemiologists has been to accept materialism and a pragmatic determinism. Epidemiologists tend to believe that one thing causes another, and they must so believe if they are to take or propose action. They do not doubt that there is a material world in which causality operates. They allow that empirical doubt surrounds the quality of evidence and the models constructed to reflect reality, but not the existence of the real world.

The pragmatic answer to the empiricists is to accept that knowledge is founded on inference and theoretical models of reality and that the best of these models represent a particular version of the truth, and to make outcomes the focus of concern. William James defined a fact as something that makes a difference. In other words, theories should be tested by the observable outcome of their application. Deficiencies in the quality and validity of observation and measurement need not falsify theory or invalidate the tests that show theory to be false.

John Stuart Mill[4] in the nineteenth century devised logical strategies from which the existence of causal relationships might be inferred. Among a number of canons, four are especially applicable. Mill named these the methods of "agreement," of "difference," of "concomitant variation," and of "residues." He described his work as a system of logic. To the eye of the epidemiologist a century later, Mill's canons seem especially appropriate to the construction and interpretation of the research designs on which he relies.

In the "method of difference," the situations compared are "alike in all variables but one." This is the case of the classic experiment. The investigator sets up identical situations and himself causes only one factor to vary among them. A close public health approximation would be a field experiment to test the effectiveness of a vaccine.

In the "method of agreement," the situations compared have "only one circumstance in common." For instance, in twenty-seven different studies of smoking as a cause of lung cancer, the populations studied, the research designs, and the methods all varied, but the association appeared in every one despite the variations in the studies.[5]

In the "method of concomitant variation," the factors under study vary in the same direction through a range of situations. A typical situation would be the variation through time of two related factors, e.g. smoking varies regularly with lung cancer in its distribution through time, among men and women, and between countries.

In the "method of residues," known causal factors are removed from the system and the reckoning in order to isolate and measure the contribution of remaining factors. Removal of variation due to known causes leaves a residue due to other causes. In the case of squamous cancer of the lung, smoking accounts for say 90 percent. Other causes account for the remaining 10 percent. A suitable approach to explaining the residue through the design of a study is illustrated by an investigation of the possible contribution of air pollution to respiratory disease.[6] Since smoking makes a major contribution to respiratory disease, the nonsmokers of a random sample of an adult urban population were identified and the frequency of their respiratory disorders was then related to their history of exposure to different urban environments.*

By means of Mill's logic, many hypothetical causes can be effectively tested and eliminated. Indeed, these forms of argument

*Another approach can be made in the stage of analysis, by the use of statistical methods. In multiple regression analysis, each independent variable (X_1, X_2, X_3, etc.) can be tested to discover how much of the variation in the dependent variable it alone can account for with the others held constant. In a contingency table analysis, a similar effect can be achieved by adding "control" variables in stacked tables. Standardization procedures offer yet another means of removing the influence of other variables to reveal the effect of the residue.

and inference provide a foundation for forming epidemiological hypotheses and designing studies; but the logic does not finally prove the causal inferences that are made. The reason is that even the more powerful among Mill's methods still require simplifying assumptions about which we cannot achieve certainty: Mill requires that the situation shall be "alike in all circumstances but one" or shall have "only one circumstance in common." There is no sure way of knowing that all the relevant factors which could influence the manifestation under study have been located and accounted for.

If the epidemiologist is to pursue the course of determinism in order to find the grounds to act, he must cope with these further sources of uncertainty. Research design and the logic of causal inference provide the means to do so.

The problem is not the same as that posed by the empirical philosophers about the quality and meaning of evidence. The uncertainty about the exact causes of observed effects arises from the complex interrelatedness of all levels of organization in the ecological systems of the real world.

Complexity in causation is a problem in all sciences. Most philosophers of science, indeed, have referred to the physical sciences for examples. Yet the physical scientist has to cope with much less variation in the phenomena he studies than does the biologist or the social scientist. The height of the physical scientist's achievement is the statement of universal laws. Above the simplest molecular level in biology and sociology, however, the variation and plasticity in manifestations is so great that universal laws tend to be reduced to somewhat banal observations about such everyday events as conception, birth, and death.

To deal with this variability of biological and social phenomena in populations and with the uncertainty of their casual inferences, epidemiologists have five broad strategies: (a) they simplify the conditions of observation by isolating and controlling a segment of reality, (b) they screen their causal models for sources of variation extraneous to the model, (c) they test and specify observed associations by elaborating their relationships in analysis, (d) they use the notions of probability to estimate the significance to be attached to the concurrence of the variables in the instances under observation and (e) they make judgments about the accumulated data on the basis of a number of criteria.

These strategies call on the particular skills and art of the epidemiologist. To apply the strategies, the epidemiologist must have substantive knowledge of the diseases he studies, he must apply the general principles of nonexperimental research, and he must use ingenuity to exploit available situations. Each strategy will be discussed in turn. We shall deal briefly with the first and the fourth strategies, which are thoroughly treated in many statistical texts, and give more attention to the second, third, and fifth strategies.

Simplifying the Conditions of Observation

The interrelatedness of all phenomena within ecological systems poses acute problems for the investigator who must select a segment of a system for observation. He can select among causes and effects from many types and levels. One kind of selection is imposed by the historical accidents of academic and scientific development. Each discipline has a frame of reference and demarcated areas of inquiry. Often a hindrance to adequate comprehension of systems, the demarcations also restrict choice among the causes and effects to be studied.

In any particular investigation, the investigator himself must impose additional and deliberate limits. His research design aims to isolate that segment of the ecological system that is most relevant to the investigation. Relevance is determined by the question asked and by the opportunities for obtaining the data to answer it. The most effective research design is that which eliminates the largest proportion of extraneous factors that might intrude on and influence the relationship we aim to establish between cause and effect. A main object of research design in epidemiology is thus to simplify the conditions of observation. Since good texts are available, the question of design can be briefly considered from the special point of view of establishing causality.

Two major approaches to research design exist in epidemiology. These are by *experiment* and by *observation.* In the classic experiment, only one factor might be introduced to make two similar situations different from one another. The test situations are created by the investigator and they are deliberately made alike. The test factor is introduced to create particular effects. But all other factors are "held constant," or "controlled."

The observational method culls and analyzes data from existing records or field surveys as the data come to hand through the uncontrolled historical experience of the study populations. Like the experiment, the observational method relies on prediction and inference to establish cause. We make an hypothesis, and we predict what effects will occur in particular situations according to the hypothesis; then we seek out groups exposed to the situations in which we are interested and, for comparison, unexposed groups; finally, we compare the effects observed in the exposed and unexposed groups.

In the observational studies of epidemiology, however, the comparison groups will differ from each other in many subtle or obvious ways that might influence the manifestation under study. The difficulty arises also in those field experiments that the epidemiologist may conduct. It is a commonplace that people cannot be manipulated as the experimenter chooses. Therefore the situations compared cannot be completely controlled and kept exactly the same.

For these reasons, the epidemiologist cannot be content with the analysis of two variables alone or, at any rate, with the consideration of two variables alone. If the epidemiologist hopes to apply Mill's canons of causal logic, he must invent methods for attaining greater comparability between groups. To do this, he tries to anticipate the variation introduced into the study situation by factors extraneous to the variables of direct interest. The variables of direct interest are those defined by the researcher as *independent* and as *dependent.**

*For our purposes, an *independent variable* is one the value of which is not affected by the outcome variable (or manifestation) within the defined area of relationship under study, i.e. the independent variable is not influenced by the manifestation, but may cause it or contribute to its variation.

For our purpose, a *dependent variable* is one the value of which is dependent upon the effect of other variables in the defined area of relationships under study, i.e. the dependent variable is a manifestation or outcome whose variation we seek to explain or account for by the influence of independent variables.

To illustrate, persons exposed to air pollution (an independent variable, X) may have an excess of lung cancer (the first dependent variable, Y_1) or an excess of chronic bronchitis and emphysema (the second dependent variable, Y_2) over those persons not exposed to heavy pollution. Convincing inferences about such an observed association cannot be made until we take account, in the population at risk, of many other factors that have a potential effect on the disease selected as possible outcomes of pollution. For instance, age and smoking both have known effects on chronic bronchitis. They could be responsible, therefore, for any observed variation in the dependent variables unless they have somehow been controlled.

Thus in well designed studies, independent variables other than the hypothetical causal variable that have potential effects on the dependent variable are brought under control. Experimental studies are prospective and control can be achieved by assigning participants to experimental and control groups in a random manner. Given large enough numbers, extraneous factors with potential influence on the dependent variable can be expected, by chance, to be evenly divided between the experimental and control groups and to cancel out. Random assignment is the preferred means by which experimental studies are structured. Because the experiments are prospective, the assignments can be made to the levels of the independent variable whose effects are to be tested. In this manner, randomization removes two kinds of bias: bias inherent in selecting subjects by attributes that might favor either test or control groups, and bias in data where foreknowledge of the outcome could have influenced the information obtained.

The method of random assignment was a technique that led to a great leap forward in medicine, a leap forward that has been compared with that which followed the introduction of the microscope. This elegant research method eliminates those errors that arise from attributing effects to particular causes without controlling other potential causes of the effect. Many other sources of error can be introduced into an experiment by inadequate design and lax execution; for instance, by crude or invalid measurement of variables, by losses from samples, and so forth.[7,8]

Often the input of the test variable is not what the experimenter imagines it to be. In a drug trial, many patients do not comply with the regimen; at the same time, the psychological and social input of the giver of the drug has effects additional to the drug. The concern of this discussion, however, is with the problems of interpreting the real world as it exists and not with the problems introduced by the researchers. We therefore proceed on the assumption that the observations made and analysed are unexceptionable.

Observational case-control studies[2] begin with cases. Independent variables with a potential effect on the manifestation under observation must be brought under control in other ways than by randomization. In case control studies the cases have happened, and random assignment is of course impossible. The comparison groups can only be constructed retrospectively since the observations are made after the event. The design is then built around the manifestation, or dependent variable. In these circumstances, the cases are given and the control group for comparison is selected from those who are not cases. Although it is not possible to assign cases and controls randomly, it is possible to match pairs or groups of cases and controls.

The method of matching on control variables eliminates certain (but not all) extraneous factors from account and from analysis by a direct approach; each case is matched with a supposedly unaffected person who has the same value on the control variables.[9-11] Thus in case-control studies, controlled comparisons between groups can be achieved through the group composition dictated by the research design.

Matched population can be drawn by various sampling techniques from the population at large or, more conveniently, from other types of patients. By taking patients, an additional series of factors that lead to the state of patienthood is automatically matched. (It must not be forgotten that for each social position and each type of health disorder the selective paths to patienthood are likely to be different.) Matching thus restricts the diversity of the population selected from the "universe" which was sampled. It reduces the number of variables which can be expected to cause differences between the comparison groups, and it therefore reduces the size of the sample needed to demonstrate the effect of the study variable. At the same time, matching reduces the generality of a result: the procedure eliminates variation between comparison groups on the matched variable, and hence the effect on the dependent variable of change in the matched variable cannot be studied. The closeness of a match, and the degree to which extraneous factors are controlled thereby, depends on the number of variables on which cases and controls can be matched and on the precision of the information from which the variables are constructed. The number of variables that can be matched, in turn, depends on the size of the population pool and the chance of finding a match within it, and on the amount of information available on the attributes of the population. Matching on many variables requires a large population with information available on all the variables for each member.

The information on which a pair is matched is often less precise than appears at first sight. For instance, characteristics of individuals may be similar at a point in time, but if they are not fixed characteristics their values may change through time in divergent directions determined by the norms of disparate groups of origin from which each individual may be drawn.[12] This difference is likely to be mistakenly attributed to the unmatched factor under test. Regression of this kind is a hazard where a matched characteristic is closely related to the independent variable. For instance, low birthweight has a strong association with low social class. In a study of the effect of low birthweight on childhood intelligence test scores, therefore, infants were matched with infants of normal weight by parental social class at birth. The differences in IQ observed between the groups at school age, however, could have been due to imprecise matching by social class, for the investigator found that in the interim the families of infants of normal birthweight had been upwardly mobile relative to those of low birthweight.[13] Thus the apparent match for parental social class did not hold up through time, and the normal birthweight of the controls was to some degree an index of their social differentiation from the cases. The difference, imperceptible at birth by the measures of social class available to the investigator, could only be detected by measuring change over time.

In observational studies that draw cases from a defined population and therefore yield incidence or prevalence rates, control can be achieved in the analysis of the data without the preliminary selection of comparison groups. This control can only be as tight as the number of influential variables known for the population. We are fortunate if much information about potential interfering variables like age, sex, or race is available for the unaffected population as a whole or for a representative sample drawn from it. Since the same set of data is available from the unaffected population as from the cases, a ready-made control group is available.

In the studies shown in Figure 2.1 and Table 2.1, lung cancer and bronchitis respectively were related to air pollution. Potential interfering variables were controlled in analysis. A control variable is held constant by analyzing the relationship between the independent and dependent variables for each specific category or value of the control variable. Thus the frequency of lung cancer within each degree of air pollution exposure was analyzed

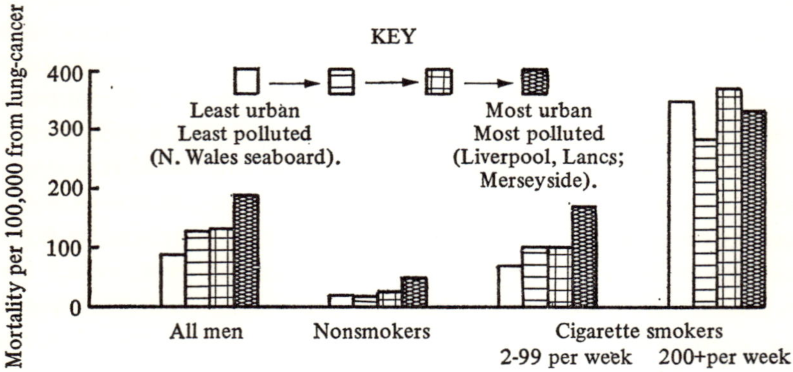

Figure 2.1. Deaths from lung cancer in N.W. England and N. Wales, by cigarette-smoking habit and "urban" environment ("air pollution") : Estimated annual death rates among men aged 35-74, *standardized* for age. From Stocks, P. *Suppl. to Part II of the 35th Ann. Rep.* of the British Empire Cancer Campaign, London, 1957.

TABLE 2.1

SYMPTOM-PREVALENCE RATIOS (PERSISTENT COUGH AND PHLEGM) *STANDARDIZED FOR AGE AND SMOKING*, BY AIR-POLLUTION INDICES:ENGLAND & WALES

Concentration (μg/cm)	Smoke		Sulphur dioxide		Douglas-Waller index		
	Males	Females	Males	Females		Males	Females
<100	97 (*82*)	93 (*35*)	87 (*11*)	*103* (*7*)	Very low	88 (*201*)	95 (*93*)
100—	112 (*90*)	120 (*45*)	96 (*59*)	110 (*31*)	Low	91 (*217*)	94 (*97*)
150—	116 (*97*)	116 (*47*)	120 (*118*)	115 (*53*)	Moderate	117 (*188*)	97 (*75*)
200+	134 (*50*)	129 (*23*)	118 (*122*)	120 (*56*)	High	118 (*169*)	115 (*81*)

Note. Figure in italic type show observed numbers of symptom-positive respondents. Smoke and sulphur dioxide concentrations are based on values at residential sites in March, 1965 (National Air Pollution Survey). From Lambert, P.M., and Reid, D.D. Smoking, air pollution and bronchitis in Britain. *Lancet, 1*:853-857, 1970.

within each smoking category, defined by amount and type of smoking. Alternatively, these interfering variables can be standardized by other statistical devices, as with age in Figure 2.1, and age and smoking in Table 2.1. By standardizing, the results observed are compared with what would be expected if the control variable were distributed in the same way in each of the comparison populations.

A single observational study usually makes a less precise test of an hypothesis than a well-conducted experiment. In an experiment, the hypothetical causal factor is under the control of the experimenter. The factor can be defined and limited; the extraneous input that is inevitably carried with the test factor (for instance, the psychological and social effects of professional interaction with a patient who is given a drug) can be controlled and the fact of acutal intake can be ascertained. In an observational study all these matters are often in doubt. Compared with an experiment, at least six disadvantages can be listed: The documentation of exposure to the hypothetical cause is less certain. The specificity with which the independent variable represents the hypothetical cause is less precise. The independent variable selected as causal factor is usually more remote from the dependent variable selected as effect. The time order and direction of relationship between independent and dependent variables is less certainly known. Assignment to exposure or control cannot be random, and thus the comparison groups are subject to selective bias and are less well matched. Finally, the efficiency of the statistics used in analysis is less.

Yet observational studies are the first resort of the epidemiologist. Experiments have their own disadvantages. An unbiased representation of the population to be studied is often difficult to achieve. By the same token, fair representation of a natural setting is also difficult to achieve; the greater the number of natural effects and interactions excluded from the experiment, the greater the number of assumptions that must be made in generalizing the results. The chief reason for the preference of epidemiologists for observational studies, however, is practicability. Observational studies permit a variety and a scale of tests of hypotheses that cannot be matched by experiments. Both variety and scale, we shall see, buttress causal inference.

Many medical experiments are ruled out from the start on ethical grounds, because people can be subjected to risk of harm neither from exposure to the test factor nor from withholding it. Many other experiments are simply impossible, because an inborn attribute is not a matter of choice and subject to manipulation. Nor is it easily possible to maintain an experimental intervention over long periods of time. The experiment has the disadvantage of a prospective cohort study in that it is difficult to follow the experimental population, without loss over decades, to observe long-term effects, and even to maintain the continuity of staff and organization to do so, while during a long observational period cumulative growth and experience dilutes the effects of the planned intervention and reduces the advantage of the experiment over the observational approach. By contrast, the opportunities for observational studies of every kind of causal factor and health disorder are manifold, and few observations need be ruled out on ethical grounds. Moreover, vast populations can often be taken into observational studies; to mobilize equivalent numbers for experiment would be impracticable.

In sum, the advantage of experiments in matters of control of extraneous factors and in the quality of their measures is offset by the advantage of observational studies in matters of representativeness of populations and of natural setting and, above all, in feasibility in the pursuit of determinants.

Screening Causal Models for Extraneous Factors

A good research design eliminates as many as possible of the extraneous variables that may intrude on the relationship we hope to establish between hypothesized cause and effect. In order to interpret the results, the analyst implicitly constructs a causal model of their relationship from the observed association. Even with the tightest designs, these models must make simplifying assumptions. All the possible variables that could explain the observed association can never be tested and controlled, and it is assumed that these unknowns do not affect the results. The possibiliity that they may do so must always be weighed when finally the effort to reach a judgment is made.

In order to obtain the data from which the causal model is constructed, further assumptions are made about the validity of the indices used to assign qualitative or quantitative values to the study variables. Records of sphygmomanometer readings are not the same thing as the pressure of columns of blood against artery walls; even less are reported occupations arranged in classes the same thing as social class. Assumptions of this type are passed over in the following discussion.

Simplifying assumptions are concealed in all unqualified equations about the real world, and they must be qualified by the local conditions to which they are applied. Even laws of gravity cannot be applied to an empirical situation without qualification. Allowances must be made for the difference from the assumed ideal conditions of the law—in this case, for atmospheric pressure. In the social and biological world, the more general and mathematical a formulation, the less likely it is to represent the parochial realities of our concern. A mathematical model that describes the epidemic spread of an infection can give insights into the process of its spread, but it cannot predict a local epidemic with precision. Any equation in epidemiology is only a model of actual relationships and contains simplifying assumptions. The equation $P_t = ID$, referred to above, makes the assumption that the disease is in equilibrium and does not change in frequency through the time period studied.

Thus general formulations hold only given the restricting conditions contained in the assumptions. For example, the formulation may assume constancy in certain extraneous variables, like age, sex, and race, that influence the relationship described. The assumption of constancy in influential extraneous factors restricts the application of the formulation. Only given constancy in these conditions can it be generalized to situations beyond the ones observed. In a general formulation, the unknown factors that exist in local situations are excluded from consideration. It is always possible that unknown local factors may produce outcomes different from those predicted by generalizing from previously observed relationships between the variables of concern.

These assumptions are made less tenuous, it has been argued above, by research designs that isolate the independent variables of concern from those of no concern and thereby reduce irrelevant variation in the dependent variable. At the same time, factors of no concern to the study that remain in the system can be controlled in a variety of ways, some of which have been discussed.

Whenever it is postulated that an observed association reflects a causal relationship, it is always necessary to review the causal model for the simplifying assumptions it contains. Sources of variation in the dependent variables that could be caused by variables extraneous to the association must be searched for. To detect the possibility that change in the dependent variable is due to extraneous variables, it can be useful to consider systematically the following types of independent variable: (a) the hypothetical causal variable, or independent study variable, (b) control variables, (c) uncontrolled variables, (d) confounding variables, and (e) moderator variables.

Hypothetical Causal Variables

The investigator hopes to discover change in the dependent variables that he can attribute to change in the hypothetical causal variable, the independent variable selected for study. This variable is the focus of research, and by design and inference the investigator aims to isolate its effect from that of all other independent variables. The sharpness of the effect that can be isolated will depend in part on the clarity with which both the independent study variable and its effects are conceived, defined, and measured. For this discussion, however, the validity, specificity and reliability of measures will be taken as given.

Control Variables

Independent variables can be called control variables if they satisfy two conditions: they are known to have a potential effect on the dependent variable and they are subject to control.[1,14] The general principles of research designs that control potential extraneous variation in the dependent variable by removing it have been referred to above. The principles of analysis that control extraneous variation by specifying and measuring it will be dealt with below, first under the heading of confounding variables and later in the section on the elaboration of associations between two variables.

Uncontrolled Variables

Change may be caused in the dependent variable by uncontrolled variables. These are independent variables whose potential effect on the dependent variable may or may not be recognized but which cannot be brought under control or assessed quantitatively. Variables of this type account for the variation in the dependent variable that remains unexplained by the analysis. For instance, with cancer of the lung, even when smoking, air pollution, age, sex, and social class are controlled, the disease will still occur among some individuals who do not have any of these high-risk attributes or exposures. Other carcinogens cause lung cancer, for example, nickel and radioactive chromium, in the absence of all the other factors listed; in addition, other unknown carcinogens may be active. Conversely, individuals with the same exposure to all the control factors do not all end with the same manifestations; they do not all get cancer. Therefore the case must differ from those unaffected in an additional unknown respect.

Residual variation in the dependent variable implies that other factors than the study and control variables are at work. There are many possibilities in addition to unknown agents in the environment. Variation may be due to the vagaries of individual development in the host, to genetic susceptibility, or to constitutional factors that render people unduly susceptible to the disease in question. Finally, there is measurement error. All these sources of variation must be considered as possible causes of an observed association.

Confounding Variables

A confounding variable is one which varies systematically with the independent study variable, so that its effects, when uncontrolled, cannot be distinguished from those of the study variable. Where the independent study variable is common, the confounding variable is also common, i.e. the two variables are statistically associated. Where the independent study variable is statistically associated with a dependent study variable, the confounding variable is also associated with it. Thus in an observed association between two variables, a confounding variable is an uncontrolled third variable that is associated with both the independent and dependent variables. The change in the dependent study variable that is apparently caused by the independent study variable initially found to be associated with it could therefore be caused by the confounding variable. By control in research design or analysis, a confounding variable can be converted into a control variable. The effects of the confounding variable are then separated from those of the independent study variable by removing or measuring them.

In the example of the association of air pollution with bronchitis, air pollution will be found to vary systematically and directly with the density of urban settlement (so much so that researchers have used this density as an index of pollution). Pollution will also vary with the overcrowding of homes and consequent respiratory infection, and with the social and economic level of residential areas. The causal model for the association of air pollution with bronchitis (see Table 2.1) would then be as follows:

Air pollution ——————————→ Bronchitis
(independent variable)   (dependent vartable)

But the truth could as well be that the overcrowding and high population density that are regularly found with the urban poverty complex confound the association. These factors could cause bronchitis by facilitating the spread of infection, on the one hand; on the other hand, quite independently of bronchitis, they could cause air pollution by concentrating the use of fuels and motor transport. In that case, crowding would be a confounding variable: air pollution and bronchitis would be in a symmetrical relationship with each other as part of a complex of factors, and the causal inference would be spurious.

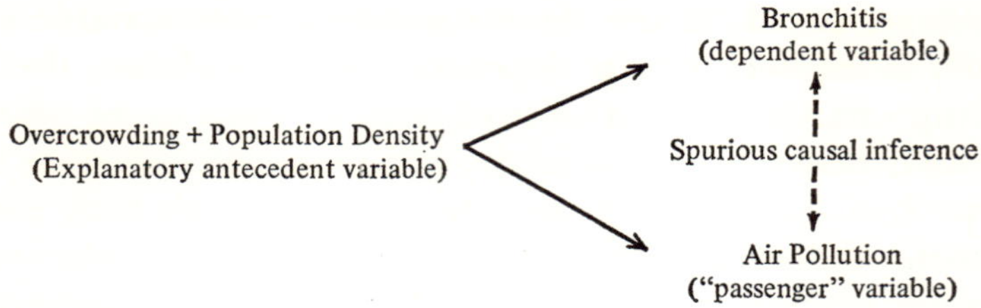

If a term is needed for the apparent independent causal variable that gives rise to the spurious inference in such an association, it might be called a "passenger" variable, for it "rides" with the dependent variable. A *passenger variable varies* systematically with the dependent variable under study without being causally related to it (most often because a particular causal factor can give rise to both).

An *explanatory antecedent variable,* as shown in the above diagram, is a confounding variable that "explains" the apparent association between two variables conceived as hypothetical cause (independent variable) and effect (dependent variable). Such a variable is antecedent in time to the hypothetical causal variable in the initial association. When a third variable of this type is controlled, whether by research design or by analysis, the initial association between the hypothetical causal independent variable and the dependent study variable disappears.

To eliminate the risk of confounding and of spurious causal inference by research design, one must search for situations in which the variation may not be systematic and where the study factor and the confounding factor might be found to diverge.

To continue with the example of air pollution effects, few opportunities present themselves in which social and economic level, overcrowding, and density of population can be disassociated from the degree of pollution of the ambient air. Situations have to be found in which, say, enough persons of high socioeconomic levels are exposed to heavy pollution while persons of low socioeconomic levels are not. Table 2.2 illustrates one attempt to analyze such a situation. If no opportune situation can be found in which to make such comparisons, then socio-economic level persists as an uncontrolled confounding variable, and it remains suspect as a potential cause of the manifestations that we wish to attribute to the independent variable we are studying—in this case air pollution.

TABLE 2.2
AVERAGE ANNUAL DEATH RATES PER 100,000 (*N* IN PARENTHESES) FOR PROSTATIC CANCER, BY INCOME* AND AIR POLLUTION LEVELS, IN TWO AGE-GROUPS: WHITE MALES, BUFFALO AND ENVIRONS, 1959-61.

Income	Air Pollution Level				Total
	1 (Low)	2	3	4 (High)	
		50-69 Years			
$3005-$6004	18 (2)	26 (8)	38 (14)	39 (6)	32 (30)
$6013-$11,792	18 (7)	23 (15)	33 (7)	51 (2)	24 (31)
		70 Years and Over			
$3005-$6004	61 (2)	143 (15)	204 (23)	356 (16)	189 (56)
$6013-$11,792	224 (18)	295 (47)	297 (16)	99 (1)	296 (81)

Source: Winkelstein, W., and Kantor, S. Prostatic Cancer: Relationship to Suspended Particulate Air Pollution. Paper presented at 96th Annual Meeting, American Public Health Assn., Detroit, Mich., 1968.
*Median family income of census tract of last residence.

In experimental studies where the experience of the group to be compared is at the researcher's choice, the confounding variable can be controlled by random allocation. For instance, low birthweight has a regular association with late and "insufficient" prenatal care. We do not know that the association is causal—that inadequate care is a cause of low birth weight—because of uncontrolled confounding variables. Low socioeconomic class is associated with low birthweight and also with late and "insufficient" prenatal care and might cause both. The same goes for poor nutrition. We can test these factors in an epidemiologic experiment, however, in which pregnant women are randomly assigned to different levels of care. If we have enough cases, the social class factor will cancel out provided we ensure equal participation of women of all classes once they enter the experiment.

In social experiments, random assignment to experimental and control groups does not remove confounding in every case where extraneous variables vary systematically with the independent study variable. Although random assignment can ensure an even distribution of the existing attributes of a study population between comparison groups, the assignment does not assure the similarity of future experience in every respect but one. For example, assume the unlikely event that one could perform an experiment in relation to air pollution and bronchitis. One might take advantage of rehousing schemes to assign households at random either to remain where they were, in an area with a high level of pollution, or to take up new housing in an area with a low level of pollution. Such factors as overcrowding and density of population would be unlikely to cancel out. While the newly housed group could escape exposure to pollution, they would also escape the crowding of those left behind. In most social experiments, the intervention exposes the experimental group not to one but to several factors. The propensity of such factors to vary systematically with each other is rich in possibilities for confounding.

Researchers have devised many ingenious variations on the theme of twin studies, and at the same time have tapped many unsuspected sources of confounding. About a century ago, Galton raised the hope that biologists could separate heredity from environmental factors by comparing the attributes of twins with those of siblings less closely related. Later, after Mendel's work was understood, came the exciting realization that monozygotic twins had an identical dose of genes, while dizygotic twins, like other sibs, shared only half their genes. Monozygotic twins, however, generally have an identical dose of experience, to a degree that psychiatrists have suggested that they have special problems of maintaining their personal identity. One tactic invented to overcome this confounding factor in the study of the effects of heredity was to search out identical twins reared apart. Even in such cases, identical twins reared apart come from, and enter, environments with unusual features. Moreover, these environments of twins reared apart are likely to be correlated with each other. An appropriate model takes account of and isolates the confounding variable in a well-known formulation:

Shared genes ——————→ Concordant inherited attributes and characteristics

Therefore, (a) MZ (identical) twins are more concordant

than DZ (fraternal) twins and sibs and (b) DZ twins and sibs equally are concordant. But

Shared experience ⟶ Concordant acquired attributes and characteristics

Therefore, (a) DZ twins are more concordant than sibs and (b) MZ twins are more concordant than DZ twins.

Distorter and Suppressor Variables

Confounding occurs in many guises. "Distorter" and "suppressor" variables give a special twist to the phenomenon.

The introduction of confounding variables into analysis of an observed association between independent and dependent study variables, we have noted, explains and reduces the size of the initial association. By the logic of arithmetic, one may predict that two other results are possible when a third variable is added to the analysis of an observed association between two study variables. First, when the third variable is controlled, it might be capable of producing the extreme effect of reversing the direction of an observed association between independent and dependent study variables. Such a third variable is a "distorter" variable. Second, when the third variable is controlled, it might reveal that an association existed between independent and dependent study variables, where initially no association or only a weak association was observed. Such a third variable may be either a "distorter" or a "suppressor" variable.

A distorter variable is associated with both independent and dependent study variables. Its association with the dependent variable, however, is opposite in direction and sign from that of the independent study variable with the dependent variable. If the independent study variable varies directly with the dependent variable, the distorter variable varies inversely with the dependent variable, and vice versa. Thus a negative association of the distorter with the dependent variable counterbalances and thereby distorts, masks, or diminishes a positive association between independent and dependent study variables. When controlled, a distorter variable is therefore capable of reversing a distorted association. If the distortion is less, control of the distorter variable may reveal an association where none seemed to exist, or strengthen a weak association.

In epidemiology, perhaps the most common distorter variable is age. Table 2.3 shows an example. In a study of all episodes of psychiatric care in an English city, rates of depressive psychosis were higher in the married than in the single. At first sight, it seemed that depression might be connected with marital strain.

TABLE 2.3
DEPRESSIVE PSYCHOSIS: AVERAGE ANNUAL RATES (PER 100,000 POPULATION) OF FIRST ENTRY TO PSYCHIATRIC SERVICES IN SALFORD 1959-63, BY AGE, SEX, FOR SINGLE AND MARRIED

			Age-Group						
		All	15—	20—	30—	40—	50—	60—	70+
Men	Single	120	7	97	204	325	278	330	85
	Married	124	0	50	125	140	142	168	81
Women	Single	261	40	204	552	605	479	440	248
	Married	278	43	177	276	278	376	338	157

Adapted from Susser M. *Community Psychiatry: Epidemiologic and Social Themes,* Random House 1968, Appendix A., A.4, A.5.

The results among both sexes, however, were distorted by the age variable. Increasing age was positively associated both with marriage and with depressive psychosis: older people were more likely to be married and were also at greater risk of depressive psychosis. Thus, when age was controlled, the rates of depressive psychosis were found to be higher among the single than the married; in fact, marriage was negatively associated with depressive psychosis. The positive association of age with marriage and depressive psychosis had overwhelmed this negative association and produced a spurious association between marriage and depressive psychosis.

Emile Durkheim, in his classic book on suicide, provided a similar example. Contrary to the predictions from his hypotheses about egoistic suicide, he found an absolute ratio of married to unmarried suicides of 1.4 in the years 1873-78. When available figures (for the years 1889-91) were analyzed by age, however, the ratio was reversed for all age and sex groups but one (Table 2.4).

TABLE 2.4
RATIOS OF MARRIED TO UNMARRIED SUICIDE RATES, BY AGE AND SEX: FRANCE 1889-91

	15—	20—	25—	30—	40—	50—	60—	70—	80+
Men	4.4	0.4	0.3	0.4	0.3	0.4	0.4	0.4	0.5
Women	0.4	0.5	0.5	0.7	0.6	0.7	0.8	1	0.6

Adapted from *Durkheim, E., Suicide,* 1897. Trans. by J.N. Spaulding and G. Simpson. The Free Press, 1966.

In both these examples age was a distorter variable associated both with the independent study variable and the dependent variable, and its association with the dependent variable was opposite in direction from that of the independent study variable. A distorter variable thus exerts a seesaw effect on the observed association under study that counterbalances and outweighs the effect of the independent study variable.

Table 2.5 illustrates how the effect of a distorter variable can lead to misinterpretation. In an anlaysis of the relationship of verbal reasoning scores with birth order, columns i and ii of Table 2.5 comprised the table referred to in the following quotation taken from the author's discussion: "The results shown in [the] table. . .suggest that the differences within each social group are also not mainly determined by variation within families. For while the difference according to birth rank in the general population of births is considerable, differences between sibs are small.[15]

On logical grounds one would not expect to find the difference noted by the author between birth ranks in the general population and in a representative sample of sibs from that population. Two effects, one caused by a family-size variable uncontrolled for lack of data, and the second by a distorter variable, contributed to the apparent differences between the results of the general population and the sib pairs. First, sib comparisons between ranks are not representative of the general population, for

TABLE 2.5
DIFFERENCES IN VERBAL REASONING SCORES OF CHILDREN IN CONSECUTIVE BIRTH RANKS

Birth Ranks Compared	i. Total Sample (*N* 35,863) standardized for maternal age		ii. Sib Pairs (5,054 Pairs)	iii. Total Sample (*N* 35,863)
1 with 2	2.9		1.5	1.8
2 with 3	3.7		0.9	2.8
3 with 4	2.8	2.7	0.5	2.2
4 with 5	2.6			2.8
6 and later	3.4			1.9

Adapted from McKeown, T. Prenatal and early postnatal influences on measured intelligence. *Brit. Med. J., 2:*63-67, 1970; Record, R.G., McKeown, T., and Edwards, S.H. The relation of measured intelligence to birth order and maternal age. *Ann. Hum. Genet., 33:*61-69, 1969.

they must differ in the distribution of family sizes. Each sib comparison, by definition, can include no families of a size less than that indicated by the highest birth rank in that comparison. In comparing the firstborn with the secondborn, for instance, sib comparisons can contain no "only" children (who usually score higher on the IQ test) among the firstborn, while the general population does include "only" children.

Second, inspection of birth-rank comparisons among both the general population and the sib pairs, in columns i and ii respectively of Table 2.5, shows that only the general population data are standardized for maternal age. In this case, maternal age is the distorter variable. Maternal age varies with birth rank and with test scores; high maternal age is associated with high birth rank and also with high verbal reasoning scores. Birth rank varies directly with maternal age and inversely with test scores; high rank is associated with high maternal age and with low test scores.

Column iii shows birth-rank comparisons for the general population when maternal age is not controlled. The differences between birth ranks in column iii are less than when maternal age is standardized as in column i. In other words, maternal age distorts the association of birth rank with verbal reasoning scores, and when maternal age is standardized the association is strengthened.

This study provided examples of some other distorter variables that were recognized and controlled in a test of the effects of low birth weight in reducing measured intelligence in later childhood. Thus female sex is associated with low birth weight but also with higher measured intelligence at 11 years of age. Primogeniture too is associated with low birth weight but also with high measured intelligence, or at the least with high educational achievement. In each of these cases, one of the associated independent variables varies directly with the dependent variable, while the other varies inversely with it; if the association of study variable with dependent variable is positive, that of the distorter variable is negative.

A suppressor variable is one which, when controlled, reveals or strengthens a suppressed association between two study variables but is not capable of reversing the association irrespective of the size of its effect. A suppressor variable has an association with the independent study variable, but unlike a distorter variable, it does not have an association of opposite sign with the dependent study variable. Few writers distinguish between distorter and suppressor variables, and some who do imply that the distinction is one of degree. In this paper, I propose to maintain the qualitative distinction made in the definition given above.

Suppression as here defined occurs because the third variable, when uncontrolled, dilutes the association of the independent variable. The third variable is irrelevant to the association under study and reduces or overwhelms it. Thus the main circumstance in which suppression occurs is one in which but a portion of the independent variable, as initially defined, has an effect on the dependent study variable, and the remainder has no effect and is irrelevant. For example, smoking in all its forms—cigars, pipes, and marijuana as well as cigarettes—might be defined as the independent study variable in a study of cancer of the bronchus. The strength of association of all smoking with cancer of the bronchus is weak compared with that of cigarette smoking alone. Cigarette smoking is an integral segment of the initial independent variable, of which it is a refinement. (This circumstance is further discussed in the section below on refined variables, p. 78) .

The irrelevant portion of the independent study variable initially defined may be a component that is not recognized or whose effects are unanticipated. For instance, a test of aptitude for carpentry (the independent study variable) was found to correlate poorly with skill in carpentry exhibited on the job (the dependent variable). Control of the variable "verbal comprehension" revealed a much stronger correlation between the aptitude test and carpentry skills. Verbal comprehension was an irrelevant component of the independent variable; high verbal comprehension contributed to high aptitude test scores but not to carpentry skill. When verbal comprehension was controlled, the suppressed portion of the aptitude test that related to carpentry skills alone contributed to and strengthened the association.*

The researcher who would avoid or uncover confounding must be vigilant. By avoiding confounding in a research design, he limits the simplifying assumptions built into his causal model and strengthens causal inference. By uncovering confounding in analysis, he obtains protection from false inferences that are not eliminated by design.

Moderator† Variables

Some independent variables that have no demonstrable effect on a manifestation when taken alone do have an effect when they act in concert with other factors. For example, concomitant causal agents, termed cocarcinogens, have been postulated in hypotheses about various cancers. To be effective, the carcinogen requires the complementary activity of a cocarcinogen. Epidemiological studies point to the mineral asbestos as a cocarcinogen; both pleural mesotheliomas and bronchial cancers have been linked with this substance. In the case of bronchial cancer, high rates have been found among workers exposed to asbestos, but so far only for the cigarette smokers among them.[16]* The risk for these workers was considerably higher than would be expected from the

---

*I am indebted to Jacob Cohen for this example.[29]

†Also called "qualifier" variables by some authors.

*Number of exposed nonsmokers is too small, however, to allow a good estimate of the risk.

predicted risks of smoking alone. Smoking is a cause sufficient in itself to produce bronchial cancer. Exposure to asbestos presumably renders the bronchial mucosa more susceptible to malignancy caused by smoking.

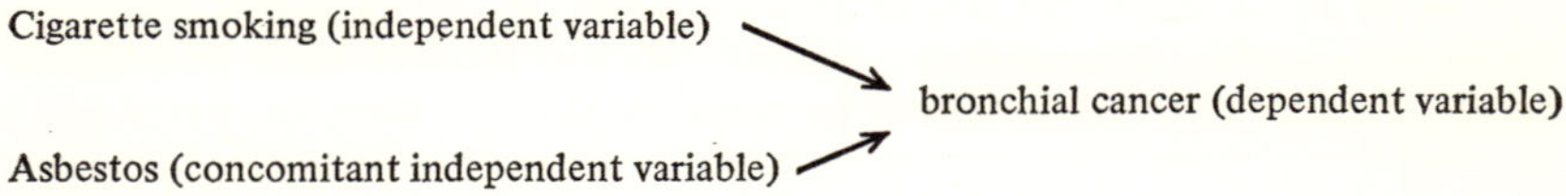

Until knowledge is further advanced, however, we will not know whether this interaction does in fact represent the effect on the disease of a configuration and not a sequence of factors.

These concomitant or synergistic causes are moderator variables. A moderator variable specifies conditions. When it is introduced into the analysis of the association between two variables, the association becomes stronger than before for certain conditions or values of the added variable; the association becomes weaker for other conditions or values and may even change direction and sign.

For example, sex is a moderator variable in relation to the effects of some infections in children; thus males suffer higher death rates than females from meningococcal infection. Nutrition is also a moderator variable in relation to infection; malnourished children suffer high death rates from measles while well-nourished children rarely suffer death from measles. Table 2.6 illustrates the specification of such conditions. A random sample of individuals who at school were classed as mildly retarded had made gains in measured intelligence when observed at ages 20 to 24 years. These gains were confined, however, to those without detectable brain disorder.

When moderator variables are quantified as independent variables, they exhibit the statistical property of interaction, or joint effect. The joint effect of the independent variables is greater than the sum of their independent effects acting separately. A moderator variable, then, can be defined as an independent variable that in combination with any other independent variables produces an effect over and above the sum of the effects each produces alone. Conversely where there is interaction, the sum of the

TABLE 2.6

IQ CHANGE OVER AN AVERAGE OF TEN YEARS (DEPENDENT VARIABLE) IN 52 PERSONS CLASSED AS MILDLY RETARDED AT SCHOOL (CAUSAL VARIABLE) BY CLINICAL STATE (MODERATOR VARIABLE) AT AGES 20 TO 24 YEARS

A moderator variable, introduced in an analysis of an association between a hypothetical causal (independent) variable and a dependent study variable, reveals a greater degree of association for some "conditions" than for others.

a.

	Diagnosis at School	
	Mildly Retarded	Normal Intellect†
Mean I.Q. Change*	+5	0

b.

	Clinical State of Mildly Retarded	
	Brain Disorder	No Brain Disorder
Mean IQ Change*	—1.2	+8.3

Adapted from Stein and Susser. *J. Ment. Sci. (London)*, *106:*1311 ff, 1960.
*S.D. ± 3.
†Inferred from known data. No comparable data available on clinical state of "normals."

effects of each of the independent variables taken alone is a weighted average of its effects when it is taken together with other independent variables, as in the hypothetical examples of Table 2.7. When a moderator variable is introduced into an analysis and reveals interaction, the process is described as "specification."[18] The relations thus specified are "conditional relations"; that is, each of the specified values of the modifier variable reveals a different level of association of the original independent variable with the dependent variable. Each of the conditions of the moderator variable thus indicates a specific effect.

In Table 2.7a, the mean effect of both levels of X_1 on Y (as seen at the margins of the table) is the same: 100 in each case. Nevertheless, when an additional variable X_2 is introduced and its levels specified, the mean values of Y for "hi" and "lo" categories of X_1 do not remain the same: differential effects are noted. In this example, interaction is symmetric and X_1 and X_2 are interchangeable in the discussion.

This symmetry is highly unlikely in actuality. Table 2.7b is a made-up example of a more likely situation. The main effect of an independent variable is the difference in the degree of variation observed in the dependent variable under different categories or conditions of the independent variable. Interaction between independent variables, or joint effect, is the mean of their main effects. In Table 2.7b, the main effect of X_1 taken alone is +7 (i.e.

TABLE 2.7

Mean Values of Dependent Variable Y for Different Values of Interacting Independent Variables X_1 and X_2

a.

		X_1 hi	X_1 lo	"Marginals" (mean X_2 averaged over X_1)
X_2	hi	150	50	100
	lo	50	150	100
Marginals (Mean X_1 averaged over X_2)		100	100	

b.

		X_1 hi	X_1 lo	Mean $\overline{X}_2$ (averaged over X_1)	Main effect X_2 (X_2 hi − X_2 lo)	$\overline{X}$ hi − $\overline{X}$ lo	Joint effect
$\overline{X}_2$	hi	16	6	11	5	10	6
	lo	8	4	6		4	
Mean $\overline{X}_1$ (averaged over X_2)		12	5				
Main effect ($\overline{X}_1$ hi − $\overline{X}_1$ lo)		7					
$\overline{X}$ hi − $\overline{X}$ lo		8	2				
Joint effect		6					

the overall mean change in Y from X_1lo to X_1hi is X_1hi–X_1lo = 12-5 = 7) and of X_2 taken alone is +5. However, their interaction or joint effect is ±6. When X_2 is hi, the effect of X_1 is 16–6 = 10. When X_2 is lo, the effect of X_1 is 8–4 = 4. The interaction between X_1 and X_2 is the difference between these two effects, 10–4 = 6, and is the same if one compares the effects of X_2 specific to levels of X_1.

In that fourfold table, the mean effect of both levels of X_1 on Y is the same: 50. Nevertheless, differential effects are noted when the level of X_2 is specified. This example is made somewhat more dramatic in that the mean effects of both X_1 and X_2 on Y are the same; interaction is symmetric and X_1 and X_2 may be interchanged in the discussion.

Interaction is a statistical concept. The behavior of the interacting variables is only a model of factors acting in the material world. This model has the properties of other mathematical models that generalize relationships; the more general the model, the greater the number of different actual sets of relationships it is likely to fit.* The path diagram illustrating the interaction of smoking and asbestos in bronchial cancer shows a complex or configuration of factors acting together and not a sequence of factors in a causal chain. The assumption of the diagram is that the factors act concomitantly on the organism, at the same point in time and at the same location, to produce the disease process.

Statistical interaction can shelter a number of different material circumstances. In itself it cannot determine which of a number of possible causal models is correct, although some can be discarded as incorrect. For example, in a British prevalence survey, smoking and age showed interaction in relation to bronchitic symptoms (Fig. 2.2a). Age had virtually no association with the frequency of symptoms in nonsmokers, but in ex-smokers and in smokers age had an association that grew stronger with each increase in smoking level in fairly regular fashion. In a prevalence

*Thus Lazarsfeld distinguishes "conditional" and "contingent" qualifier variables. Both types show joint effects, and both types are each associated with the independent and the dependent variable of the initial association. In his terms, the conditional type, however, is antecedent to the independent variable; the contingent type is interposed between independent and dependent variables.[18]

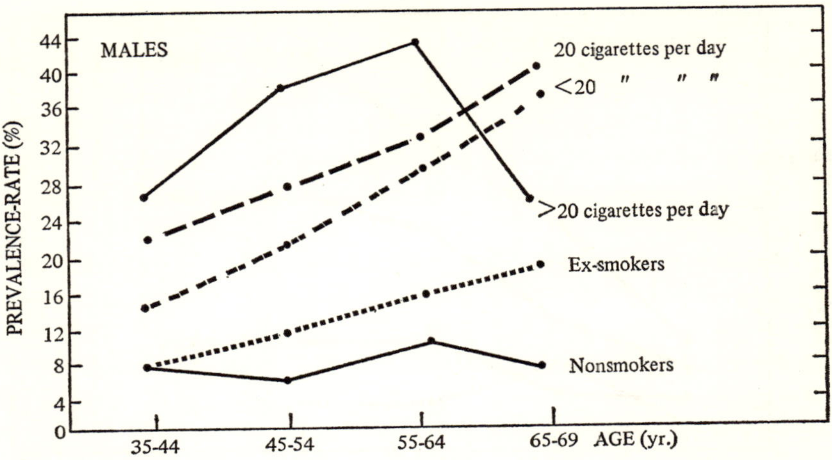

Figure 2.2a. Prevalence of persistent cough and phlegm production in sex, age, and smoking groups.

survey, the frequency distributions by age could reflect the survival and cumulation in higher age-groups of sufferers from chronic nonfatal disorder caused by smoking. The distribution could also reflect an increasing vulnerability to smoking caused by intrinsic aging processes, or by the effects of continuing life experiences whose duration (or "dose") must necessarily be greater the longer people live.

The presence of such an experiential factor is suggested by Figure 2.2b. Even among nonsmokers, high pollution was associated with a distinct if slight increase in the frequency of symptoms in older age-groups. Among smokers high pollution was associated with a quite sharp increase in the frequency of symptoms. In order to know whether smoking and air pollution act at the same time and the same location, or whether they act in sequence or at different locations, however, a more detailed knowledge of pathogenesis is needed.

Whatever the pathogenesis that underlies statistical interaction may be, the discovery of interaction supports causal inference by specifying the conditions under which a hypothetical cause contributes most, and least, to an effect. The recognition of

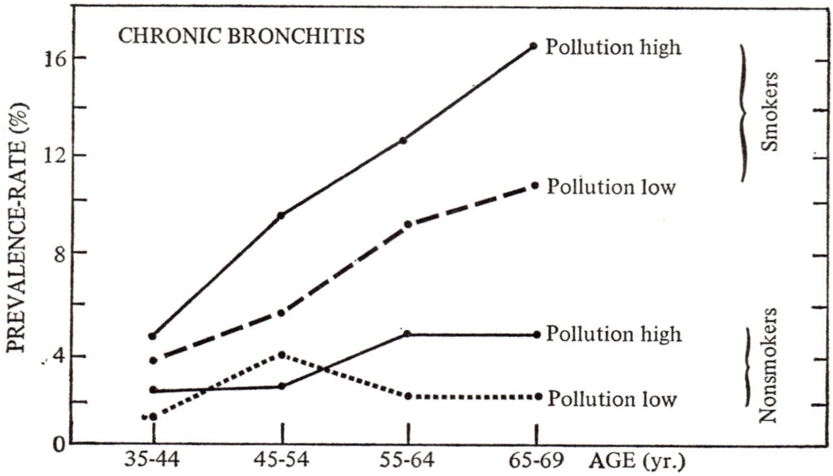

Figure 2.2b. Age-trends in respiratory disease in relation to smoking and air pollution. Source: Lambert, P.M., Reid, D.D. Smoking, air pollution, and bronchitis in Britain. *Lancet, 1*:853-858, 1970.

conditions is one way of identifying the "high-risk" or "vulnerable" groups so important to defining targets for prevention. Relationships are clarified, and concealed relationships may be revealed.

Elaborating the Association Between Variables

> . . .one of the five basic Confucian texts was the I Ching, or book of Changes, made up of sixty-four hexagrams which exhaust all possible arrangements of six broken or whole lines. One of the diagrams, to give an example, consists of two whole lines, of one broken line, and of three whole lines laid out one above the other. A prehistoric emperor is supposed to have discovered them on the shell of one of the sacred tortoises. Leibniz thought he saw in the hexagrams a binary system of numbers; others, a secret philosophy; others, like Richard Wilhelm, a scheme for looking into the future, since the sixty-four figures correspond to the sixty-four phases of any given enterprise or process; others again, the vocabulary of a certain tribe; still others, a calendar. I remember my friend Xul-Solar, the painter and mystic, laying out the diagrams with toothpicks or matchsticks. To outsiders, the Book of Changes runs the risk of seeming a mere piece of chinoiserie, but generations of scholars have read and studied it with reverence for

thousands of years, and generations will go on reading and studying it. Confucius told his disciples that if fate were to grant him another hundred years of life, he would devote fifty of them to studying the Book of Changes and its commentaries, or wings.[20]

The hypothesis that a demonstrated association between two variables is causal can be subjected to certain tests by further analysis. The essence of the tests is to elaborate the association by introducing additional variables into the analysis. When a third variable is introduced into an association between independent and dependent study variables, the initial association can alter in a variety of ways. In what follows, the procedures of elaboration and its effects on an association between two variables will be dealt with more systematically than in the preceding pages.

This discussion does not aim at systematization for its own sake. For many epidemiologists there is at present an unbridged gap between the well-tried technique of contingency table analysis and the newer statistical techniques of multivariate analysis. Since electronic computers have provided the capacity to handle these analyses with facility, it has become possible to deal simultaneously with a large array of control variables. The introduction of multiple control variables into the analysis of observed associations has already altered the strength of a number of causal hypotheses that have had currency. To take the dependent variable birth weight as an example, its long-recognized associations with maternal age and with maternal height both disappear upon the introduction of multiple controls. The whole of these observed associations can be acounted for by other variables, principally maternal prepregnancy weight and maternal weight gain during pregnancy.[21]

Yet some epidemiologists are ill at ease with the results of multivariate analysis by computer. The facile electronic procedures of computer programs all too readily allow one to lose one's grasp of real data, whereas the plodding procedures of contingency table analysis reinforce that grasp. To plod can also be to ponder and to probe.

Some of this unease may be due, however, to the different ways in which associations are conceived in these different approaches. In what follows, I attempt to set out, in words and diagrams, the forms of association between variables in a manner that may make for easier passage from the language of contingency tables and the syntax of rates to the language of multiple regression analyses and the syntax of variance.

For an epidemiologist a first step is to comprehend the kinds of associations that may cloud or clear his view of causal relationships. The most general categories of *associated variables* are independent and dependent variables. In an observed association of such variables the most general categories of *additional variables* are controlled, uncontrolled, confounding, and moderator variables. These variables may lie concealed within the simplifying assumptions of causal models, and the role of additional variables in strengthening causal inferences about the relationship of two associated variables has been discussed in that context. The relationships between variables that emerge when we turn from screening for extraneous factors to analysing them differ according to specific properties of the additional variable. Some of these have been noted, but in this section a more systematic classification and review of the properties of additional variables will be made.

Several possible relationships may exist between two variables, and many more relationships between three variables, if among them no restrictions are imposed either of time-order or direction of effect. We shall first rehearse possible causal sequences among variables neutral in regard to time-order and direction, and label them in the terms that have emerged from the previous discussion.

Three relationships between *two* associated variables must be distinguished from each other in order to proceed towards causal inference:

1. A symmetrical relationship: $X \leftrightharpoons Y$
2. An asymmetrical relationship: X may cause Y, $X \rightarrow Y$
3. An alternative asymmetrical relationship: Y may cause X, $Y \rightarrow X$

Once a *third* variable, Z, is associated with the other two, the forms of their possible relationships are multipled,* as illustrated in Figure 2.3.

*It has lately been pointed out that a system of ten free variables can give rise to more than 3 million orderings.[19,32]

Sequences 1, 3, 4, 10, and 13 will serve for illustration. In these sequences, the labeling of the variables is as follows: In the linked casual sequence 1, *X* is the independent hypothetical causal variable under study, *Y* is the dependent variable under study, and *Z* is an intervening variable.

In sequence 3, *X* is a single independent causal variable that gives rise to variation in two dependent variables (*Y* and *Z*) associated in a symmetrical relationship, since they are the outcome of a common cause. Where *Z* is a hypothetical causal variable and

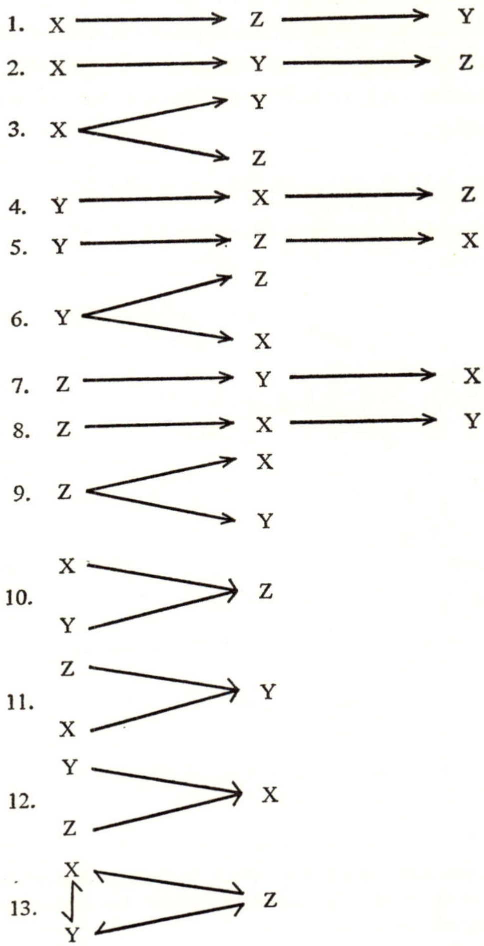

Figure 2.3 Possible causal sequences between three unrestricted variables.

Y the dependent variable under study, a variable like *X*, before it is controlled, acts as a confounding variable. Once it is controlled, *X* is seen to be an explanatory antecedent variable; *Z* turns out to be a passenger variable and not the independent causal variable initially hypothesized.

In sequence 4, if *X* is the independent study variable, then *Y* is an antecedent variable. *Y* produces variation in *X*, and *X* produces variation in *Z*. The difference between sequence 4 and sequence 1 is determined merely by which independent variable was initially selected for study and named as such.

Sequence 10 is an example of a pair of concomitant variables acting on a single dependent variable. Sequence 13 illustrates some of the variety of possible reciprocal relationships between the three variables.

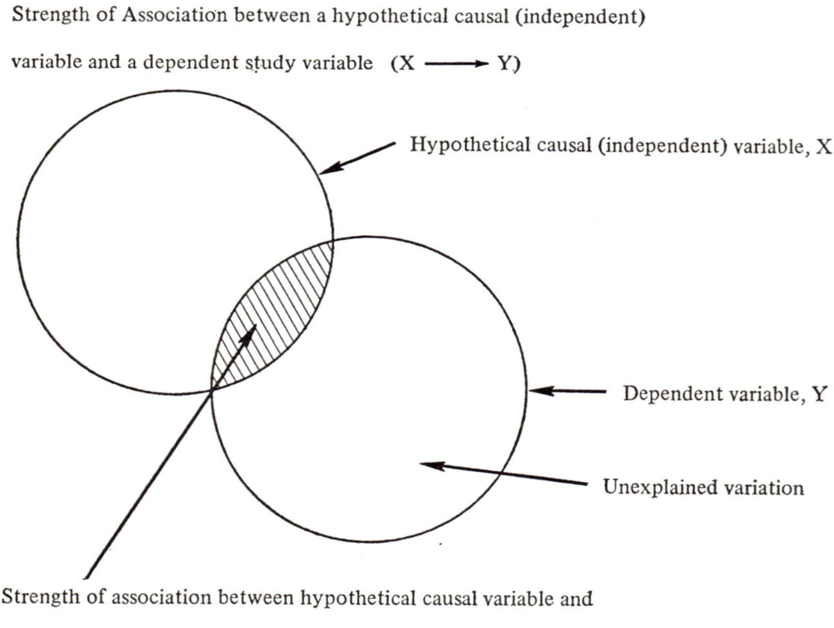

Figure 2.4

***This relationship can also be conceptualized and measured as correlation (*r*), or as the proportion of variance (r^2) in the dependent variable accounted for by the hypothetical causal variable.**

Figure 2.4 is a Venn diagram that illustrates the association between two variables. Each circle represents one variable, and the area of the circle is equivalent to the variance of that variable. Variance describes variation in quantitative terms; it is a measure of the degree of dispersion of the values of a given variable. The association between the variables is represented by the overlap between the circles; the greater the overlap, the stronger is the association, the greater the correlation (r), and the larger the proportion of variance (r^2) that the independent variable accounts for in the dependent variable. Figure 2.5 illustrates in the same terms the effect of the introduction, into an analysis of an observed association between an independent and dependent variable, of a third variable, unassociated with the independent vari-

Association between a hypothetical causal (independent) variable, a "third" unassociated independent variable, and a dependent variable ($X \rightarrow Y$, $Z \rightarrow Y$)

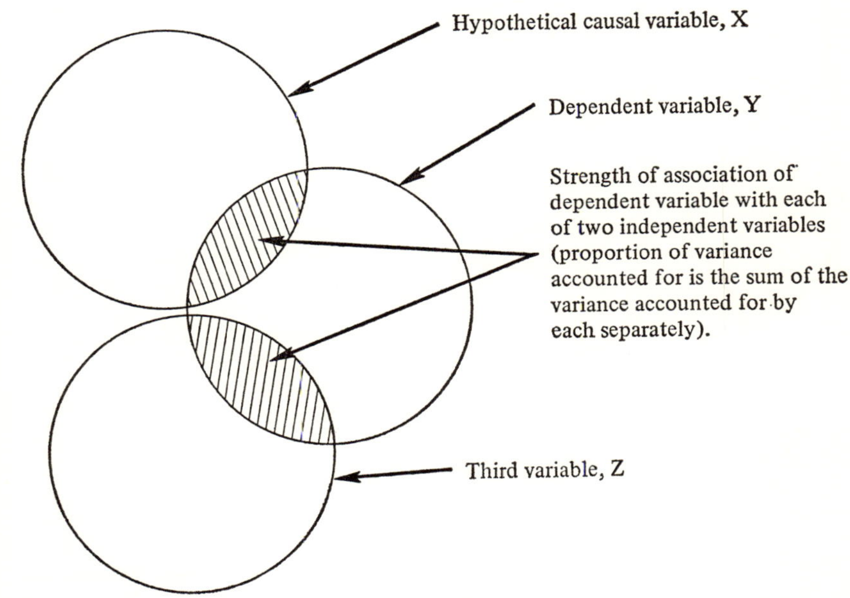

Figure 2.5

able. The third variable makes a simple additive contribution, as an additional cause of variation in the dependent variable, but does not affect the initial association between hypothetical causal and dependent variables.

Figure 2.6 illustrates the introductions into the analysis of two associated variables, of a third variable, *associated* with the independent variable. The contribution of the control variable to variation in the dependent variable is not simply additive. Its intro-

Strength of association between a hypothetical causal (independent) variable, an associated control variable, and a dependent study variable (X → Z → Y, or Z → X → Y, X⇅Z → Y)

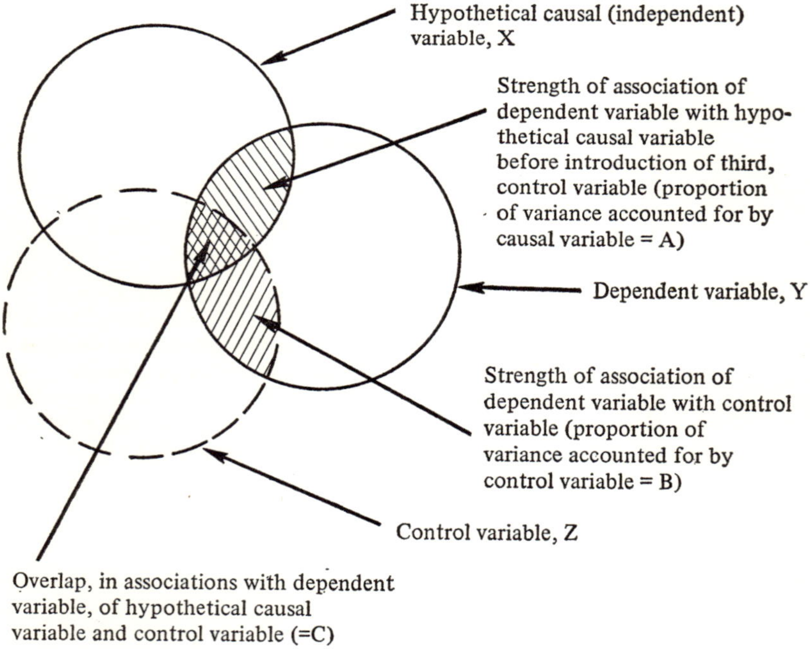

Figure 2.6

Note. **Variance uniquely accounted for by hypothetical causal variable, when the variance B contributed by Z is controlled, = A—C. (In the case of *distorter* and *suppressor* variables, the arithmetic value of the overlap, C, may be negative).**

duction alters the strength of association between the hypothetical causal and dependent variables. The change in the initial association varies with the special properties of each variable, including its time order and whether it strengthens or weakens the initial association, and the causal hypothesis is affected accordingly.

The additional variables that appear in the elaboration of associations between two variables include at least five types with distinctive properties of time-order and effect on the strength of the association: (a) simple antecedent,* (b) explanatory,† (c) intervening, (d) component, and (e) refined. Two types of additional variables are antecedent to the independent variable: simple antecedent and explanatory. An intervening variable falls between the independent and dependent study variables. A component variable contributes to the independent study variable and is concurrent with it. A refined variable is a subvariable of either the independent or dependent variable and is therefore concurrent with one or the other.

The naming of these variables is something of a Talmudic exercise, with due semantic byplay. In the literature of surveys, epidemiology, and biostatistics, many writers have developed their own special terminology for variables without regard to previous usage, others have appropriated terms used in one way for their own special use, and many terms have been used loosely or without any definition at all. Hyman and Kendall[22] and Lazarsfeld[18] had used well-defined terms in developing their excellent accounts of the analysis of the third variable, but they left off their task before completing the formal systematization of their analysis. Recently Rosenberg[3] took this systematization a further step forward. Some of the labels he chose to use lack cogency or precision and with reluctance I have sometimes used other terms than his.

Simple Antecedent Variables

A simple antecedent variable is antecedent in time to the independent study variable, and adding it to the analysis of an as-

*In the terminology of Rosenberg and some others, an "extraneous" variable.[3]

†In the terminology of Rosenberg, an "antecedent" variable.[3]

sociation between a hypothetical causal variable and a dependent variable traces the causal sequence backward in time.

> For want of a nail, the shoe was lost,
> For want of a shoe, the horse was lost,
> For want of a horse, the rider was lost,
> For want of a rider, the battle was lost,
> For want of a battle, the kingdom was lost
> And all for the want of a horseshoe nail.

For instance, one of the strongest known associations with birth weight is the mother's prepregnancy weight. The causal model would be:

Mother's weight ⟶ Birth weight
(independent variable, X) (dependent variable, Y)

The mother's diet, however, is an antecedent cause of the mother's weight, thus:

Mother's diet ⟶ mother's weight ⟶ birth weight
(simple antecedent variable, Z) → (independent variable, X) → (dependent variable, Y)

Each succeeding variable is associated with the preceding one: $Z \rightarrow X \rightarrow Y$, and any two variables of the three are associated with each other. When the simple antecedent variable Z is controlled, the initial association between independent and dependent variables does not disappear, but remains the same for each category or level of the control variable. This result is called internal replication (Fig. 2.7). (After the antecedent variable has been added to the causal sequence, it can be seen that, were Z conceived as the initial study variable, then the independent study variable X has precisely the same position as an intervening variable. We shall see that if an intervening variable is controlled, the initial association disappears. In this sequence, therefore, if the initial association were between Z and Y, and variable X were to be controlled, the association between the simple antecedent variable Z and the dependent variable Y would disappear).

While the addition to an analysis of a simple antecedent variable extends the causal chain ever backwards in time, it does not explain any more of the variation in the dependent variable than does the independent variable of the initial association.

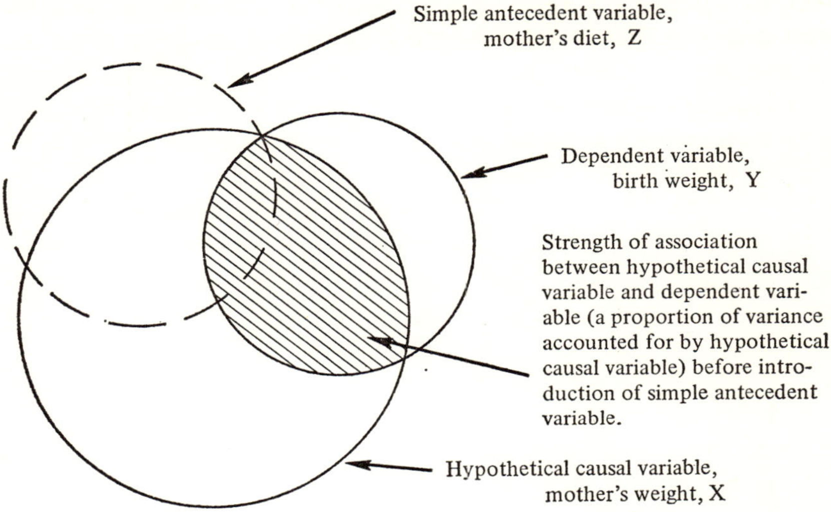

Figure 2.7. Introduction of a simple antecedent variable, in an analysis to test the association between a hypothetical causal (independent) variable and a dependent study variable, does not affect the initial association nor explain more variance.

Explanatory Variables

An explanatory variable is always antecedent in time to the hypothetical causal variable. We have noted that the apparent initial association between the hypothetical causal and dependent variables disappears when the explanatory variable (*Z*) is controlled. The third variable, *Z*, "explains" the association between *X* and *Y*, and the hypothetical causal variable (*X*) then becomes a "passenger" variable. The discovery of such explanatory variables disposes of any causal inferences that are likely to be made.

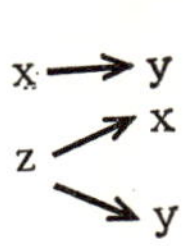

An example of confounding attributed to an explanatory variable appears in a study of the effect of the mother's diet during pregnancy on birth weight. A. M. Thompson[24] found that the mother's calorie intake was correlated with birth weight, a result that gave plausible support to the hypothesis that diet was an independent causal factor in birth weight: i.e.

Mother's calorie intake ⟶ Birth weight
(independent variable, *X*) (dependent variable, *Y*)

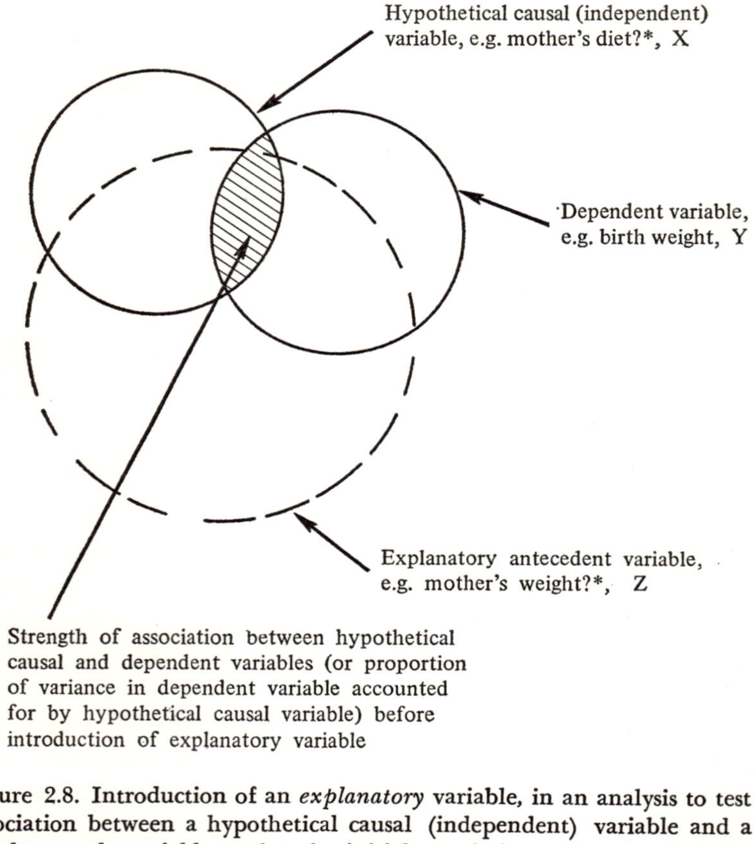

Figure 2.8. Introduction of an *explanatory* variable, in an analysis to test the association between a hypothetical causal (independent) variable and a dependent study variable, makes the initial association under test disappear.
***The question mark indicates the existence of another interpretation, discussed under the heading of intervening variables.**

The correlation virtually disappeared, however, when maternal body weight was held constant. The actual correlation was then reduced to $r = 0.05$. On the other hand, when caloric intake was held constant, the correlation between maternal body weight and birth weight persisted ($r = 0.29$). Thompson therefore discounted the correlation between calories and birth weight as spurious; he considered that it was "explained" by the correlation of an antecedent factor, "maternal body size," with both caloric intake and birth weight.

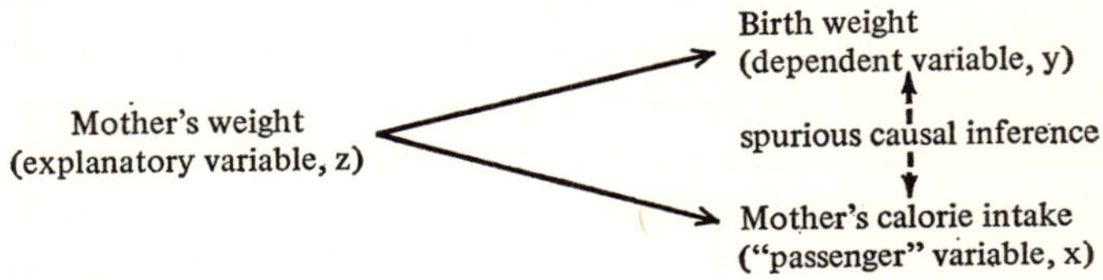

Figure 2.8 illustrates the causal model in diagrammatic form.

Intervening Variables

An intervening variable occurs in a linked causal sequence between associated independent and dependent study variables; it causes variation in the dependent variable under study, and itself is caused to vary by the independent variable under study. Like an explanatory variable, therefore, an intervening variable is statistically associated with both the independent and dependent study variables. The effect on an association between two variables of introducing an intervening variable is called "interpretation":[18] intervening links in the chain between the observed cause and effect are revealed.

When an intervening variable is controlled in an analysis, the initial association between the independent and dependent study variables disappears, or is markedly reduced, just as in the case of an explanatory variable. A causal chain of those variables formed by adding an intervening variable to an observed association has the same properties, in principle, as one formed by adding an explanatory variable. Thus analysis alone cannot settle the question of whether a third variable is an antecedent variable that explains an association, or whether it is an intervening variable that specifies further links in a causal chain. The answer must be obtained from other sources, either from the logical priority in time of the variables, or from further research.

To illustrate further from the association between diet, maternal weight, and birth weight, Thompson weighed his prenatal sample of women at the twentieth week of pregnancy. Part of the weight gain during pregnancy takes place before the twentieth week of pregnancy, and subsequent studies have shown that weight gain during pregnancy is related to birth weight. Maternal diet could thus have been a causal variable that was *antecedent* to and determined the mother's weight at the twentieth week of pregnancy, rather than that the mother's weight determined her diet. Maternal weight would then be a variable intervening, in a linked causal sequence, between maternal diet and birth weight:

Mother's diet (independent variable, X)	→	Mother's weight (intervening, Z)	→	Birth weight (dependent variable, Y)

This causal model of the initial association can be illustrated

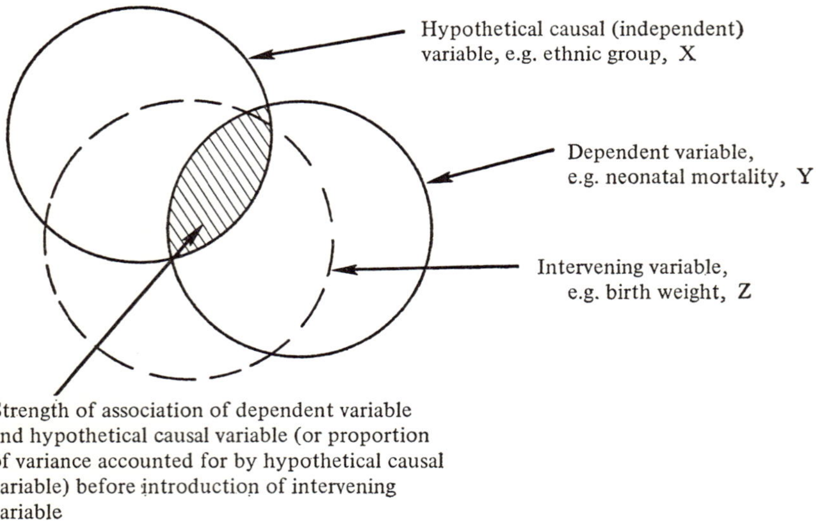

Figure 2.9. Introduction of an *intervening variable,* in an analysis to elaborate the association between a hypothetical causal (independent) variable and a dependent study variable, reduces the initial association under test or makes it disappear.

from Figure 2.8 by simply transposing the variables "mother's diet" and "mother's weight."

An example of the effect of an intervening variable on an association, and of its contribution to causal analysis, is given in Figure 2.9 and Table 2.8. In New York City in 1965, the neonatal death rate was 29 for nonwhites, 16 for whites. Low birth weight is a crucial intervening variable in this relationship. The high mortality associated with low birth weight accounts for the whole of the difference between ethnic groups.[25] When birth weight is introduced into the analysis of the association of ethnic group and neonatal deaths, the death rates of each group are seen to be equal above birth weights of 2501 gm, and actually lower among nonwhites below 2507 gm. The high neonatal death rate of nonwhites can thus be explained by the two to threefold risk of low birth weight among them.

TABLE 2.8

INTRODUCTION OF INTERVENING VARIABLE ILLUSTRATED IN CONTINGENCY TABLE ANALYSIS

Neonatal death rates per 1000 live births (dependent variable) for whites and nonwhites (independent "causal" variable), by birth weight (intervening variable): New York City, 1965.

	All	<1001	1001—	1501—	2001—	2501—	3001—	3501—	4001—	4501—
Nonwhites	29	845	333	84	19	17	5	3	4	16
Whites	16	918	480	140	31	7	4	3	3	8
All	19	879	408	115	26	7	4	3	3	9

Taken from *Summary of Vital Statistics for New York City, 1965*. New York City Health Department.

In this case the intervening variable is a distorter variable. When introduced into the analysis of the initial association, it reverses the direction of the initial relationship between ethnicity and neonatal death. Birth weight is associated with ethnicity, and with the dependent variable neonatal death, but the associations of birth weight and of ethnicity with neonatal death are in opposite directions.

The discovery of intervening variables particularizes understanding of the sequence of events in a causal chain. The analysis of intervening variables may thus elucidate pathogenesis; their analysis may also remove confounding and clarify the relationships between different levels of organization.

Component Variables

Component variables describe the components combined in global independent variables. Analysis of these variables specifies how much of the original association with the dependent variable is contributed by particular components of the global independent variable. For instance, social class is an independent global variable that can be defined in terms of occupation, education, and place of residence, each of which would constitute a component variable. All the effects of a component variable are not encompassed by the global independent variable under study. In fact, a component variable, as well as having effects quite separate from the dependent variable under study, may have effects on the dependent variable separate from those it contributes as part of the global independent variable. An example is occupation used as an index of the global independent variable, social class, and related to the dependent variable, measured intelligence. As a component of social class, occupation influences IQ. Apart from its influence through social class, occupation can independently influence IQ through the performance of certain occupational roles.

A component variable, insofar as it may cause variation in the dependent variable separate from that subsumed in the global independent variable, resembles any other control variable (see Fig. 2.6). Some effects of any control variable may in part overlap with the effects of the independent study variable; therefore, when the variable is controlled, the total proportion of variance in the dependent variable accounted for by the independent study variable may be reduced. Other effects of the control variable may be separate; their effects do not overlap with the effects of the independent study variable, and account for a unique portion of the variance in the dependent variable.

The characteristic that distinguishes the component variable from other control variables is its integration, often by definition, with the global independent variable under study; the component variable is coincident and concurrent with the global independent variable. Except for its time relations, the term is somewhat redundant, for component variables comprise elements similar to two other types of variable, namely, explanatory and moderator variables.

An example of a component variable given by Rosenberg[3] is of the explanatory type. Pearlin and Kohn showed an initial association of child-rearing values held by fathers in Italy (and the United States) with the father's social class position (Table 2.9) ; social class appeared to determine the value placed on self-

TABLE 2.9
SPECIFICATION OF COMPONENT VARIABLES OF HYPOTHETICAL CAUSAL (INDEPENDENT) VARIABLE: *EXPLANATORY TYPE*
(Illustrated by Standardizing for the Component)

Per cent of fathers selecting each characteristic in child (taken as index of childrearing values) as one of three most important characteristics among several: (a) by social class and (b) by social class standardized for independence of fathers' work.

	a.		b.	
	Initial Association		Standardized For Independence of Father's Work	
Child Characteristic	Middle Class	Working Class	Middle Class	Working Class
Self-control	52	35	41	41
Obedience	22	40	25	35
Neither	26	25	34	24

Adapted from Rosenberg, M. *The Logic of Survey Analysis.* New York, Basic Books, 1968, pp. 43, 44.

control and on obedience in children. "Independence of father's work" is a factor in the rating of occupations by social class, however, and its contribution to social class explains much of the initial association. Thus, when the association between social class and these two child-rearing values is standardized for independence of father's work, the association of social class with self-control disappears and that with obedience is lessened. In other words, independence of father's work explains the high values the middle classes placed on self-control and the lower values they placed on obedience that appeared in the initial association with social class.

Table 2.10 illustrates a second example of a component variable. The social class difference in the distribution of mild mental retardation with or without detectable handicaps to learning is apparent in classes I and II, using a conventional classification. This difference is "explained," and indeed revealed to its full extent, by an explanatory component variable, namely family type. These families were defined by their potential for vertical social mobility, and the classification by type separated families that were socially immobile (demotic) from those that were mobile or potentially mobile (aspirant). These dichotomous family types helped differentiate the characteristics of a syndrome of cultural retardation from other forms of mild mental retardation.

TABLE 2.10
SPECIFICATION OF COMPONENT VARIABLES OF HYPOTHETICAL CAUSAL (INDEPENDENT) VARIABLE

a.

Percent distribution of mildly retarded school children, with and without detectable handicaps to learning (dependent variable), by social class as defined by father's occupation (hypothetical causal variable).*

	Social Class				
Clinical State	*I & II*	*III*	*IV*	*V*	*Total*
Clinically Normal (N 283)	0.35	8.8	54.0	36.7	100
Detectable Handicap (N 37)	2.7	8.1	51.4	37.8	100

b.

Percent distribution mildly retarded school children, with and without detectable handicaps to learning (dependent variable), in each family type (component variable: explanatory type) as defined by occupation and education of all family members (component variables: moderator type).*†

Clinical State		*Family Type*	
		Aspirant	Demotic
Clinically Normal	(*N* 30)	0	100
Detectable Handicaps	(*N* 22)	25	75

Stein, Zena A., and Susser, M. In Redlich, F.C. (Ed.) *Social Psychiatry* Res. Publ. A.R.N.M.D. *47*:62-85, 1969, and other papers.

*I have taken some liberties with these data, without violating their sense, in order to construct a satisfactory example. For actual data refer to the original papers.

†Proportions have been weighted to correct for the stratification of the subsample.

The "family type" variable, however, was itself created by combining the contributions to social class of two components, namely the occupational and educational status of all family members. In relation to family type, occupation and education are component variables of the moderator kind. With such variables, discrete types are created among the categories of the independent variable by combining specified values or categories of the component variables with each other. Each component of the global variables, i.e. the type created by the component variables, is analogous to a moderator variable, for unless there was interaction between components, there would be little use in creating a fixed type.

Another example of the creation of types from moderator component variables appears in the development of the concept of status crystallization, or status consistency. Categories of status crystallization have been defined by determining the degree to which the statuses of individuals, with respect to education and occupation or income, were consistent with each other. The effects of status inconsistency, considered as a stressor, have been studied in terms of such manifestations as psychiatric symptoms, entry to psychiatric care, ischemic heart disease, and hypertension.[26]

With component variables of moderator type, then, the contributions of the components to the global independent variable can be conceived as fixed for each of the categories of independent variable. With component variables of explanatory type, their contributions in determining the values or categories of the global independent variable can be conceived as though they were scaled and weighted together with other scaled factors. The proportionate contribution of a single component variable to any particular value or category of the independent variable would therefore vary in relation to the values of the array of factors that contributed to that particular combined score.

By analyzing the component variables subsumed by a hypothetical causal variable, we learn what proportion of the association with the dependent variable each component of the global variable explains. We therefore identify ever more particular causal factors. By this means too, as by specifying antecedent conditions, we may identify high-risk groups and types.

Components of an independent study variable may be ill defined, or ill chosen. The researcher who aims to construct a measure or a type as independent variable will hope to avoid adding irrelevant variance to it. If for lack of knowledge or foresight irrelevant variance is included in his definition of the independent study variable, the result will be to suppress or damp down any association that in fact may exist between it and the dependent study variable. Such a result was illustrated in the discussion of suppressor variables on p. 51.

Refined Variables

Refined variables may be defined as variables created by the subdivision of any study variable, either independent or dependent, into mutually exclusive segments. Refined variables are not true additional variables; they belong to a different logical and analytic category from all the other types described above. Unlike control variables, they are subvariables, all of whose effects are encompassed by the global variable of which they form a part. Thus refined independent variables account for part of the variation in the dependent variable that the global variable contributes, but cannot add to it.

Refined independent variables are like component variables in that they are coincident with the global independent study variable. But they differ from component variables in that they exert no effects separate from those of the independent variable under study and bring no additional source of variation into the association under analysis.

Unlike component variable analysis, successful refinement of a study variable into meaningful subcategories strengthens the initial association unless each subcategory happens to account for exactly half of the effect of the study variable. As with component variable analysis, however, the effect of refining the independent study variable is to reveal the proportion of the initial association accounted for by the refined variables (Fig. 2.10 and Table 2.11).

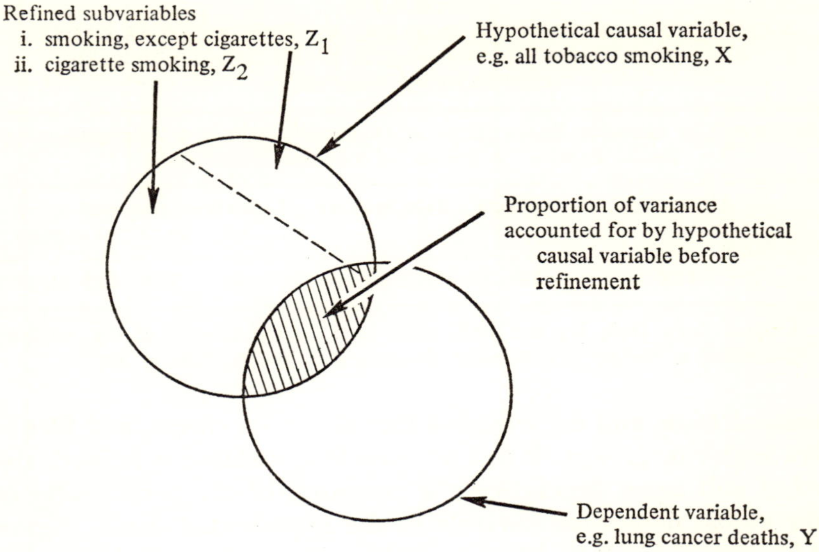

Figure 2.10. ***Refinement of hypothetical causal (independent) variable*** **to strengthen its association with the dependent study variable.**

The global independent variable accounts in all for a greater proportion of the variance in the dependent study variable than the refined variable; no segment can be greater than the whole. Thus in Figure 2.10, all smoking combined accounts for more variance than any particular kind of smoking. This variance is divided between tobacco smoking excluding cigarette smoking and cigarette smoking. But although the refined variable "cigarette smoking" accounts for less variance in all than the global variable "all tobacco smoking," this refinement makes the association of cigarette smoking with lung cancer deaths stronger in terms of relative risk than the association of all tobacco smoking with lung cancer deaths. As Table 2.11 shows, the relative risk of the global independent variable is a weighted average of the risks associated with each of its segments; some segments have higher risks (heavy cigarette smoking), others lower (other forms of smoking).

Refinement of an independent variable particularizes homogeneous causal factors, specifies the relevant elements of the hypo-

TABLE 2.11
REFINEMENT OF TOBACCO SMOKING AS HYPOTHETICAL CAUSAL VARIABLE IN ASSOCIATION WITH LUNG CANCER DEATHS (DEPENDENT VARIABLE)

(Illustrated by Mortality Ratios [Ratio of Observed Deaths in a Subpopulation to Deaths Expected in a Standard Reference Population])

All Smokers	Ex-smokers	Pipe Smokers	Cigarettes per day 1-9	Cigarettes per day 10-19	Cigarettes per day 20 or more
12.8	5.0	5.4	4.4	10.8	43.7

Adapted from Doll, R., and Hill, A.B., cited in the Report of the Advisory Committee to the Surgeon General, *Smoking and Health*, 1964, p. 164.

thetical cause and the elements that dilute its effects, and identifies high-risk groups. When a dependent variable is refined, the effect will again depend on the relevance of the partitioning of the global dependent variable to the hypothetical cause. Figure 2.11 and Table 2.12 illustrate refinement and strengthening of the association of the hypothetical causal variable "tobacco smoking" with the dependent variable "lung cancer deaths." Meaningful refinement not only strengthens the association in terms of rel-

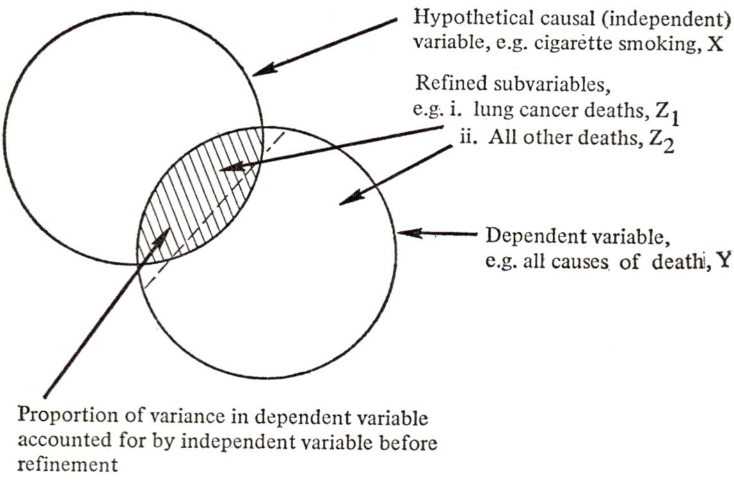

Figure 2.11. Refinement of a dependent variable in order to strengthen its association with a hypothetical causal variable.

ative risk but also, in the usual case, allows the hypothetical causal variable to account for a greater proportion of variance in the refined dependent variable than it did in the global dependent variable. For instance, Figure 2.11 shows that refinement is likely to reduce the amount of variance in the dependent variable that has to be accounted for (i.e. it reduces the size of the denominator in the association), while it hardly affects the amount of variance accounted for by the causal variable (thus it hardly reduces the numerator of the association) so that the proportion of variance accounted for must rise. The refinement of the dependent variable thus particularizes homogeneous effects in the dependent variable. The process specifies the most relevant of these effects; it removes those effects that are unrelated to the hypothetical cause and dilute the association; and it helps to reveal the full impact of a cause of a health disorder.

TABLE 2.12
MORTALITY RATIOS, IN SEVERAL STUDIES OF CURRENT CIGARETTE SMOKERS (HYPOTHETICAL CAUSAL VARIABLE), FOR ALL CAUSES OF DEATH (DEPENDENT VARIABLE), AND CANCER OF LUNG (REFINED DEPENDENT VARIABLE)

Cause of Death	British Doctors	Men in 9 States	U.S. Veterans	California Occupations	California Legion	Canada Veterans	Men in 25 Sstates	Total
All causes	1.4	1.7	1.8	1.8	1.6	1.7	1.6	1.7
Cancer of Lung	20.2	10.0	12.0	15.9	4.9	11.7	11.7	10.8

Adapted from Report of the Advisory Committee to the Surgeon General, *Smoking and Health,* 1964, p. 149.

Table 2.13 illustrates the use of refinement in an analysis that helped establish a syndrome of mental retardation. Identification of the syndrome was aided by refining the dependent variable "backwardness in school." A first refinement was achieved through the research design: severe mental retardation was excluded from the sample, and only mild mental retardation (defined as referrals for backwardness in school) was selected for inclusion in the dependent study variable. In the analysis, the condition of mild retardation was refined by specifying IQ levels and clinical characteristics. The refined dependent variable, the syn-

TABLE 2.13
REFERRAL FOR INVESTIGATION OF BACKWARDNESS IN SCHOOL (DEPENDENT VARIABLE) BY IQ AND CLINICAL STATE (REFINED DEPENDENT VARIABLES) AND SOCIAL CLASS OF SCHOOLS (INDEPENDENT VARIABLE)

(Average Annual Rates per 1000 Salford School Children 7 to 10 Years of Age, 1955-59)

Refinement of Referrals	Social Standing of Schools Low	High	Relative Risk of Referral Low/High S.C.
All	10.0	4.0	2.5
IQ 90+	1.4	1.5	0.9
IQ 80-89	1.7	0.	—
IQ 50-79	4.3	0.5	8.6
*IQ 50-79 clin. norm	3.8	0.26	15.*
IQ 50-79 with lesions	0.5	0.26	1.9

Adapted from Stein, Z.A., and Susser, M. In Redlich F.C. (Ed.) *Social Psychiatry* Res. Publ. A.R.N.M.D., *47*:62-85, 1969.
*The syndrome of mild mental retardation.

drome of mild mental retardation without detectable brain damage, showed distributions by social class* that diverged sharply from the distribution of the other elements of the dependent variable. Thus by refining a dependent variable we may identify syndromes, or we may identify the particular manifestations of a disorder that relate most closely to the causal variable.

The strength of logical inference is much enhanced by the application of systematic analysis. Where an association is found between two variables, the hypothesis that the association is causal is tested by introducing data on additional relevant variables. By this means, an analysis is elaborated.

*Table 2.10 illustrates further procedures used to identify the syndrome of mild mental retardation without brain damage. In this analysis the component conditions—family types—under which the syndrome occurs were specified. The high specificity of the association of the syndrome with family type legitimized the descriptive label of "cultural mental retardation."

Table 2.6 illustrates further refinement of the syndrome of mild mental retardation. In this analysis the syndromes were specified as antecedent conditions. A distinctive characteristic of the syndrome of cultural retardation emerged, namely, a rise in IQ level during adolescence and young adulthood. A next step in elaborating the causal chain would be to elucidate intervening variables between family types and the manifestation of the syndrome.

The advantages that the elaboration of the analysis of associations by the addition of variables confers may be summarized as follows:

1. Elaboration tests the association between two variables for confounding factors. Possible confounding variables are controlled and their influence on the initial association is made visible.

2. Elaboration specifies the conditions under which an association between two variables is stronger or weaker, and reveals associations between two variables is stronger or weaker.

3. Elaboration helps to identify intervening links that may exist between associated independent and dependent variables.

4. Elaboration refines the association between the independent and dependent variables and specifies which elements contribute most to their association. Irrelevant components which dilute an association are removed or controlled.

These extensions of knowledge about the associations between variables give leverage to judgment and logic.

Notions of Probability

The fourth epidemiologic strategy that deals with extraneous sources of variation in the dependent variable is statistical. Uncontrolled variables always exist in the real and complex world outside the isolated conditions set up for experiments or observational studies. Hence some variation in the dependent variable that cannot be explained by specified independent variables always remains. In epidemiologic analysis, but *not* in inference, it makes little difference whether this unexplained variation is attributed to unknown factors still to be elucidated or to chance variation. In either case, the unknown is treated the same way, by introducing the notion of probability.

The law of falling bodies holds only if ideal conditions are assumed. If the law is to be used in empirical situations, without the simplifying assumption of a vacuum, it must be stated in statistical terms. One cannot say that bodies will fall at thirty-two feet per second per second; one can state the probability of a body falling at rates dispersed around 32 ft/sec./sec given specified conditions.

The basic statistical procedure assigns to chance the variation in the dependent variable that is due to unknown extraneous sources of variation. This degree of variation is taken as the norm, and becomes a base line for expected values. It can then be determined whether observed values depart from the expected to a degree that does or does not fall within the limits set for chance events.

Statistical method thus enables the epidemiologist to handle unexplained variation by attributing it to chance. The probable frequency with which the association of independent and dependent variables can be ascribed to chance is estimated; from this estimate the statistical "significance" of a result can be stated.

At the same time, statistical method helps the epidemiologist to handle variation that can be explained and is not due to chance. Thus it provides the means to estimate the power of a research design.[27] This is the probable frequency with which an effect that is not due to chance can be expected to appear (with a given true magnitude, a given sample size, and a given significance level). Whether for the purpose of assessing the results of research or preparing a research design, statistical method thus enables us to derive the quantitative conditions, numbers needed in numerators and denominators, under which the test of a hypothesis can be expected to reveal a positive result that is present.

Apart from these estimates of probabilities, statistics also provides the means to estimate how much of the variation in a dependent variable could be accounted for by a particular independent variable, either uniquely or when taken together with an array of other independent variables. This is effectively done by multiple regression techniques. These estimates of the amount of variance accounted for by independent variables can assist epidemiologists in making judgments about cause by pointing to the strength of associations.

Still another contribution of statistics is to test causal models quantitatively. The fit of the values predicted from the model under different conditions is examined against observed statistics values. Where the fit is poor, the model can be discarded. Imaginative use has been made of these methods recently in developing path analysis.[19,31] This mode of analysis proceeds on the basis of simplifying assumptions about the direction of relationships between linked sequences and configurations of variables. These assumptions permit the analyst to construct a model of the causal relationships that may exist between the array of variables he had included in the finite system he has chosen to study. Observed values are then assigned to each variable. The source and amount of variance that can be accounted for in each variable under the assumptions of the model can then be quantitatively expressed.[1,29,30] Regression analysis helps identify the less probable sequences of causal relationships, which may then be eliminated from consideration.[19,32] These complex models, however, introduce assumptions about distributions, reliability of measurement, and direction, including all the assumption made by regression analysis, that demand wariness of the user.[31] Where longitudinal data based on repeated observations of the same phenomena on the same people are available, approaches similar in principle provide stronger grounds for the inference that change in an independent variable has produced change in a dependent variable.[8,34-36]

Probability and statistics, by giving numerical values to procedures and assumptions, prop the simplifying and elaborating strategies for strengthening causal inference. Thus chance variation can be handled, the conditions under which an hypothesis can be accepted or rejected can be specified, the strength of associations can be quantified, and the contribution to variation of each known variable can be calculated. For the thorough and professional exposition of all these questions, I leave the reader to turn to appropriate texts.

Criteria of Judgment

The fifth and final strategy available to the epidemiologist for making inferences about causal relationships depends on his own subjective judgments. These judgments are reached by weighing the available evidence; there are no absolute rules, and different judges often reach conflicting conclusions. A number of criteria can be used that assist judgments about whether associations found to be statistically significant on testing also have causal significance. One must of course scrutinize the methods used to obtain the data whose relationships are under analysis, but here we take as given the array of criteria regarding sound method. The *Report of the Advisory Committee to the Surgeon General*[5] has provided a framework for what follows. Five separate criteria for judging causal relations will be discussed: (a) time sequence of variables, (b) consistency of associations on replication, (c) strength of association, (d) specificity of association, and (e) coherent explanation.

Time Sequence

Knowledge of the temporal relationship of associated variables is a basic condition to be satisfied if one variable is to be established as the cause of another. We have to establish which variables are antecedent in the relationship and which subsequent.

In an analysis of two associated variables elaborated by the introduction of a third variable (to extend the causal sequence, or to test, control, or specify the association between the two variables), we have seen that the effect on the status of the causal relationship differs according to whether the third variable precedes or follows the independent variable in time. In either case the strength of the association between the two initial variables may be increased or reduced, but the inference to be drawn from an increase or decrease differs according to the precise location in time of the added variable.

The knowledge about the actual time sequences that is needed to classify variables, however, may not be easily come by. The time relationship is not difficult to establish in the case of acute diseases caused by some specific agent. It can be much more difficult to establish with conditions that are chronic, especially those of insidious onset. In such cases an ascribed status or a fixed attribute can assist in analysis. In a relationship between sex, or birth cohort, and some manifestation, there will be no questions about what is antecedent. An attribute that alters with time, like marital state, can greatly complicate analysis, and leave uncertain which is antecedent and cause and which is subsequent and effect.

The association of mental illness with the divorced state is one of many examples where the question of which came first is difficult to answer. A second example is the association between coronary disease and personality type. In one study a particular set of personality traits was found with undue frequency in individuals who had coronary disease. Further analysis, in persons who had not yet developed coronary disease, but had high-risk attributes for it, revealed no association with these same personality traits. The inference drawn was that the personality traits developed in response to the disease.[33]*

The association of schizophrenia with poverty and low social class has presented even greater difficulties of interpretation. The disease was first found to be concentrated in deteriorated urban areas by Faris and Dunham[37] in 1937, in a study of hospitalized schizophrenic patients in Chicago. It took almost thirty years to get a reasonably clear view of the time sequence of events which lead to this finding, a consistent one in large cities. Many studies have been made around the question of whether deteriorated social conditions breed schizophrenia, or whether the schizophrenics drift down into deteriorated social conditions because of their illness or because of their predisposition to the illness, and the question is not closed.

Predisposition presents a considerable analytic problem. When the event of schizophrenia is elaborated into a process which may be preceded in time by the tendency to the condition, the problem of ordering variables in time becomes complicated. It can be complicated even in acute disease with a clearly defined onset and an obvious agent. A death by suicide is an acute event with usually an obvious agent. But a predisposition to suicide may long precede the event. The existence of a predisposition is suggested by the high risk of successful suicide among persons who have previously attempted suicide. Predisposition therefore complicates the question of what factors precede the origin of the tendency to suicide and what factors are subsequent to it.

In schizophrenia, many studies of large cities confirm the con-

*Since the data came from a prevalence study, however the inference was still open to challenge.[35]

centration of the condition among the lower socioeconomic classes. For lack of a clearly defined criterion of onset, however, it remained difficult to say that the condition or the predisposition to it had not preceded the social class position of the patient. Eventually an investigation which showed that drift down the social scale almost certainly does operate was based on the birth certificates of patients. From these certificates the patients could be assigned a social class position according to the occupations of their fathers, which was recorded on the certificates. The social class position undeniably antedated the onset of the disease, and it could be compared with the patient's own social class position according to his own occupation. (However, drift down the social scale demonstrated in this manner probably does not account for the whole of the excess of schizophrenia in the lower social classes.) These examples illustrate the difficulties of establishing temporal sequences with insidious onsets, and even more with predispositions. Figure 2.12 is a simplified diagram of a few of the possible time relations of schizophrenia with social factors.

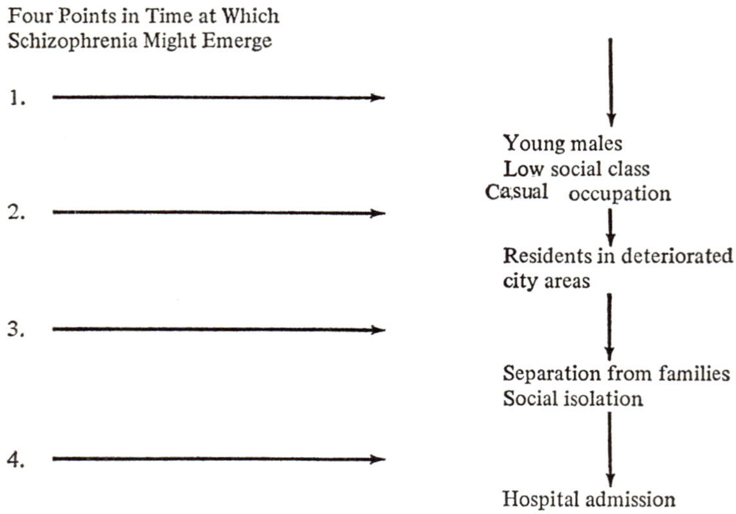

Figure 2.12. Time sequence. Possible time sequence of social factors associated with schizophrenia. Source: Susser, Mervyn. *Community Psychiatry: Epidemiologic and Social Themes.* New York, Random House, 1968.

Consistency and Replication

The epidemiologist is denied the opportunities for exact replication which are available to the physical scientist. In epidemiology, variation in the conditions of study is for all practical purposes a constant. An epidemiologic alternative to exact replication is to seek for consistency of a finding on repeated tests.

The criterion of consistency depends on the replication of results in many studies or many analyses. The strength of the argument rests on the fact that diverse approaches produce similar results. John Snow piled up evidence that the cause of cholera was an invisible water borne agent by the consistency of repeated tests of his hypotheses. This criterion is much the same as J.S. Mill's "method of agreement": all the situations are different but they have one circumstance, or association, in common. In addition to the nineteen retrospective and seven prospective studies reported in *Smoking and Health*,[5] all of which found an association between smoking and health and roughly the same relative risks, the classic studies of Durkheim on suicide at the end of the nineteenth century are worth mentioning in this context. He carried out these studies with the object of testing, in terms of a specific phenomenon, general sociologic hypotheses about social structure and social cohesion.

Durkheim tested the official statistics of the nations of western Europe for correlations between suicide rates and such factors as age and sex, religion, occupation, marital status, and economic cycles. He found a high rate of suicide in Protestant countries, a low rate in Roman Catholic countries, and moderate rates in countries with mixed populations of Catholics and Protestants. To show that this association was independent of the many other associated differences between Catholic and Protestant countries, he broke the figures down into groups and regions: in Switzerland the association with religious persuasion held for each language group, in Prussia and Bavaria for each province, and in all for seventeen essentially independent comparisons.*

*The principles involved in replication are discussed by Selvin.[38] By applying a probability test to the chances of attaining replications of the result in all these independent comparisons, Selvin concluded that the result has a much higher degree of significance than could be attributed to it from any one study.

Consistency does not entirely rule out confounding variables. In the case of the association of suicide with religious persuasion, such a confounding variable could be the inaccurate reporting of causes of death. Suicides among members of religions which deny burial rights to those who die by their own hand, and generally strongly disapprove of suicide, might be attributed to other causes in order to assure decent burial. Although such a contingency lacks organic connection with the causal sequence resulting in suicide, it can be treated as an intervening variable between the death and the enumerated rate:

Deaths from suicide → Certification of death → Suicide rates

In the case of the associations between smoking and health disorders, which are also strongly shored up by their consistency, it is difficult to conceive that any hidden, unknown confounding variable could be responsible for the results. The confounding variable would have to be present nine times as frequently in all smokers, and twenty times as frequently in heavy smokers, as in nonsmokers. Confounding variables rarely account for so large a risk. Indeed, a statistical test has been devised to determine the probability that a factor could be confounding that depends on the proportion of the variation for which it could account.[39,40]

Strength of Association

The stronger an association, the more likely it is to be causal. The strength of an association means the degree to which phenomena are in close association.* Figure 2.4 through 2.11 and Tables 2.8 through 2.13 illustrate the effects, on the strength of association between independent and dependent study variables, of introducing different types of third variables. These effects of third variables, taken together with their time-order, have clear import for causal inference.

Relative risk is one of the most useful ways of stating the strength of association in epidemiology. The relative risk de-

*It is almost a biostatistical cliché that the strength of an association and its statistical significance should not be confused. An association may be weak and yet highly significant. Tests of significance are necessarily closely related to the numbers of cases being studied. Differences that are proportionately quite small can be made highly significant by large numbers.

scribes the ratio of the incidence of a condition in those exposed to a risk or causal factor to the incidence in those not so exposed. Thus the relative risk of lung cancer for smokers is the ratio of the rates of lung cancer in smokers to the rates of lung cancer in nonsmokers. Stated in another way, this relative risk is the ratio of the observed incidence in smokers to the incidence to be expected among them had they experienced the rates of nonsmokers (Fig. 2.10). *Attributable risk* indicates the absolute incidence of a health disorder that can be attributed to the causal factor. It is derived by substracting the incidence of the disorder among persons not exposed to the causal factor from its incidence among persons who were exposed.[2]

Another approach to estimating the strength of association is to calculate either a correlation coefficient or a regression coefficient. The *correlation coefficient* indicates the degree to which a hypothetical causal factor varies with a manifestation of disease. The *regression coefficient* expresses the mean change to be expected in the dependent variable for a unit change in the value of the independent variable. *Multiple regression* analysis indicates how much of the variation exhibited by a dependent variable can be accounted for by one variable or a subset of variables, also how much of that variation can be accounted for by many independent variables together, and finally how much of the variation in the dependent variable can be accounted for uniquely by one variable, or a subset of variables, when other independent variables are held constant.

Figure 2.13 illustrates the application of such analysis to a study of social and family factors in psychiatric impairment. A large number of items of social, family, and psychiatric information was collected. These items were analysed and grouped into factors by the method of factor analysis. The factors were then treated as independent (or predictor) variables in the separate areas of demographic background, parental relationships, and parent-child relationships. The psychiatric information was also combined into dependent (or criterion) variables in a number of separate areas of psychiatric functioning.

In Figure 2.13, the triangle represents the total variance in the

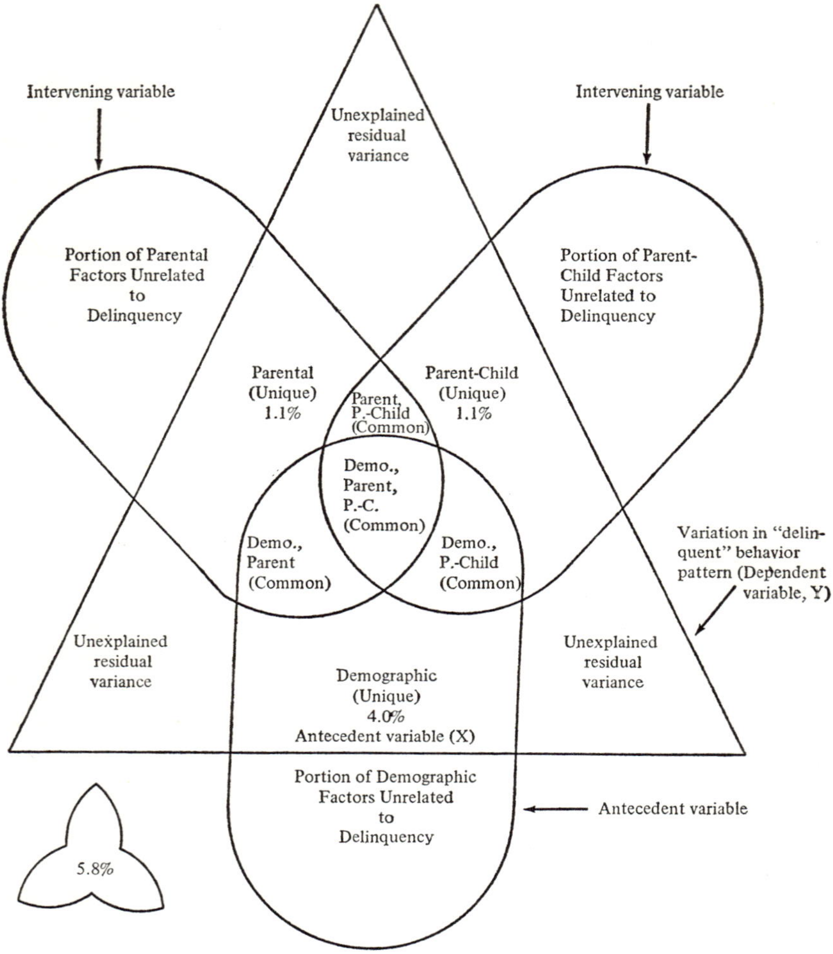

Figure 2.13. Proportion of variance in "delinquent" behavior pattern accounted for by three sets of hypothetical causal variables, (namely, demographic factors, parental relationships, parent-child relationships) in a random sample of about 1000 Manhattan children aged 6-18 years. 5.8 percent = Portion of delinquency related jointly to demographic, parental, and parent-child factors ("common criterion-related variance"). Total variance explained by demographic factors, parental relationships, and parent-child relationships combined = 12 percent. Taken from Langner, T. Progress Report on Psychiatric Impairment in Urban Children, 1970.

single dependent factorized variable "delinquent behavior pattern." Each ellipse-like area shows the amount of variance in each factorized set of independent variable taken separately. The combined area of all the ellipse-like figures within the triangle represents the total amount variance in the dependent variable that the factorized independent study variables account for jointly (12%). The area of each ellipse-like figure in the triangle that does not overlap with other ellipse-like areas represents the variance in the dependent variable uniquely accounted for by that factorized independent variable. The cloverleaf-shaped area of overlap in the center of the triangle represents the amount of the variance in the dependent variable that is jointly accounted for by the independent variables together and cannot be attributed to anyone.

Specificity of Association

By the term "specificity" we attempt to describe the precision with which the occurrence of one factor or variable will predict the occurrence of another. The ideal is a one-to-one relationship, in which a cause is both necessary and sufficient. The more closely the relationship resembles the conditions of being both necessary and sufficient the more specific it will be. Thus if a particular manifestation followed only one particular cause, it would be specific to that cause.

Generally, specificity is increased by the research design focusing on the variables of concern, or in analysis, by the introduction of additional variables. An association gains in specificity from the elaboration of an analysis, procedures illustrated in the preceding discussion. Thus we have seen that moderator variables, component variables, intervening variables, and refined subvariables add specificity to an association.

In the case of smoking as a cause of disease and death the report *Smoking and Health*[5] begins with an analysis of smoking in relation to mortality. This analysis shows that the risk of death from *all* causes is increased among smokers. The *dependent* variable was refined, and a much greater specificity was attained, when smoking was related to deaths from particular causes, subvariables of the overall death rate. Still greater specificity was attained when broad causes of death such as cancer were broken down into its subcategories at specific sites (Fig. 2.11 and Table 2.12).

In this analysis the independent variable was refined into components by dividing smokers into those who smoked by different methods, that is, cigarette, cigar, and pipe smokers. The independent variable was further refined by classifying smokers according to the amount they smoked, according to the duration of their smoking, and according to whether they had discontinued smoking. In this way the causal factor was made much more specific. Cigarettes in particular were incriminated. In addition, the plausibility of the association was enhanced because it was found that the risk for ex-smokers was lower than for smokers.

In another perspective, all additional variables are used for control and thereby add to specificity: they reveal confounding and remove irrelevant components of the association from further consideration. In the report *Smoking and Health*,[5] age and sex were introduced as control variables in many of the analyses. At various points in the report such factors as geographic variation, urban/rural variation, income, social class, occupation, and ethnic group were also examined, although they were not regularly introduced as control variables.

At the outset, when an association is shown between the independent study variable and the dependent variable, we will always find that we have not explained the whole phenomenon. There will not be a one-to-one correspondence between cause and effect; therefore, the variation cannot be attributed wholly to the operation of the cause we hypothesize and pursue in the investigation. In other words, some of the variation in the dependent variable remains unexplained.

But in the degree to which each independent control variable contributes to the disease manifestation and explains some of the variation in it when introduced into the analysis, so there remains less unexplained variation, and the proportion of the remaining variation explained by the independent study variable increases. By increasing the number of detailed investigations of independent variables, a fairly weak empirical association between the causal factor and disease manifestation can be moved towards greater specificity. In this manner, design and persistence in research, and analytic procedures (holding constant in contingency tables, standardization, multiple regression), enable the researcher to seek out the unique and specific contribution of a hypothetical causal variable to the variation in the dependent variable.

Coherent Explanation

A final criterion by which we may judge a causal association is its coherence, as an explanation, with other known facts about the disease, and also with the other known facts about the causal factor under study. We ask ourselves whether all the known facts about the disease fall into place in relation to this cause. If they do not we must have due pause. We do not expect the whole phenomenon to be explained by a cause we have adduced. But if some features appear inconsistent with that hypothesized cause, either another explanation must be found for the facts as they stand, or another explanation can be tested in further studies, or the inconsistency can be filed until some better explanation is developed.

In the case of the studies on lung cancer, one such inconsistency was the early finding of Doll and Hill that among those who smoked, inhalation did not increase the risk of lung cancer. The reasonable expectation would be that it should increase the risk of lung cancer, because inhalation would bring the presumed carcinogen into closer contact with the target tissues.

There were several possible explanations for the inconsistency, including the fact that smokers' histories of inhalation are unlikely to be accurate. It is a subjective and ill-defined piece of information. There have been other inconsistencies in the smoking and lung cancer studies, but the coherence of the findings in other respects overrides most of these.

In addition to other coherent findings, the association between smoking and lung cancer is congruent with the histopathology of the disease. Smoking is associated with squamous changes in the epithelium and with the squamous type of malignancy. This type of pathological change is that usually found with a recurring injury to epithelial tissue. Other types of lung cancer, such as adenocarcinoma, have not been found to be associated with smoking. Thus, the attribution of lung cancer to smoking by studies of the exposure of individuals to tobacco was found to be congruent (a) with the rise in mortality parallel with the rise in tobacco consumption (b) with the higher male mortality parallel with higher tobacco consumption of males in each cohort, (c) with the urban/rural differences in mortality, (d) with the socioeconomic differences in mortality, (e) with the histopathology of the disease, and (f) with the linear relationship between amount of smoking and lung cancer.

Linear relationships between independent and dependent variables confer ostensive coherence on hypotheses derived from them. Thus, a response proportional to dose is highly persuasive of a causal relationship. In the case of smoking and lung cancer, an increase in the dose of cigarettes was associated with an increase in the incidence of lung cancer (see Fig. 2.14). The dose-response relationship was consistent with the amount smoked, with the duration of smoking, with the age of starting to smoke, and with discontinuance.

Linear relationships, however, are by no means invariable with causal relationships. Some cause-effect relationships are curvilinear; they may not increase beyond a certain threshold. Others may be U-shaped parabolas, or S-shaped, or exponential.

The relationship of cholesterol levels to dietary intake provides an example of a probable threshold phenomenon. In surveys that include poorly nourished groups of people, cholesterol levels have varied with dietary intake. These results were consistent with the dietary hypothesis of the etiology of coronary heart disease, in which blood cholesterol level was considered an intervening variable. In surveys of people all of whom were well fed, however, no relationship could be found between the intake of fats and calories and the level of cholesterol. It seemed as if, above a threshold level of cholesterol and dietary intake, the blood was saturated and added fat intake no longer affected the cholesterol level in the blood.

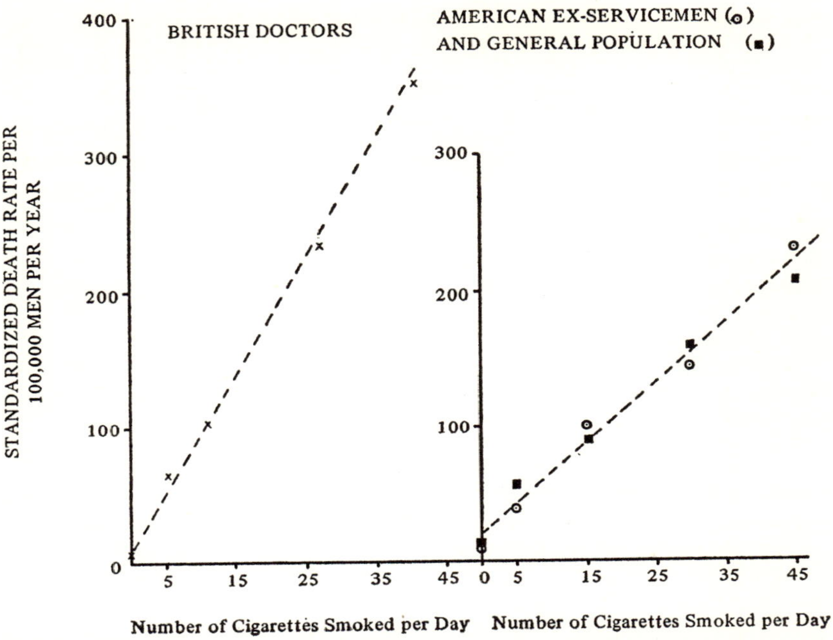

Figure 2.14. Relationship observed between lung cancer mortality and number of cigarettes smoked per day in British and American studies. Doll, R. *Prevention of Cancer: Pointers from Epidemiology*. Nuffield Provincial Hospital Trust, 1967.

In another example of a saturation threshold, during World War II strategic bombing did not seem to have the effect of increasing anxiety and lowering morale among those who were bombed (Table 2.14 cols. 1 and 2). There was little difference in the analysis between those exposed to moderate bombing and those exposed to very heavy bombing. The threshold value, for an effect of bombing on morale, was any bombing at all (Table 2.14 col. 3). After the effect on morale caused by any exposure to bombing, there was practically no added effect on morale from heavier bombing.

More often, perhaps, thresholds below which effects do *not* occur have been postulated, especially in such matters as the setting of safety standards for exposure to environmental hazards. Thus controversy surrounds the assumption that a safe threshold

TABLE 2.14
SELECTED FINDINGS FROM THE UNITED STATES STRATEGIC BOMBING SURVEY OF GERMANY BEARING ON THE RELATIONSHIP BETWEEN MORALE AND EXPOSURE TO BOMBING

Percent of each group exhibiting following Indices of morale	Moderate Bombing (6000 tons) (%)	Heavy Bombing (30,000 tons) (%)	Light Bombing (500 tons) (%)
Expressing anxiety	12	12	9
Showing increased fear	36	33	18
Showing war weariness	62	62	48
Listening to Allied broadcasts	35	36	38
Change in opinion that Germany could win the war	47	47	45
Showing willingness to surrender	59	59	54
Belief that leaders had best interests of people at heart	44	48	52

Source: *The Effects of Strategic Bombing on German Morale.* U.S. Strategic Bombing Survey, Morale Division. U.S. Gov't. Printing Office, 1946, Vol. I, Ch. 3. Cited in Hyman, Herbert. *Survey Design and Analysis.* New York, The New Press, 1955.

exists for irradiation, an assumption which laws and regulations have tended to use. A good deal of evidence shows the contrary, namely that the effects of irradiation are linear (Fig. 2.15).

Examples of U-shaped curves can be found in the relationship of birth weight and fetal age to perinatal mortality. In the case of both birth weight and fetal age (assessed from duration of pregnancy), mortality is high both among light babies and among heavy babies, but not among those centrally distributed (Figs. 2.16a, 2.16b).

CONCLUSION

Judgments that apply the criteria outlined above to rigorous analysis carry our understanding beyond the level of intuition. The discipline needed to achieve rigor is rewarded by the precision of the hypotheses generated, by economy in the pursuit of further investigations, and by the avoidance of many traps and culs-de-sac. In epidemiology and the social sciences, turbulence, wilfulness, and low levels of predictability are manifest characteristics of the subjects of study. In this discussion I have sought

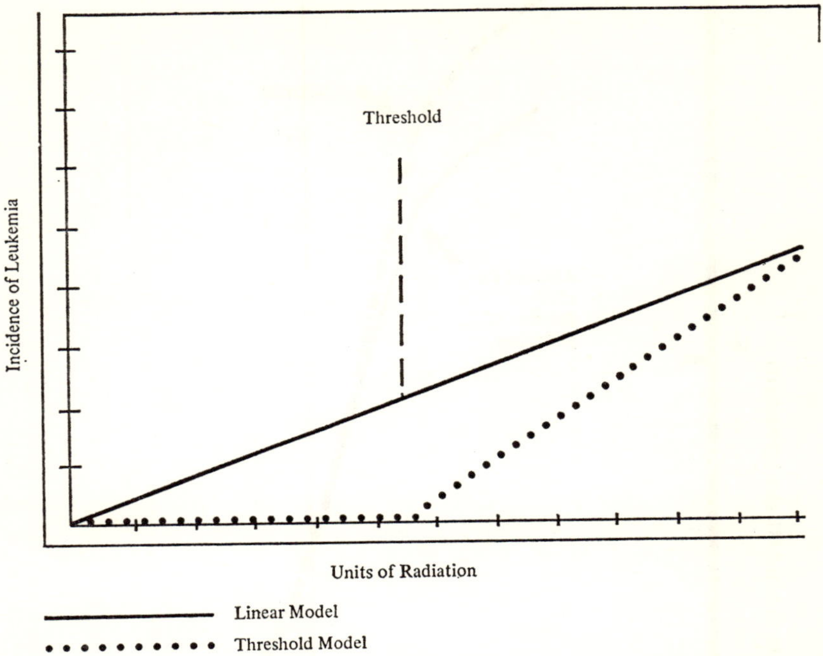

Figure 2.15.Simple models of relationship in a population of leukemia to radiation.

ways of structuring and organizing observations that can lead to sound inferences about causal relationships. The process of causal analysis, central to all science, is most crucial where the subjects of study are least biddable. Where land mines are everywhere, one should not venture without a mine detector. Here I have tried to show how one might make a systematic sweep of treacherous ground.

ACKNOWLEDGMENTS

The analysis I have made, it is proper to note, draws mainly from the work of a few writers and teachers from whom I have freely borrowed. These key sources are J.S. Mill,[4] P. Lazarsfeld,[18] H. Hyman,[22] B. MacMahon, Pugh, and Ipsen,[2] the Surgeon General's Committee on Smoking and Health,[5] H.M. Blalock,[1] M. Rosenberg,[3] and J. Cohen.[29]

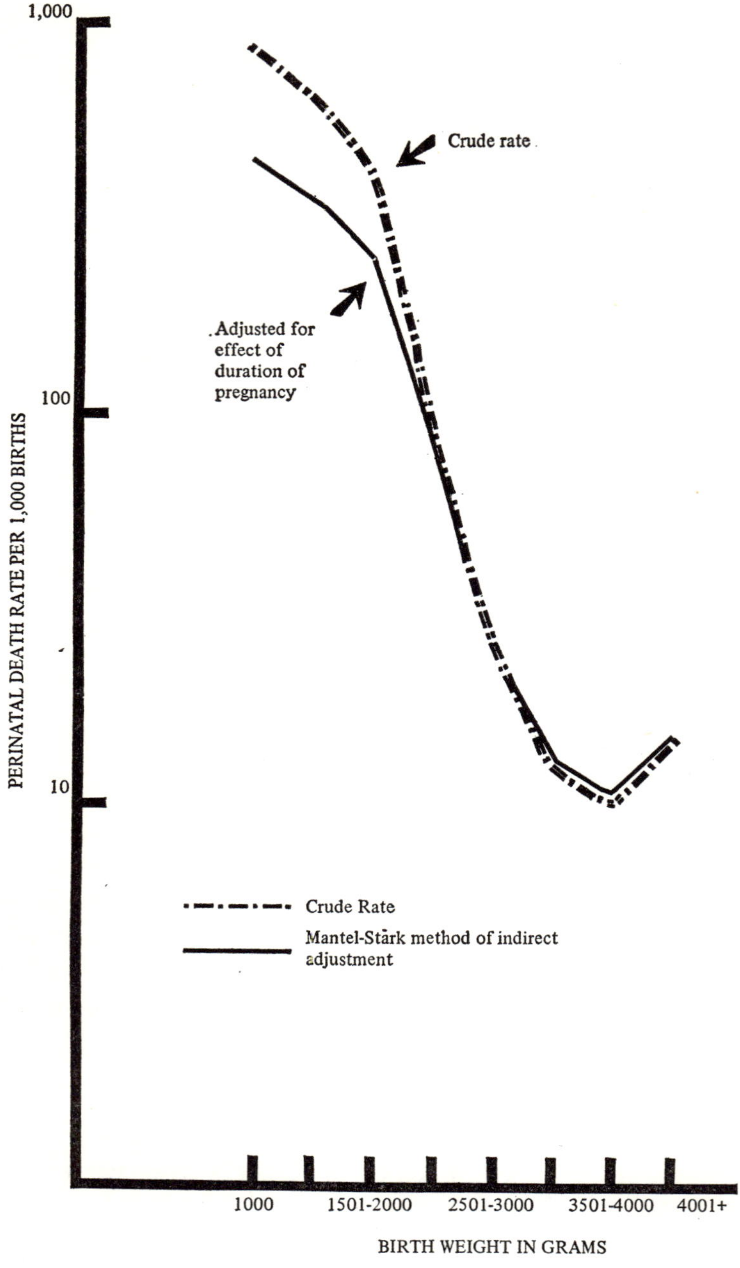

Figure 2.16a. Perinatal death rates by birthweight, crude and adjusted for duration of pregnancy. Data from British Perinatal Mortality Survey, 1958.

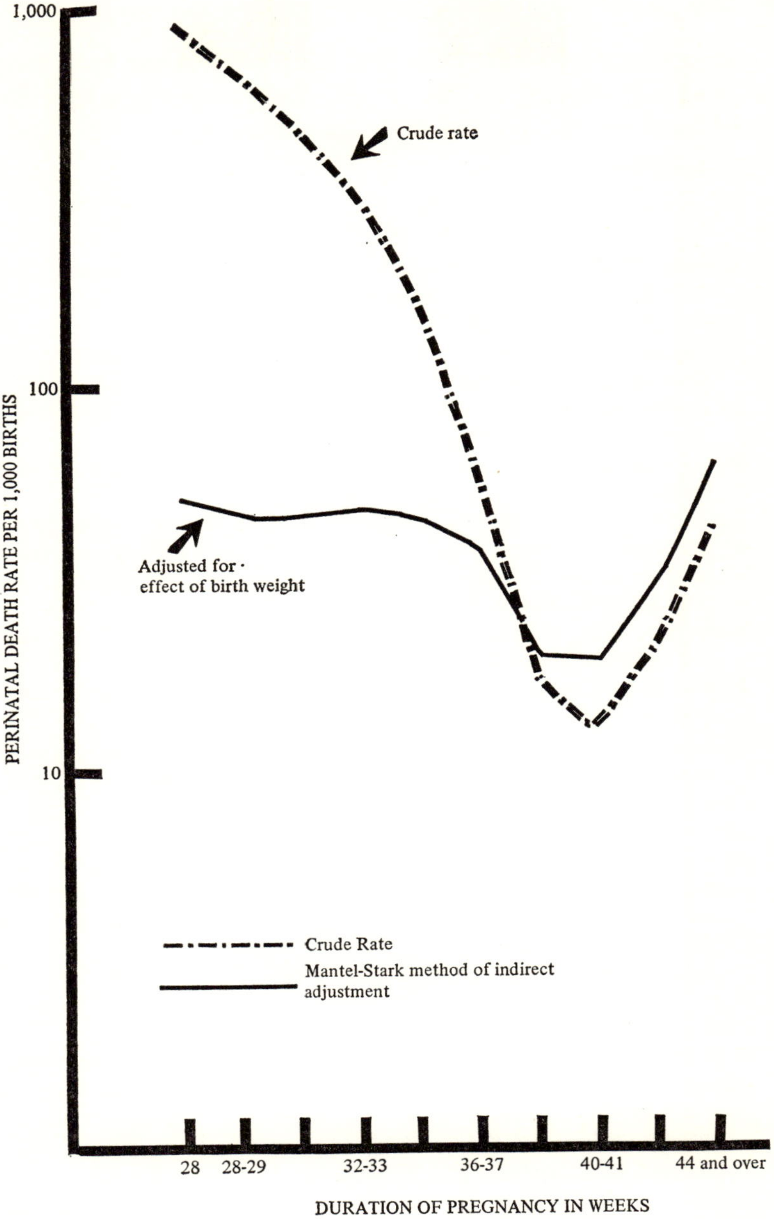

Figure 2.16b. Perinatal death rates by birthweight, crude and adjusted for duration of pregnancy. Data from British Perinatal Mortality Survey, 1958.

Jacob Cohen, Joseph Fleiss, and Elmer Struening have kindly read and commented on the paper. Zena Stein has, as always, turned over all these ideas with me many times and supplied several examples.

REFERENCES

1. Blalock, H.M. *Causal Inference in Non-experimental Research.* Chapel Hill, University of North Carolina Press, 1964.
1a. Simon, H.A. *J. Amer. Stat. Ass., 49:*467, 1954.
2. MacMahon, B., and Pugh, T.F. *Epidemiology: Principles and Methods.* Boston, Little, Brown & Co., 1970.
2a. Susser, M. W. *Community Psychiatry:Epidemiologic and Social Themes.* New York, Random House, 1968, Chap. 5.
3. Rosenberg, M. *The Logic of Survey Analysis.* New York, Basic Books, 1968.
4. Mill, J.S. *A System of Logic.* London, Parker, Son & Bowin, 1856.
5. U. S. Dep't. of Health, Education, and Welfare. *Smoking and Health: Report of the Advisory Committee to the Surgeon General.* Washington, D. C., Public Health Service, 1964.
6. Stebbings, J.H. Urban Residence and Pulmonary Function. Unpublished Ph.D. thesis, Johns Hopkins University, 1969.
7. Fisher, R.A. *The Design of Experiments.* 8th ed., New York, Hafner, 1966.
8. Campbell, D.T., and Stanley, J.C. *Experimental and Quasiexperimental Designs for Research.* Chicago, Rand McNally, 1963.
9. Miettinen, O.S. *Biometrics, 24:*339, 1968.
10. Bross, I.D.J. *Amer. J. Epidem., 89:*359, 1969.
11. Miettinen, O.S. *Amer. J. Epidem., 91:*111, 1970.
12. Campbell, D.T., and Erlebacher, A. In Hellmuth, J. (Ed.) *The Disadvantaged Child,* Vol. III, *Compensatory Education.* New York, Brunner-Mazel, in press.
13. Douglas, J.W.B. *Brit. Med. J.,* p. 1008, 1960.
14. Kish, L. *Amer. Sociol Rev, 26:*328, 1961.
15. McKeown, T. *Brit. Med. J., 2:*63, 1970.
16. Selikoff, I. J., Hammond, E.C., and Churg, J. *J.A.M.A., 204:*106, 1968.
17. Kendall, P.L., and Lazarsfeld, P.F. In Merton, R.K., and Lazarsfeld, P.F. (Eds.) *Continuities in Social Research.* Glencoe, Fress Press, 1950.
18. Lazarsfeld, P.F. *Daedalus, 87:*120, 1958.
19. Heise, D.R. In Borgatta, E. (Ed.) *Sociological Methodology.* San Francisco, Jossey-Bass, 1969, p. 38.
20. Borges, J. L. *N.Y. Review of Books,* August 13, p. 3, 1970.
21. Rush, D., and Susser, M.W. *Progress Report of the Prenatal Study to*

the National Institute of Child Health and Human Development. National Institute of Health Contract No. 692180, 1970.
22. Hyman, H. *Survey Design and Analysis.* New York, Free Press, 1955.
23. Reference deleted.
24. Thompson, A.M. *Brit. J. Nutr., 13:*509, 1959.
25. Bergner, L., and Susser, M.W. *Pediatrics, 6:*946, 1970.
26. Susser, M.W., and Watson, W. *Sociology in Medicine,* 2nd ed. London, Oxford, 1971, Chaps. 5 and 6.
27. Cohen, J. *Statistical Power Analysis for the Behavior Sciences.* New York, Academic Press, 1969.
28. Wright, S., *J. Agric. Res., 20:*557, 1921.
29. Cohen, J. *Psychol. Bull., 70:*426, 1968.
30. McNemar, Q. *Psychological Statistics.* 4th ed., New York, John Wiley & Sons, 1969.
31. Land, K.C. in Borgatta, E. (Ed.) *Sociological Methodology.* San Francisco, Jossey Bass, 1969, pp. 3-37.
32. Linn, R.L., and Werts, C.E. *Psychol. Bull., 72:*307, 1969.
33. Ibrahim, M.A., Jenkins, C.D., Cassel, J.C., McDonough, J.R., and Hames, C. G. *J. Chronic Dis, 19:*255, 1966.
34. Lipset, S. M., Lazarsfeld, P.F., Barton, A.H., and Linz, J. In Lindzey, G. (Ed.) *Handbook of Social Psychology.* Cambridge, Mass., Addison-Wesley, 1954, p. 1124.
35. McFarland, D.D., and Cobb, S. *J. Chronic Dis., 29:*393, 1967.
36. Pilz, D.C., and Andrews, F. *Amer. Sociol. Rev., 29:*836, 1964.
37. Faris, R.E.L., and Dunham, H.W. *Mental Disorders in Urban Areas: An Ecological Study of Schizophrenia and Other Psychoses.* Chicago, University of Chicago Press, 1939.
38. Selvin, H.C. *Amer. J. Sociol., 63:*607, 1958.
39. Bross, I.D.J. *J. Chronic Dis., 19:*637, 1966.
40. Bross, I.D.J. *J. Chronic Dis., 20:*487, 1967.

Chapter 3

THE APPLICATION OF GENETICS TO EPIDEMIOLOGY

EDMOND A. MURPHY

TO THE LAY mind and to much of the medical profession the term "epidemiology" has infectious disease as its object. This belief can be attributed to the historical beginnings of the subject and, until perhaps the last twenty-five years, the epidemiologist was concerned with little else. Now that the epidemiological principles for studying infectious disease have been defined if not entirely solved, the research epidemiologist has directed his attentions to other chronic diseases. The success of this endeavor is less evident and has had correspondingly little impact on medicine generally.

Epidemiology has been most successful and has commanded the greatest respect where three conditions have been fulfilled:

1. A causal factor for a disease is being traced, not sought.
2. A good experimental model is available.
3. There is an adequate theory.

It would, perhaps, be unwise to infer that the endeavor has been successful because these conditions have been fulfilled. For instance, the development of a good theory might be a result of the fact that the object of study is accessible to methods of high resolution. It might well be argued, for example, that the mathematical theory of epidemics did not start before the 1920's, half a century after the discovery of bacteria and eighty years after the classic researches of Snow. However, it is, perhaps, misleading to identify all theory with mathematics, and Koch's celebrated postulates, imperfect though they were, constituted a substantial contribution to epidemiological theory.

The new epidemiology represents a departure from classical

infectious disease epidemiology, a departure which is much more extensive than might be at first apparent. In the first place, in studying, for example, atherosclerosis, the epidemiologist is not tracing an agent which has either been already identified or been proved to exist. Rather, his endeavor is directed to trying to *find* specific causes by the study of populations. As to the opportunity for experiment, he is impeded by the prolonged course of the disease, which makes experiment extremely expensive and indeed gives rise to more or less serious ethical and legal problems. Moreover, there is still nothing like a consensus over the relevance of the experimental atherosclerosis in animals to the clinical disorder encountered in man despite an enormous body of data.

But what is the most profound departure, though one which has only slowly been realized, is of an epistemological nature. In exploring the etiology of typhoid there is very good reason to believe that we are dealing with a specific disease. On the other hand, it is far from obvious that this is true of atherosclerosis. If it is true that atherogenesis is a heterogeneous problem, the prospect of finding a homogeneous answer must be faint indeed.

Though such criticism comes ill from someone who is not an epidemiologist, I cannot resist expressing the opinion that the greatest enemy of modern epidemiology is the habit of taking over holus-bolus the notions of clinical medicine as the terms for rigorous study. Every branch of medicine, not excepting the study of infectious disease, has done much to foster spurious groupings and factitious divisions.

Every five years or so, an editorial is written pointing out that the granular contracted kidney has diverse etiologies: that the unity of morphology does not reflect unity in cause but the limited repertoire of the kidney's responses, and that perhaps the same is true of atherosclerosis. Expressing such comments appears to provide a catharsis and the epidemiologist immediately goes back to exploring hypotheses predicated on homogeneity. But the criticism is to the point: if the phenomenon is heterogeneous then the etiology must be heterogeneous. But it is fatally easy to confuse a *heterogeneous* with a *composite* etiology (Fig. 3.1). The multifactorial approach to the granular contracted kidney would sug-

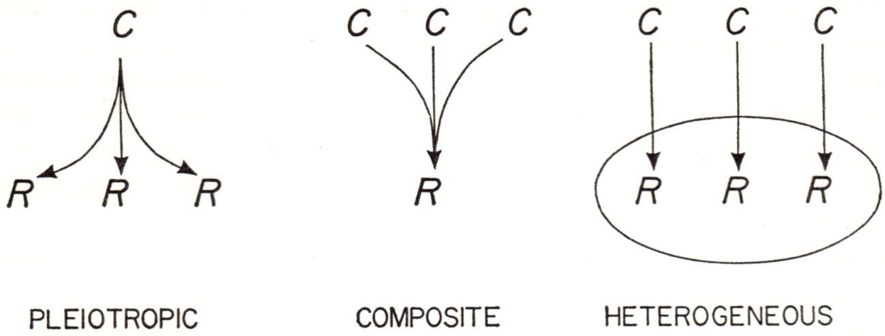

Figure 3.1. Some complex patterns of caustality. Three patterns must be distinguished: (1) pleiotropic (multiple effects from a single cause), (2) composite (in which a result occurs only from the conjunction of multiple causes), and (3) heterogeneous (in which the causes are distinct but the results are indistinguishable).

gest that the outcome is best predicted by a weighted combination of the number of streptococcal infections in the throat, the dietary intake of lead, the stiffness of the joints, the number of white cells in the urine, and various other factors. The confusion of the outcomes would unearth a multiplicity of causes, but this is not (as is so easily supposed) attributable to the need for interactions between the causes; it is an artifact of thought which fails to distinguish glomerulonephritis, lead poisoning, amyloidosis, gouty kidney, pyelonephritis, and so forth, pathogeneses between which there is little relationship.

A celebrated controversy in recent years,[1-4] that over the nature of so-called "essential" hypertension, has thrown these problems into high relief. It is much to the point that the motivation for this controversy was a genetic one. The matter at issue is whether this putative disorder is inherited as an all-or-none characteristic or whether it represents the combined effects of many factors, some or all of which might be genetic. In a word, the central question is whether this disorder is genetically unilocal or multilocal. Much has been made in this argument of the pattern of distribution, as to whether it is bimodal or not. This argument involves a treacherous enthymeme. Apart from the problems that arise from the limited size of the samples and from errors of measurement, it is by no means so obvious as has been supposed that bimodality of a distribution implies genuine heterogeneity.[5-8] Conversely, the absence of bimodality in the distribution of some measurable characteristic cannot be taken as a refutation of the single-locus hypothesis.[8] This realization comes as a disappointment to those investigators who have an inexhaustible faith in the ability of statistics to resolve scientific questions. (Indeed, no statistical technique can resolve questions unless certain axioms are fulfilled. But these axioms, in turn, are formulated in the light of scientific belief which is itself sustained by the statistical analysis of previous information. The paralysis of endeavor which this circularity could too easily generate can be confronted with two considerations, one pragmatic, one logical. Firstly, that science has in spite of it made progress; and secondly, that scientific truth may be pursued in stages in which first approximations are successively refined by an iteration between experiment and analysis.)

The question then arises: What is meant by a cluster in a nosological sense? If a peril of investigation is to mistake a composite question for a simple one, what safeguards are possible? The answer to this question has been, and perhaps necessarily, pragmatic. In fact, the notion of a completely homogeneous problem is an abstraction which we cannot expect to encounter in the real world. If the large majority, say 70 percent, of the variance of a characteristic can be accounted for by a single factor, then for practical purposes we could treat it as a homogeneous problem. But it is necessary to recognize that there is no sharp dividing line between a "single-factor" disorder and a "multifactorial" disorder, any more than there is a sharp division between a monarchy and a democracy.

Some of the characteristics that have this quasi-unifactorial quality have been mentioned and comprise the subject matter of classic epidemiology. They include infectious disease, industrial intoxication, and specific vitamin and other dietary deficiencies.

One area, however, which meets nicely this requirement of single-factor etiology is Mendelian genetics. It may be noted that it fulfills unusually well those conditions which we have listed as favoring epidemiologic studies. In the first place, a single factor is being traced, not sought. The definition of this factor varies with the condition being considered. Sometimes, as in Huntington's chorea, it is a somewhat shadowy clinical picture, shrouded in equivocations and calling for the exercise of judgment which even among the experienced is fallible. Sometimes, as in specific enzyme deficiencies, the resolution is better but still not beyond reproach. But when seen to best advantage, as in the hemoglobinopathies, the resolving power of genetics far transcends any other source in the entire range of biology. Then secondly, genetics, par excellence, is the branch of biology which has been amenable to cogent and precise experimentation in species other than man. Finally, there has been no branch of biology which has lent itself to such an extensive theoretical development. A number of standard texts may be consulted for a didactic treatment of this subject in greater detail.[9-14]

In view of these obvious advantages it may seem rather strange that genetics has been so neglected by epidemiologists (or, for that matter, that epidemiology has been so neglected by the geneticist). It seems to me that three major explanations may be given for this estrangement.

Firstly, it is not true that genetics has been neglected by epidemiologists. There can be no doubt that from time to time excellent studies of a genetic character have been carried out by epidemiologists. But apart from that it might be argued that studies such as those by Neel and Schull, by Morton, by McKusick, and many others ordinarily considered to be within the domain of population genetics are, in fact, epidemiology just as the theory of mathematical genetics as developed by Fisher, Haldane, Wright, Bailey, Crow, Kimura, and others is properly a branch of statistics or applied mathematics. This comment has substance. It is all the more mysterious that such studies are not ordinarily included in epidemiological training.

Secondly, it might be answered that the domain of the epidemiologist has been environment—that the subject of paramount importance to him is the interaction between members of a society and their individual and collective reactions to the physical world.

Certainly, the epidemiologist who conducts his studies with an eye to preventive medicine is much more likely to be concerned with environmental factors which can be readily manipulated, if necessary by law, than with genetics, where intervention would touch close to sensitive areas. We shall see, however, that certain recent developments may have changed this aspect.

Then thirdly (and this consideration is likely to be most telling to the epidemiologist concerned with public health), genetical problems, however important to theoretical knowledge, from a practical standpoint tend to be of rather trivial dimensions. Dahlberg's principle *(vide infra)* and the unsatisfactory nature of multilocal disease from an analytical standpoint have jointly made it unlikely that the four following conditions will all be satisfied simultaneously:

1. That the disease be common.
2. That the harm it inflicts in the population be other than trivial.
3. That it be unilocal.
4. That the effects of prevention will be rapidly evident.

Now for preventive medicine and public health to win at once the enthusiasm of the epidemiologist and the support of the legislature, these four conditions, in general, require to be fulfilled. There are some exceptions. For example, legislation on the early diagnosis of phenylketonuria (a rare disease, the cause of which may not, despite early hopes, be preventable) was very easily effected. The recent prohibition of cyclamates and DDT has been achieved on scanty evidence of doubtful relevance. Nevertheless, such legislation is, perhaps, exceptional and certainly has differed from what has been achieved in the past.

Despite the weight of the foregoing considerations from every point of view, I believe it true that genetics has much to contribute to the furtherance of all branches of epidemiology: investigative, preventive, and social.

It will be necessary to pay some attention to principles of genetic theory.

FOUR CARDINAL PRINCIPLES

Mendel's Laws

These laws are so well known as to call for little elaboration. If need be, the reader can consult standard genetic texts.[9-14] They may be restated in modern terms very briefly as follows.

Firstly, certain characteristics are transmitted in their entirety or not at all, being undiluted by transmission over many generations. Whether or not the characteristic is inherited depends on which of two (or more) alternative genes at a particular locus is transmitted from parent to child. This law is commonly stated by the principle that "alleles segregate," in which the term "alleles" is used for genes which may occupy the same part of the chromosome ("locus"). Characteristics so determined we shall refer to as "unilocal."

Secondly, which of two homologous chromosomes is inherited at one locus is in no way influenced by the choice at any other. The inheritance of a gene on one chromosome is stochastically independent of the inheritance of a gene in another chromosome. In general, this "random assortment" of genes is not true for two genes at different loci on the *same* chromosome. Such genes are said to be "linked," and the shorter the physical distance between linked loci the more likely genes are to be transmitted together. This nonindependence, or "linkage," will probably have an important bearing on genetic counseling in the future.

Galtonian Inheritance

While there is as yet no compelling evidence that Galtonian inheritance is qualitatively different from simple Mendelian inheritance, it is worth while to keep it separate, not only for historical reasons but also because it gives rise to analytical methods which are quite different in character. Galton[15] studied a class of characteristics (height and so forth) which, in his terminology, "blend." Such characters lack the discrete all-or-none quality of Mendelian characters. Thus, a man and woman might have many progeny exhibiting a wide variety of heights. This outcome is in striking contrast to Mendel's classical studies on the height of the pea plant, in which the progeny fall into two distinct classes: tall and short. It was shown in a classic paper by R.A. Fisher in 1918 (recently reissued with comments by Moran and Smith[16]) that a system behaving like a Galtonian character can be constructed by supposing that many loci contribute in more or less equal degree to the control of the character. Thus, intelligence might depend on the aggregate of a large number of the components of the brain, each under separate genetic control. Such a genetic system we shall refer to as "multilocal." The control of height is unilocal in peas, multilocal in man. The distinction between the unilocal system and the multilocal system is somewhat arbitrary since it is most unlikely that any phenotypic character is entirely under the control of a single locus and unmodified in any way by other genetic information in the system. As we have remarked above, the term "unilocal" is appropriately applied to those systems in which the *major* part of the genetic variance can be ascribed to one locus.

The Hardy-Weinberg Principle

This is the axis of reference of all population genetics. In its simplest form it may be stated in the following terms: In a *large* population of which the allele frequencies at *one* locus are *equal in the two sexes* and are *unperturbed by outside influences,* in *one* generation of *random* mating the frequencies of the genotypes for that locus are the same as if the gametes had been assembled at random from the gene pool.

The Hardy-Weinberg principle will not in general operate for X-linked loci or pairs of loci taken jointly, whether linked or non-linked, where the genetic composition of the population is subject to change as a result of mutation, selection, migration, or probabilistic drift, or where random mating is violated by either the encouragement or discouragement of consanguineous marriages or by the tendency of people of either similar or dissimilar genotypes to mate. The expected proportions will not be realized if the population is small and the variances of the proportions large. Population genetics concerns itself in a large part with departures from the Hardy-Weinberg principle.

Dahlberg's Law

Consider the dynamics of an unusual but transient type in a population. For instance, we might consider the number of medical students in a university. It is obvious that if there is a stable system, the number at any one time will be the product of two things: the number of medical students entering the university each year and the average length of time for which they stay in medical school. Thus, if 90 students are admitted each year and the average duration of the course is four years, then at any time, including students of all degrees of seniority, there will be 360.

This simple consideration is of fundamental importance in population genetics. It has been stated in a well-known formula of Dahlberg's as $f = \mu p$ where f is the frequency of some genetic condition, μ is the mutation rate, and p is the "persistence," that is, the average time between appearance of a new genetic line and the generation at which all the descendants bearing that particular mutant line become extinct.

The persistence of a gene can be shown to be the reciprocal of the fitness where the fitness is defined as the ratio of the average size of family of people bearing the mutant gene to that for the average in the population. Thus, if the average size of family is 2.8 and people bearing the mutant gene have an average of 1.4 children, then the fitness for the gene is 50 percent and the reciprocal of this, 2, is the average number of generations for which this line will persist in a stable population.

Despite its simplicity both conceptually and mathematically, Dahlberg's law is of great value. The frequency of some genetic character is, for the most part, easily determined, though for rare diseases sampling methods of some complexity may be necessary. Thus the mutation rate may be solved for in terms of the fitness or vice versa. Numerous estimates by this method and by direct counting, in many organisms including man, suggest that new mutation is an event occurring with a probability of the order of 10^{-5} per locus per generation. The variation in the individual estimates might be largely eliminated if the mutation rate could be expressed per unit length of DNA—it seems not unreasonable that a larger gene should be more liable to the copying accidents which cause mutation than a smaller one. But this refinement must be ignored at this stage.

It is clear that any reasonable frequency of a disease could be maintained either by a high mutation rate, by low selection pressure, or by both. By far the greatest source of variation in frequency, however, is selection. In the light of these facts we can now establish a conclusion stated previously. A unilocal disorder, with which the Dahlberg law deals, must either be rare or be subject to little selection. Selection in the genetic sense simply depends on the number of descendants the subject has; and reproductive capacity is generally expressed in the early part of life, say before the age of 45. Overt coronary disease, for instance, is comparatively rare before this age, so that its high prevalence is not in itself conclusive proof that the disorder is not unilocal. Such a disease may lead to little selection in the genetic sense and yet be a serious clinical and public health problem, but both these facts will in general be true only where the disease is one of later life. It would be difficult to think of an example of such a disorder which has been established to everyone's satisfaction to be unilocal. Huntington's chorea has this late pattern of onset (though cases in the mid-twenties are not uncommon), but it is a rare disorder. Diabetes is common and there have been many claims that it is a unilocal disorder; certainly there are many rare unilocal conditions which produce it, but no such claim for the common type can bear close scrutiny. Color blindness is common and each type is unilocal but gives rise to no grave disorder.

The lack of good examples may tell us something about the fitness of these conditions even in the larval stage. But also there may be an ascertainment problem. In the first place, as is well known (particularly for dominant disorders), a long-established mutant line tends to accumulate genes which modify the phenotype at the locus of interest, and thus diagnosis becomes elusive. And secondly, the unambiguous tracing of a trait through a pedigree is easiest for rare disorders. If a character is common, there may be multiple sources of the gene in a pedigree and confusing features (such as apparent father-to-son transmission of an X-linked character) may be present. A third feature, of course, is age dependence. Genetic patterns are traced with far greater confidence vertically than horizontally. A disease distributed horizontally, e.g. in a sibship, may easily be attributed to an environmental factor; recurrence generation after generation in one pedigree but not in others is much less easily accounted for by nongenetic mechanisms. But if the trait occurs over the age of 50 only, and especially if the diagnosis depends on some subtle diagnostic procedure only recently devised, vertical tracing may fail for scarcity of data.

These three features, variable phenotype, multiple sources of the gene, and age dependence, all conspire to obscure the character of unilocal diseases, and perhaps we often give up the search too easily. The problems of studying the genetics of coronary disease have been discussed in some detail elsewhere.[17]

However, the application of Dahlberg's principle calls for a clear recognition of the underlying assumptions. In particular, it is assumed (a) that the population is of constant size; (b) that it is in a steady state; for example, that its genetic composition is fixed, and (c) that the environment is fixed, since the fitness of a population is a function of the environment with which it has to contend.

Some of the most interesting recent developments in the impact of population genetics on epidemiology have stemmed from an exploration of departures from these assumptions. First and foremost it is, of course, obvious that the very notion of evolution is at variance with a steady state. The distinction between selection against a gene and the replacement of one gene by another is a fine one indeed and perhaps illusory. Then again the assumption of a stable population size can hardly be sustained, for the human species at least.

An intriguing idea that has emerged in the last twenty years or so is that chronic disease represents an anachronism. It may well be that a genotype which has been favored by one set of environmental circumstances in the past may now be the subject of extensive selection. For instance, it has been suggested that diabetes is the manifestation in an affluent and overfed society of a stringently economical gene selected for in times of recurrent or even persistent famine.[18] A similar notion has been put forward to account for coronary disease.[19]

It has been pointed out before[20] that the multifactorial system should be favored over the unilocal for the following reasons:

1. It allows a larger number of possible phenotypes and hence more genetic adaptability to changing environment.

2. The distribution of outcomes for traits controlled by multiple independent factors has a smaller variance than those for unilocal characters and hence it promotes clustering of genotypes about the optimal.

3. By providing a large number of genotypes with the same phenotype it allows for selection in the other pleomorphic effects of the participating genes.

These considerations and the assumption of a steady state are the rational basis for the identification of the normal with the average. There are two points of interest, however, which arise. Firstly, since the variance of the phenotype is a function of the number of loci involved, it may well be an inevitable price for the stability of such a system that outlying values be subjected to selection. But with a highly heterotic population there will be an inexhaustible genetic source for the production of outliers. If so, then the notion of eugenics as a practicable system for eliminating undesirable multilocal characters is inevitably doomed to failure.

The second point is that, ignoring the anachronism theory of chronic disease, the centralizing tendency for the distribution of the phenotype and a stable mean for this distribution can be maintained only by selection against both extremes. For instance, the maintenance of the blood cholesterol level is effected by an elaborate system which combats vigorously any attempt at reduction by dietary privation. Genetically speaking, then, we may be confident that so elaborate and so active a mechanism must have major advantages; otherwise, the selective effect of disease that is associated with hypercholesterolemia would eliminate this mechanism from the species. If the cholesterol-synthesizing system in the liver is not an anachronistic one, then it seems inescapable that there must be selection against low as well as high cholesterol values. The same argument seems to suggest that there should be selection against low blood pressures, low uric acid levels, and high intelligence. The curious thing is that these reciprocal extreme states do not seem to be well-established clinical disorders. The lack of evidence incriminating them may be due to the fact that it does not exist, but much might be due to failure to look for it. It seems strange that so much attention has been paid to high cholesterol levels as a risk factor and virtually none to low levels (excepting a few notes on hypocholesterolemia secondary to wasting disorders such as ulcerative colitis, which are the objects of selection in their own right). Of course, it may be, as in the case of intelligence, that evolution is taking place, that the "center of gravity" is slowly being shifted. But it seems unlikely that this explanation accounts for all such instances. One would then expect "quantitative" diseases to occur in pairs, one representing an excess and one a defect of the particular phenotype.

HEREDITY AND ENVIRONMENT

The point has been made above that, with some exceptions, the concern of epidemiology has been with environmental factors whereas that of population genetics has been with inheritance. The fashion is growing for those interested in the interaction between the two to call themselves "evolutionists." But it is far from obvious that the distinction between heredity and environment is real. Thought in this area is still dominated by nineteenth-century physical determinism, a philosophy which the physicists themselves abandoned fifty years ago. If indeed all behavior is unambiguously determined by the genetic endowment and the environment, then the sharp distinction between heredity and environment will stand. But if it be conceded that there is an indeterminate element in behavior (whether we understand this indeterminancy in the physical or the psychological sense), then the dividing line becomes hazy. For habits, perhaps acquired by chance, can obviously be a basis for selection, and they resemble genetic endowment in being authochthonous but differ in not being, as such, genetically transmissible. It seems, then, that such habits cannot be classed as either hereditary or environmental. And one is tempted to see genetic stock as a long-term conservation of characteristics which have arisen by chance, and habit as a short-term conservation. This notion is reminiscent of that of Koestler,[21] that we can think of structure as a function with a long half-life.

The rapprochement between these ideas may be illustrated by reference to a heuristic diagram (Fig. 3.2). Consider the behavior of blood pressure. Experience with many experimental approaches, notably the use of the more powerful hypotensive drugs, shows that attempts to change the blood pressure meet strenuous opposition from body mechanisms. Such systems as these are commonly used as illustrations of the concept of homeostasis. The interesting feature is that the adjusting mechanisms operate to restore blood pressure to its untreated level even if this level is so high as to threaten immediate disaster, and the greater the experimental displacement the more vigorous the homeostasis. Certainly the patient with a blood pressure of 220/140 mm Hg *feels* better at that pressure than he does if it is halved. Of course, sometimes, as in the common fainting attack or perhaps in hypertensive encephalopathy, the distortion takes the measurement outside "the zone of convergence" and the homeostatic mechanism is abandoned.

The analog at a genetic level of this "homing" tendency is the source of stabilizing selection (Fig. 3.2). Certain levels of blood pressure are more conducive to long survival than others; and insofar as the regulation of blood pressure is hereditary, optimal levels will tend to be selected for. The "tails" of the distribution will be subject to constant attrition.

These two mechanisms, then, tend to promote optimum levels. On an evolutionary scale, homeostasis operates quickly to deal with emergencies for the benefit of the individual; selection operates slowly and does much to maintain stability and structure to the benefit of the population, sometimes at the expense of individuals. The relationship is like that of the enactments of a parliament to a written constitution. The reaction to a cold climate, for example, on a homeostatic scale will be dealt with by vasoconstriction, shivering, increased appetite, and a sensation of cold; on a genetic scale it is met by such devices as the formation of blubber and the development of body hair.

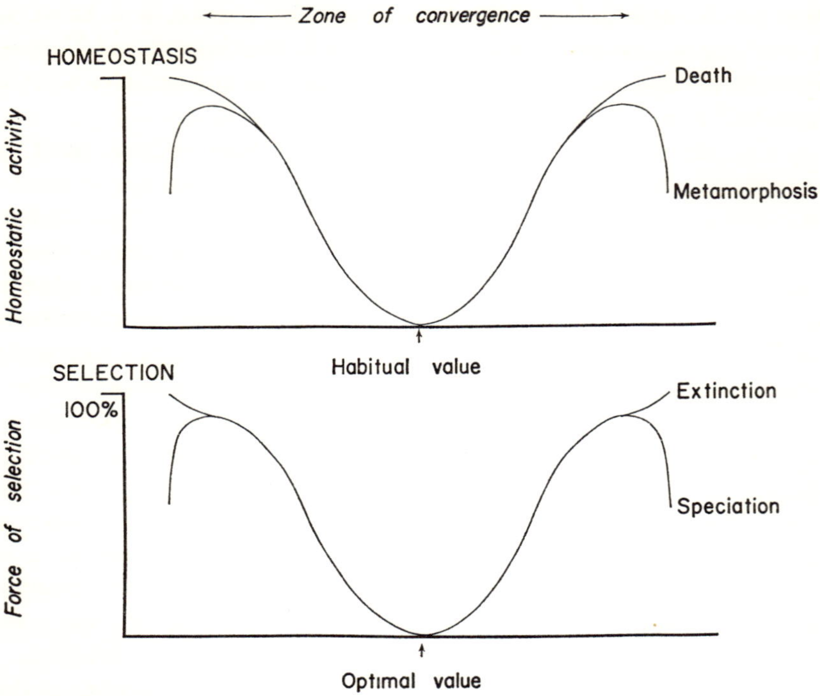

Figure 3.2. The analogy between homeostasis and selection. For the individual there is some habitual state (which may or may not be optimal) displacement from which is actively resisted. Beyond certain limits ("the zone of convergence") either the individual dies (as in shock) or he undergoes metamorphosis (as in hibernation). For the species there is an optimal value departures from which are met with selection. Beyond the zone of convergence either the species becomes extinct or a new species with a different local optimum is formed ("speciation").

If now disease be thought of as a substantial departure from the optimal, it is far from clear that the separation of heredity and environment is a useful one. If, for example, the metabolic rate is in large part under genetic control, a genetic endowment with a high rate may be adapted to a hot climate by excessive sweating.

A favorite question is whether some characteristic is "hereditary or environmental." Such a question is too vague to serve any useful purpose. Any conceivable phenotype must represent a mixture of the two. A genetic trait can be expressed only in an environment, and environment is pertinent to the fitness of a particular organism, the nature of which is determined largely by genetic factors. Indeed, genetics and heredity are not strictly commensurable. The *milieu intérieur* is a subset of the environment organized by genetic factors which comprise not matter but an ordering of matter.

A notion extensively employed is heritability, which is the proportion of the total variance of the phenotype transmissible from parent to child. Heritability, conventionally denoted by the symbol h^2, may clearly take on any value between zero and unity

We make use of the following simple relationships:

$$\text{Var}\ (X + Y) = \text{Var}\ (X) + \text{Var}\ (Y) + 2\ \text{cov}\ (XY)$$

Should X and Y be uncorrelated (for example if they are independent) the covariance is zero and the variance of the sum is the sum of the variances. In genetic terms we would then say that X and Y do not interact. A positive covariance means that X and Y interact positively and vice versa.

The pattern can conveniently be represented by a diagram (Fig. 3.3). Let a triangle be drawn such that BC is proportional to the standard deviation of the trait in organisms of identical genotype in the environment. Let CA be proportional to the standard deviation of the trait in organisms in an identical environment, and let it be drawn so that the cosine of the angle ACD is the correlation coefficient, thus:

$$\rho = \frac{CD}{AC}$$

Finally, we let the area of the triangle ABC represent the "total phenotypic variance." Then this variance can be partitioned by the following device. If lines CE and CF are drawn such that the angles they form with the sides of the triangle correspond to the angles of the main triangle in the manner shown, then three subtriangles result (Fig. 3.2). The triangles BCE and ACF correspond to the environmental and the genetic variances, respectively, while the triangle interposed between them, CEF, represents the component of variance due to interaction. The case shown at the top right is where interaction is positive. However, the inter-

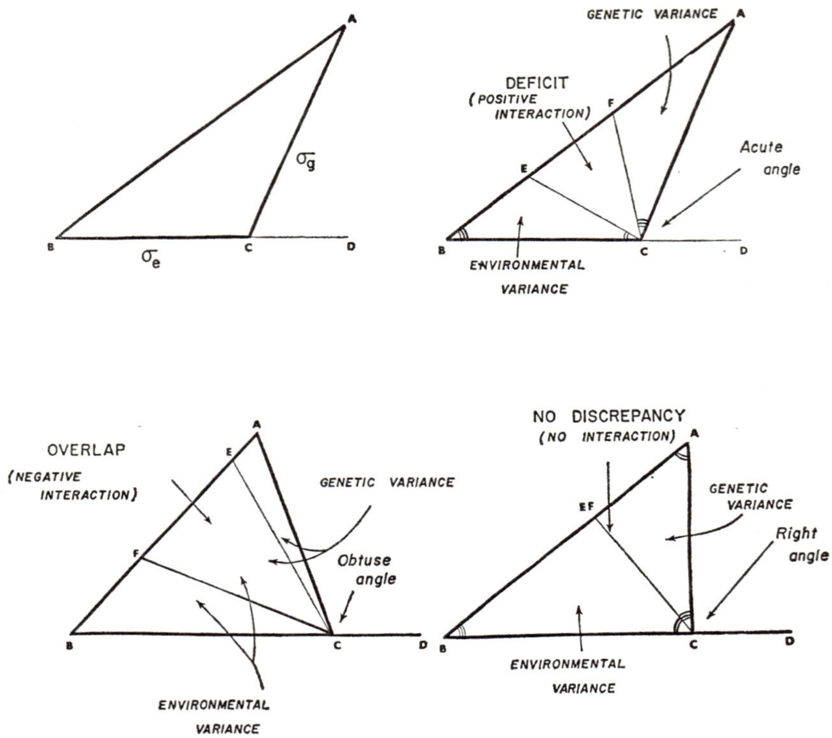

Figure 3.3. The partition of total phenotypic variance. The component of variance is, in each case, proportional to area. In each diagram the triangles *ABC, BCE,* and *ACF* representing, respectively, total, environmental, and genetic variance are similar. The degree of correlation between the two components is represented by the angle between the two lines marked σ_e and σ_g which are the standard deviations of the phenotype under uniform genetic and uniform environmental conditions, respectively. Where the two components are uncorrelated (bottom right) the lines are at right angles and the interaction is zero.

action area may be negative (bottom left). The area corresponding to interaction is zero if the total triangle is right-angled as at bottom right (hence the term "orthogonal"). Any or all of these triangles can be further partitioned into principal components with or without interactions.

Thus genetic variance can be divided into additive, dominance, epistatic, and so forth components; environmental variance might be divided into those for nutrition, infection, radiation, and so on. The subject is simply but extensively dealt with by Falconer.[10]

Without going in detail into the possible partitions of the total phenotypic variance and the methods which the quantitative geneticists employ to estimate them, it will be evident that the notion of heritability is an inadequate one. Of course, from the point of view of preventive medicine it may have value in indicating the most remunerative point of attack. Coronary artery disease, for instance, might conceivably be attacked by elimination of the environmental factors or by eugenic measures. If estimation of heritability showed that 90 percent of the variance is due to genetic factors, then preventive medicine would be far better to concern itself with genetic counseling than with production of dietetic foods—not, of course, that either should be neglected.

But how the phenotypic variance is composed is not an intrinsic property of the disease but an accident of the population under study. The recognition of a genetic component by classical genetical analysis depends intimately on the existence of heterosis. A hypothetical Negro in a remote part of Africa with access to all modern knowledge except that he was kept ignorant of the existence of the white man would not by genetic analysis recognize that skin color is genetically determined unless the very rare accident of albinism occurred. To the contrary, he might find that those exposed most to sunlight have the darkest skins and vice versa; this would lead him to the conclusion that skin color is determined exclusively by the environment and in this context he would be correct. If an entire population suffered from von Willebrand's disease, it would be impossible by studying it to recognize any genetic component. Conversely, if every member were protected from all sources of trauma, then inevitably the common bruise would emerge as an exclusively genetic disorder. Now these extreme cases are unlikely to occur in practice, but the two components may be mixed in highly variable proportions. This fact gives point to the definition of genetics as the science of variation. Thus, heritability and (what is much more to the point) answering the question of which it is the mathematical formulation is a notion of limited utility in epidemiology.

COMMON APPROACHES TO THE EXPLORATION OF THE GENETIC FACTOR

When the geneticist attempts to explore the genetics of a disorder which has perhaps been empirically defined, he may be fortunate enough to be confronted with a problem in which not only a single major locus is involved but also the phenotypes produced are clearly separable. Most often, however, one or both conditions are violated. It then becomes difficult to identify the segregation pattern at the major locus, if indeed it exists. Now in broad terms the segregation of the phenotypes depends on the difference in mean values, the scatter of individual cases about these means, and the relative sizes of the phenotypic populations. (If the phenotype is measurable and the measurements are normally distributed, then no other factors are relevant; in the general case, other properties of the distribution are probably only of minor importance). If study of the empirical distribution does not make it possible to identify the phenotypes and to classify individual cases with confidence, something may be done to enhance the separation by attention to these three factors. For instance, the means may be separated by the use of provocation tests; the variances may be reduced by directing attention to measurements close to the site of gene action and by punctilious attention to method of measurement and standardization in the circumstances of the tests; and the relative frequencies of the genotypes may be made as nearly equal as possible by examining children of matings of suitable type. The methods involved and some of the logical difficulties in interpretation are dealt with elsewhere.[6,7,17,22]

But such devices commonly fail and the question then arises as to how the problem is to be dealt with. Where inferences have to be made from data which the geneticist can observe but over which he has no control—this is almost always the case in human populations—the geneticist is hard put to distinguish similarities among relatives which are properly attributable to genetic factors from those which are purely cultural. Lilienfeld,[23] for instance, has produced evidence which he obviously does not intend to be taken seriously but which nonetheless is formally compelling, that the decision to become a physician is determined by the homozygous state of a recessive gene.

Once single-locus models have been abandoned, cogent tests of the origin of such similarity are even more difficult to devise. Winklestein and his associates[24,25] have found that much of the apparently genetic component in blood pressure control may in fact be environmental since spouses who are not blood relatives have correlated blood pressures much as blood relatives do. The possibility that this similarity represents assortive mating, i.e. a preference for a spouse of similar physique or temperament, is considerably weakened by the fact that this correlation is a function of the time for which the marriage has lasted.

The first maneuver then is to see if the single-locus model can be salvaged in the particular case by the application of modifications of classical Mendelian theory such as incomplete penetrance. The next approach is to explore not the genetics of the entire disease but of some facet of it. Thus, approaches to the problem of the genetics of coronary disease having been inconclusive,[17] investigators have examined mechanisms believed to contribute to its pathogenesis, such as blood cholesterol levels, blood pressure, or platelet function. The utility of this approach depends on several factors and results must be interpreted with caution.

In this specific problem, for instance, in spite of much careful epidemiological work and experimentation on various laboratory animals, it is far from clear that cholesterol is a causative mechanism. If one could show that cholesterol is regulated exclusively by genetic factors, this would be at best persuasive evidence of the genetic nature of coronary disease. Furthermore, the easiest genetic studies to do are those in which there is a conspicuous phenotype. Over the last thirty-five years there have been many studies suggesting that there is a disorder, hypercholesterolemia, which segregates as a Mendelian character in sibships.[26-28] Segregation patterns almost always have shown some degree of irregularity such that sooner or later each investigator has been driven to "putting patches" on the single-locus model. But even had the claims for this genetic model been substantiated, its pertinence to coronary disease would be in question. Certainly a prominent feature in many such pedigrees has been overt coronary disease, often at an early age, but the majority of people who develop coronary disease have neither this early onset nor these excessively high blood cholesterol levels. It seems then that the most ambitious claim that could be made is that there is a small group of people with very high blood cholesterol, in some of whom precocious coronary disease occurs. Whether or not this has any bearing on coronary disease which is commonly encountered is a different matter.

To take an example from another field, there is no doubt of the existence of intestinal polyposis commonly associated with soft-tissue masses and complicated by carcinoma as a manifestation of Gardner's syndrome,[29] which appears to be inherited as a regular autosomal dominant. But it would be perilous to infer from this that the commonplace carcinoma of the bowel is genetically determined.

NONSEGREGATIONAL METHODS

If all attempts to demonstrate a genetic component in some disorder by classical Mendelian methods fail, with or without adjustments for epistasis, incomplete penetrance, and bias of ascertainment, the investigator has recourse to other methods which we may call "nonsegregational." They are more inductive in character and therefore less compelling. Nevertheless, they have been used extensively by animal breeders with considerable empirical success. They fall into three broad groups: racial studies, multilocal analysis with or without dichotomous expression, and twin studies.

Racial Studies

Often the epidemiologist analyzing the distribution of a disease in a population has no information about family history. Such is indeed usually the case where the source of information used is vital statistics. It is possible to keep track of relationships in members of a population as the various studies on isolates and record linkage have demonstrated,[30,31] but such systems are beyond the scope of routine demography. However, one feature which can be, and often is, recorded is race. The existence of several races in a population implies that there is incomplete genetic mixing, and this should be reflected by differences in genetically determined diseases. By analogy, the animal breeder exploits the virtues of different varieties of the same species. One breed of cattle is distinguished by its production of milk, another by the quality of its meat.

In this approach "there is something but not much." Where the data have been routinely recorded, what information there is may as well be extracted as not, and it may provide some clues as to what may be genetic. But to push inferences beyond this is to court disaster. It may well be, for example, that what is observed may be attributable to cultural factors rather than genetic. The traditions of cooking, for instance, may well explain different cholesterol levels or peptic ulcers; and such instances could be multiplied. Even such studies as that of Keys *et al.*,[32] in which the prevalences of coronary artery disease in Japanese in three locales are compared, have too glibly been used as evidence that the environment is responsible for the differences; the results could as well be attributed to differences between the personality which migrates and that which does not or to the effects of genetic admixture in the migrant population.

But even apart from the effects of confounding with cultural factors, the value of racial studies may be called into question. Several attempts have been made to assess the extent of the racial admixture between white and Negro Americans. They suggest that the figure in Baltimore is something like 30 percent.[33,34] But it can be seen that this figure is probably incorrect, for undoubtedly there must be some scatter in the phenotype: even people who have the same ancestry will differ in the proportion of genes of Negro origin which they inherit, and some will undoubtedly have phenotypes which will lead them to be classed as white. Thus the estimate is based on a truncated population. Moreover, there are no well-defined criteria as to who will be classed as a Negro. A more sophisticated mathematical approach is being developed.[35,36]

Again, there will be much genetic variance, especially among Negroes, and yet the notion of classifying people implies that the variance among groups is very large compared with that within groups. The danger of treating a heterogeneous group as homogeneous is well known in statistics.

Multilocal Analysis

We have already considered the Galtonian pattern of inheritance. Such a system will under certain well-known conditions produce a phenotype which follows the normal distribution more or less closely. This genetic model has been the basis of a considerable body of theory well covered by Falconer[10] and by Kempthorne.[11] Test crosses in general provide evidence of an inductive nature, i.e. they provide an opportunity for the hypothesis to be disproved. The more tests the hypothesis survives, the more sure we are that it is correct. But the coercive character of tests for single-locus hypotheses is lacking.

It is a fair statement that these methods are difficult to apply to man because of the impossibility of appropriate test crossing and cross fostering.

The general nature of the tests is to examine the similarities among relatives. Is the height of a son correlated with that of his father? In interpreting the results we are obliged to be careful about two points. In the first place, confounding is a major factor. Height is known to be influenced by heredity in some degree, if for no other reason than that there are many well-known forms of hereditary dwarfism.[37,38] It is also certainly influenced by diet and by general state of health. But diet itself will show family influence for economic reasons. Thus we are obliged to be careful that the intrafamilial correlation is not a reflection of a common culture. The second cause for caution concerns the reference set. The extent to which height is genetically determined will depend on whether we are considering the human species or all species. In the latter case the herditary component would be much higher. This extreme case is chosen by way of making a point but, for example, in exploring heredity in man it would make a difference whether racial isolates were included or not. Heredity would contribute less to height if we considered pygmies alone than if we combined members of several different races.

We may distinguish from the foregoing the group, so far small, in which the mechanism of the trait is much more clearly understood. The outstanding example is the behavior of finger-ridge counts, which were the subject of classical studies by Sarah Holt.[39] There are few, if any, better examples to be found in the literature about any species. The formation of the fingerprints occurs quite early in embryonic life and thereafter they do not change, so that any environmental factors must operate at this early stage. In particular, they are not, like height or intelligence, age dependent. Observations on the similarity of ridge counts in relatives conform with surprising exactness to the predictions of theory for purely genetical conditions.

Threshold Phenomena

In the past it has been too easily assumed that categorical characters are necessarily Mendelian. Yet it is obvious that the phenotype, though dichotomous, might reflect some underlying mechanism which is multifactorial. For example, let us make the somewhat naive assumption that the syndrome of gout is due to crystallization of uric acid with the exciting of a foreign-body reaction. Suppose that the level of uric acid in the blood is multifactorial. Crystallization is a process which starts when some critical concentration of uric acid is exceeded. Human beings will fall into two groups—those in whom the uric acid is below this critical level and who will have no gout and those in whom it is exceeded and who will. The mechanism is multifactorial but the expression dichotomous. But further, suppose that there is (for whatever reason) a high correlation among relatives in the levels of uric acid. Then if one member of the family is above the threshold, others will tend to be also. Some of the relatives may be just above the threshold and affected and some just below it and unaffected, and the pattern of inheritance may quite easily be mistaken for that produced by an autosomal dominant disorder at one locus; occasional anomalies are readily explained away by invoking sampling error, incomplete penetrance, epistasis, or illegitimacy. It is perhaps mechanisms such as this which have led some investigators to suppose that xanthomatosis and gout are autosomal dominant disorders. Two clues should suggest that a character is not unilocal but multilocal with dichotomous expression.

A true dominant will tend to persist intact over an indefinite number of generations. In investigating the genetics of a dominant disorder, "vertical" data are better than "horizontal." There are many examples from animal genetics of disorders the pattern of which for one or two generations behaves faithfully like a dominant but which in subsequent generations disintegrates.

The second clue is that if a disorder is multifactorial but dichotomous, consanguinity will promote the occurrence of the disorder in the offspring, whereas for dominant unilocal disorders consanguinity has no effect (except, of course, where as a result both parents are affected).

The threshold model has been used by many investigators. Some of its statistical properties have been explored by Edwards.[40] A practical application to genetic counseling problems has been worked out by Falconer[41,42]; this latter subject has by no means been exhausted.

In Falconer's model, the underlying variable (e.g. uric acid) is referred to as the "liability," a somewhat unfortunate term since liability (in the usual sense) is either zero or one. More recently, Edwards[43] has suggested a modification. He proposes that the idea of a threshold be replaced by a probability of getting the disease, which is a function of the underlying factor. Thus those with low levels of uric acid would have a small chance of getting gout and vice versa. This latter elaboration seems somewhat more realistic than the sharp threshold model in the general case; for example, in liability to coronary disease. It is doubtful that the present state of knowledge is sufficient to support and exploit it. Much of the success of developing a good model depends on identifying and studying precisely what the nature of the underlying cause is.

Twin Studies

There is a long tradition, dating back to the studies of Galton, of exploring the genetic component of a characteristic by studying the similarities among twins. The argument is that if twins are identical they have the same genetic content and therefore any differences between them must be environmental in origin. Nonidentical twins, on the other hand, are no more closely related genetically than any pair of sibs. They are, however, more similar than ordinary sibs by being coeval, sharing the same uterine environment, and, particularly if they are of the same sex, having a similar upbringing. It is felt that comparisons of the variability between these two kinds of twins should lead to a method of assessing the genetic component. It has been common experience that nonidentical twins are often much less similar than identical twins. However, there has been some uneasiness that this discrepancy may, at least in part, be attributable to cultural factors. For example, some parents tend to exploit the similarity of identical twins by dressing them alike, providing them with the same toys, and so forth. It is not clear what impact this may have on the development of their identities.

It is the opinion among geneticists that considerable care must be exercised in deciding whether or not twins are identical. The common practice is to examine a large number of marker phenotypes such as blood groups. It seems then that there may be some considerable probability that on the basis of physical appearance alone, nonidentical twins of the same sex may be taken for identical. If this is indeed the case, then there is a very simple means available for looking at the sources of variation more critically. If it is true that the way in which parents behave towards twins is influenced by whether or not they believe them to be identical, then whatever impact this may have on their phenotypes of the twins should, in the absence of interaction, be independent of zygosity. It would seem useful then in such studies to subdivide both identical and nonidentical twins according to what their parents believe them to be. By this means it would be possible to apportion variances into those due to environment, those due to genetics, and those due to the parents' belief about zygosity. Such a scheme would be by no means above criticism. For instance, it takes no account of interaction between these components, but it would go some way toward eliminating some of the spurious genetic opponents.

But there are other respects in which many proponents of the twin method have failed to keep up-to-date. Galton knew nothing of the biological mechanisms of heredity, which though then discovered had not been widely publicized. His methods have been somewhat amended to encompass this knowledge but little of recent discoveries has been incorporated into these methods.

We may, if we please, insist that twins are not to be reckoned identical if they differ in any character known to be genetically determined. Represented in these terms, we then have the unassailable, but rather useless, tautology that twins that differ are not identical. But at a biological level the word "identical" is taken in a different sense to mean that the twins are both derived from a single ovum fertilized by a single sperm. This criterion is to take the term from the domain of the arbitrary to that of the empirical. It thus becomes liable to error. There is nothing in the nature of things which demands that descendants from a single cell should be identical in genetic content, let alone in phenotypic expression. The phenomenon of mosaicism has been repeatedly documented in animals, including man; that is, two different cell lines in the individual may have different karyotypes. But difference in karyotype represents the grossest of indications that the genetic content differs. It has been possible in animals in which fine structure in chromosomes can be studied to demonstrate the extent to which homologous and even nonhomologous chromosomes may break with cross-union between the fragments. As a result of such crossings-over or translocations (as the case may be), there may be considerable differences in the daughter cells. For all we know at a biochemical level such oddities may be very frequent indeed. But further, it is now thought that "point mutations," i.e. base pair substitutions in the DNA, are due to coyping errors, and these may therefore arise any time that a mitotic division occurs.

It seems a priori most unlikely that all the cells in the adult body should have the same genotype. There seems little reason then for demanding that identical twins should be identical in any particular respect. From time to time, cases have been reported in which the karyotypes of twins determined to be identical nevertheless differ; for example, one twin may have Down's syndrome and the other not. If such gross discrepancies may arise, to say the least, it seems a trifle precious to deny the possibility that blood groups would differ. For example, an ovum which at the ABO blood group locus had genotype AO could give rise to an offspring of phenotype O by deletion of the A gene. Such an accident for any one particular locus is unlikely; but when a large number of loci are considered, the probability of such an accident in one of them, at least, might be reasonably large.

A decision whether or not any particular pair of twins is monozygous will thus be probabilistic. Such a state of affairs is a familiar one in genetics. It differs in that conceptually, at least, there is no final court of appeal as to zygosity except, of course, whether or not the twins were derived from a single fertilized ovum; this information will be lost beyond hope of recovery by the time the real problem has arisen. Graft acceptance by one twin from another is the most stringent proof of monozygosity, but does not solve the problem in principle. For instance, I know of no data on mosaic animals as to whether a graft from one tissue will be accepted by other tissues of different karyotype.

STUDIES IN GENETIC ISOLATES

In recent years there have been many studies on groups who for one reason or another have been genetically isolated. Some, the Amish, Dunkards, and Mormons, and to a lesser extent Jews, are isolated by religion. Others have been isolated by tribal or other social influences (for example, the We Sorts and the Pima and Papago Indians). Yet others have been isolated by geography and by primitive means of transport (for example, in the Swiss cantons). Good genealogies are commonly maintained either as a matter of family pride or in accordance with ecclesiastical requirements, notably in Catholic countries (for example, in the French-Canadian and Italian isolates), where restrictions on consanguineous marriages operate.

These populations provide excellent opportunities for study of an entire community where the genetic composition of the population is distinctive. It has even been possible to construct complete or nearly complete pedigrees for the study of inbreeding. Complicated pedigrees of this kind call for computer assistance in analysis.[44-46]

Much of what has been done with these populations, however, are not orthodox epidemiological studies. The writings of McKusick, of Jackson, and of others have been concerned largely with exploiting the inbred character of these populations. By this means many autosomal recessive conditions which under ordinary circumstances are rare and even previously undescribed have been brought to light. As such, it might appear that the orientation is primarily nosologic. However, two aspects of these discoveries bring the results more into line with the classical preoccupations of epidemiology. In the first place, the recognition of a syndrome is essentially probabilistic.

A syndrome, a "running together," can only be identified when two or more characters appear together more commonly than could be accounted for by chance. Recognition of this probabilistic relationship necessarily depends on a multiplicity of cases, and in unselected populations it may be difficult to find cases even in haphazard fashion. In an isolate, cases may be abundant and the reference population is precisely known. If a cardinal prerequisite for an epidemiologic study is the identification of a condition for study, then this property of isolates may be valuable indeed.

The other respect in which studies of isolates conform in content to classic epidemiology is that they may show a hitherto unexpected genetic component to a disease. The Amish studies, for instance, have furnished good evidence that hydrometrocolpos (transverse vaginal septum) is inherited as an autosomal recessive.[47]

Isolates have many other advantages which McKusick and his colleagues[48] have listed. For instance, they tend to be geographically stable, to have uniform environment, and they may have an unusual interest in disease.

ASSOCIATION OF BLOOD GROUPS AND DISEASE

Much effort has been expended in the last fifteen years in exploring associations between certain common diseases (coronary disease, hypertension, cancer, and so on) and certain single-locus characters which are not apparently harmful in themselves. These harmless single-locus characteristics usually exhibit polymorphism, that is, there are several alleles of roughly equal frequencies. They are commonly referred to as marker genes, a term which carries over from linkage analysis. The most widely used markers are the blood groups; such studies should not be undertaken lightly because competent blood grouping, especially for the minor and more recently discovered groups, is technically demanding. It should also be emphasized that association between marker genes and any other characteristic must not be confused with genetic linkage. Genetic linkage can only be demonstrated from pedigree studies extending over at least two generations and only clearly demonstrated for single-locus characteristics. As we have seen, single-locus etiology has not been demonstrated in these diseases nor is it likely that it will be. Moreover, except where linkage is very close and the data derived exclusively from one source, we cannot expect genetic linkage to give rise to permanent association except perhaps as a result of peculiar epistatic interactions.

The association between a disease and a blood group is difficult to demonstrate except where it has reached extraordinary dimensions. All manner of subtle traps lie in the way of evaluating any published data, some of which have been discussed recently by Wiener.[49] He does not mention what is not the least of these: that investigators tend to publish, and editors tend to accept for publication, studies which show positive, rather than those which show negative, results. Biases of this kind are in no way mitigated by large numbers of published studies. It is hard to say offhand how much impact this bias may have. But even granted that the true frequency of gastric carcinoma in people of blood group A is 20 percent higher than that in people of blood group O, it must be wondered whether this discovery is of much importance and whether it is likely to lead to much elucidation of pathogenesis.

STUDIES ON CHROMOSOME ANOMALIES

The foregoing discussion has dealt with anomalies of the apparatus of inheritance studied by genetic analysis, that is, ultimately by the study of the resemblances among relatives. This approach is basically functional. However, there is an alternative approach, to study the anatomy of the system. Here the subject of study in man is at present on a much grosser scale—the chromosome. The anomalies which may occur in the number of chromosomes (aneuploidies), in their shapes (translocations and deletions), and in the bizarre forms they may assume during synapsis (star forms, rings, loops, and the like) can be usefully studied even where there is no family history. Needless to say, light may be thrown on their etiology by a study of relatives and the environment, but it is possible to do surveys on population frequency from data collected in a systematic, though perhaps rather restricted, fashion.

There are three broad classes of methods by which epidemiological surveys may be carried out.

1. On a defined population, karyotypes may be done on all individuals. This is the only irreproachable method, though that is not to say that there are not sources of serious errors. However, a great deal of work and expense is involved. Since the yield for any one kind of anomaly is likely to be small, it is reasonable that studies of this sort should be diffusely directed to the detection of all kinds of anomalies.

2. Abnormal numbers of X chromosomes may be detected by the study of Barr bodies in cells from an appropriate source. The specimens are usually taken from the epithelium of the buccal mucosa ("buccal smear"). This approach has been of the greatest value in Turner's and Klinefelter's syndromes. But it is not suited to detection of aneuploidies for the autosomes and it may fail to detect mosaics if the tissue sampled is part of the normal tissue. One of the most promising developments in recent months is the recognition that parts of the chromosomes may be made to fluoresce when stained with atebrine and other fluorochromes.[50,51] The parts which fluoresce appear to be quite distinctive and consistent. This method provides a welcome addition to the means of observing distinguishing characteristics of chromosomes. In particular, the Y chromosome has a characteristic fluorescent spot so that there is prospect of being able to detect aneuploidies of it by

the comparatively simple screening procedure of examining buccal smears. However, the details of this technic have not yet been worked out.

3. In certain cases the phenotype associated with the anomaly may be distinctive. Such instances are Down's syndrome ("mongolism") and the *cri-du-chat* syndrome (deletion of the short arm of chromosome 5). In competent clinical hands these conditions can be diagnosed as well as other disorders which are more controversial. Many of the sex-chromosome anomalies can also be detected, but they are, of course, readily picked up by buccal smear examination. One feature which is disturbing from an epidemiological standpoint, however, is that when this approach is used it is possible to verify how many of the clinical diagnoses are correct, i.e. what proportion of false positives there is; but there is no means of determining the proportion of false negatives except by complete surveys (by whichever of the first two methods is appropriate). Studies of this kind have not been done. The present state of ignorance about the XYY karyotype admirably illustrates these shortcomings.

One aspect of the phenotype which deserves special mention is the use of dermatoglyphics, including handprints and soleprints. For reasons which are not understood, patterns are disturbed in a characteristic way in many of these chromosome anomalies, notably in Down's syndrome and in the aneuploidies of sex chromosomes. Quite elaborate methods of diagnosis of Down's syndrome, using discriminant analysis, have been worked out.[52] It may be noted that these changes are in a special tissue; thus in mosaic subjects, they may yield positive results when the buccal smear may be normal.

Epidemiological Aspects

Much of the geneticist's interest in screening for chromosome anomalies is simply with the collection of cases; in this way he can attempt to define the distinctive phenotype, and in certain cases—for instance, Down's syndrome, due to translocation but with a normal number of chromosomes—the information is of value in genetic counseling. An epidemiologist looking at this problem would be much more concerned with evidence that the distribution of cases was not uniform. The frequency of aneuploidies depends on the age of the parents, especially on the mother; there is well-known evidence from Jenkins[53] and Penrose[54] on this point, evidence which has been repeatedly confirmed. There are grounds for believing that certain virus infections promote aneuploidies, and since infections are seasonal it seems reasonable that aneuploidies show a seasonal variation in birth date. There is a study under way at Denver by Puck and Robinson[55] in which evidence of clustering in time is being sought, so far with equivocal results. Lilienfeld[56] lists the previous studies published.

There is some interest in racial distribution of these disorders, but the evidence is mostly in the form of case reports. It may be said that such-and-such a disorder is "not unknown" in a particular race, but epidemiologically satisfactory evidence is wanting. In the first place, such cases have not been picked up in a systematic survey so that there is no denominator in the fraction; but also the technical difficulties of doing karyotypes and the opportunities for misinterpretations are so great that the frequencies observed are as likely to reflect the skill and preoccupations of the observer as they are the peculiarities of the population.

Despite a large literature, the population aspects of none of these chromosomal aberrations can be said to have been adequately worked out. One extensive study has been published.[57] An excellent account of the present state of knowledge in Down's syndrome, the first such syndrome to have been identified clinically or explained by karyotype, is provided in a recent review by Lilienfeld.[56]

GENETIC COUNSELING

One of the areas of genetics which may soon be of major importance in preventive medicine is genetic counseling. Quite a considerable body of theory has been developed for this subject, which is reviewed elsewhere.[58,59] Many newer advances in the detection of the carrier state, by methods of biochemistry and tissue culture, are gaining popularity. Amniocentesis is a recent approach which holds great promise of success as a means of antenatal diagnosis. Finally, after a long, slow period of development, genetic linkage analysis is expanding rapidly; the larval stage of such disorders as Huntington's chorea may soon be detectable by observing the inheritance of readily detected marker genes, of which the coupling phase in the parents is known.

Two major questions arise. The first is how adequately the information so obtained can be transmitted to the consultands, i.e. the persons whose future reproductive activities are under question. If we tell them that the probability of some disorder in their children is 10 percent, what does this really convey to them? Childs and Leonard[60] have explored this to some extent, and their impression is that only a minority of people have any practical grasp of what a probability means. Closely related to this is the matter of what impact counseling is likely to have on the reproductive behavior of persons counseled. Here the published data are very scanty indeed and rather discouraging from the standpoint of the eugenicist.[61]

The second question is what the impact of modifying the reproductive behavior of affected persons or carriers may be on gene frequencies. This is an area in which intuition serves badly. To give one example only, consider a population of fixed size with an autosomal condition lethal in homozygous state, carriers of which are allowed to marry normal people only; the number of deaths from the disorder would not be changed and the frequency of the gene will be very little increased over that with random mating unless the heterozygotes are themselves fully fit. Details are given elsewhere.[62]

REFERENCES

1. Hamilton, M., Pickering, G.W., Roberts, J.A.F., and Sowry, G.S.C. the Aetiology of essential hypertension: Arterial pressure in the general population. *Clin. Sci., 13*:11, 1954.
2. Platt, R. The nature of essential hypertension. *Lancet, 2*:55, 1959.
3. Morrison, S.L., and Morris, J.N. Epidemiological observations on high blood pressure without evident cause. *Lancet, 2*:864, 1959.
4. Pickering, G.W. *High Blood Pressure,* 2nd ed. London, Churchill, 1968.
5. Baker, G.A. Transformations of bimodal distributions. *Ann. Math. Stat., 1*:334, 1930.

6. Murphy, E.A. One cause? Many causes? The argument from the bimodal distribution. *J. Chronic Dis., 17:*301, 1964.
7. Murphy, E.A., and Bolling, D.R. Testing of single locus hypotheses where there is incomplete separation of the phenotypes. *Amer. J. Hum. Genet., 19:*322, 1967.
8. Harris, H., and Smith, C.A.B. The sib-sib age of onset correlation among individuals suffering from a hereditary syndrome produced by more than one gene. *Ann. Eugen., 14:*309, 1949.
9. Li, C.C. *Population Genetics.* Chicago, University of Chicago Press, 1955.
10. Falconer, D.S. *Introduction to Quantitative Genetics.* New York, Ronald Press, 1960.
11. Kempthorne, O. *An Introduction to Genetic Statistics.* New York, John Wiley & Sons, 1957.
12. Neel, J.V., and Schull, W.J. *Human Heredity.* Chicago, University of Chicago Press, 1954.
13. Malécot, G. *The Mathematics of Heredity.* San Francisco, Freeman, 1969.
14. Crow, J.F., and Kimura, M. *Population Genetics.* New York, Harper & Row, 1969.
15. Galton, F. *Natural Inheritance.* London, Macmillan, 1889.
16. Moran, P.A.P., and Smith, C.A.B. Commentary on R.A. Fisher's paper on the correlation between relations on the supposition of Mendelian inheritance [originally published in *Transactions of the Royal Society of Edinburgh 52:*399, 1918]. *Eugenics Laboratory Memoirs 41.* London, Cambridge University Press, 1966.
17. Murphy, E.A. Some difficulties in the investigation of genetic factors in coronary artery disease. *Canad. Med. Ass. J., 97:*1181, 1967.
18. Neel, J.V. Diabetes mellitus: A "thrifty" genotype rendered detrimental by "progress"? *Amer. J. Hum. Genet., 14:*353, 1962.
19. McKusick, V.A., and Murphy, E.A. Genetic factors in the etiology of myocardial infarction. In James, T.N., and Keyes, J.W. (Eds.) *The Etiology of Myocardial Infarction.* Boston, Little, Brown & Co., 1963.
20. Murphy, E.A. A scientific viewpoint on normalcy. *Perspect. Biol. Med., 9:* 333, 1966.
21. Koestler, A. *The Act of Creation.* New York, Dell, 1964.
22. Murphy, E.A. Incomplete penetrance and the ascertainment of recessive characters in man I. Introduction and distribution theory. *J. Chronic Dis., 23:*9, 1970.
23. Lilienfeld, A.M. A methodological problem in testing a recessive genetic hypothesis in human disease. *Amer. J. Public Health, 49:*199, 1959.
24. Chazan, J.A., and Winkelstein, W. Household aggregation of hypertension: Report of a preliminary study. *J. Chronic Dis., 17:*9, 1964.
25. Winkelstein, W., Kantor, S., Ibrahim., M., and Sackett, D.L. Familial aggregation of blood pressure. *J.A.M.A., 195:*160, 1966.
26. Wilkinson, C.F., Hand, E.D., and Fliegelman, M.T. Essential familial hypercholesterolemia. *Ann. Intern. Med., 29:*676, 1948.

27. Stecher, R.M., and Hersh, A.H. Note on the genetics of hypercholesterolemia. *Science, 109:*61, 1949.
28. Khachadurian, A.K. The inheritance of essential familial hypercholesterolemia. *Amer. J. Med., 37:*402, 1964.
29. Gardner, E.J. Follow-up study of a family group exhibiting dominant inheritance for a syndrome including intestinal polyps, osteomas, fibromas and epidermal cysts. *Amer. J. Hum. Genet., 14:*376, 1962.
30. Newcombe, H.B. Present state and long-term objectives of the British Columbia population study. In Crow, J.F., and Neel, J.V. (Eds.) *Proceedings of the Third International Congress of Human Genetics.* Baltimore, Johns Hopkins Press, 1967.
31. Acheson, E.D. *Medical Record Linkage.* New York, Oxford University Press, 1967.
32. Keys A., Kimura, N., Kusukawa, A., Bronte-Stewart, B., Larsen, N., and Keys, M.H. Lessons from serum cholesterol studies in Japan, Hawaii and Los Angeles. *Ann. Intern. Med., 48:*83, 1958.
33. Glass, B., and Li, C.C. The dynamics of racial admixture—an analysis based on the American Negro. *Amer. J. Hum. Genet., 5:*1, 1968.
34. Steinberg, A.G., Stauffer, R., and Boyer, S.H. Evidence for a Gm^{ab} allele in the Gm system of American Negroes. *Nature, 188:*169, 1960.
35. Reed, T.E. Critical tests of hypotheses for race admixture using Gm data on American Caucasians and Negroes. *Amer. J. Hum. Genet., 21:*71, 1969.
36. Workman, P.L., and MacLean, C.J. Intermixture and the study of genetic difference between populations. Abstract. *Proceedings of the Annual Meeting of the American Society of Human Genetics.* Indianapolis, 1970.
37. Smith, D.W. Compendium on shortness of stature. *J. Pediat., 70:*463, 1967.
38. McKusick, V.A. *Mendelian Inheritance in Man,* 3rd ed. Baltimore, Johns Hopkins Press, 1971.
39. Holt, S.B. Inheritance of dermal ridge patterns. In Penrose, L.S. (Ed.) *Recent Advances in Human Genetics.* Boston, Little, Brown & Co., 1961.
40. Edwards, J.H. The simulation of Mendelism. *Acta Genet. (Basel), 10:*63, 1960.
41. Falconer, D.S. The inheritance of liability to certain diseases, estimated from the incidence among relatives. *Ann. Hum. Genet., 29:*51, 1965.
42. Falconer, D.S. The inheritance of liability to diseases with variable age of onset, with particular reference to diabetes mellitus. *Ann. Hum. Genet., 31:*1, 1967.
43. Edwards, J.H. Familial predisposition in man. *Brit. Med. Bull., 25:*58, 1969.
44. Hoen., K., and Grandage, A.H.E. Calculation of inbreeding in family

selection studies on the IBM-650 data processing machine. *Biometrics, 16*:292, 1960.
45. Mange, A.P. Growth and inbreeding of a human isolate. *Hum. Biol., 36:* 104, 1964.
46. Edwards, J.H. Analysis of pedigree data, In Harris, H., and Hirschhorn, K., (Eds.) *Advances in Human Genetics 1*. New York, Plenum Press, 1970.
47. McKusick, V.A., Bauer, R.L., Koop, C.E., and Scott, R.B. Hydrometrocolpos as a simply inherited malformation. *J.A.M.A., 189*:813, 1964.
48. McKusick, V.A., Eldridge, R., Hostetler, J.A., and Egeland, J.A. Dwarfism in the Amish. *Trans. Ass. Amer. Physicians, 77*:151, 1964.
49. Wiener, A.S. Blood groups and disease. *Amer. J. Hum. Genet., 22*:476, 1970.
50. Caspersson, T., Farber, S., Foley, G.E., Kudynowski, J., Modest, E.J., Simonsson, E., Wagh, U., and Zech, L. Chemical differentiation along metaphase chromosomes. *Exp. Cell Res., 49*:219, 1968.
51. Pearson, P.L., and Bobrow, M. Technique for identifying Y chromosomes in human interphase nuclei. *Nature, 226*:78, 1970.
52. Borgaonkar, D.S., Davis, M., Bolling, D.R., and Herr, H.M. Evaluation of dermal patterns in Down's syndrome by predictive discrimination. Abstract. *Clinical Research, 16*:296, 1968.
53. Jenkins, R.L. Etiology of mongolism. *Amer. J. Dis. Child, 45*:506, 1933.
54. Penrose, L.S. The relative effects of paternal and maternal age in mongolism. *J. Genet., 27*:219, 1933.
55. Robinson, A., Goad, W.B., Puck, T.T., and Harris, J.S. Studies on chromosomal nondisjunction in man III. *Amer. J. Hum. Genet., 21:* 466, 1969.
56. Lilienfeld, A.M. (with the assistance of C.H. Benesch) *Epidemiology of Mongolism*. Baltimore, Johns Hopkins Press, 1969.
57. Ratcliffe, S.G., Stewart, A.L., Melville, M.M., Jacobs, P.D., and Keay, A.J. Chromosome studies on 3500 newborn male infants. *Lancet, 1*:121, 1970.
58. Murphy, E.A., and Mutalik, G.S. The application of Bayesian methods in genetic counseling. *Human Heredity, 19*:126, 1969.
59. Murphy, E.A. Genetic counseling. In *Medicine in the University and Community of the Future*. Halifax, N.S., Faculty of Medicine, Dalhousie University, 1969, pp. 143 *et seq*.
60. Childs, B., and Leonard, C.O. Personal communication.
61. Carter, C.O. Prospects in genetic counseling. In Emery, A.E.H. (Ed.) *Modern Trends in Human Genetics—1*. New York, Appleton-Century-Crofts, 1970.
62. Murphy, E.A. Why monitor? In *Monitoring, Birth Defects, and Environment—The Problem of Surveillance*. Academic Press, 1971.

Chapter 4

PSYCHOLOGY IN EPIDEMIOLOGY: THE GROWING EDGE

C. DAVID JENKINS

THE ROOTS of epidemiology can be traced as far back as the writings of Hippocrates.[1] For the Hippocratean writers, the study of human behavior was an important component in the investigation of medicine—and of what was to become epidemiology. In the essay "On Airs, Waters, and Places," the writer lists variables essential "to investigate medicine properly." "One should consider," he states, "the mode in which the inhabitants live, and what are their pursuits, whether they are fond of drinking and eating to excess, and given to indolence, or are fond of exercise and labor." A much later talent in the history of epidemiology, John Snow,[2] revealed his sensitivity to the psychology of human behavior in the anecdotal evidence he cited to support his explanation of the London cholera epidemics. We recall his mention of the arrogant landlord who drank his tenant's water to prove the supply was not contaminated and forthwith contracted cholera and died; or the sick woman who lived far from the Broad Street well but had sent her son that distance to fetch the water which tasted best to her.

Rapid development and amazing success of the germ theory in subsequent decades turned the view of medical scientists away from studying the host of disease and towards the infectious agent. One cannot question the great scientific progress and improvement in the public's health brought about by the efflorescence of laboratory medicine. Epidemiology followed medicine in turning from *in vivo* concerns to *in vitro* measurements, and, in exchange for a season of rapid advance, sustained a serious loss in perspective.

A reawakening of interest in human behavior is now taking

place in medicine. The introduction of the scientific study of behavior into epidemiology has begun, but is still being ignored by many leaders of traditional epidemiology, though there are several notable exceptions.

The concept of "cause" has undergone drastic reformulation in recent years. The once-popular teaching device, the epidemiological triangle, labeled host, agent, and environment at its apices, is generally regarded as too simplistic to depict the multicausal circumstances now recognized to stand behind most diseases. An excellent discussion of the multicausal matrix is found in Morris,[3] who relabels the epidemiological triangle to emphasize (a) the causes in the host, (b) external-environmental causes, and (c) personal behavior. He points out the role of personal habits and behavior in modifying the impact on health exerted both by causes intrinsic to and extrinsic to the host organism. I should like to supplement this by pointing out the following:

1. The probabilities of coming into contact with most infectious agents are a function of the behaviors of an individual or a group.

2. Host resistance is left undeveloped, acquired, or even exhausted by previous behaviors. Host resistance is also found to be correlated with certain measurable psychological traits.

3. The environment of modern urban man has been importantly shaped by human behavior. Human behavior writ large, accumulated over time, is referred to as culture, and culture has without doubt altered environment drastically—in some ways promoting man's health and in other ways undermining it. The intrusion of way of life, behaviors, and emotions into the development of chronic noninfectious diseases is even better documented.

Inasmuch as psychology is one field of scientific study of human behavior, it follows from the above that psychology has a great potential contribution to make to the scientific study of health and disease in human communities—that is, to modern epidemiology. The remainder of this chapter attempts to amplify and specify the emerging contributions of psychology to the health sciences.

What form might these contributions of psychology take? Three forms immediately come to mind: theories, concepts, and techniques. Over the years psychologists have developed a variety of theories to explain and predict human behavior. Certain of these serve as useful frames of reference for initiating study of the interrelation of behavior and health. Different theories would be selected depending on whether the issue under study was psychophysiological, dealt with habit formation, or involved health-relevant behaviors of groups. The array of concepts which the field of psychology has developed derives from, but often is only loosely related to, theory. These concepts provide the health scientists with an established symbolic system for describing and analyzing behavior and for planning the exploration of problems. The third contribution is the methodology which has developed over the decades for gathering, measuring, and analyzing information regarding knowledge, attitudes, feelings, personality structure, and overt behavior. A wide variety of psychological tests and techniques are available whose validity, reliability, implications, and limitations are known. This material is too extensive to be covered in a single chapter or book, but rather could fill an entire professional career.

Psychology and the other behavioral sciences contribute to several frontiers of epidemiological research: (a) studies of the etiology of disease, (b) studies of psychological and behavioral concomitants of physiological changes, (c) studies of the "sick role" and seeking of medical care, (d) studies of the course of disease: recovery versus fatality, (e) the measurement of mental health, and (f) psychological and social determinants of public response to health programs. There are additional health frontiers at which psychology can make important contributions; for example, evaluation of the impact of health programs on human well-being and research into changing health policies of the "body politic" (i.e. social engineering). The present chapter will limit itself, however, to a more intensive examination of the first six frontiers listed.

INCORPORATION OF PSYCHOLOGICAL VARIATES INTO THE STRATEGY OF EPIDEMIOLOGY

Studies of the Etiology of Disease

When the epidemiologic elucidation of the etiology of disease is pursued in a programmatic fashion, investigators are soon confronted with the need to take psychological factors into account in their studies. Epidemiologists studying lung cancer have considered many possible causal variables: heredity, aspects of the environment (particularly atmospheric pollution), but the strongest of risk factors has proven to be a behavioral one—cigarette smoking. Epidemiologic studies of lung cancer continually lead back to the behavior of cigarette smoking.[4] Researchers should not stop at this point, but should seek to push back the veil of the unknown one step further by studying the epidemiology of cigarette smoking. Most workers acknowledge the feasibility of applying the epidemiologic method to investigation of health-related variables other than disease, but few epidemiologists actually pursue it. Studies of the epidemiology of smoking have revealed two domains of variables to be associated with this behavior: host factors and environmental factors. A recent study of a large group of employed males from a variety of industries revealed that heavy cigarette smokers differed from those who had quit smoking, or those who had never smoked, in serum lipids, hematocrit, type of occupation, level of income, and amount of schooling.[5] Studies of the smoking habits among adolescents have revealed the importance of the social environment. Young people who smoke are more likely to associate with a peer group in which smoking is the norm. This is in sharp contrast to nonsmoking adolescents in the same schools.[6-8]

We now turn to a very different disease, paralytic poliomyelitis. Epidemiologic studies of polio have shown that individuals most at risk of a paralytic attack are those who failed to obtain a natural immunity as a result of exposure to polio virus at a very early age and who have further failed to obtain an artificial immunity through receipt of an effective polio vaccine. Thus the epidemiology of paralytic polio is reduced to the epidemiology of the absence of appropriate antibodies. Serological surveys conducted in various parts of the world before the mass distribution of polio vaccines revealed the importance of environment. It was first thought that tropical environments favored the dispersion of polio virus, the early acquisition of natural immunity, and hence reduced risk of paralytic polio in later childhood and adulthood.[9] Later studies showed that the social class of the neighborhood (a sociological concept) and not its latitude was the key factor associated with early acquisition of serologic immunity.[10] A later study by Backett[11] pursued this association to more specific levels of "cause," and these were found to be behavioral in nature, such as the play habits of children and habits of personal hygiene.

With the development and distribution of safe, long-lasting live polio vaccines, it is no longer necessary, for practical purposes, to pursue a study of behavioral influences on the acquisition of natural immunity. For most administrative purposes, in an environment where sanitation level is high, infant mortality rate is low, and the natural spread of polio virus is minimal, the epidemiology of susceptibility to polio (lack of antibodies) can be reduced to the epidemiology of nonacceptance of polio vaccine. The nonacceptance of polio vaccine has been studied intensively using epidemiologic methods.[12] Standard epidemiologic variables like age, race, and sex have been associated with rate of vaccine acceptance.[13] In addition, sociological and psychological variables have proven to be even more potent predictors of vaccine acceptance.[14] Characteristics found strongly associated with the acceptance of polio vaccine, like the perception that most of one's friends have already taken vaccine, or the possession of personality traits of planning ahead, trust in medical experts, ability to postpone gratification, and a generally "productive" orientation, can, in turn, be studied in a community in terms of their distribution and determinants. That is, they can be studied epidemiologically.[12] Unlike age, race, and sex, many of these dynamic behavioral variables have the potential of being changed by programs of health motivation and education.

Psychological and social factors have also been found to relate quite directly to the dynamics of respiratory infections. Holmes's studies[15] argue for the complicity of life change and life crisis in timing the clinical emergence of tuberculosis. Hinkle and colleagues[16] have shown the temporal clustering of life stress and illness in a retrospective study covering a long time period. In a series of studies by Stewart, Voors, Jenkins, and others, it was first shown that the shared experience of particular human environments generates different levels of nonspecific susceptibility of sickness. Mathematical analyses implicated the social environment as a stronger contributor to differences in sickness rates between platoons of military recruits than such specific causes as spread of an infectious organism or exposure to a common hazard.[17] It was then found that incongruity in social status (that is, simultaneously having attributes of contrasting social levels) was associated with higher risk of respiratory infection.[18] Incongruities and discontinuities in one's social standing appear to be a better predictor of brief upper-respiratory infections in military recruits than are the various scales of the Minnesota Multiphasic Personality Inventory.[19] These and other aspects of behavior as it affects communicable disease are discussed further in Chapter 9.

Coronary heart disease, the pandemic of the modern world, is a disease of complex etiology. Part of the reason for the slow progress of the epidemiologic study of coronary heart disease (CHD) may be epidemiologists' traditional reluctance to consider systematically the involvement of behavior in many facets of predisposition to and precipitation of clinical manifestations of coronary disease. CHD has both behavioral and biological risk factors, and many of its biological risk factors are demonstrably influenced by psychological factors.

Most cardiovascular epidemiologists agree that the best-established risk factors for CHD are cigarette smoking, elevated serum cholesterol, elevations of other lighter-density serum lipids, and elevated blood pressure.[20] Excess weight has been found associated with CHD by some investigators[21] but not by others.[22] Diets rich in fats have been found associated with coronary disease when whole nations are compared, but diet has not been found associated with coronary risk[23,24] and often diet is not even related to serum cholesterol levels when free-living populations within a nation are studied.[25,26]

Evidence is accumulating from studies in various parts of the world that various social and psychological factors may also predispose to CHD.[27] Foremost among these is the "coronary-prone behavior pattern," an overt syndrome which includes excessive haste and impatience, exaggerated drive for achievement, competitiveness, and unusual investment of energy in one's occupation.[28] Let us consider, in turn, the role of behavior in each of these risk factors.

Cigarette smoking is obviously a learned behavior. Initiation of the habit is through imitation of desired role models, and maintenance of the habit is reinforced in part pharmacologically and in part psychologically. Most effective procedures for discontinuing the habit involve the learning of incompatible responses, substitutions of other oral gratifications, or deconditioning through aversive reinforcement. Much has been learned about these complex issues, and the reader is referred to the appropriate psychological literature.[29]

Blood lipids are unquestionably important risk factors for CHD. Despite considerable experimental and clinical literature on the influence of psychological responsiveness on serum lipid levels, epidemiologists have tended to assume that the level of fat in the blood is controlled exclusively by diet and exercise. The literature suggests that somewhat different emotional parameters may be involved in altering the level of serum cholesterol, a fairly dense lipid, as contrasted with those factors influencing lighter-density lipids such as serum triglycerides and beta and prebeta lipoprotein fractions.[30] In brief, it seems that serum levels of these lipids are elevated either when the individual is in a state of excitation or when he is actively suppressing his impulses. It is not known whether these behavioral factors operate through alteration of diet or exercise or act directly through the central nervous system or the endocrine system to affect the mobilization or degradation of these constituents of the blood. Some studies favor the latter explanation.[31] These issues are discussed further in the next section.

It is common clinical knowledge that excitement raises the blood pressure. Clinicians take this into account when measuring the blood pressure of "normal" individuals and in recommending a regimen for their hypertensive patients. The next section of this chapter cites clinical and laboratory studies of behaviorally caused alterations in blood pressure.

Three additional risk factors which have received much emphasis in some quarters are diet, exercise, and obesity. Dietary practices are influenced by social and cultural background, as well as by current economic state. Psychoanalytic theory holds that early childhood experience, particularly the child's relationship to the mother and the feeding situation, make a lifelong imprint on character structure. Even without accepting the bulk of psychoanalytic theory, it is hard to deny that early childhood eating experiences influence dietary habits and the role of food in the psychic economy. The psychodynamics supporting the overeating in specific groups of cases have been elucidated by Hamburger,[32] and the social and psychological forces which may be brought to bear in weight reduction programs have been reviewed and synthesized by Dwyer.[33]

Recent epidemiologic studies have thrown considerable doubt on the utility of dietary data as a predictor of CHD risk within any one population.[23,24] If further study should confirm the finding of the New York Anti-Coronary Club[34] that a dietary modification can alter coronary risk, a more depth-oriented psychological approach to altering eating habits should be utilized than the present practice of merely communicating nutritional information.

The amount of physical exercise engaged in has been shown to be related both to CHD risk and to CHD mortality.[35] Much of the average person's daily physical exertion occurs in his or her occupation. However, now that even blue-collar occupations are becoming largely sedentary, voluntary (nonoccupational) physical activity stands as the major opportunity for physical exertion for most people. Sheldon[36] has asserted that the propensity for active physical sports is, in part, constitutionally determined. It is also likely that habits of physical activity can be learned, and, if socially reinforced, will be maintained. Psychologically oriented studies of the epidemiology of voluntary physical activity could isolate and specify the personality characteristics of persons having highest and lowest likelihood of participating in physical activity, and could delineate the social circumstances most conducive to promoting healthful physical activity. Indeed studies are now under way of characteristics of persons entering and continuing in coronary-prevention programs involving regular exercise sessions and maintenance of a prudent diet.[37]

The result of excess dietary intake coupled with inadequate physical exercise is usually obesity. This condition has been found to be a risk factor of coronary disease. In a recent study, however, a variety of measures of obesity were made and the best of these was only a weak predictor of CHD. Most of the predictive strength of all weight-based variables was eliminated when level of blood pressure was taken into account in the regression equation predicting risk of CHD.[22] The role of personality and emotions in the development and maintenance of obesity has been studied by workers in psychosomatic medicine.[38] These findings will not be reviewed here.

In addition to all these traditional CHD risk factors, in which social and psychological forces play a role, there is an additional risk factor, recently established, which is purely behavioral. By this we mean that its observation and measurement are at the level of overt behavior. Its role in the pathogenesis of CHD, however, is no doubt mediated by neurophysiological or biochemical mechanisms. We are referring to the "coronary-prone behavior pattern." This pattern is an overt style of living characterized by extremes of competitiveness, striving for achievement, aggressiveness (yet sometimes stringently repressed), haste, impatience, restlessness, hyperalertness, explosiveness of speech, tenseness of facial musculature, and feelings of being under the pressure of time and under the challenge of responsibility. A recent volume by Friedman[39] traces the historical development of this concept from the writings of Osler, Dunbar, and more recent workers. A broad array of studies carried out by psychologists, cardiologists, and workers in many other specialities in such locations as Australia, Holland, Sweden, Israel, and the United States, converge in finding that one or more aspects of the above-described symptoms are correlated with presence of CHD.[40] The work of Rosenman and Friedman and their colleagues[41] has shown that the coronary-prone behavior pattern, "Type A," is associated both with CHD prevalence and with CHD incidence in a prospective study of a large industrial population. These findings have been confirmed in the prevalence survey of Benedictine and Trappist monasteries reported in papers by Caffrey[42,43] and by Quinlan and associates.[44] More complete discussion of the psychological and social precursors of coronary disease is found in the review paper by Jenkins.[27] This review also specifies the psychological tests and sociologic indices which have shown significant associations with coronary disease.

The Minnesota Multiphasic Personality Inventory, particularly the hypochondriasis and hysteria scales, have been repeatedly found associated with coronary disease, especially when it manifests itself as angina pectoris. Other psychometrically derived scales of anxiety or "stress" have registered higher scores among coronary-disease patients, but in general, these scales have not been used in replication studies, so the generality of the findings remains untested. It should be noted, however, that in studies where the stress-anxiety issue was approached both by use of one or two obvious interview questions and by use of a psychometrically validated scale, only the latter showed a significant association with coronary disease.

The cardiologists who have developed the concept of the coronary-prone behavior pattern and directed the laboratory research of the Harold Brunn Institute and the epidemiologic Western Collaborative Group Study have called upon psychologists and psychometricians to make a wide variety of scientific contributions. The interview procedure for determining the coronary-prone behavior pattern was subjected to content analysis. Clusters of items having similar content were studied in terms of their relationship to myocardial infarction and to levels of blood lipids.[45] A psychologist also conducted reliability studies of the interview procedure to determine the degree of interjudge agreement and the stability of behavior type over time.[46] Other psychologists learned the procedures for behavior typing and applied them in other studies of coronary disease.[42,47] Still another psychologist has developed new methods for ascertaining behavior type: a battery of performance tests[48] and a short, self-administered rating scale.[49] A cardiologist and electrical engineer using a laboratory approach involving advanced electronics developed a method for analysis of patterns of changes in voice amplitude which has been found associated with the behavior type and with existing CHD.[50]

An intensive program of research into questionnaire techniques for more precise measurement of the coronary-prone behavior pattern was initiated at the University of North Carolina in 1964. Since the beginning of these efforts by psychologically trained epidemiologists, the following progress has been made.

An intensive observational study was done of the cardiologists' clinical criteria for judging behavior type. This observational work included participation in hospital rounds, co-interviewing of coronary disease patients with the cardiologists, and detailed discussions of specific major and minor signs and symptoms of the coronary-prone behavior pattern. This firsthand "soaking in the situation" enabled the psychologists to share the frame of reference of the cardiologists to a large degree. This provided the basis for a more sensitive approach to developing psychological measures of the coronary-prone behavior pattern.

A pool of questionnaire items was written and administered to men who had previously been rated as being Type A (having the coronary-prone behavioral characteristics). This pool of items was then subjected to empiric validation procedures according to accepted psychometric methodology. Inadequate items were discarded and marginal items were revised, and new items were added to the pool. The entire list was subjected to cross-validation on a new sample of subjects. These procedures have been described in detail elsewhere.[51] The result was a self-administered test questionnaire whose items are scored by computer, optimally weighted, entered into a discriminate function equation, and adjusted to population constants. The final scores for each individual are then punched into a card bearing his identification number and/or printed in a listing. Thus, through the efforts of psychometrics and computer science, a clinical procedure which originally resulted in only a dichotomous judgment (a person was rated either Type A or Type B) has now been transformed into a relatively automatic procedure not involving professional personnel which results in a calibrated score reflecting the degree to which an individual possesses characteristics of the coronary-prone behavior pattern. The technical improvement is comparable to that achieved in the measurement of blood pressure when digital palpation of an artery was replaced by the cuff-and-mercury manometer. It remains to be demonstrated, however, whether this technical improvement in measurement properties is accompanied by an equivalent gain in medical usefulness of the measurement thus obtained.

The usefulness or value of numbers obtained from a measurement system is referred to as "validity." Efforts to establish the validity of this test for the coronary-prone behavior pattern are currently under way. Thus far it has been shown that higher Type A scores (i.e. higher scores on the A-B scale of the Jenkins Activity Survey) are found in patients having coronary disease as compared to nondiseased individuals in the same population.[52] It has also been observed that patients with coronary disease who subsequently sustain a recurrent episode of disease (such as another myocardial infarction) have higher scores on the A-B scale than do those patients who continue without further infarctions. Persons with multiple infarctions are found to have higher scores than persons without coronary disease or with only one coronary episode, whether their second coronary event occurs before or after they complete the test questionnaire. Thus it would seem that the elevated scores are not the result of retrospective bias triggered by the coronary episode. Preliminary study of a limited sample of men who develop their initial coronary attack after taking the JAS questionnaire does not show them to have scored significantly higher than their fellows who remained healthy. This raises the possibility that this test in its present form may not be able to predict the CHD candidate, even though it has modest success in distinguishing between the behavior traits of men already having coronary disease and those without this disease.[53] Further study and refinement of this test is needed.

This detailed description of a psychometric approach to the study of behavioral factors in coronary disease is not offered as a resolution of issues about the etiology of coronary heart disease;

rather, its methodological approach illustrates the potential contribution of psychometric measurement and psychologic study, clinical and social, to the study of any health problem which has antecedents or concomitants of a behavioral nature.

Studies of Psychological and Behavioral Concomitants of Physiological Changes

Alterations in physiological function commonly accompany changes in the life situation or in the individual's interpretation of his situation. Such alterations may be physiologically adaptive or maladaptive. Sustained deviations of certain biochemical and physiological parameters have been implicated as risk factors for a number of diseases. For these reasons it is not only justifiable but important for epidemiology to study the distributions of physiological parameters in communities and the factors associated with abnormal values of these parameters.

The serum lipids, particularly serum cholesterol, have been implicated as risk factors in coronary heart disease and cerebrovascular accident for several decades. To date, the comprehensive epidemiology of lipid distributions has not been worked out, but such community studies as those conducted in Framingham, Massachusetts, Tecumseh, Michigan, and Evans County, Georgia, have laid the groundwork by providing demographic associations. Parallel with this development, a number of smaller studies have searched out the behavioral and emotional correlates of alterations in serum lipids. One of the earliest of these studies was that conducted by Friedman, Rosenman, and Carroll.[54] They observed cyclical changes in the serum cholesterols of a group of accountants they were studying throughout the year. Many of the accountants showed a sharp rise in serum cholesterol late in March and during most of April. This led to the hypothesis that stress of income tax preparation increased as the April 15 deadline approached and was accompanied by an elevation of serum cholesterol. The hypothesis was further strengthened when it was discovered that many of the men who did not show this rise in cholesterol during April were corporate accountants whose period of deadlines coincided with the closing of the fiscal year, December

31. Subsequently a wide variety of studies have corroborated this association of work pressure and elevated cholesterol. Many of these studies have been conducted on medical students awaiting crucial examinations. Additional cross-sectional studies of larger samples of people have used either psychiatric interviews[55] or psychological tests[56] to ascertain differences in personality traits within a group. Certain of the psychological differences have been found to coincide with differences in levels of serum cholesterol or serum triglicerides. The general thrust of these findings is that more active, aggressive, outgoing, stimulated people have higher cholesterols, as do those persons who are conscientious, suppress their impulses, show high levels of self-control and propriety, and are self-critical.[30] The implications of these findings were discussed above in connection with coronary disease.

Psychosomatic research for many years has examined the personality of the hypertensive patient.[57] In addition, the roles of anxiety and hostility in raising blood pressure levels have been demonstrated.[58] Recently, Hokanson[59,60] has shown that experimental manipulation of hostility also influences blood pressure. Hokanson's experiment placed college students in a game situation where they could give or receive electric shocks to the finger. Blood pressures rose in subjects receiving many shocks. If these subjects were then allowed the opportunity to retaliate by shocking the experimentor, their blood pressures declined to base-line levels. If this opportunity for revenge was withheld, it was then observed that blood pressure remained elevated for much longer periods of time. In another approach,[61] adults have been "trained" to alter their heart rate through operant conditioning procedures. Both increases and decreases of heart rate can be elicited, and these changes are independent of rate of respiration or overt body movement. A variety of other laboratory experiments and observations of natural situations have also shown the connection of psychological factors to blood pressures. These studies were reviewed by McGinn and colleagues.[62] It may be pointed out here that most of this experimental evidence deals with transient alterations in blood pressure level and not sustained hypertension. In reply, it should be noted that epidemiologic studies have shown that a single casual reading of elevated blood pressure has predictive value as a risk factor for CHD.

Serum uric acid is a compound which is invariably at high concentration in persons with gout. It has occasionally been suggested as a risk factor in coronary heart disease, but most large-scale studies have not found it to be valid predictor. The folklore has long held that gout is the result of extravagant living, particularly the consumption of rich food and drink. Studies have shown that indeed serum uric acid levels are higher, on the average, in upper and middle classes than in lower social class. High serum uric acid levels have also been noted in geniuses and in high-achieving individuals.[63] Psychologists entering this area of research sought to distinguish amongst these three correlated concomitants of elevated serum uric acid by use of intelligence tests, scales measuring drive for achievement, and a social class index. Each of these three variables could be measured on a continuous scale and its relation to serum uric acid studied with other statistically controlled variables as inclusions. The work of Brooks and Mueller[64] and of Kasl and colleagues[65] suggest that drive for achievement is the more important correlate of serum uric acid levels among these three factors.

This research problem regarding uric acid has been debated by physicians and epidemiologists for decades. The contribution of behavioral scientists was to introduce methods for the measurement, on continuous scales, of intelligence and drive for achievement. In addition, the techniques for statistical analysis used in these studies, such as partial correlation, while known to statisticians and epidemiologists, are seldom used by them. These are everyday tools of psychologists. The presence of a quantitatively oriented psychologist on an epidemiologic research team serves to broaden not only the range of explanatory concepts being considered and the techniques for measuring behavior and attitudes, but also enlarges the armamentarium of techniques for data analysis.

Studies of the "Sick Role" and Seeking of Medical Care

As epidemiology moves into the study of the utilization of health services, it must be aware of the various factors which influence a person to seek the help of a health professional. Certainly the presence of disease brings a person to the doctor, but not all people with disease will seek medical help. Similarly, physiological changes may promote the seeking of medical care, particularly if they give rise to symptoms. However, many persons present themselves at clinics and doctors' offices without detectable disease and without detectable physiological abnormality. The use of professional time and facilities by these people is substantial and must be included in the epidemiologist's purview.

Medical sociologists have defined as the "sick role" that set of attitudes toward the self which lead one to claim the privileges afforded to the "sick" and lead one to seek medical care. Understanding the utilization of medical services necessitates understanding how the sick role is learned and used. If we could learn how it is developed and used inappropriately, we could reduce the load on medical care facilities. If we could learn how it is denied inappropriately, we could bring into earlier care those people whose denial and delay make subsequent curative medicine more difficult. While the "sick role" is a concept developed by medical sociologists, effective measurement of its properties through use of questionnaires or interviews is a psychometric problem. A useful discussion of the "sick role" is found in the chapter by King.[66]

Closely related to the "sick role" is the way in which culture and learning alter the modes of experiencing and expressing physical symptoms. This is nicely illustrated by Zola's study[67] of outpatients at an ear, nose, and throat clinic in Boston. He found that patients of Italian descent described their symptoms in expansive terms with vivid and dramatic language, implying the involvement of the entire body. In contrast, the patients of Irish descent reported localized symptoms in rather laconic terms and did not seem to be suffering unduly. Analysis of the medical charts revealed that the two groups had essentially the same distribution of diagnoses for their respective ailments. The interrelation of culture, personality, and health is obvious.

Studies of the Course of Disease: Recovery versus Fatal Outcome

There is evidence to suggest that *different* processes are involved in primary resistance to disease than are involved in recovery after a disease or injury has occurred. In psychosomatic research, also, somewhat different variables have been found to predict good recovery than were found associated with primary host resistance. A rather broad variety of precursors were reported earlier in this chapter as being associated with risk of specific diseases. In contrast, the research literature on recovery from disease and disability coalesces around two major factors in the psychological realm which are associated with good recovery: high ego strength and lack of depression.

Recovery from mononucleosis and from brucellosis was found in retrospective studies to be associated with high scores on the ego strength scale of the Minnesota Multiphasic Personality Inventory (MMPI) and on other objective scales which have the same basic meaning.[68,69] One might properly ask whether delayed recovery might encourage patients to report complaints and inadequacies consistent with low scores on the ego strength scale. To answer this question of which came first, Imboden *et al.*[70] did a prospective study of recovery from Asian influenza. The MMPI scores were not associated with who became ill with the flu and who remained free of disease, but the ego strength score was again significantly higher in those who recovered from the flu in less than the median time for the entire group of patients.

Recovery from gastric ulcer has also been studied psychologically. The Bender Gestalt test was evaluated by a technique which gives scores indicative of high ego strength and impulse control. Those persons with intractable ulcer scored much more poorly on these variables.[71] In a replication study, similar findings were observed.[72]

The course of cancer in humans has also been studied psychologically. Physicians and nurses working on hospital wards containing numbers of terminal cancer patients have been known to comment that the friendly, cooperative patients seemed to die more quickly, while the complaining resistive, cantankerous patients seemed to survive longer. It would be easy to assert that it just *seems* that the difficult patients survive longer and dismiss the whole hypothesis. Bruno Klopfer[73] was one investigator who decided to test this issue empirically. He found that the observation of the clinical personnel was indeed true. In a well-controlled prospective study, Klopfer found that certain indices on the Rorschach inkblot test discriminated between patients with fast-growing and slow-growing tumors. Klopfer also discusses previous studies, one of which used the MMPI, showing similar findings.

Personality attributes and tests of flexibility of thought processes have been found to discriminate between survivors and nonsurvivors in a longitudinal study of an aging population. K. F. Riegel *et al.*[74] found seven test scores in his lengthy battery which predicted which persons between ages 55 and 64 would die in the ensuing five-year period. His predictions were significantly better than chance but, of course, far from perfect.

Two prospective studies of open heart surgery, performed at about the same time in different medical centers, agreed in showing that fatal outcome of surgery is far more frequent in patients who are depressed or hopeless before the operation. Anxiety and other psychological symptoms did not correlate nearly as strongly with risk of fatal outcome. In a study by Kimball[75] at Yale University, 80 percent of the patients depressed before the operation had fatal outcomes. In a study by Tufo and Ostfeld[76] in Chicago, following one hundred patients undergoing open heart surgery, all twelve of the patients who showed severe preoperative depression and inability to discuss plans for the postoperative period experienced fatal outcomes. This is in contrast to a 20 percent mortality for the total patient group.

Measurement of Mental Health

The mental health field has, of course, seen the greatest use of psychological measurement, both for purposes of diagnosis and estimation of prognosis. A variety of different kinds of tests have been established as useful in the measurement of mental deficiency, in preliminary screening, for neurological damage, in preliminary psychiatric diagnosis, and in elucidating the psychodynamic problems in persons coming for psychotherapy. Several major approaches to psychological testing have evolved. Projective tests consist of relatively unstructured stimuli such as inkblots or pictures. The subject's task is to report what he sees or to tell a story about it. Both the stimulus and the nature of the response expected are left relatively undefined. A number of semiprojective tests have been developed. This is perhaps a peculiar term, but it indicates those tests which have more structured stimulus and response modalities than the ones mentioned above, while still leaving much more flexibility to the respondent than is the case with personality inventories. Word association tests, sentence completion tests, and tests calling for the drawing of pictures are included in this category. As with the projective devices, the semiprojective devices depend for their validity and reliability upon the training and sensitivity of the interpreter. As a result, these tests are expensive to obtain and cumbersome for large studies.

Questionnaires and inventories containing specific questions and precoded answers, usually true-false or multiple choice, are rigidly structured both in terms of the stimulus presented and the response expected. For this reason they are of limited usefulness among the very young, persons with limited reading ability, short attention span, or severe emotional problems. They also may fail to reflect unusual problems or atypical situations to the examiner. Their structure, however, makes them particularly useful for mass administration and screening of relatively average individuals. They can be administered and scored quickly and cheaply by clerical personnel. In many instances machine scoring is available. Hundreds of such objective tests have been developed for a wide variety of uses ranging from psychiatric screening to vocational guidance to recreational interests and personality differences between the subcultures. Many of these tests are inadequate in their validation and lead all too often to erroneous decisions. Lengthy descriptions and critiques of many projective, semiprojective, and objective procedures as well as individually and group-administered intelligence tests and special aptitude measurements are contained in *The Sixth Mental Measurements Yearbook,* edited by O. K. Buros.[77]

Standard objective tests also pose dangers. Because they can be administered and scored so automatically, the patient or client can be relatively ignored by professional personnel. Extreme scores on these tests may not be due to extreme lack or extreme presence of the trait supposedly being measured, but rather be simply an artifact of a failure to understand the directions, poor reading levels, or active resistance to the test-taking situation. There are also many factors which bias these tests results in less obvious ways. Group-administered tests, both of intelligence and of personal traits, often have spurious correlations with respondents' education, socioeconomic status, or cultural group—or even age or sex —operating by means of biased contents, "response set," or social desirability set. Many objective tests and inventories are easy to purchase and the test manual contains guidelines for interpretation. This opens the door to use of these instruments by personnel agencies, health departments, or medical research teams who do not retain professional behavioral scientists to consult with them on test selection, administration, and most of all, interpretation. This is a danger to be avoided.

We have described some of the general forms of psychological tests and some limitations to their usage. They also have great *potentiality* for research and practice in health, and often advantages over alternative procedures for gathering personal data.

Individual diagnosis of psychological and emotional problems is most often based on the psychiatric interview. This procedure consumes too much time of highly trained manpower for large-scale studies and screening programs. Well-selected, well-interpreted psychological tests, however, can lead to diagnostic decisions which closely approximate psychiatric findings. They have the added advantage of permitting a more objective means of rank-ordering people in terms of their degree of mental illness or wellness. As screening procedures, psychological tests can take the same role in mental health programs as the chest x-ray has done in TB programs and the Schick and Dick tests have done in communicable disease control.

Recent social psychiatry surveys, such as the Stirling County Study by the Leightons[78] and the Midtown Manhattan Study,[79] have used brief psychologic questionnaires for quick estimation of the mental health of large samples of people. The advantage of these procedures is that larger populations of persons can be studied, quantitative analyses can be introduced, and findings from different samples can be compared. Comparisons can rarely be made between samples rated by different psychiatrists because of great interobserver variability.[80] Since comparisons are the heart of the strategy of epidemiology, objective psychological procedures seem essential in the epidemiologic study of mental health.

While psychologic procedures are commonplace in psychiatric screening, they are less frequently used in screening of neurologic disorders. Yet there is a firm research basis for their use. A number of tests can be competently administered by psychometrists which are sensitive to both acute and chronic brain syndromes. For example, diffuse EEG slowing of a degree the effects of which are not apparent to the observer is often marked by deteriorated performance on visual motor tests even though language and reasoning are not impaired.[81] Various patterns of impairments on mental tests have been associated with the extent and localization of brain pathology and with the acuteness of its progression.[82,83]

Psychological tests have also been used to measure a number of capacities and personal qualities which are important in everyday life and yet not usually included as variables in medical or psychiatric research. The Vineland Social Maturity Scale scores information gathered on the self-care habits of retarded children and adults. It is not an intelligence test but is often a better predictor of how well a retarded individual can adjust to life outside of an institutional setting.[84] The ability to plan ahead and use good judgment is well predicted by scores on the Porteus Mazes. This test has also been widely used in cross-cultural studies and appears to be relatively free of cultural bias. A procedure for obtaining an "impulsiveness" score from the Porteus Mazes has been found to be associated with delinquency and also with recidivism among reformatory inmates.[85] The California Psychological Inventory is a lengthy true-false test which has well-standardized scales for such traits as responsibility, self-acceptance, achievement through independence, and other traits which seem to be important in the prediction of social adjustment.[86] These are but a few of the tests which have the potential for making major contributions to understanding the relations of psychological and social factors to health. They await the call of the ingenious hypothesis and the careful researcher.

Psychological and Social Determinants of Public Response to Health Programs

Most major current health problems depend for their solution more on changing the personal and social behaviors of people than on inventing new medical technologies. Preventive or risk-reducing measures are known, and successful control depends primarily upon public cooperation for such diverse maladies as poliomyelitis, rubella, diphtheria, lung cancer, coronary heart disease, overpopulation, tuberculosis, malaria, many types of childhood poisoning, and dental caries. This list of diseases serves as an honor roll to the ingenuity of biological researchers, yet it also dramatizes the underdevelopment of the "public" or behavioral aspects of public health. There are barriers in programs and problems in people which keep the two from getting together in effective preventive health activity.

What scientific approach might be used to study these issues in health-related behavior? May I suggest that epidemiology is singularly fitted to study the distribution and determinants of health-related behavior, in much the same way that it has effectively studied the distribution and determinants of disease.

As in the study of the causes of disease, epidemiologic studies of public response—or nonresponse—to health programs begin with hypotheses. These hypotheses would, of course, derive from behavior theory rather than germ theory. Key variables in such hypotheses are psychological and social concepts regarding the forces which shape behavior.

Behavioral epidemiologists can study public response either in the local situation, such as in tracking down the causes of an epidemic of noncooperation, or at the level of "arm-chair epidemiology," where field reports and data from large surveys are analyzed to the accompaniment of whirring computers. In the former instance, the behavioral epidemiologist will proceed in a roughly similar manner to his colleague who deals with infectious outbreaks. He will confirm the diagnosis by interviewing both persons who participated and persons who refused to participate in the health program. He will orient the public response as to time and space by attempting to discover trends in amount of cooperation and to find those places where the health program has obtained its best and worst participation. As a third step, these data will be studied in a search for those cultural, social, and psychological differences which adhere to the same temporal-spatial patterns. On the basis of the resulting diagnosis, a decision will have to be made by the program administrators whether it is most feasible to attempt to change the respondent population or to change the approach and emphasis of the health program itself. Barnes and Jenkins[87] have reported a detailed case history of a behavioral epidemiological analysis of noncooperation with a malaria eradication program in a tribal society. Mass surveys of public response to health programs have also made major contributions to our knowledge of how to study health behavior and how to maximize the effectiveness of preventive health activities.

An early theoretical formulation of the determinants of health behavior was developed by Hochbaum and Rosenstock[88] of the U.S. Public Health Service in the early 1960's. This model has been refined and elaborated in recent years by Rosenstock[89] and his students at the University of Michigan. This theory of health-related behavior derives from Gestalt approaches to social psychology. The theory is limited in that it focuses almost exclusively on the respondent's perceptions of the disease being attacked and his perceptions of the utility of the recommended health behaviors. By reason of this concentration, the theory underestimates the influence of social factors on behavior and takes little account of the fact that many health-related actions are instigated by perceptions and motivations which are quite unrelated to health. A more comprehensive theoretic formulation has been offered by Edward Suchman.[90] He used the epidemiologic model of host, agent, and environment to construct a theoretic framework for the study of health-related behavior. This framework takes into account sociological indices, the social pressure of peers, the individual's perception of the health problem, and the suggested preventive behavior as well as features directly related to the circumstances of the particular program under study. But even this theory fails to alert health program planners to the importance of unconscious impulses and motives not logically related to health as determinants of the behaviors of large numbers of people.[91] The American advertising industry is fully aware of these issues and knows how to capitalize on them.

Two studies with less theoretical structure but very broad empirical coverage of social and psychological variables were conducted in Florida in connection with oral polio vaccine programs.[12,14] The findings from these studies showed that a wide variety of demographic, social, and psychological characteristics were associated with acceptance of both oral and injected polio vaccines. The significant variables included the following:

1. Knowledge about the program, its sponsors, and the vaccine.
2. Convenience of obtaining vaccine.
3. Sources of information regarding the program.
4. Perception of susceptibility to polio.
5. Worry about getting polio.
6. Acquaintance with a polio patient.
7. Knowledge of cause of polio and of how to prevent it.
8. Record of previous polio injections.
9. Personal attributes such as sex, ethnic group, religious preference, and particularly social class.
10. Amount of group interaction, including number of organization memberships, number of friends, and family composition.
11. General personality factors, based on items estimating the emotional maturity and "productivity" of the respondent.

This wide array of significant correlates of this particular health-related behavior suggests the need for a multidisciplinary theory to understand the dynamics of individual and community response to health programs, As one can see from the listing above, effective studies of these variables requires reliable measurement of many social and psychological phenomena. We come again to a major point of this chapter: the need for a "hard numbers" behavioral science approach to develop reliable and valid techniques for measuring those social and psychological variables which are now becoming so important to modern epidemiology.

SUMMARY

In this chapter we have looked back to the early sources of epidemiology, noting that at its birth the science was intimately involved with "way of life" and human behavior. We then traced the science through its *in vitro* phase, wherein rapid progress, mechanization, and to some degree, a retreat from the whole person and the whole community took place. We now stand looking into the future, our vision no doubt strongly colored by our personal hopes. Yet we cannot but anticipate that epidemiology as a science and as an art will undergo a rehumanization without sacrificing its rate of movement toward understanding and overcoming the barriers to health. We feel that the social and behavioral sciences have an important contribution to make at this growing edge of epidemiology because, as this chapter has shown, thinking, feeling, and behaving are intimately involved with the etiology of disease. We have given illustrative findings for the role of behavior in both infectious and chronic diseases, with particular emphasis on coronary heart disease. The chapter has also documented the role of psychological factors in altered physiological responses, some of which are risk factors for the endemic chronic diseases of our time. The social definition of sickness and the rights and obligations of the sick person (the "sick role") were next discussed. These are defined by one's social group, and social change alters these definitions. Psychological factors also play an important role in the course of disease—whether the patient recovers rapidly, remains sick, or suffers a fatal outcome. The role of psychologic tests in the definition and measurement of emotional health and mental retardation, and in screening for neurological disorders, was then outlined. We then briefly listed several other useful data gathering procedures used in studying psychological and sociological aspects of health problems. Finally, the chapter described the contributions of psychology and behavioral epidemiology in the study of public response to health programs.

The intimate involvement of behavioral issues in these six problem areas now confronting medical science and public health underscores the need for the greater inclusion of behavioral sciences in the epidemiology of the future.

REFERENCES

1. Hippocrates. On air, water, and places. Cited by Brian McMahon *et al.* in *Epidemiologic Methods.* Little, Brown & Co., Boston, 1969.
2. Snow, J. On the mode of communication of cholera. In *Snow on Cholera: A Reprint of Two Papers.* New York, Hafner, 1936.
3. Morris, J.N. *Use of Epidemiology.* London, E.S. Livingston Ltd., 1967, p. 188.
4. U.S. Public Health Service. *The Health Consequences of Smoking.* U.S. Public Health Service Publication No. 1696. Washington, U.S. Dep't. of Health, Education, and Welfare, 1967.
5. Jenkins, C.D., Rosenman, R.H., and Zyzanski, S.J. Epidemiologic Study of Cigarette Smokers and Nonsmokers. Submitted for publication, 1971.
6. Horn, D., Courts, F.A., Taylor, R.M., and Solomon, E.S. *Amer. P. Public Health, 49:*1497, 1959.
7. Bajda, L. *Amer. J. Public Health, 54:*441, 1964.
8. Salber, E.J., and McMahon, B. *Amer. J. Public Health, 51:*1768, 1961.
9. Paul, J. In *Clinical Epidemiology.* Chicago, University of Chicago Press, 1958.
10. Melnick, J.L., Walton, M., Isaacson, P., and Cardwell, W. *Amer. J. Hyg., 65:*1, 1957.
11. Backett, E.M. *Lancet, 2:*778, 1957.
12. Johnson, A.L., Jenkins, C.D., Patrick, R.C., and Northcutt, T.J. *Epidemiology of Polio Vaccine Acceptance: A Social and Psychological Analysis.* Jacksonville, Florida State Board of Health Monograph No. 3, 1962.
13. Sirkin, M.G., and Brenner, B. *Public Health Monographs, 61,* 1960.
14. Northcutt, T.J., Jenkins, C.D., and Johnson, A.L. Chapter IV in Neill, J.S., and Bond, J.O. (Eds.) *Hillsborough County Vaccine Program.* Jacksonville, Florida State Board of Health Monograph No. 6, 1964.
15. Holmes, T.H. Multidiscipline studies in tuberculosis. In Sparer, P. (Ed.) *Personality, Stress, and Tuberculosis.* New York, International Universities Press.
16. Hinkle, L., *et al. Ann. Intern. Med., 49:*1373, 1957.
17. Stewart, G.T., Voors, A.W., Jenkins, C.D., *et al. Amer. J. Epidem., 89:* 254, 1969.
18. Voors, A.W., Stewart, G.T., Gutekunst, R.R., *et al. Amer. Rev. Resp. Dis., 98:*800, 1968.
19. Voors, A.W., Rytel, M.W., Jenkins, C.D., *et al. Amer. Rev. Resp. Dis., 99:*420, 1969.
20. Epstein, F.H. *J. Chronic Dis., 18:*735, 1965.
21. Shurtleff, D. Section 26 in Kannel, W.B., and Gordon, T. (Eds.) *The Framingham Study.* Washington, U.S. Gov't. Printing Office, 1970.

22. Pascarella, E.A. *An Analysis of the Relationship between Two Measures of Obesity Derived from Selected Anthropometric Dimensions and the Occurrence of Coronary Heart Disease.* Ph.D. dissertation, Dep't. of Epidemiology. Chapel Hill, University of North Carolina, 1969.
23. Zukel, W.J., Lewis, R.H., Enterline, P.E., *et al. Amer. J. Public Health, 49:*1630, 1959.
24. Epstein, F.H. Chapter 5 in Stewart, G.T. (Ed.) *Trends in Epidemiology.* Springfield, Thomas, 1971.
25. McDonough, J.R., Hames, C.G., Stulb, S.C., *et al. J. Chronic Dis., 18:*443, 1965.
26. Kahn, H.A. Medalie, J.H., Neufeld, H.N., *et al. Israel J. Med. Sci., 5:*1117, 1969.
27. Jenkins, C.D. *New Eng. J. Med., 284:*244 and 307, 1971.
28. Rosenman, R.H., Friedman, M., Straus, R., *et al. J.A.M.A., 189:*15, 1964.
29. Marson, A.R., and McFall, R.M. *J. Consult. Clin. Psychol., 36:*153, 1971.
30. Jenkins, C.D., Hames, C.G., Zyzanski, S.J., Rosenman, R.H., and Friedman, M. *Psychosom. Med., 31:*115, 1969.
31. Wolf, S., McCabe, W.R., Yamamoto, J., Adsett, C.A., and Schottstaedt, W.W. *Circulation, 26:*379, 1962.
32. Hamburger, W.W. *Bull. N.Y. Acad. Med., 33:*771, 1957.
33. Dwyer, J.T., Feldman, J.J., and Mayer, J. *J Health Soc. Behav. 11:*269, 1970.
34. Christakis, G., Rinzler, S.H., Archer, M., *et al. J.A.M.A., 198:*597, 1966.
35. Frank, C.W., Weinblatt, E., Shapiro, S., *et al. J.A.M.A., 198:*1241, 1966.
36. Sheldon, W.H. *The Varieties of Temperament: A Psychology of Constitutional Differences.* New York, Harper, 1944.
37. Heinzelmann, F., and Bagley, R.W. *Public Health Rep., 85:*905, 1970.
38. Glucksman, M.L., Hirsch, J., McCully, R.S., *et al. Psychosom. Med., 30:* 359, 1968.
39. Friedman, M. *Pathogenesis of Coronary Artery Disease.* New York, McGraw-Hill, 1969.
40. Myocardial infarction and other psychosomatic disturbances. Special Issue, *Psychother. Psychosom., 16:*189-292, 1968.
41. Rosenman, R.H., Friedman, M., Straus, R., *et al. J. Chronic Dis., 23:*173, 1970.
42. Caffrey, B. *J. Chronic Dis., 22:*93, 1969.
43. Caffrey, B. *Amer. J. Public Health, 60:*452, 1970.
44. Quinlan, C.B., Barrow, J.G., Hayes, C.G., *et al.* The Association of Risk Factors and Coronary Heart Disease in Trappist and Benedictine Monks. Paper presented at the American Heart Association Conference on Cardiovascular Epidemiology, New Orleans, Louisiana, 1969.
45. Jenkins, C.D. *J. Chronic Dis., 19:*599, 1966.
46. Jenkins, C.D., Rosenman, R.H., and Friedman, M. *Brit. J. Prev. Soc. Med., 22:*16, 1968.

47. Keith, R.A., Lown, B., and Stare, F.J. *Psychosom. Med., 27*:424, 1965.
48. Bortner, R.W., and Rosenman, R.H. *J. Chronic Dis., 20*:525, 1967.
49. Bortner, R.W. *J. Chronic Dis., 22*:87, 1969.
50. Friedman, M., Brown, A.E., and Rosenman, R.H. *J.A.M.A., 208*:828, 1969.
51. Jenkins, C.D., Rosenman, R.H., and Friedman, M. *J. Chronic Dis., 20*: 371, 1967.
52. Jenkins, C.D., Zyzanski, S.J., Rosenman, R.H., *et al. Psychosom. Med., 33*:193, 1971.
53. Jenkins, C.D., Zyzanski, S.J., Rosenman, R.H., *et al. J. Chronic Dis.,* in press.
54. Friedman, M., Rosenman, R.H., and Carroll, V. *Circulation, 17*:852, 1958.
55. Sloane, R.B., Habib, A., Evenson, M.B., *et al. J. Psychosom. Res., 5*:183, 1961.
56. Harlan, W.R., Oberman, A., Mitchell, R.E., *et al. Ann. Intern. Med., 66*: 540, 1967.
57. Oken, D. *A.M.A. Arch. Genl. Psychiat., 2*:441, 1960.
58. Moses, L., Daniels, G.E., and Nickerson, J.L. *Psychosom. Med., 18*:471, 1956.
59. Hokanson, J.E., and Edelman, R. J. *Abnorm. Soc. Psychol., 3*:442, 1966.
60. Hokanson, J.E., Willers, K.R., and Koropsak, E. *J. Personality, 36*:386, 1968.
61. Levene, H.I., Engel, B.T., and Pearson, J.A. *Psychosom. Med., 30*:837, 1968.
62. McGinn, N.F., Harburg, E., Julius, S., *et al. Psychol. Bull., 61*:209, 1964.
63. Stetten, D., Jr. *Perspect. Biol. Med., 2*:185, 1959.
64. Brooks, G.W., and Mueller, E. *J.A.M.A., 195*:415, 1966.
65. Kasl, S.V., Brooks, G.W., and Rodgers, W.L. *J.A.M.A., 213*:1158, 1970.
66. King, S.H. In Freeman, M.E., Levine, S., and Reeder, L.G. (Eds.) *Handbook of Medical Sociology*. Englewood Cliffs, N.J., Prentice-Hall, 1963, see esp. pp. 111-116.
67. Zola, I.K. *Amer. Sociol. Rev., 31*:615, 1966.
68. Greenfield, N.S., Roessler, R., and Crosley, A.P. *J. Nerv. Ment. Dis., 128*: 125, 1959.
69. Imboden, J., Canter, A., Cluff, L., *et al. A.M.A. Arch. Intern. Med., 103*: 406, 1959.
70. Imboden, J.B., Canter, A., and Cluff., L. *A.M.A. Arch. Intern. Med., 108*: 393, 1961.
71. Lothrop, W.W. *Psychosom. Med., 20*:30, 1958.
72. Pascal, G.R., and Thoroughman, J.C. *Psychosom. Med., 20*:625, 1964.
73. Klopfer, B. *J. Project Techn., 21*:331, 1957.
74. Riegel, K.F., Riegel, R.M., and Mayer, G. *J. Personality Soc. Psych., 3*: 342, 1967.
75. Kimball, C.P. *Psychosom. Med., 30*:552, 1968, abstract.

76. Tufo, H.M., and Ostfeld, A.M. *Psychosom. Med., 30*:552, 1968, abstract.
77. Buros, O.K. *Sixth Mental Measurements Yearbook.* Highland Park, N.J., Gryphon, 1965.
78. Leighton, D.C., Harding, J.S., *et al. The Character of Danger.* New York, Basic Books, 1963, see esp. Chapter VII and Appendix E.
79. Srole, L., Langner, T.S., *et al. Mental Health in the Metropolis: the Midtown Manhattan Study.* New York, McGraw-Hill, 1962.
80. Beck, A.T. *Amer. J. Psychiat., 119*:210, 1962.
81. Jenkins, C.D. *J. Nerv. Ment. Dis., 135*:162, 1962.
82. Vega, A., Jr., and Parsons, O.A. *J. Consult. Psychol., 31*:619, 1967.
83. Zimet, C.N., and Fishman, D.B. In Mussen, P.H., and Rosenzweig, M.R. (Eds.) *Annual Review of Psychology.* Palo Alto, Annual Reviews, Inc., 1970, vol. 21, pp. 113-154 (esp. 133 ff.).
84. Doll. E.A. *Measurement of Social Competence.* Princeton, Educational Testing Services, 1953.
85. Porteus, S.D. *The Porteus Maze Test and Intelligence.* Palo Alto, Pacific Books, 1950.
86. Gough, H.G. *Manual for the California Psychological Inventory.* Palo Alto, Consulting Psychologists Press, 1957.
87. Barnes, S. T., and Jenkins, C.D. *Soc. Sci. and Med.,* in press.
88. Rosenstock, I.M., Hochbaum, G.M., and Kegeles, S.S. Determinants of Health Behavior. Golden Anniversary White House Conference on Children and Youth, 1960.
89. Rosenstock, I.M. *Milbank Mem. Fund. Quart., 44*:94, 1966.
90. Suchman, E.A., *J. Health Soc. Behav. 8*:197, 1967.
91. Jenkins, C.D. The Epidemiology of Public Response. *Proceedings of the Sixth Annual Immunization Conference, U.S.P.H.S.* National Communicable Disease Center, Atlanta, Georgia, Mar. 1969, pp. 115-118.

Chapter 5

CORONARY HEART DISEASE EPIDEMIOLOGY

Current Aspects of Research, Prevention, and Community Programs

FREDERICK H. EPSTEIN

IN THIS CHAPTER, the epidemiology of coronary heart disease will be reviewed as it presents at this point in time. The look will be briefly backward and surveying the present to gain perspective, but mostly forward. Thus, it will be a view, personal in part, rather than a review. The observations and facts have been presented and discussed[1-7] and no attempt at full documentation or description will be made. The need, instead, is for assessment in terms of application of current knowledge and avenues toward further research. These needs must be seen in the context of the demands for health in the community—epidemiology forming, as it does, a bridge between field, clinical, and laboratory research and community medicine. Surely, there is no chronic disease at present which can be predicted with as high a degree of probability as coronary heart disease, which is to say that those susceptible to the further development of manifest illness can be identified with unprecedented precision. This development is, in fair measure, the result of epidemiological studies. Those who are concerned about the expense of such epidemiological research should reflect how much has been bought for a quite modest proportion of the total research expenditure. Yet, much remains to be done. Now is the time to take stock because a new strategy built upon current achievements is required to exploit and extend what is now known. Since most coronary heart disease is due to atherosclerosis, the two terms will be used interchangeably as appropriate.

PAST AND PRESENT

Lessons from International Epidemiology

The conviction that atherosclerosis constitutes a disease caused in large part by exposure to a multitude of detrimental environmental influences is based mostly on the wide variation in the frequency of the lesions and their clinical consequences in different parts of the world. This evidence comes both from pathological observations[8] and from population surveys.[1,2,4,9,10] It is unlikely that much of this variation is due to genetic differences. Whenever ethnically similar populations in different environments have been compared, such minority groups seem to acquire the characteristics of the majority as far as the frequency of coronary heart disease is concerned.[11] It is quite likely that there are genetic isolates which are particularly resistant or susceptible to atherosclerosis or the factors predisposing to it; the discovery of such groups is important for the elucidation of etiology but their discovery would not negate in any way the importance of the environment as a paramount modifier.

By and large, populations in which coronary disease is rare have eating patterns which rely on carbohydrates, mostly complex, rather than fats; what relatively little fat there is tends to be of vegetable rather than animal origin (i.e. it is low in saturated fatty acids and cholesterol). Such populations also tend to be more physically active and less obese; if they smoke cigarettes, the consumption is not likely to be heavy. Their life is "simple." By contrast, a high frequency of atherosclerosis occurs where the food is rich in fats, particularly of animal origin, rich in calories, and where people are more sedentary. All this is so well known that mention of it is made somewhat apologetically. Yet, there still are some who seem to question the relevance of these observations to the problem of coronary heart disease prevention in the so-called "Western culture"! It is argued that Western man cannot revert to a more primitive and "idyllic" mode of life. This is true. Also, it is by no means certain that there may not be hitherto intangible sociocultural influences which elevate such coronary heart disease risk factors as serum cholesterol above and beyond levels which can be accounted for by diet alone.

Discussions of this kind are scientifically interesting but their practical value is limited. The public health aim is not to reduce the community burden of coronary heart disease to the level in primitive societies but to postpone it in time of onset. Toward this end, the evidence from international comparisons—circumstantial though it is—suggests that the changes in the mode of life need not be very drastic in order to make a significant dent in the shocking mortality and morbidity presented by this disease in the United States and a good many other countries.[2] There is no reasonable doubt that coronary heart disease has become much more common over the past few decades.[4] The reason must obviously be inherent in recent changes in the environment. More people eat more of the foods which elevate serum lipids, an accompaniment of coronary disease. People smoke more and are more sedentary. The onus of proof that these changes in habits are unrelated to the current epidemic of coronary disease must be primarily on those who question their importance; but even most of those who believe in their importance look for firmer support based on the results from preventive trials, as will be discussed. There are very few diseases of which the etiology is fully understood; yet they are being treated by whatever means are available. Why should preventive therapy be withheld until all etiological pathways are completely grasped?

Lessons from Studies Within Countries

Data from international studies have a profound bearing on preventive health strategy at home, as was mentioned. These studies do not derive from a taste for travel but are carried out primarily for "home protection" though they are of benefit to other countries as well. Studies at home, on the other hand, are less well suited to investigate environmental factors unless there is a fairly wide variation in the factor (like smoking habits) or community exposure (like "water hardness"[12,13]). In regard to eating habits, there are indeed countries in which these are sufficiently varied to permit their study,[8,10] but in the United States the spread of nutrients appears to be too narrow to allow study of dietary factors in regard to coronary heart disease. Specifically, a number of investigations have shown that there is little correlation in this country between fat intake and serum cholesterol level;[14-17] this is to be expected in view of the uniformity of eating habits and the ubiquity of high fat intake. If it were not for the evidence from international comparisons, the significance of variation in eating patterns could not have been assessed. It is not proposed that all international differences in serum cholesterol level are explained in terms of fat and cholesterol intake alone.[18]

Intranational studies, on the other hand, have made a truly vital contribution to the knowledge concerning what are now universally called "risk factors." Epidemiological studies, largely but not exclusively, have provided the means to identify, say, 20 or 30 percent of the male, overtly "healthy" middle-aged population among whom the subsequent risk of developing coronary heart disease is at least two or three times greater than among the remainder of the population; some two-thirds of new events occur among the minority of the population so identified.[19-21] This, as mentioned before, is a predictive power which is unequalled for any other chronic disease. At the extreme of the scale, the gradient of risk for the highest and lowest 10 percent of the population, classified in terms of scores from multivariate risk function, is of the order of tenfold![22] All this is all the more remarkable because most of the predictive power is based on such simple and simply measured variables like serum cholesterol and blood pressure level and the cigarette-smoking habit.

Intranational studies have also revealed marked regional differences in reported mortality from coronary heart disease within the same country, both in the United States and elsewhere.[1] Moreover, regions with a low mortality from cardiovascular disease have a low mortality from all causes, and vice versa,[23,24] suggesting strongly that there are environmental forces which promote or impair health in general. Intranational studies of coronary heart disease mortality over time have shown striking increases in some countries in the recent decade or so.[4] International comparison of national trends in terms of mortality, morbidity, and risk factor associations should eventually provide an important means for the identification of the factors responsible for the phenomena under discussion.

The Advent of Preventive Trials

Once epidemiological studies had suggested, in concert with clinical, experimental, and pathological evidence, that serum lipids (especially cholesterol) and blood pressure levels, cigarette smoking, and lack of exercise are associated with coronary heart disease, it became imperative to set up preventive trials to demonstrate whether intervention on these factors could reduce the risk of disease. Some such trials have been completed and others are still in progress; some have been among survivors from myocardial infarction, while others have been on the level of "primary prevention." The mode of intervention has been through changes in dietary and other habits or by means of drugs; double-blind designs have sometimes, but not always, been used; subjects have come from open and closed populations or from clinics; some studies have been confined to high-risk subjects. In view of what has just been said, it might be thought that a large number of controlled trials, using these various approaches in a variety of combinations, have been done or are in progress. Actually, few trials have been or are being carried out; moreover, all have had shortcomings in design or number of subjects, so the results cannot be taken at face value. Nevertheless, whatever information there is on the effectiveness of lowering serum cholesterol levels by dietary changes shows a trend which is usually in favor of the treated group.[25,26] Needless to say, such trials are very difficult, time and effort consuming and expensive. Being critical of some of the results does not indicate a lack of appreciation or respect for the work that has been done. The issues which have just been discussed have all been summarized in some detail in a number of papers.[25-29]

It may be questioned whether preventive trials of the kind which are feasible and possible in regard to coronary heart disease will ever be "definitive" in the sense of "proving" a causal relationship in the same way as a vaccine can be proven to be effective. There is a need to set up criteria for a level of success which will justify the institution of preventive programs in the community. A good deal of the present controversy over whether the evidence (both circumstantial from observational studies and from the limited number of trials) is adequate to advocate a full-scale national prevention program stems from a lack of agreement on what constitutes "adequate evidence." Trials of this nature move into a hitherto uncharted area of medical research, and the guide posts for statistical significance and inference applicable to clinical and laboratory situations require adaptation for these new needs. This is not to suggest that scientific standards be lowered; the call is for scientific criteria and methods which can be applied realistically to a new problem. Future directions as regards preventive trials will be considered further in a subsequent section.

The Advent of Heart Attack Registers

An exciting recent development in Europe has remained almost unnoticed in the United States—the development of "ischemic heart disease register." Such a register is in full operation in Gothenburg, Sweden, and a pilot study was successfully carried out in Edinburgh, Scotland. Several such registers are now being set up in Europe with the help and coordination of the World Health Organization.[30] How many heart attack patients die before they reach the hospital? How many might be saved and how? What are the characteristics of such patients in terms of premonitory symptoms and signs at a time when preventive action might be taken? How many such patients had seen a physician recently? Of the patients reaching hospital, how many have a verified diagnosis of myocardial infarction? How do those who do differ from those who do not? What is the experience and prognosis of *all patients* in a *community* over a period of time, as compared to what has been learned from coronary-care units in selected hospitals? How many of such patients had previous heart disease? How can medical services be improved? What role can the physician in the community play in the way of spotting victims early and providing preventive aftercare? Above all, how can the "susceptibles" in the community be detected and protected before a heart attack supervenes?

These are but some of the questions to which answers must be found—answers which can come *only* from a systematic, comprehensive, and continuing surveillance of coronary heart disease in the total community. Among all else, such operations will monitor whether the attack rate is rising or falling, giving danger signals or suggesting reasons for observed improvements. Registers will also provide the base for a valid assessment of preventive and curative medical care. There is much current concern about community medicine. In the field of coronary heart disease, with answers to so many of the key questions enumerated above outstanding, it is hard to see what community cardiology can mean without the establishment of coronary heart disease registers in several carefully chosen areas.

Screening for "Risk Factors"

As mentioned, one consequence of the recognition of risk factors was the realization of the need for preventive trials; another is the need for screening programs. Clearly, these matters are linked. There is no point in identifying high-risk individuals unless they can be protected by preventive measures,[31] and there is no real assurance of effective prevention without the evidence from preventive trials. Moreover, lacking preventive measures, a high-risk person is better off if he does not know his status! Thus, advocating screening programs is linked with the belief that circumstantial evidence for a causal relation between risk factors and coronary heart disease is sufficiently strong to justify an intervention program even before more conclusive support will come from controlled intervention trials. It would seem that a majority of workers in this field find the total evidence for a causal association sufficiently compelling to be "activists."

From a pragmatic and practical point of view, any measure which has a fairly high probability of doing good (and even "antiactivists" would usually concede this) and is unlikely to do harm should not be withheld from a person whose risk of developing coronary heart disease is two or three times higher than that of his counterpart devoid of enhanced risk. On this basis, even those who are convinced that more conclusive preventive trials are imperative can, in good conscience, advocate screening programs.

Large-scale screening programs present a formidable task. It is quite unlikely that they can be carried out on a national scale except within the context of a reorganized system of preventive and curative medical care. In the meantime, pilot and demonstration projects are much needed to work out the logistics and cost effectiveness of such programs. It cannot be stressed sufficiently that screening programs are not "one-shot" affairs but a continuing operation where those screened "positive" must get help and advice and be reexamined to ensure that the preventive regimen is effective. This requires, among much else, the creation of a new generation of health workers. Optimally, such pilot projects should be designed in such a way that there is a comparison group, *less* actively treated rather than *un*treated, to be ethically acceptable, in order to rule out a "placebo effect" resulting from "tender, loving care" rather than specific therapy.

FUTURE TRENDS

Consolidating Gains

Identification of Susceptibility; Multiple Risk Factors

The development of methods for the identification of susceptibles for the purpose of instituting preventive measures is a major purpose of epidemiology. In the case of coronary heart disease, this is now possible in terms of single and multiple risk factors. In general, a major single risk factor will "pick up" about 10 to 20 percent of the population at risk (in this case middle-aged men in the United States, the best and most studied group) at levels where the probability of future clinical disease is, perhaps, twice as high as among the remainder of the population. Using two or three risk factors presenting simultaneously in the same man, the risk of future disease (the "risk ratio") will increase to three or fourfold, but the proportion of persons at such risks in the total population of middle-aged men will go down to 5 percent or less.[19-21] Thus, inevitably, the number of persons at a given risk in the community is inversely related to the risk ratio.

These considerations present no particular problem in designing screening programs from the point of view of detecting high-risk individuals, because it is obviously advantageous to know one's risk level even if it is "only" twice as high as that in the "lower range." The problem arises when one looks at the proportion of the population at risk on account of *one or more* risk factors. Taking again middle-aged men in this country, at least half will harbor one or more risk factors in the "upper range"! The other half is by no means "immune," because a substantial number of cardiac events will occur among them, the sensitivity and specificity of the tests being what they are.[19,20] Does it make sense to set up enormously expensive screening programs in the full knowledge that every second person will "screen positive"? This, again, is an entirely new problem in public health and it has not been given enough thought. The matter is raised not to deprecate screening programs; the opposite is the case. The call is for proper consideration of the issue. One consequence, however, is clear: the prevention of premature coronary heart disease in the community cannot possibly rely only on screening programs as long as the sensitivity and specificity of predictive tests remain what they are today. The screening of susceptibles must be coupled with a national program toward alteration of the detrimental features in the environment. Then the *total* population will be less exposed to nutritional and other habits which are likely to be harmful and to other and more all-pervading influences such as, perhaps, trace substances in water, air, and soil. All this must be even more true when it is considered that atherosclerosis starts well before middle age,[8,32] so prevention also must start much earlier. These are really truisms but the obvious is so apparent that it sometimes seems to escape notice!

Causality and the Need for Preventive Trials

The matter of preventive trials has been running like a red thread through all the previous discussions. It is unlikely that the *full* force of a national strategy toward prevention[26] can ever be made to bear upon the public, the public health agencies involved, and industry until acceptable scientific evidence from controlled trials is available. Moreover, as already mentioned, preventability and screening programs are closely interlinked, and here again, the results from preventive trials would lend much needed strength. Problems connected with such trials have been discussed in an earlier section. It might be added here that such trials not only serve the practical need of providing the base for public health and community action; they also constitute the only means to establish directly, rather than through circumstantial evidence, whether an association is causal (e.g. the relationship between serum cholesterol level and the clinical consequences of atherosclerosis). Thus, from every point of view, preventive trials represent a priority of the first order.

Community Programs

In this section, which is concerned with the consolidation of gains in the past and present, as discussed before, it is appropriate to close with the subject of community programs. Such programs are not, of course, limited to screening, about which enough has already been said except to repeat that screening is only the first phase in setting the stage for preventive care. In fact, "screening programs" is an unfortunate term, failing to convey the all-important matter of follow-up. It would be better to speak of "community programs" and "screening" to emphasize that the latter is but one ingredient of the program.

Apart from the detection and protection of susceptible, high-risk persons, community programs should include educational services. Professional education should provide continuing information on recent advances in the care of coronary heart disease patients in and out of the hospital, with further regard to "pre-coronary care"[33] and primary prevention. Public education should deal with risk factors, sensible living habits, and early warning signals for seeking medical attention. Heart attack registers, as already discussed, would provide much of the needed scientific base for community programs, including ways to prevent death prior to hospital admission and delays in hospitalization.

Who will be responsible for community programs in the way of initiating and maintaining them? Presumably, these will be joint undertakings between public and private agencies and the health professions. The full realization of the potential for community programs, as already stated in connection with screening, depends on a broader reorganization of preventive and curative medical care services.

Searching for Causes and Mechanisms

The Future of Observational Field Studies

It has been frequently stated in recent times that observational studies have largely outlived their usefulness and that the emphasis should be on preventive trials to test whether the associations based on observational studies are, in fact, causal in nature. Such a view would seem to presuppose either that coronary heart disease can already be adequately "explained" in terms of currently established risk factors or that, even if it cannot, there are no new hypotheses which need testing and no old ones which have not been tested fully. In order to make a case for preventive trials, it is not necessary to belittle the need for further observational research! There is a current need for both. Preventive trials have already been justified. The need for continuing observational studies derives from the view that there *are* new hypotheses and that not all those in existence for some time have been adequately explored.

Among metabolic factors predisposing to atherosclerosis, there have appeared two major entities which show only a limited degree of overlap and, as such, would seem fairly distinct. The first revolves around cholesterol and is exemplified, at the uppermost end of the distribution, by Fredrickson's Type II abnormality.[34] The other is exemplified incompletely by Fredrickson's Type IV,[34] which represents one of the expressions of a broader complex including elevation of triglycerides, carbohydrate intolerance, hyperinsulinemia, and obesity in various combinations. Only fragmentary information exists on the distribution of these variables, singly and in combination, in the population and their relation to coronary disease. Yet it is very likely that a good many people who experience a heart attack "unexplained" by serum cholesterol, blood pressure, smoking, and other factors have a metabolic abnormality of the general nature just described.

Even though there is reason to think that massive coronary thrombosis is more often the result rather than the cause of coronary occlusion, it does occur. Moreover, some persons presumably develop atherosclerosis in part because of some predisposition to thrombosis or a defect in the ability to lyse thrombi or fibrin. Yet, virtually nothing is known about this as a risk factor, largely on account of the lack of appropriate tests usable in the field.

Why do people die suddenly? In other words, what are the factors which predispose to ventricular fibrillation? Ventricular premature beats are one, but what is *their* cause? It has long been suspected that there must be intrinsic myocardial factors aside from the myocardial damage caused by coronary atherosclerosis which make the heart vulnerable to electrical instability. The study of these factors must be an important aim of future epidemiological research. Looking for mechanisms, catecholamines and electrolytes immediately come to mind.

If some kinds of psychosocial stress antecede coronary heart disease, better definition and identification of the pathways involved between the brain and the arterial wall is needed. Catecholamines are likely to play a role, but the mechanisms involved are certainly more subtle and complex than this.

Other opportunities for novel observational studies arise among populations in rapid transition from simple to more complex modes of living or from one country to another. These provide a unique but often fleeting chance to observe the total impact of an "atherosclerosis-promoting" environment on the several risk factors which determine individual susceptibility.[4]

Is the absolute risk of developing coronary heart disease the same for two groups of men, one living in a country of higher and the other in a country with lower mortality from coronary disease, matching for blood pressure, serum cholesterol, and smoking? This type of information would provide insight into some of the risk factors and environmental influences which still remain unknown. That not all that there is to know is known must be apparent from the fact that the predictive power, specificity, and sensitivity of currently available "tests" are not as high as one would wish them to be, even though much better than for any other chronic disease. Having yet more to learn is no excuse for not trying to apply what is known! Conversely, having learned so much is no excuse for not trying to do better still!

Clinical-Epidemiological and Laboratory Research

In the search for causes and mechanisms, there remains a good deal of room for observational studies in the field, as already mentioned. Such studies need to be supplemented by the development of new methods of clinical investigation applicable to epidemiological studies. Yet, it is not impossible to do fairly sophisticated examinations as part of epidemiological research, involving, for example, standard glucose tolerance tests[35] or treadmill exercise coupled with complex monitoring.[36] This assumes that, in population studies, it is not always necessary to do "everything in everybody," but to use, instead, carefully defined subsamples in order to reduce the need for examining excessively large numbers of persons. A further requirement for observations of this type is the availability of laboratory support to carry out more than "routine" determinations.

Some Special Approaches

Leads may sometimes come from unexpected sources. From the point of view of practical approaches to prevention, it is of major importance to search for less harmful foods. The meat of animals from woodlands and bushlands contains more unsaturated fatty acids than that of animals from water-rich grasslands, which resemble domestic cattle.[37] Some types of cattle produce leaner milk than others.[26] There must be more integration between experts in farming and food production and epidemiologists studying human health. World population problems have stimulated research in increasing food production. In the developed and developing countries, the quality rather than the quantity of food is of greater concern.

Epidemiology was called "human ecology" quite a long time before "ecology" became a household word. If trace and other metals may play a role in atherosclerosis,[13] the study of soil, water, and air in collaboration with environmental scientists will become a concern of cardiovascular epidemiologists.

Some studies cannot be done on human beings. For instance, do the food patterns now advocated in the prevention of atherosclerosis affect growth and development? Data of this kind will have to come from observations on primates, in preference to animals less similar to man.

These examples have been given to illustrate the potential for scope and imagination in finding new ways to search for causes and mechanisms. Needless to say, the cardiovascular epidemiologist must keep in close touch with atherosclerosis research at all levels—clinical, experimental, and in pathology—in order to try at all times to find a breach in the wall which will permit the testing of new findings by epidemiological means.

Some Specific Needs

Atherosclerosis: A Problem of Pediatrics and Family Medicine

There is now no serious doubt that atherosclerosis is a slowly progressive disease, largely preventable in its premature form, having its origins in childhood. It must be admitted that geographic differences in the extent of lesions which constitute a cornerstone in the concept of preventability are not yet marked, in the coronary vessels at least, at younger ages.[8] It must be concluded that lesions below the age of 15 or 20 either have a different etiology from those at older ages or that the ability to "cope" with harmful environmental stresses, such as large amounts of saturated fats, is adequate until puberty and shortly thereafter but then declines. In either case, there is no question that eating, exercise, and other habits are acquired early, within the family setting, and that they are "unlearned" with much difficulty when the need arises later, and against heavy odds in terms of established personal patterns of preferences and social pressures. Thus, from the viewpoint of habit formation alone, there is no doubt that acquisition of sensible living habits should take place early in life, taught by example and practice. This is clearly a family matter. It is neither feasible nor psychologically sound if mother and children go their own way while father, approaching middle age, "goes on a diet" (i.e. gets his meals cooked separately) and stops all kinds of habits which are considered perfectly acceptable for the rest of the family. This is so patently wrong, if not rather ridiculous, that it is hard to see how the concept of prevention as a family matter could be seriously questioned.

The word "premature" has been used reluctantly in the previous paragraph because it invites the question below what age clinically manifest coronary heart disease becomes "premature." Yet, it is a useful term because it focuses attention on the fact that coronary disease is a tragedy because it so often kills early. A third of all the deaths from the disease among men in the United States occurs prior to age 65, not counting those whose well-being is impaired because of having to live with this illness. In our kind of society, death or clinical disorder prior to age 65 or 70, in most instances, is surely premature! After that, it is more difficult to tell when it is too early for the bell to toll, because so much depends on the kind of life individual men or women have been able to make for themselves. Certainly, given the choice, one would rather die of a heart attack than cancer. Perhaps death is "premature" when it occurs before it is welcomed.

Speaking of coronary heart disease prevention as a family matter raises the question whether and to what extent the disease clusters in families.[38-42] Probably, having a close relative who died of a heart attack after the age of 55 or so does not in itself increase one's own risk as long as one does not harbor high-risk factor levels oneself. Earlier death in a first-degree relative increases individual risk but it is unknown how much of this is mediated through familial resemblance in risk factors. The study of families is a prime need in coronary heart disease research, not only to assess the risk associated with a "positive family history" but as a means to determine causative factors of environmental and genetic origin, which are investigated, in their interactions, with particular advantage in kindreds and households.

Clinical Methods of Detection

It almost goes without saying that one major obstacle to epidemiological research in coronary heart disease is the unavailability of methods to detect early and, sometimes, even more advanced disease. So-called "nonspecific" electrocardiographic changes, ECG changes following exercise, and demonstration of cardiac calcification by x-ray all have their usefulness. However, all lack sensitivity, specificity, or both. Coronary cineangiocardiography is not an acceptable research procedure and, where it has been done, the subjects have of necessity been highly selected on account of symptoms. With present technology, it is not at all impossible that some entirely new approaches may make their appearance. In the meantime, the shortcomings of presently available methods make it all the more surprising how much has been achieved by their use. Conversely, considering their successful use, they cannot be as deficient as one sometimes thinks.

Biostatistical Methods

The advances made in cardiovascular disease epidemiology would not have been possible without the close collaboration of biostatisticians. New approaches to study design and analysis were developed in response to specific needs, for both observational and intervention studies. It is not the current purpose to enumerate all remaining and unresolved problems. Instead, attention will be drawn to two areas of current interest and need: multivariate methods and the use of "interval data."

Individual risk toward future disease is determined by the interaction and combination of a variety of risk factors. Looking at one risk factor at a time is useful to see if there is any association at all. Beyond this, the coexistence of other risk factors and influences has to be taken into account. As a matter of fact, even the search for any association at all in regard to one risk factor may require taking into account others, because the *overall* correlation between the risk factor and the disease could be nonsignificant but there may yet exist small-risk factor clusters in which the factor in question plays a key role. This exploration for "clusters" is a neglected field, there being much scientific and intuitive reason to think that a given risk factor may have to be "conditioned" by others in the same way as drugs may enhance each other synergistically. Thus, the search for clusters of risk factor constellations requires one new type of biostatistical approach.

The calculation of total "scores," incorporating a series of risk factors, constitutes another area of need in which much progress has already been made.[20,22] Such scores have much usefulness in screening and the assessment of individual risk, and they may also be used in selecting subjects for controlled clinical trials. It has been calculated that the traditional epidemiologic-biostatistical method of multiple cross-classification for 10 variables studied at only three levels (low, medium, and high), would generate 59,049 cells![22] The need for more realistic multivariate methods is apparent.

A problem which has hardly been touched relates to the question whether interval information about risk factors adds predictive power. Almost all analyses of prospective epidemiological studies in coronary heart disease have used only the base line characteristics of the cohorts, i.e. readings which may be removed in time from the new event of coronary heart disease by a good many years. Intuitively, one would assume that risk factor readings closer to the event might be more telling or, coronary atherosclerosis being a chronic, slowly progressive condition, that multiple readings over time would be more predictive than a single reading taken several years earlier. Furthermore, changes or fluctuations in level over time may have predictive value of their own. These questions have two practical implications: (1) Is it necessary, in epidemiological studies, to repeat risk factor measurements at relatively frequent intervals or is it enough (which is much easier and cheaper to do) to monitor clinical events? (2) In risk factor screening, how often should measurements be made? Biostatistical techniques applicable to these problems must be developed.

Monitoring Mortality Trends

Monitoring mortality trends should be particularly important in countries in which the rates were hitherto low, as in developing countries, or relatively low but increasing.[4] In parts of the world where rates now are high, will there be a decline in mortality, as would be anticipated, if the environment were improving in subtle and insidious ways or if the most highly susceptible persons were to "die out"? Rates among women, in contrast to men, have almost universally been declining.[4] This is, perhaps, unexpected because women have been engaged more and more in doing "men's jobs."[5] Are there countries where rates in women are rising? Monitoring of this kind is, of course, an essential part of public health surveillance; national and international trends should provide important etiological leads and guide health policy.

SUMMARY—A STRATEGY FOR PREVENTION

Coronary heart disease epidemiology was shown to have made important strides in regard to identifying susceptibles and predicting risk. The causal importance of the environment in making the disease such a threat has been stressed, pointing the way toward preventive environmental changes. The need for preventive trials has been explained.

The importance of establishing "heart disease registers" toward the practice of community cardiology and the prediction and prevention of sudden death was discussed. Community programs and screening were considered within the context of community medicine. Future trends in research and its applications have been outlined.

Coronary heart disease will remain a major health problem until a strategy for prevention, control, and further research as a national priority has been developed.[26] Countries in which coronary disease is not yet as common as in the United States and several other nations will face an issue of the same magnitude unless they give attention to this matter while there is still some time left. The solution involves not only medical and scientific but also socioeconomic and cultural considerations. The ultimate thrust of the strategy must be toward prevention.

ACKNOWLEDGMENT

The author was fortunate enough to discuss with a good many colleagues here and abroad over the years the problems which are the substance of this report. In the course of working together, listening, and reading, he has learned much of what he has written. Their help and stimulation is acknowledged and greatly appreciated.

REFERENCES

1. Epstein, F.H. The epidemiology of coronary heart disease; a review. *J. Chronic Dis., 18:*735, 1965.
2. Stamler, J. *Lectures on Preventive Cardiology*. New York and London, Grune & Stratton, 1967.
3. Simborg, D.W. The status of risk factors and coronary heart disease. *J. Chronic Dis., 22:*515, 1970.
4. Epstein, F.H., and Krueger, D.E. The changing incidence of coronary heart disease. In Jones, A. Morgan (Ed.) *Modern Trends in Cardiology*. London, Butterworths, 1969, pp. 17-35.
5. Fejfar, Z., and Morris, J.N. A look at the future; the broad approach. *World Health: The Magazine of The World Health Organization, 39,* Aug.-Sept. 1970.
6. Epstein, F.H., and Ostrander, L.D., Jr. Detection of individual susceptibility toward coronary disease. *Prog. Cariod. Dis., 13:*324, 1971.
7. Epstein, F.H. Epidemiologic aspects of atherosclerosis. *Atherosclerosis, 14:*1, 1971.
8. McGill, H.C., Jr., *et al.* The geographic pathology of atherosclerosis. *Lab. Invest., 18:465,* (No. 5) 1968 (See also entire issue).
9. Fejfar, Z. Prevention and control of the epidemics of ischaemic heart disease. *Arch. Klin. Med., 216:*184, 1969.
10. Keys, A. (Ed.) *Coronary Heart Disease in Seven Countries.* American Heart Association Monograph No. 29. New York, American Heart Association, Inc., 1970, pp. 1-199.
11. Gordon, T. Further mortality experience among Japanese Americans. *Public Health Rep., 82:*973, 1967.
12. Schroeder, H.A. The water factor. Editorial. *New Eng. J. Med., 280:*386, 1969.
13. Masironi, R. Trace elements and cardiovascular diseases. *Bull. W.H.O., 40:*305, 1969.
14. Adelson, S.F., and Keys, A. Diet and some health characteristics of 123 business and professional men and methods used to obtain the dietary information. U.S. Dept. of Agriculture, Agricultural Research Service, Publication ARS *62-11,* Sept. 1962.
15. Paul, O., Lepper, M.H., Phelan, W.H., Dupertuis, G.W., MacMillian, A., McKean, H. and Park, H. A longitudinal study of coronary heart disease. *Circulation, 28:*20, 1963.
16. Stulb, S.C., McDonough, J.R., Greenberg, B.G., and Hames, C.G. The

relationship of nutrient intake and exercise to serum cholesterol levels in white males in Evans County, Georgia. *Amer. J. Clin. Nutr., 16:*238, 1965.

17. Gordon, T. The Framingham diet study: Diet and the regulation of serum cholesterol (Section 24). In Kannel, W.B., and Gordon, T. (Eds.) *The Framingham Study.* U.S. Public Health Service, National Institutes of Health, 1970. U.S. Gov't. Printing Office, Washington, D.C. 20402.
18. Kahn, H.A., Medalie, J.H., Neufeld, H.N., Riss, E. Balogh, M., and Groen, J.J. Serum cholesterol: Its distribution and association with dietary and other variables in a survey of 10,000 men. *Israel J. Med. Sci., 5:*1117, 1969.
19. Epstein, F.H. Predicting coronary heart disease. *J.A.M.A., 201:*795, 1967.
20. Epstein, F.H. Multiple risk factors and the prediction of coronary heart disease. *Bull. N. Acad. Med., 44:*916, 1968.
21. Stamler, J., and Epstein, F.H. Risk factors and the detection of susceptibles. In Symposium on Coronary Heart Disease Prevention. *Preventive Med.,* to be published.
22. Truett, J., Cornfield, J., and Kannel, W. A multivariate analysis of risk of coronary heart disease in Framingham. *J. Chronic Dis., 20:*511, 1967.
23. Sauer, H.I., and Enterline, P.E. Are geographic variations in death rates for cardiovascular diseases real? *J. Chronic Dis., 10:*513, 1959.
24. Syme, S.L. Is There a Future for the Epidemiologic Study of Cardiovascular Disease? Paper presented at the 96th Annual Meeting of the American Public Health Association, Detroit, Mich., 1968.
25. Stamler, J. Acute myocardial infarction—progress in primary prevention. *Brit. Heart J., 33* (Suppl.) : 145, 1971.
26. The primary prevention of the atherosclerotic diseases: Position paper for the Intersociety Commission for Heart Disease Resources prepared by the Atherosclerosis Study Group (J. Stamler, Chairman) and the Epidemiology Study Goup (A.M. Lilienfeld, Chairman). *Circulation, 42:*A55, 1970.
27. The national diet-heart study: Final report National Diet-Heart Study Research Group, with the Approval of the Executive Committee on Diet and Heart Disease. *Circulation, 37* (Suppl. 1), (No. 3) 1968.
28. *Mass Field Trials of the Diet-Heart Question: Their Significance, Timeliness, Feasibility and Applicability.* American Heart Association Monograph No. 28. New York, American Heart Association, Inc., 1969.
29. Cornfield, J., and Mitchell, S. Possible effects on coronary heart disease of intervention on selected risk factors. *A.M.A. Arch Environ. Health, 19:*382. 1969.
30. World Health Organization, Regional Office for Europe. Report of a

Working Group, Copenhagen, May 1968; Working Group on Ischaemic Heart Disease Registers. Parts I and II. Copenhagen. May 1969.

31. Epstein, F.H The value of screening examinations in identifying high-risk individuals in coronary heart disease prevention programs. (Presented at the 4th Asian-Pacific Congress of Cardiology. Jerusalem and Tel-Aviv, Sept. 1968.) In Eliakim, M., and Neufeld, H.N. (Eds.) *Cardiology—Current Topics and Progress.* New York and London. Academic Press, 1970, pp. 92-95.
32. Epstein. F.H. Studies on the Epidemiology of Atherosclerosis in Youth. Paper presented at the Symposium on "Atherosclerosis and its Prevention: A Pediatric Responsibility," 39th Annual Meeting of the American Academy of Pediatrics, San Francisco. Cal., Oct. 1970. To be published.
33. Lown, B., Klein, M.D., and Hershberg, P.I. Coronary and precoronary care. *Amer. J. Med., 46:*705, 1969.
34. Fredrickson, D.S., Levy, R.I., and Lees, R.S. Fat transport in lipoproteins—an integral approach to mechanisms and disorders. *New Eng. J. Med., 276:*32, 94, 148, 215, and 273, 1967.
35. Ostrander, L.D., Jr., Neff, B.J., Block, W.D., Francis, T., Jr., and Epstein, F.H. Hyperglycemia and hypertriglyceridemia among persons with coronary heart disease. *Ann. Intern. Med., 67:*34, 1967.
36. Montoye, H.J., Cunningham, D.A., Welch, H.G., and Epstein, F.H. Laboratory methods of assessing metabolic capacity in a large epidemiologic study. *Amer. J. Epidem., 91:*38, 1970.
37. Shaper, A.G. Current developments in atherosclerosis studies in Africa. In Jones, R.J. (Ed.) *Atherosclerosis: Proceedings of the Second International Symposium.* New York, Heidelberg, and Berlin, Springer Verlag, 1970, pp. 314-320.
38. Epstein, F.H. Hereditary aspects of coronary heart disease. *Amer. Heart J., 67:*445, 1964.
39. Epstein, F.H. Risk factors in coronary heart disease: Environmental and hereditary influences. *Israel J. Med. Sci., 3:*594, 1967.
40. McKusick, V.A. Genetic factors in arteriosclerosis, with particular reference to atherosclerosis of the coronary arteries. In Blumenthal, H.T. (Ed.) *Cowdry's Arteriosclerosis: A Survey of the Problem,* 2nd ed. Springfield, Thomas, 1967, pp. 551-575.
41. Murphy, E.A. Some difficulties in the investigation of genetic factors in coronary artery disease. *Canad. Med. Ass. J., 97:*1181, 1967.
42. Bloor, C. Hereditary aspects of myrocardial infarction. *Circulation, 39* and *40* (Suppl. IV)130-135, 1969.

Chapter 6

THE PROSPECTIVE STUDY OF CARDIOVASCULAR DISEASE

TAVIA GORDON *and* WILLIAM B. KANNEL

THE EPIDEMIOLOGIC approach to the study of a disease in essence involves an investigation of the circumstances under which it arises and evolves in a population sample rather than an individual. Among other things, it aims to delineate differences between those who go on to develop disease and those who remain resistant to it. Epidemiologic studies usually evaluate spontaneously occurring and interacting factors in a population rather than those which emerge under precisely defined and controlled conditions. Clinical experience is particularly useful in suggesting hypotheses of causation by determining in what particulars those who are clearly ill differ from those who are well. However, preselection of symptomatic persons, absence of suitable controls, paucity of rigorously objective observations, and lack of information on the population from which the patient comes render such information difficult to interpret. Also, clinical impressions or retrospective studies alone are not sufficient to ascertain with assurance the risk of acquiring a disease in relation to personal attributes, living habits, and other possible precursors at a time relatively early in the course of a chronic disease process. Findings are often confounded by the presence of the disease and its management.

Prospective studies appear to provide the soundest epidemiologic information available. They provide a clearer picture of the nature of the problem and the total spectrum of the disease in all who have it, including those not hospitalized or under care. It may be possible to discern the chain of events leading to the disease, including its precursors. Especially vulnerable subgroups may be identified and a profile of likely candidates for the disease can eventually be constructed from estimates of the risk associated with each factor. Clues to pathogenesis are provided, hypotheses tested, and on occasion, new hypotheses suggested.

In 1948, the U.S. Public Health Service initiated a long-term study of cardiovascular disease in the town of Framingham, Massachusetts. A sample of adults resident in the town were invited to participate. Those who agreed to join were invited to receive a standardized medical examination and every two years thereafter were asked to return for reexamination. By characterizing persons when they were free of cardiovascular disease and determining what characteristics were associated with its subsequent incidence, it was hoped to discern factors related to the development of cardiovascular disease and to measure the strength of any relationships that appeared.[1,2,11]

The chief characteristics of this study were these: (1) It was based on a sample of the general population, including both sick and well persons. (2) It was prospective in nature. (3) It entailed repeated standardized medical examinations for the purpose both of determining habits and physiologic and biochemical characteristics that might be factors in the development of cardiovascular disease and also of determining cardiovascular status. (4) It was long-term.

By 1956, it was possible to report the initial findings from the study together with those from two others similar in nature.[6] A year later, it was possible to assemble investigators from at least seven similar studies to discuss common concerns. In another decade, it was possible to undertake the pooling of incidence findings from six American studies, and there were at least as many other studies of similar design under way around the world.

It might seem improbable that the long-term prospective study of cardiovascular disease could become so fashionable. The career commitments required, the large amount of work and money entailed, the long wait for results, and the uncertainty that anything substantial would be learned from the effort would all seem to conspire against the popularity of these studies. Why was this not the case? One explanation lies in the stimulus and support given this approach by the National Heart Institute. Without that it would have been impossible. But it went deeper than that. In 1945, nearly half of all deaths in the United States were assigned to cardiovascular causes and the percentage was rising. In current thinking, most of these deaths would be considered to arise from atherosclerotic or hypertensive processes. It is in this perspective of urgent need for information that we should view the sudden multiplication, about that time, of prospective studies of cardiovascular disease.

In some respects the dominance of the cardiovascular diseases as a force of mortality is a tribute to the success of previous epidemiological investigations. The revolution in our understanding and control of the infectious diseases is certainly a most remarkable accomplishment. This, together with the discovery and control of diseases arising from nutritional deficiency, led to a radical alteration of the pattern of disease and death. Mortality in infancy, childhood, and early adult life dropped sharply. As more people lived to older ages, the population was increasingly subject to the influence of the chronic and degenerative diseases. Even at older ages the effect of the reduction in the incidence of infectious and nutritional-deficiency diseases was felt. Thus the chronic diseases, like some bedrock of mortality, were uncovered as the layers of infectious and nutritional diseases were scraped away.

Concurrently other changes were occurring. During the first third of the twentieth century, the incidence of coronary heart disease began to rise. This disease, which was recognized only late in the nineteenth century, initially had only a minor impact on public health; by the third or fourth decade of the twentieth century, it began to hit increasingly in the population as a whole, especially affecting the male, with a particularly dramatic impact on the middle-aged male. Gradually it dawned on investigators that they were face-to-face with an intractable, lethal epidemic. Neither the causes nor the cure of this disease were apparent.

In 1948, responding to the pressing public health program posed by these cardiovascular diseases, the U.S. Public Health Service launched in the town of Framingham, Massachusetts, the then novel long-term prospective study of cardiovascular diseases, focusing in particular on the hypertensive and atherosclerotic diseases. In the decade that followed, a succession of other prospective studies of these diseases got under way and, more recently, new studies have been undertaken. Now, with the apparent curtailment of the Framingham Study some twenty years later, it may be useful to look back over this period of investigation to consider what has been accomplished.

No doubt that there are nearly as many rationales for prospective studies as there are investigators using the method. When the Framingham Study was initiated, the underlying philosophy of the prospective approach was expressed in this manner:

> That pathological change in, or disordered function of, the intimate structures of the cardiovascular system resulting from stresses and insults of various types is reversible up to a degree or point which is inherent in the individual, and
>
> That pathological or physiological change beyond that degree probably results in minute residual changes which are immeasurable by methods now available, and
>
> That continuous accretion of such residual changes results finally in a clinically recognizable abnormality, and
>
> That there is a wide variety in the individual response to many stresses and insults,
>
> It is hypothesized that the age of onset of degenerative cardiovascular disease is a function of three variables:
>
> (1) Constitutional factors (including hereditary factors)
> (2) Conditioning factors (including external environmental factors) and,
> (3) The time factor or length of time the conditioning factors must act on the constitutionally determined characteristics or interact with them to result in clinical cardiovascular disease.
>
> The Framingham Heart Disease Epidemiology Study is designed to measure certain selected constitutional factors and certain of the conditioning factors in a large number of "normal" persons selected at random and to record the time during which these selected factors act and interact before clinical cardiovascular disease results.

THE IMPERCEPTIBLE PROCESS

It may indeed be argued that if the underlying disease process proceeds by imperceptible steps, the rationale for repeated reexamination to redefine the precursive characteristics disappears. To take a specific example: At each biennial examination two or three casual blood pressure determinations were obtained on each examinee. Blood pressure is one of the chief factors found to be related to coronary heart disease incidence. It is also the index used to assess the presence or absence of hypertension. Thus, it is a key factor in both atherosclerotic and hypertensive disease processes. Since these repeated measurements are highly correlated, it is reasonable to ask whether any more information is gained from a series of blood pressure measurements than from one.

The most prevalent atherosclerotic process accessible to study is coronary heart disease (CHD), and an analysis of the relationship between this clinical event and the antecedent measurements of systolic blood pressure from the first five examinations has been undertaken. The statistical model used has been described in an unpublished paper by Truett and Sorlie. It shows that while there was a clear relationship between blood pressure (averaged over all five examinations) and the subsequent development of CHD, this relationship is essentially the same for blood pressure measured at entry or any subsequent examination. Furthermore, the CHD event was not associated with any specified blood pressure trend prior to the CHD event. In short, so far as analysis to date has shown, there is no evidence of any gain in the ability to predict the incidence of CHD from repeated blood pressure measurements over time.

It is difficult to look at blood pressure as an indicator of the hypertensive process since the hypertensive process is ultimately defined by the blood pressure. In that sense the process is completely perceptible. Moreover, it has been shown that, on the average, blood pressure rises in a linear fashion as people get older. In that sense, also, the hypertensive process is perceptible over time and it is necessary to obtain blood pressure determinations at repeated intervals to delineate this process. Since systolic "hypertension" is arbitrarily said to exist when the systolic pressure is 160 mm Hg or greater, it is possible to predict the incidence of systolic hypertension in a group of persons if their initial systolic pressure is known. A similar statement can be made with respect to diastolic hypertension, which is considered to be present if the diastolic pressure is 95 mm Hg. or more. Furthermore, the number of persons who will undergo abrupt increases in their blood pressure in a short period of time can be predicted from a relatively straightforward statistical model. Few persons were found to change from a "normotensive" (less than 140 systolic and less than 90 diastolic) pressure to a "hypertensive" pressure in the two years between successive examinations. To date, we have been singularly unsuccessful in discerning the characteristics that distinguish persons with large increases in blood pressure from persons with moderate or no increases in the same period. In short, it seems fair to say that, to date, the longitudinal study of cardiovascular disease has not done much to reveal the pathological processes underlying the atherosclerotic or hypertensive diseases.

In a more obvious sense, familiar to clinical medicine, the study has examined a number of disease processes quite successfully. For example, persons who develop ECG-LVH, a prominent sequela of hypertension, have been shown thereupon to come at greater risk of a variety of cardiovascular diseases—CHD, atherothrombotic brain infarction (ABI), and intermittent claudication (IC). Persons developing IC are at enhanced risk of subsequently developing CHD or ABI. The study has been quite successful in delineating and quantitating this kind of process. The more basic processes which (as ordinarily construed) would require intrusive procedures and extended observations using complicated techniques are probably more appropriate to clinical research than to field epidemiology.

INITIAL RESPONSE AND FOLLOW-UP

In a study which purports to describe what happens in the general population, it is important to examine the affidavits for such a claim. The choice of the town for study was largely a matter of convenience. It is impossible to represent any town as constituting a sample of the population of the United States. The best that can be said for the town of Framingham is that with respect to overall mortality it has been similar to the United States as a whole and the town has no obvious peculiarities that might be suspected to lead to unusual morbidity. Nonetheless, it is probably more precise to describe Framingham as *a* general population rather than as representative of *the* general population. However, it is patently impossible to examine prospectively a population representative of mankind in general. The biologic validity of the findings must be validated by other studies, including other ethnic groups.

More critical is the question of initial response. Two things can be said respecting this. The first is that it was poor. The second is that it was biased. A sample of two-thirds of the Framingham residents aged 30 to 59 was drawn, this appearing to be the most practical age range to study. This produced a drawn sample of roughly 6600. Only 4469 of these were examined (Table 6.1). It has been shown that this group had a better mortality experience than the nonrespondents from the outset, suggesting that the respondents were healthier than the nonrespondents. This bias was enhanced by the addition of 740 volunteers to the cohort. These were nonsample residents who had received an examination during the initial period of the study and returned for reexamination when requested. Their mortality experience has been somewhat better than that for the respondent sample and again, by this token, this group must be regarded as biased.

TABLE 6.1
RESPONSE OF DRAWN SAMPLE AND NONRESPONSE BY REASON

	Number of persons	*Percent of Drawn Sample*	*Percent of Nonrespondent*
Total	6532	100.0	———
Examined	4494	68.8	———
Not examined	2038	31.2	100.0
Moved from Framingham	426	6.5	20.9
Died	74	1.1	3.6
Ill or incapacitated	74	1.1	3.6
Refused	1464	22.4	71.8

It is clear, then, that were this an investigation of prevalence, there would have had to be considerable reservations as to the conclusions one could draw from it. The extent to which this constitutes a source of difficulty in a prospective study is moot. Insofar as events are related to prior characteristics, the initial response bias might be manageable analytically were all the characteristics related to differential incidence measured and entered into the analysis. To the degree that this is not true, then, the question is unresolved. In any event, the ultimate validation of the findings must lie in the corroboration by other studies. To the limited degree that such corroboration has been sought, it has been found to be fairly good.

Follow-up has been undertaken by two methods. One is clinic examination. Loss of interest and dispersion of the cohort have led to a gradual erosion of the reexamination rate, but even on the tenth examination 81.6 percent of the cohort still alive appeared for examination. At the time of the ninth examination, fully 84.5 percent of those examined had received all nine examinations. Thus, the clinic examination has been a powerful source of completeness and uniformity of clinical evaluation (Tables 6.2 and 6.3) .

The other sources of follow-up information are death notices, hospital admission records, and physicians' and families' reports. For those not appearing for reexamination, these are, of course, critical. Mortality follow-up has been essentially complete, with few persons disappearing from view. Morbidity follow-up has

TABLE 6.2
NUMBER SURVIVING IN COHORT AND NUMBER RECEIVING EXAMINATION AT EACH OF THE FIRST TEN EXAMINATIONS

Exam	*Number Surviving*	*Total*	*Sample*	*Volunteers*
1	5209	5209	4469	740
2	5177	4792	4052	740
3	5125	4416*	3935	481*
4	5073	4541	3843	698
5	4990	4421	3750	671
6	4895	4259	3593	666
7	4803	4191	3551	640
8	4678	4030	3402	628
9	4552	3833	3225	608
10	4403	3593†	3011	582

*The indicated drop is an artifact arising from the arbitrary decision that volunteers would not be followed if they did not take Exam 2. Some 237, however, were recalled so late for Exam 2 they were not called for Exam 3.
†Because routine examination was suspended as of July 1970, the usual year's grace period with not available for continued follow-up of Exam 10.

TABLE 6.3
NUMBER OF PERSONS ACCORDING TO EXAMINATION STATUS AT EXAM 9 AND THE NUMBER OF BIENNIAL EXAMINATIONS RECEIVED: THE FRAMINGHAM STUDY

Number of Exams Received	*Received Exam 9*			*Did Not Take Exam 9* *Alive or Dead*			*Alive at Exam 9*		
	Both	*S*	*SX*	*Both*	*S*	*SX*	*Both*	*S*	*SX*
1	—	—	—	174	174	—	107	107	—
2	10	10	—	182	165	17	105	100	5
3	7	7	—	156	139	17	80	74	6
4	26	24	2	156	136	20	72	66	6
5	30	28	2	175	154	21	75	68	7
6	56	51	5	150	127	23	61	52	9
7	93	80	13	185	166	19	95	85	10
8	373	171	202	198	183	15	124	115	9
9	3238	2854	384	—	—	—	—	—	—
Total	3833	3225	608	1376	1244	132	719	667	52

Note. S = sample, SX = volunteers

been enhanced by the fact that Framingham has only one hospital, which has cooperated fully with the study. The extraclinic information is also important for evaluating the clinical status of persons routinely reexamined and has been vigorously sought throughout the study.

PREVALENCE AND INCIDENCE

One of the raisons d'être for a prospective study is the persuasion that this is a possibly unbiased method for studying the relation of characteristics to clinical experience, whereas retrospective studies are more likely to be biased and all too often their bias is impossible to assess. There are a number of concerns about a cross-sectional or retrospective study. Not everybody who is ill will come in. Are they the same or different from those who do? Some persons who become ill die during their illness; a sizable number developing coronary heart disease or atherothrombotic brain infarction die almost immediately. Are they the same as the survivors? Does the event affect the characteristic, either directly by some physiological process inherent in the event or indirectly by leading to some change in habits?

These questions have been examined a number of times and

in different ways during the course of the Framingham study and we will say something about the findings presently. But before we do, we must point out that such an inquiry is essentially academic. If we find that serum cholesterol levels are unaffected by the event, can we be sure that serum triglyceride levels also will be unaffected? If serum cholesterol levels are unaffected by the event in the Framingham cohort, can we be sure that they will be unaffected in some other group? The answer to these questions is clearly no, but the methodological issues are nonetheless interesting.

At exam 4 some of these questions were evaluated.[11] It was found that the men who died were distinguished from those who did not by higher blood pressures and a higher prevalence of cardiovascular disease and x-ray and electrocardiographic abnormalities. For most comparisons the contrast was even stronger for women. In addition, women who died had an elevated serum cholesterol level and there was a small (but statistically not significant) elevation of relative weight. Those men who moved from the area appeared to be slightly healthier on the average than those who remained; for women there appeared to be no difference. Persons who remained in the town but declined to return for reexamination appeared to have slightly more physiological and clinical abnormalities.

With respect to the effect of the event itself, the data were much more neutral. Weight, blood pressure, and serum cholesterol levels seemed to be little different after the appearance of CHD than before in persons surviving, and these three characteristics seemed to differ little among those surviving the disease and those dying during the acute stage. On the other hand, similar statements could not be made respecting cigarette-smoking habits which are changed by the event and do differ before the event between decedents and survivors of CHD.

Such a direct examination of characteristics must be interpreted carefully, however. By and large the characteristics related to CHD are not powerfully related to the disease; in general we are dealing with factors that tend to enhance the probability of CHD rather than factors that are overpoweringly evocative of

CHD. Thus, it may be more revealing if we compare directly a prevalence analysis and an incidence analysis.

Consider the following factors: serum cholesterol level, systolic blood pressure, left ventricular hypertrophy on the electrocardiogram, cigarette smoking, and blood glucose. We restrict our consideration to men aged 45 to 64 at that time, since this is the group with the largest number of CHD cases available. Prevalence is defined as of the fourth biennial examination and includes all persons who took that examination and at that time were known to have definite CHD. (It should be made clear that not all of these persons would be considered to have definite CHD on the basis of the fourth examination alone but that all the antecedent clinic and extraclinic information is taken into account in making the diagnosis. Thus, we are not talking of prevalence diagnoses in the ordinary sense, but they are prevalence cases in the sense that they all took the fourth examination.) The characteristics, also, are those measured at the fourth examination (Table 6.4).

TABLE 6.4
MULTIVARIATE DISCRIMINANT FUNCTION FOR DISTINGUISHING CASES OF CHD FROM NONCASES IN MEN 45-64: THE FRAMINGHAM STUDY, PREVALENCE AT EXAM 4.

	*Men 45-54**		*Men 55-64**	
Characteristic	β	$t(\beta)$	β	$t(\beta)$
Systolic blood pressure	.00424	0.39	.00696	1.07
Serum cholesterol	.00905	1.70	—.00022	—0.06
Blood glucose	.00710	1.00	.01206	2.52
Cigarette smoking	.02314	1.53	.00046	0.04
LVH on ECG	.11176	0.16	1.01159	2.64
Number of cases	25		48	

*Age at Exam 4.

As a contrast, we consider the same characteristics determined prior to the event in relation to CHD developing *de novo* prior to the fourth examination. This includes persons who never took the fourth examination (Table 6.5).

The method of analysis used is linear discriminant analysis (as devised by R.A. Fisher). The tables show the multivariate discriminant coefficients for these. Also shown is the test of sig-

TABLE 6.5
MULTIVARIATE DISCRIMINANT FUNCTION FOR DISTINGUISHING BETWEEN THOSE LIKELY AND UNLIKELY TO DEVELOP CHD IN MEN 45-64: THE FRAMINGHAM STUDY, INCIDENCE TO EXAM 4.

	*Men 45-54**		*Men 55-64**	
Characteristic	β	$t(\beta)$	β	$t(\beta)$
Systolic blood pressure	.00031	0.03	0.1278	1.98
Serum cholesterol	.01494	2.94	.01109	2.98
Blood glucose	.00002	0.00	.00894	1.36
Cigarette smoking	.02571	1.68	.02077	1.77
LVH on ECG	—.81957	—0.86	1.30293	3.08
Number of cases	24		49	

*Age at Exam 4.

nificance for these coefficients characteristics. The two sets of data certainly do not appear to give the same results. The failure to show statistically significant relationships on the basis of prevalence analysis for blood pressure or serum cholesterol is particularly striking, but the apparently strong relation shown for blood glucose in one age group is also surprising. It would be unwise to make too strong a statement on the basis of these data alone, since the number of cases involved is not overwhelming, but they do suggest that retrospective studies of CHD must be treated very cautiously. A previous inquiry comparing CHD incidence and prevalence as of exam 6 found a similar discrepancy between incidence and prevalence for serum cholesterol and also noted a weaker association of CHD with blood pressure in the prevalence series than in the incidence.[25]

STUDY RESULTS

What, then, has been the upshot of the twenty years of buzzing and stirring at Framingham? First of all, a clearer picture of the natural history of the hypertensive and atherosclerotic diseases has gradually emerged. Secondly, a more concrete and quantitative assessment of factors related to the onset of these diseases is now available. The literature of results is too large to encompass in this report; a review of the bibliography may suggest its scope. However, a discussion of one development arising from the Framingham study might be in order.

Early in the study, it became evident that categorical analysis of the relation of characteristics to clinical events was foredoomed. For example, if five characteristics are each divided into three levels (a crude partition, indeed), the resulting table would include 243 cells. There are simply not enough clinical events of interest to distribute over 243 cells.

It was suggested that it might be possible to use a modification of discriminant analysis to graduate the incidence of events over the range of pertinent characteristics. Initially, this was applied to two variables, then extended to any number.[60,65,66] Since then, a more robust but computationally more difficult approach to the same problem has been developed and come into use.[58] From this has come a statistic called the "risk function." In mathematical terms, if χ_i is any characteristic and p is the probability of the event occurring to any individual, then it is assumed that

$$p = \frac{1}{1 + e^{-(a + \Sigma b_i \chi_i)}}$$

The method used for estimating a and b_i is either a modification of the discriminant function or a least squares fit by maximum likelihood.

The logistic curve has been found to fit the data reasonably well, and the assumption of simple additivity of the independent variables also seems to be reasonably consistent with the data. It must be emphasized, however, that the model used is a pragmatic one. It is not an effort to express any presumed structural relations between the independent variables (factors) and any disease outcomes.

In a pragmatic sense it works. It has been shown (in a limited exploration) that it predicts events; that is, if the parameters b_i are estimated from one set of data and another set of data are looked at, those persons with larger estimated values for p are more likely to develop disease than persons with lower values. In all likelihood, for the purpose of ordering persons from lower to higher risk, precision in estimating b_i is not critical. This is particularly important if data from one population are to be used to predict events in another population.

Procedures for choosing an optimum subset of variables from a large set of possible candidates do not lead to unique choices. Table 6.6, which lists nineteen different variables which might be considered for predicting CHD cases and noncases, might serve as an example. The data are from the sixteen-year follow-up for men 45 to 54. The table shows univariate regression coefficients for each of these variables on the two-year incidence of CHD.

TABLE 6.6
REGRESSION COEFFICIENTS OF SPECIFIED VARIABLES ON THE INCIDENCE OF CHD IN MEN 45-54: THE FRAMINGHAM STUDY, SIXTEEN-YEAR FOLLOW-UP.

	β	*S.E.* (β)	*t*
Systolic blood pressure	.01479	.00411	3.60
Diastolic blood pressure	.02310	.00726	3.18
Serum cholesterol	.00914	.00179	5.11
Hemoglobin	.01021	.00826	1.24
Phospholipid	.00560	.00145	3.86
Blood sugar	.00563	.00263	2.14
Uric acid	.01354	.00925	1.46
Framingham relative weight	.01641	.00667	2.46
Vital capacity	—.03283	.01439	—2.28
Alcohol consumed	.00122	.00242	0.50
Cigarettes smoked	.26717	.08049	3.32
Albumin in urine	.46437	.23762	1.95
Sugar in urine	.39424	.25690	1.53
Heart enlargement by X-ray	.31022	.13737	2.26
Left ventricular hypertrophy by electrocardiogram	.38578	.21144	1.82
Definite nonspecific T-wave abnormality by electrocardiogram	.54800	.37200	1.47
Diabetes mellitus	.64300	.42700	1.51
Hypertension	.42613	.11714	3.64
Glucose intolerance	.79500	.30000	2.65

Note. β is the regression coefficient, *S.E.*(β) is the standard error, and *t* is $\beta/S.E.(\beta)$, which has a normal distribution with mean *0* and standard deviation *1.*

The strength of each variable taken by itself as a "predictor" is indicated by the size of the t-statistic. The strongest variables by this criterion are systolic blood pressure, diastolic blood pressure, serum cholesterol, phospholipid, cigarettes smoked, and hypertension. Analytically, systolic and diastolic blood pressures are highly correlated with hypertension. There is no point in entering both for the analysis, and our preference is for the continuous blood pressure variables as containing more information. Serum cholesterol and phospholipid also are highly correlated. If entered together in a multivariate discriminant function, phospholipid would turn out to have a nonsignificant coefficient. We therefore omit it. Thus, of this set of variables, the best statistical set would include systolic and diastolic blood pressure, serum cholesterol, and cigarettes smoked. Consideration of data from other age groups indicated the value of adding glucose intolerance and LVH by ECG to the roster. Adding any of the other specified variables to this subset improves discrimination little, if at all. Moreover, the variables chosen describe a range of factors that are clinically distinct and each of interest in its own right.

If we now consider the other major atherosclerotic events, specifically atherothrombotic brain infarction and intermittent claudication, we find that the same variables are also "predictive." We next proceed to calculate multivariate logistic functions for each clinical event and each sex separately for each of the groups: 45-54, 55-64, and 65-74. On the basis of this, we obtain for each person in each age-sex group a probability for that event. Persons are then ranked from lowest to highest according to these probabilities and the population is then divided into deciles. The persons in decile 1 should have the lowest risk of the event and the person in decile 10 the highest risk (Table 6.7).

There are two interesting observations to be made about these data. The first is this: we now apparently know how to identify a small subgroup of the population from whom a sizable percentage of CHD, ABI, or IC will come—roughly 25 percent of the CHD cases, 40 percent of the IC cases, and 50 percent of the ABI cases. All that is necessary to identify this subgroup is a blood pressure determination, an electrocardiogram, a blood specimen, and a simple smoking history plus estimates of the parameters to be used in the appropriate risk function. The second fact is this: despite the lower incidence of CHD and IC in women, our ability to predict incidence in women is at least as great as our ability to predict incidence in men.

As our ability to alter risk factors increases and our confidence

TABLE 6.7

DECILES OF RISK FOR CHD, ABI, AND IC BY SEX: THE FRAMINGHAM STUDY, SIXTEEN-YEAR FOLLOW-UP

Sex and Decile of Risk	*CHD Incidence*		*ABI Incidence*		*IC Incidence*	
	Smoothed	*Actual*	*Smoothed*	*Actual*	*Smoothed*	*Actual*
Men						
Total	320.4	320	39.1	39	80.2	80
1	13.5	9	0.4	0	1.6	2
2	16.6	13	0.6	3	2,4	3
3	19.1	25	0.9	0	3.1	0
4	21.5	14	1.1	0	3.7	4
5	24.2	34	1.5	1	4.6	4
6	27.6	25	1.9	2	5.7	5
7	31.5	34	2.5	2	7.3	8
8	36.9	37	3.5	3	9.3	11
9	46.9	47	5.7	7	12.8	12
10	82.6	82	21.0	21	29.7	31
Women						
Total	183.9	184	40.5	41	38.2	38
1	6.2	4	0.7	0	1.0	1
2	8.2	8	1.0	1	1.3	0
3	9.8	12	1.3	1	1.4	1
4	11.2	14	1.6	0	1.6	1
5	12.9	8	2.0	1	1.9	2
6	14.8	13	2.3	4	2.2	1
7	17.4	13	2.9	2	2.7	3
8	20.8	23	3.7	7	3.5	3
9	27.5	37	5.3	7	5.3	8
10	55.1	52	19.7	18	17.3	18

Note. Decile of risk derived from multiple logistic function in which the variables are systolic blood pressure, diastolic blood pressure, serum cholesterol, cigarette smoking, left ventricular hypertrophy by electrocardiogram, and glucose intolerance, using the method of Duncan-Walker.

in the efficacy of such alteration becomes established by clinical experience or clinical trials, the value of the risk function for screening persons who warrant special prophylaxis will become more generally recognized. Up to this point, the prospective epidemiological study of cardiovascular diseases has served to pin down a variety of factors antecedent to these diseases. It has served to clarify various aspects of their natural history. When the time comes for increasingly active programs of intervention, it is likely that these studies will provide the framework of information within which these programs can operate most effectively.

REFERENCES

1. Dawber, T.R., Meadors, G.F., and Moore, F.E., Jr. Epidemiological approaches to heart disease: The Framingham Study. *Amer. J. Public Health, 41*:279-286, Mar. 1951.
2. Dawber, T.R., and Moore, F.E. Longitudinal study of heart disease in Framingham, Massachusetts: An interim report. In *Research in Public Health,* papers presented at the 1951 Annual Conference of the Milbank Memorial Fund. New York, Milbank Memorial Fund, 1952, pp. 241-247.
3. Dawber, T.R., Kannel, W.B., Love, D.E., and Streeper, R.D. The electrocardiogram in heart disease detection: A comparison of the multiple and single lead procedures. *Circulation, 5*:559-566, Apr. 1952.
4. Vander, J.B., Gaston, E.A., and Dawber, T.R. Significance of solitary nontoxic thyroid nodules: Preliminary report. *New Eng. J. Med., 251*:970-973, Dec. 1954.
5. Stokes, J., III, and Dawber, T.R. Rheumatic heart disease in the Framingham study. *New Eng. J. Med., 255*:1228-1233, Dec. 1956.
6. Dawber, T.R., Moore, F.E., and Mann, G.V. Coronary heart disease in the Framingham study. *Amer. J. Public Health, 47*:4-24, part 2, Apr. 1957.
7. Dawber, T.R., and Kannel, W.B. An epidemiologic study of heart disease: The Framingham study. *Nutr. Rev., 16*:1-4, Jan. 1958.
8. Kannel, W.B., Dawber, T.R., and Cohen, M.E. The electrocardiogram in neurocirculatory asthenia (anxiety, neurosis or neurasthenia): A study of 203 neurocirculatory asthenia patients and 757 health controls in the Framingham study. *Ann. Intern. Med., 49*:1351-1360, Dec. 1958.
9. Stokes, J., III, and Dawber, T.R. The "silent coronary": The frequency and clinical characteristics of unrecognized myocardial infarction in the Framingham study. *Ann. Intern. Med., 50*:1359-1369, June 1959.
10. Kagan, A., Gordon, T., Kannel, W.B., and Dawber, T.R. Blood pressure and its relation to coronary heart disease in the Framingham study. In *Hypertension: Drug Action, Epidemiology and Hemodynamics.* Proceedings of the Council for High Blood Pressure Research, American Heart Association, Nov. 1958. New York, American Heart Association, 1959, Vol. VII, p. 53.
11. Gordon, T., Moore, F.E., Shurtleff, D., and Dawber, T.R. Some methodologic problems in the long-term study of cardiovascular disease: Observations on the Framingham study. *J. Chronic Dis., 10*:186-206, Sept. 1959.

12. Dawber, T.R., Kannel, W.B., Revotskie, N., Stokes, J., III, Kagan, A., and Gordon, T. Some factors associated with the development of coronary heart disease: Six years' follow-up experience in the Framingham study. *Amer. J. Public Health, 49:*1349-1356, Oct. 1959.
13. Dawber, T.R. Summary of recent literature regarding cigarette smoking and coronary heart disease. *Circulation, 22:*164-166, July 1960.
14. Dawber, T.R., Kannel, W.B., Pearson, G., and Shurtleff, D. Assessment of diet in the Framingham study: Methodology and preliminary observations. *Health News, 38:*4-6, Jan. 1961.
15. Dawber, T.R., and Kannel, W.B. Susceptibility to coronary heart disease. *Mod. Conc. Cardiov. Dis., 30:*671-675, July 1961.
16. Kannel, W.B., Dawber, T.R., Kagan, A., Revotskie, N., and Stokes, J, III. Factors of risk in the development of coronary heart disease—six year follow-up experience: The Framingham study. *Ann. Intern. Med., 55:* 33-50, July 1961.
17. Kahn, H.A. A method for analyzing longitudinal observations on individuals in the Framingham heart study. Proceedings of the Social Statistics Section of the American Statistical Association, 1961.
18. Doyle, J.T., Dawber, T.R., Kannel, W.B., Heslin, A.S., and Kahn, H.A. Cigarette smoking and coronary heart disease: Combined experience of the Albany and Framingham Studies. *New Eng. J. Med., 266:*796-801, Apr. 1962.
19. Dawber, T.R., Kannel, W.B., Revotskie, N., and Kagan, A. The epidemiology of coronary heart disease—the Framingham enquiry. *Proc. Roy. Soc. Med. 55:*265-271, Apr. 1962.
20. Kagan, A., Dawber, T.R., Kannel, W.B, and Revotskie, N. The Framingham study: A prospective study of coronary heart disease *Federation Proceedings, 21,* Part II, Aug. 1962.
21. Kahn, H. Use of computers in analyzing Framingham data. *Circ. Res. 11,* Sept. 1962.
22. Dawber, T.R., and Kannel, W.B. Application of epidemiology of coronary heart disease to medical practice. *Modern Science,* Sept. 1962.
23. Dawber, T.R., Pearson, G., Anderson, P. Mann, G.V., Kannel, W.B., Shurtleff, D., and McNamara, P. Dietary assessment in the epidemiologic study of coronary heart disease: The Framingham study. *Amer. J. Clin. Nutr., 11,* Sept. 1962.
24. Mann, G.V., Pearson, G., Gordon, T, Dawber, T.R., Lyell, L., and Shurtleff, D. Diet and cardiovascular disease in the Framingham study. *Amer. J. Clin. Nutr., 11,* Sept. 1962.
25. Dawber, T.R. Coronary heart disease: Morbidity in the Framingham study and analysis of factors of risk. *Bibl. Cardiol. 13:*9-24, 1962.
26. Dawber, T.R., and Kannel, W.B. Computers in epidemiologic research: Uses in the Framingham study. *Circ. Res., 11,* Sept. 1962.
27. Dawber, T.R., and Kannel, W.B. Atherosclerosis and you: Pathogenetic

implications from epidemiologic observations. *J. Amer. Geriat. Soc. 10,* Act. 1962.

28. Kannel, W.B., Kagan, A., Dawber, T.R., and Revotskie, N. Epidemiology of coronary heart disease: Implications for the practicing physician. *Geriatrics, 17*:675, Oct. 1962.
29. Kannel, W.B., Dawber, T.R., Glennon, W.E., and Thorne, M.C. Preliminary report: The determinants and clinical significance of serum cholesterol. *Mass. J. Medical Technology, 4,* (No. 3) Fall, 1962.
30. Dawber, T.R., Kannel, W.B., and Friedman, G.D. The use of computers in cardiovascular epidemiology. *Progr. Cardiov. Dis., 5,* Jan. 1963.
31. Dawber, T.R., and Kannel, W.B. Coronary heart disease as an epidemiologic entity. *Amer. J. Public Health, 53,* Mar. 1963.
32. Kagan, A., Kannel, W.B., Dawber, T.R., and Revotskie, N. The coronary profile. *Ann. N.Y. Acad. Sci., 97*:883-894, Aug. 1963.
33. Kannel, W.B., Barry, P., and Dawber, T.R. Immediate mortality in coronary heart disease: The Framingham study. Proceedings of 4th World Congress of Cardiology, 1963.
34. Dawber, T.R., Kannel, W.B., and Lyell, L. An approach to longitudinal studies in a community: The Framingham study. *Ann. N.Y. Acad. Sci., 107*:539-556, May 1963.
35. Dawber, T.R., Kannel, W.B., and McNamara, P.M. The Prediction of Coronary Heart Disease. Paper read at 72nd Annual Meeting of Assoc. of Life Insurance Medical Directors of America, Oct. 1963.
36. Kannel, W.B. Cigarette smoking and coronary heart disease. *Ann. Intern. Med., 60*:1103-1106, June 1964.
37. Kannel, W.B., Dawber, T.R., Friedman, G.D., Glennon, W.E., and McNamara, P.M. Risk factors in coronary heart disease; an evaluation of several serum lipids as predictors of coronary heart disease. *Ann. Intern. Med., 61*:888-899, Nov. 1964.
38. Doyle, J.T., Dawber, T.R., Kannel, W.B., Kinch, S.H., and Kahn, H.A. The relationship of cigarette smoking to coronary heart disease. *J.A.M.A., 190*:886-890, Dec. 1964.
39. Kannel, W.B., Widmer, L.K., and Dawber, T.R. Cefahrdung durch coronare herzkrankheit; folgerungen für die praxis aus 10 jahren Framingham studie. (Susceptibility to coronary heart disease; preventive implications of 10 years of observation in the Framingham study.) *Schweiz. Med. Wschr., 95*:18-24, Jan. 1965.
40. Higgins, I.T.T., Kannel, W.B., and Dawber, T.R. The electrocardiogram in epidemiological studies; reproducibility, validity, and international comparison. *Brit. J. Prev. Soc. Med., 19*:53-68, Apr. 1965.
41. Kannel, W.B., Dawber, T.R., Thomas, H.E., Jr., and McNamara, P.M. Comparison of serum lipids in the prediction of coronary heart disease. *Rhode Island Med. J., 48*:243-250, May 1965.
42. Dawber, T.R. Heart attack—what's the risk? *Today's Health,* Aug. 1965.

43. Kannel, W.B., Dawber, T.R., and McNamara, P.M. Vascular disease of the brain—epidemiologic aspects: The Framingham study. *Amer. J. Public Health, 55:* 1355-1366, Sept. 1965.

44. Kannel, W.B., Dawber, T.R., and McNamara, P.M. Detection of the coronary-prone adult: The Framingham study. *J. Iowa Med. Soc.,* pp. 26-34, Jan. 1966.

45. Friedman, G.D., Kannel, W.B., Dawber, T.R., and McNamara, P.M. Comparison of prevalence, case history and incidence data in assessing the potency of risk factors in coronary heart disease. *Amer. J. Epidem., 83,* (No. 2) 1966.

46. Thomas, H.E., Jr., Kannel, W.B., Dawber, T.R., and McNamara. P.M. Cholesterol-phospholipid ratio in the prediction of coronary heart disease. *New Eng. J. Med., 274:*701-705, Mar. 1966.

47. Friedman, G.D., Kannel, W.B., and Dawber, T.R. The epidemiology of gallbladder disease: observations in the Framingham study. *J. Chronic Dis., 19:*273-292, 1966.

48. Kahn, H.A., and Dawber, T.R. The development of coronary heart disease in relation to sequential biennial measures of cholesterol in the Framingham study. *J. Chronic Dis., 19:*611-620, 1966.

49. Dawber, T.R., and Kannel, W.B. The Framingham Study; an epidemiological approach to coronary heart disease. Editorial. *Circulation, 34:*553-555, Oct. 1966.

50. Dawber, T.R., Kannel, W.B., and Friedman, G.D. Vital capacity, physical activity and coronary heart disease. In Raab, W. (Ed.) *Prevention of Ischemic Heart Disease: Principles and Practice.* Springfield, Thomas, 1966, pp. 254-265.

51. Kannel, W.B. *Habits and Coronary Heart Disease: The Framingham Study.* U.S. Dep't. of Health, Education, and Welfare, Public Health Service Publ. No. 1515. Washington, D.C., U.S. Gov't. Printing Office, 1966.

52. Kannel, W.B. An epidemiologic study of cerebrovascular disease. In Millikan, C.H., Siekert, R.G., and Whisnant, J.P. (Eds.) *Cerebral Vascular Diseases. Transactions of the Fifth Conference Held under the Auspices of The American Neurological Association and The American Heart Association, Princeton, New Jersey, January 5-7, 1966.* New York, Grune & Stratton, 1966, pp. 53-66.

53. Hall, A.P., Barry, P.E., Dawber, T.R., and McNamar, P.M. Epidemiology of gout and hyperuricemia; a long-term population study. *Amer. J. Med., 42:*27-37, Jan. 1967.

54. Kannel, W.B. Habitual level of physical activity and risk of coronary heart disease: The Framingham Study. *Canad. Med. Ass. J., 96:*811-812, Mar. 25, 1967.

55. Kannel, W.B., LeBauer, E.J., Dawber, T.R., and McNamara, P.M. Relation of body weight to development of coronary heart disease: The Framingham Study. *Circulation 35:*734-744, Apr. 1967.

56. Kannel, W.B., Troy, B.L., and McNamara, P.M. *Epidemiology of Stroke.* U.S. Dep't. of Health, Education, and Welfare, Public Health Service Publ. No. 1607. Washington, D.C., U.S. Gov't. Printing Office, 1967.

57. Friedman, G.D., Kannel, W.B., Dawber, T.R., and McNamara, P.M. An evaluation of follow-up methods in the Framingham Heart Study. *Amer. J. Public Health, 57:*1015-1024, June 1967.

58. Walker, S.H., and Duncan, D.B. Estimation of the probability of an event as a function of several independent variables. *Biometrika, 54:*167-179, June 1967.

59. Kannel, W.B., Brand, N., Skinner, J.J., Jr., Dawber, T.R., and McNamara, P.M. The relation of adiposity to blood pressure and development of hypertension: The Framingham Study. *Ann. Intern. Med., 67:*48-59, July 1967.

60. Truett, J., Cornfield, J., and Kannel, W. A multivariate analysis of the risk of coronary heart disease in Framingham. *J. Chronic Dis., 20:*511-524, July 1967.

61. Dawber, T.R., Kannel, W.B., Kagan, A., Donabedian, R.K., McNamara, P.M., and Pearson, G. Environmental factors in hypertension. In Stamler, J., Stamler, R., and Pullman, T.N. (Eds.) *The Epidemiology of Hypertension. Proceedings of an International Symposium Sponsored by the Chicago Heart Association and the American Heart Association, Chicago, Illinois, February 3-7, 1964.* New York, Grune & Stratton, 1967, pp. 255-288.

62. Dawber, T.R., and McNamara, P.M. Coronary heart disease: Identification of susceptible individuals. In Brest, A.N., and Moyer, J.H. (Eds.) *Atherosclerotic Vascular Disease. A Hahnemann Symposium.* New York, Appleton-Century-Crofts, 1967, pp. 130-146.

63. Thomas, H.E., Jr., Kannel, W.B., and McNamara, P.M. Obesity: A hazard to health. *Med. Times, 95:*1099-1106, Oct. 1967.

64. Kannel, W.B., Castelli, W.P., and McNamara, P.M. The coronary profile: 12-year follow-up in the Framingham Study. *J. Occup. Med., 9:*611-619, Dec. 1967.

Addenda

65. Cornfield, J., Gordon, T., and Smith, W.W. Quantal response curves for experimentally uncontrolled variables. Tokyo, *Bulletin of the International Statistical Institute, 38:*97-115, Part III, 1961.

66. Cornfield, J. Joint dependence of risk of coronary heart disease on serum cholesterol and systolic blood pressure. *Federation Proceedings, 21* (Suppl. 11) :58-61, Part II, July-Aug. 1962.

67. Revotskie, N., Kannel, W., Goldsmith, J.R., and Dawber, T.R. Pulmonary function in a community sample. *Amer. Rev. Resp. Dis., 86:*707-711, 1962.

68. Hall, A.P. Correlations among hyperuricemia, hypercholesterolemia, coro-

nary disease and hypertension. *Arthritis Rheum., 8:*846-852, Part 1, Oct. 1965.

69. *The Framingham Study: An epidemiological investigation of cardiovascular disease.* National Heart Institute Monograph, Sections 1-8, June 1968; Sections 9-22, Sept. 1968.
70. Dawber, T.R., and Kannel, W.B. Presymptomatic detection and early diagnosis. In Sharp, C.L.E.H., and Keen, H.S. (Eds.) London, Pitman Medical Publ. Co., 1968, pp. 257-281.
71. Kannel, W.B., Castelli, W.P., and McNamara, P.M. Cigarette smoking and risk of coronary heart disease. Epidemiologic clues to pathogenesis: The Framingham Study. In Wynder, E.L., and Hoffman, D. (Eds.) *Toward a Less Harmful Cigarette. A Workshop Held at the World Conference on Smoking and Health, September 11-13, 1967.* National Cancer Institute Monograph No. 28, U.S. Dep't. of Health, Education, and Welfare, Public Health Service. Washington, D.C., U.S. Gov't. Printing Office, June 1968, pp. 9-20.
72. Kannel, W.B., Castelli, W.P., and McNamara, P.M. Epidemiology of acute myocardial infarction: The Framingham Study. *Medicine Today, 2:56-71,* Aug.-Sept.-Oct. 1968.
73. Vander, J.B., Gaston, E.A., and Dawber, T.R. The significance of non-toxic thyroid nodules: Final report of a 15-year study of the incidence of thyroid malignancy. *Ann. Intern. Med., 69:*537-540, Sept. 1968.
74. Dawber, T.R., and Thomas, H.E. Prophylaxis of coronary heart disease, stroke, and peripheral atherosclerosis. *Ann. N.Y. Acad. Sci., 149:*1038-1057, Nov. 21, 1968.
75. Kannel, W.B., Pearson, G., and McNamara, P.M. Obesity as a force of morbidity. In Heald, F.P. (Ed.) *Adolescent Nutrition and Growth.* New York, Appleton-Century-Crofts, 1969, pp. 51-71.
76. Damon, A., Damon, S.T., Harpending, H.C., and Kannel, W.B. Predicting coronary heart disease from body measurements of Framingham males. *J. Chronic Dis., 21:*781-802, Apr. 1969.
77. Hall, A.P. Observations in Subjects Developing a Positive Test for Rheumatoid Factor in a Prospective Study. Paper presented at the Annual Meeting of the ARA, June 1969.
78. Kannel, W.B., Schwartz, M.J., and McNamara, P.M. Blood pressure and risk of coronary heart disease: The Framingham Study. *Dis. Chest, 56:*43-52, July 1969.
79. Kannel, W.B., Gordon, T., and Offutt, D. LVH by ECG: Prevalence, incidence, and mortality in the Framingham Study. *Ann. Intern. Med., 71:*89-105, July 1969.
80. Kannel, W.B., and McNamara, P.M. The evidence for excess risk in coronary disease. *Minnesota Med., 52:*1197-1201, Aug. 1969.
81. Kannel, W.B., Castelli, W.P., and McNamara, P.M. Serum lipid fractions and risk of coronary heart disease: The Framingham Study. *Minnesota Med., 52:*1225-1230, Aug. 1969.

82. Gerende, L.J. *Some Methodological Problems in the Study of the Natural History of Blood Pressure: An Examination of the Framingham Study Data.* Ph.D. dissertation. University of Michigan, 1962.
83. Cicchinelli, A.L. *The Composite of Two Gaussian Distributions as a Model for Blood Pressure in Man.* Ph. D. dissertation. University of Michigan, 1962.
84. Kannel, W.B., Castelli, W.P., McNamara, P.M., and Sorlie, P. Some factors affecting morbidity and mortality in hypertension: The Framingham Study. *Milbank Mem. Fund Quart., 47*:116-142, part 2, July 1969.
85. Kannel, W.B., McNamara, P.M., Feinleib, M., and Dawber, T.R. The unrecognized myocardial infarction: Fourteen year follow-up experience in the Framingham Study. *Geriatrics, 25*:75-87, Jan. 1970.
86. Kannel, W.B. The epidemiology of coronary heart disease: Methodologic considerations The Framingham Study. *Aktuel. Prob. Angiol., 7*:25-42, 1970.
87. Kannel, W.B. Coronary heart disease epidemiology: Implications for practice. *Aktuel. Prob. Angiol., 7*:82-97, 1970.
88. Kannel, W.B., Skinner, J.J., Jr., Schwartz, M.J., and Shurtleff, D. Intermittent claudication: Incidence in the Framingham Study. *Circulation, 41*:875-883, May 1970.
89. Kannel, W.B., Gordon, T., Castelli, W.P., and Margolis, J.R. Electrocardiographic left ventricular hypertrophy and risk of coronary heart disease. *Ann. Intern. Med., 72*:813-822, 1970.
90. Gordon, T., and Kannel, W.B. The Framingham, Massachusetts Study twenty years later. In Kessler, I.J., and Levin, M.L. (Eds.) *The Community as an Epidemiologic Laboratory: A Casebook of Community Studies.* Baltimore, Johns Hopkins Press, 1970, pp. 123-146.
91. Kannel, W.B., Wolf, P.S., Verter, J., and McNamara, P.M. Epidemiologic assessment of the role of blood pressure in stroke: The Framingham Study. *J.A.M.A., 214*:301-310, Oct. 1970.

Chapter 7

MULTIFACTOR PREVENTIVE TRIALS (MPT) IN CORONARY HEART DISEASE

HENRY BLACKBURN

IN THE INTRODUCTION to this volume about trends in epidemiology, Gordon Stewart clearly sets the high priority due preventive trials in chronic disease. In Chapter 5 of this same volume, Frederick Epstein provides the background and rationale for such trials in the prevention of coronary heart disease (CHD).

All the available evidence about the frequency and the nature of CHD compels the conclusion that a major reduction in premature death and disability from this disease will be achieved only through a strategy of primary prevention. Most physicians and official bodies in the United States accept the strategy that CHD patients and those at very high CHD risk, based on certain characteristics, should receive the benefit of potential though unproven preventive measures. Nevertheless, two sharply conflicting bodies of opinion exist about whether public health application of the available knowledge on coronary risk factors should be made as a primary preventive approach in the population as a whole. This lack of unity applies particularly to the question of a qualitative change in the diet and, to a lesser degree, to the question of treatment of mild hypertension. Unity of opinion is likely to come about only through the results of an adequately designed and executed preventive trial, the "inevitable ordeal." A definitive, positive, and major effect in a preventive trial would likely set in motion the considerable changes—personal, socio-

Note: Some of the data herein were obtained by support through the following grants from the National Heart and Lung Institute: National Diet-Heart Study, HE 07381; The Collaborative Physical Activity Program, 5R01-CD-00118; The University of Minnesota Cardiovascular Center Grant, HE 06314.

cultural, and economic—requisite to a substantial reduction in the national burden of CHD.

With respect to such a definitive trial, a trend is now in progress in cardiovascular epidemiology toward the Multifactor Preventive Trial (MPT). A body of thought, developed over the past few years, has led to the design, planning, and recent institution of such trials, the aim of which is to test whether intervention on the multiple major CHD risk factors will in fact influence the incidence and risk of CHD.

This body of thought, these plans, and the protocols already developed merit critical attention. They may offer the most rapid and efficient evaluation of the possibility of CHD prevention. They embody a concept which is highly appropriate and widely applicable to chronic diseases associated with multiple risk factors. They apply an approach which is compatible with the experience and precepts of clinical medicine.

The MPT concept is a simple one. In the case of CHD, the risk is firmly related to multiple characteristics. Several of these risk factors measured in health, i.e. serum cholesterol and blood pressure level and cigarette-smoking habit, have consistently and independently been shown to explain much, though by no means all, of subsequent CHD experience. It has been found that their individual effects are at the least additive.[1-3] In addition to the multiple factors influencing CHD, it has been found impossible, practically, to modify single CHD risk factors in trials which involve giving health advice, without at the same time modifying other CHD risk factors. Thus, a great deal of evidence, as well as logic, supports the attempt to simultaneously modify the major CHD risk factors in a MPT. The results will concern the practical question whether, and to what degree, the incidence of CHD may be influenced by simultaneous intervention on multiple risk factors. The MPT is therefore a pragmatic public health approach rather than an explanatory research one.[4]

The purpose of this presentation is to expose briefly the historical development of the thinking on, the evidence in support of, and the developing plans of this trend to MPT in cardiovascular epidemiology.

HISTORICAL DEVELOPMENT OF THE MPT IN CHD

The MPT in CHD is a relatively recent and a truly international development. Much of the early thinking and design grew out of the direct experience of investigators in the major first-round preventive trials. Included, among others, were members of the Diet-Heart Study,[5] the Collaborative Study on Physical Activity,[6] the Chicago Coronary Prevention Evaluation Program,[7] and the Coronary Drug Project.[8] A planning group met during the period 1966-69 and prepared a detailed design and protocol for a MPT in CHD.[9]

Concurrently, a series of international discussions was instituted to consider the need, priorities, and methods for clinical trials in CHD and hypertension. The first of these, the Makarska Conference on Clinical Trials,[10] was held in Yugoslavia in September 1968 under joint sponsorship of the International Society of Cardiology, the American Heart Association, and the U.S. Public Health Service. Subsequent discussions were carried out in conjunction with successive Cardiovascular Epidemiology Seminars of the Council on Epidemiology and Prevention, International Society of Cardiology.

Participants in this series of discussions proceeded to prepare careful and detailed protocols. The first, for a MPT in the U.S., using a partially factorial design among randomly allocated high-risk individuals, was submitted in 1969 as a grant application to the National Heart and Lung Institute. There it was rejected. In contrast, two unique European protocols have been effectively implemented. One is in London and involves randomization among industrial units[11] and the other in Gothenburg, with randomization of individuals from a population sample of that city.[12] These studies are well into the screening and run-in periods.

In November 1970, the European office of W.H.O. assembled a working group to consider the design and possible extension of these MPT to other countries.[13] Subsequently, steps have been taken to integrate other units into those protocols.

Meanwhile, in 1971, decisions have been made in the U.S. and in France to initiate controlled trials and community programs for hypertension. During 1971, a recommendation is expected from the National Heart and Lung Institute Task Force on Atherosclerosis about implementation of U.S. trials in CHD. The task force has been provided with expert testimony on all aspects of such trials, blind and nonblind, in open and in closed populations, and involving intervention on single or on multiple risk factors.

MULTIPLE CHD RISK FACTORS AS A BASIS FOR THE MPT

"Important" Risk Factors

Within populations, the individual risk of CHD is strongly related to the number and the levels of multiple characteristics. Serum cholesterol and blood pressure levels and cigarette smoking are considered risk factors of major importance because of (a) their strong individual-independent and combined predictive relationship to CHD morbidity and mortality, (b) the consistency of this relationship in many studies among differing cultures, (c) the great frequency of their presence in elevated form in middle-aged men in prosperous countries, and (d) the concordance of the evidence about the role of these particular factors between the major methodologies of clinic, laboratory, and population studies[1,2,7,14] (see also Chap. 5 of this volume). A number of other important and interesting predictors of risk will not be considered here because they are not as fully documented or have lesser predictive power or lower frequency of occurrence.

Multivariate Risk Functions

Simple cross-classification of combinations of the major CHD risk factors allows discrimination between men with an eightfold difference in CHD risk.[2] Their combination in multivariate analyses such as that of Cornfield[3] (see also Chap. 6 of this volume) discriminates those having CHD events from others with considerable precision, within the populations from which the regression coefficients were themselves derived. Much more important is the fact that this logistic function has also been found to rank individuals successfully, from lower to higher risk, in other populations, including those with greatly differing absolute risk of CHD.[1,15,16]

The risk function explains a significant part, clearly not all, of the population and individual differences in CHD risk. It indicates the potential for prevention, but, of course, cannot prove whether a population or an individual, after a generation or a lifetime of exposure to a given risk, will experience a change in risk predicted from a given reduction of the level of risk characteristics. The evidence from trials so far provides also a crude estimate of the reduction of incidence possible and the time it may take to achieve any reduction in CHD incidence.

The risk function provides a useful base on which to predicate the possible effects of multiple risk factor reduction. This is illustrated in Table 7.1, reproduced from Cornfield,[17] and indicates a potential reduction of 12-year CHD incidence from about 200 to about 50 per 1000 at age 45.

In sum, the evidence suggests that multiple risk factors operate in CHD, that they operate at least in an additive fashion, and that their simultaneous modification in a MPT would allow a more efficient test of prevention, in terms of time and sample size required, than reduction of single factors, one at a time.

TABLE 7.1
TWELVE-YEAR RISK OF CORONARY HEART DISEASE FOR DIFFERING LEVELS RISK FACTORS BY AGE, FRAMINGHAM MEN, 1948-60

Serum Cholesterol Value	Systolic Blood Pressure	Relative Weight	Smoking	Entrance Age (yr) and New Events per 1000		
				35	45	55
250	150	110	1 pack	67	209	261
220	150	110	1 pack	35	175	212
220	130	110	1 pack	23	152	164
220	130	100	1 pack	20	120	154
220	130	100	0 pack	6	54	95

Note. Age group at exam 1:30-39y $= \log_2 [P/(1—P)] = —17.6 + 0.023 \times_1 + 0.022 \times_2 + 0.014 \times_3 + 0.598 \times_4 + 0.092 \times_5$; 40-49 y $= \log_2 [P/1—P)] = 13.7 + 0.0.007 \times_1 + 0.09\times_2 + 0.027\times_3 + 0.434\times_4 + 0.120\times_5$; and 50-62 y $= \log_2 [P/(1—P)] = —11.1 + 0.009\times_1 + 0.016\times_2 + 0.008\times_3 + 0.272\times_4 + 0.072\times_5$. From Cornfield and Mitchell, 1969, with permission of the authors and publisher.

THE POPULATION FREQUENCY OF CHD RISK FACTORS

The frequency of CHD risk factors in a population, as well as the degree of concentration of eventual cases within risk categories, determines the efficiency of the risk factor approach. Roughly 10 percent of middle-aged men in the United States have *three or more* risk factors elevated.* These men are at far greater relative risk than those having only a single factor elevated, but, in fact, they produce only about 20 percent of the eventual CHD cases, a rather small fraction of the total population disease burden.

At the other extreme, approximately 80 percent of the male U.S. population has *one or more* risk factors elevated, and they account for something over 90 percent of future CHD events. This emphasizes the need for the broadest social approach in order to significantly reduce the disease. Between these extremes is the fraction of the population "carrying" *two or more* of the major CHD risk factors, i.e. something under 40 percent, and which "produces" about 60 percent of the new events. This is the proportion which it is perhaps reasonable and surely desirable to identify and among which to concentrate preventive efforts.

Despite these limitations encountered in prosperous countries where the society as a whole is at great risk, multifactor risk detection has, in fact, brought us to a level of prediction of CHD which is unequaled for any other major disease entity.

The combinations of risk factors and their associated mortality have been summarized from the Pooling Project.[1] (Fig 12) This provides another basis for a crude estimate of the potential for prevention. For example, let us assume that the 10-year CHD incidence for middle-aged men with two or more elevated risk factors (about 100 per 1000) were "converted" to the observed rate for men having no elevated risk factors (about 20 per 1000). There would have been 56 deaths from CHD instead of 280 in the 2773 Pooling Project men with two or more risk factors (38% of the total population). This would result in a decrease of 47

---

*"Elevated"—based on a level for each factor associated with twice the expected disease of the remainder of the population.

percent in total mortality from "correcting" high risk in the total pooling group (224 expected fewer deaths per 479 observed total deaths).

Finally, multiple intervention "according to the need" is a concept quite compatible with traditional clinical therapy. The individual "need" is determined by the presence and level of one or more risk factors. The population "need" is determined by the frequency of risk factors and their combinations in the population.

"PURE" SINGLE-FACTOR PREVENTION TRIALS

While the multiplicity of risk factors in CHD provides the main conceptual basis for MPT, a compelling practical reason for the MPT is the difficulty of modifying single risk factors selectively. When intervention involves health advice, it is apparently impossible, outside a double-blind design, to intervene on one risk factor without affecting others.

As examples, we will consider the National Diet-Heart Study[5] and the Minnesota contribution to a collaborative physical activity project.[6] These attempts at intervention on diet and on physical activity in free-living, middle-aged U.S. men resulted in the unintended modification of other characteristics related to CHD risk.

The National Diet-Heart Study

A common protocol was adopted in five U.S. metropolitan centers for modification of the amount and composition of dietary fat. The primary endpoint studied was the change in serum cholesterol level, but other risk factor changes were monitored. The design was double-blind, the randomization process was successful, and the double-blind was unbroken. The volunteers, men 45 through 54 years of age, were recruited by letter from the U.S. Census Bureau and encouraged by local advertising.

The volunteers differed in several respects of health and health attitude from the general population. Intervention was on diet alone and the subjects were specifically requested, for the sake of the experiment, not to change their mode of life otherwise. Because of the integrity of the double-blind, no bias in respect to diet or nondiet changes is likely between diet and control groups.

Later in the study a nonblinded diet and nonblinded control group were added to test the feasibility of an open study. The overall dropout rate for the one-year period was 9.7 percent.

The results showed a similar and significant reduction of 11 percent in the serum cholesterol level among the blind and the nonblind diet groups at the end of one year. There was a fall of 3 percent in serum cholesterol level in the blind control group and of zero percent in the nonblind controls. Specific instructions were given to the nonblind control group in order to avoid diet and habit changes.

Specific instruction was also given in the double-blind group to encourage no change in energy expenditure or smoking habits, but some got advice on calorie restriction. Nevertheless, at the end of one year, these changes were recorded:

1. Twenty-five percent of cigarette smokers had stopped smoking and another 25 percent had reduced the amount smoked.
2. A rapid and significant weight loss occurred in all groups, and the final loss in both blinded groups was a mean of 2 kg.
3. There was a significant fall in blood pressure, up to 5 percent, which could not be adequately accounted for by weight loss but which might be, at least in part, attributable to familiarization.

In sum, it appears to be impossible, even in a double-blind diet trial involving highly motivated subjects and staff, to intervene on diet habits without influencing other variables related to CHD. The double-blind design, of course, assures that there is no bias in the influence of confounding variables. But the open trial which is recommended by all of the diet-heart investigators and which is an essential aspect of conducting any mass prevention program may not allow secure conclusions whether effects of intervention on diet are in fact due to diet change, to other changes, or to combined changes. This is a key problem for a MPT as well.

Physical Activity Program

A collaborative feasibility study on physical activity among sedentary men ages 45 through 54 was carried out at the Universities of Minnesota, Wisconsin, and Penn State. The Minneapolis volunteers were recruited by a letter and telephone survey in the southern and western urban-suburban areas. Intervention consisted of one-hour progressive group exercise programs three times a week for fifteen months. The primary endpoints studied were work capacity and heart rate, but other risk factor changes were monitored.

The eventual Minneapolis volunteers differed little in characteristics from those of the general population. Their high CHD risk status was determined by a screening examination in schools near their homes, and the men and their physicians were unequivocally informed of the detected high-risk status. Risk class was based on serum cholesterol and blood pressure levels and on cigarette-smoking habit. The men were then offered a preventive program based on regular physical activity. All men were specifically requested, for the sake of the experiment, to avoid other changes in mode of life. The randomization process was generally successful. Both exercise and control groups were examined and tested every three months, and the following changes refer only to Minneapolis subjects.

The exercise group followed the program with an adherence rate around 50 percent of the "ideal," based on full participation in three weekly sessions.

The exercise group showed highly significant increases in work capacity and in cardiovascular efficiency at a given submaximal work load. The control group showed no change in these measurements.

During the course of the study there was a significant weight loss in experimental and control groups, up to 1.6 kg on the average the first year, but the weight loss was insignificant by the end of the study.

Systolic blood pressure fell by about 3 mm Hg in exercise and control groups by the end of the program.

Serum cholesterol fell by 6 mg/deciliter in exercise and control groups, but reached a significant level of fall only at one period in the study.

There was an association between serum cholesterol reduction and weight loss in the exercise group.

Four of 28 regular smokers in the exercise group stopped smoking during the course of the study.

This feasibility trial on physical exercise demonstrated that vigorous intervention on physical activity habits, an important factor in the mode of life, is accompanied by expected changes related to exercise and by unexpected changes in other habits and factors of risk.

Since it is quite impossible to conduct blinded experiments on exercise, or for that matter on smoking habit, it may never be possible to avoid entirely, or to estimate closely, the influence of associated changes in confounding risk factors on the final results of prevention trials in the open population.

EXPERIMENTAL RESULTS OF A MPT

More information is provided by a long-term study which purposely attempted to modify five major CHD risk factors, the Coronary Prevention Evaluation Program of Chicago.[2,7] The findings are useful, though the conclusions are limited by the small numbers of subjects and the absence of a randomly assigned control group.

Five hundred and nineteen volunteers to a general community campaign were identified to have two or more elevated risk factors (or a serum cholesterol alone of ⩾ 325 mg%). Intervention in these men, aged 40 to 59, was in an intensive, well-organized, and continuing program.

Skilled diet advice was given to subjects and to their families for diets moderate in calories and unsaturated fat and low in saturated fat and cholesterol. Reasonable personal programs of physical exercise were proposed. Management of elevated blood pressure and glucose intolerance was carefully coordinated with the attending physician. Continuing advice and support was given to help the subjects stop cigarette smoking.

The general experience of this multifactor risk factor program is summarized as follows:

The majority of men, free-living urban volunteers, remained in the program (37% dropped out in seven years).

Significant measurable change occurred in eating habits, and there was a 7 percent average weight loss early, which has been maintained.

Serum cholesterol was reduced 19 percent and the reduction largely maintained (15% mean fall after five years).

Over the years, about 50 percent of original cigarette smokers who continued as active participants stopped completely or successfully switched to pipe or cigars in moderation.

Heart rate was slowed at rest and in response to a standard exercise load on the bicycle ergometer.

Age-adjusted seven-year total mortality rate was 30 per 1000 in the CPEP. In 2900 closely matched men from similar groups involved in the American Heart Association Pooling Project, the rate was 50 per 1000.

PROBLEMS OF THE MPT

The MPT presents a number of special considerations in design, execution, and interpretation.

Sample-size Questions in the MPT

For example, there remain some conceptual questions about sample size in the MPT having "factorial" design (see below); i.e. How much expansion of the estimated sample size is required if risk factor subgroups are employed in an attempt to study the individual contributions and interaction of these factors? In general, the sample-size requirements for the MPT are estimated to be smaller than those for single-factor trials because of the greater theoretical potential of multifactor risk intervention in reducing CHD incidence.

MPT sample-size estimates from the U.S. group are modest[9] compared with others in single-factor trials of primary prevention.[18] Nine thousand "high-risk" subjects in each of the control and treatment groups were estimated to be sufficient to detect a 25 percent treatment effect on total mortality in a seven-year study experiencing a control group total mortality rate of 63 per 1000, with an estimated 45 percent total seven-year dropout rate, and with an δ of 0.05 and a β of 0.10.[19] Moreover, it was estimated that several important interactions, and particularly the relative effect of diet change, could be studied in a factorial design based on an estimated 50 percent treatment effect on *all CHD incidence* with a study among the same number of individuals, with the same drop-out rate and error limits.

Execution Problems

Certainly the design and conduct of a MPT is more complex and the staff and organizational requirements greater than for a single-factor prevention trial. A wider team approach and competence are required. The various approaches necessary to modify multiple factors in large groups may attenuate the effectiveness of the trial. For example, eminence and experience of the investigator in management of lipid disorders or hypertension may not suffice to persuade free-living men to change habits of eating, exercise, or smoking. The W.H.O. group[13] states: "There is a real danger that a negative outcome to the MPT may indicate not necessarily the failure of [disease] incidence to respond to changes in risk factors, but merely the failure of subjects to do as they were advised."

The problems of standardization in selecting the several cohorts and in administering the multiple treatments are obvious. The greater difficulty in securing homogeneous treatment groups has important implications in the interpretation of results. These points all suggest the greater requirement for organization and experience. This experience is best gained in a well-planned initial run-in phase of a larger trial.

Organizational Structure of the MPT

The greater complexity of the MPT led the U.S. group to recommend the organizational structure tested in the Coronary Drug Project.[9] This structure includes a Policy Board, a Steering Committee, a Coordinating Center, individual Research Centers, a Data and Safety Monitoring Committee, an Electrocardiographic Center, Central Laboratories, a Drug Distribution Center, and a National Heart and Lung Institute Liaison Office. The detailed function of each of these components is worthy of consideration.[8]

Problems of Interpretation and Application of MPT

Perhaps the greatest problem of and the strongest argument against the MPT concerns the interpretation and application of trial results. This problem hinges on the fact that most MPT designs do not allow definition of the relative contribution of a particular treatment to the final result. Since most investigators now agree on the "desirability" and "acceptability" of reducing body weight, hypertension, and smoking habits, the argument is posed primarily by those concerned with the diet-heart question.

The researcher argues that the MPT fails to disclose the relative causal influence, if any, of diet. The administrator argues that national habits and the food economy should not be deranged by public health action leading from possible MPT results when, in fact, the real contribution of diet is not disclosed in a MPT. This problem and these arguments are indeed important and may be considered in several lights.

In the first place, the MPT is not meant to replace the single-factor trial in CHD and is clearly not a suggested alternative to trials already in operation. The MPT simply offers the chance of greater efficiency in answering the primordial question on CHD prevention. The MPT should properly be carried out *in parallel* with existing single-factor trials, especially those which obviate the confounding problem by double-blind design in closed populations.

Diet-heart investigators call for an open trial in the free-living population. They and their review commission[18] also recommend a double-blind diet trial in closed institutional populations, such as the Minnesota Study and the VA Domiciliary Study. Therefore, in multifactor and single-factor trials, double-blind and non-blind, in open and closed populations, each provides information which complements that from the other, in respect to causes and to the universality of application. Thus, the question may be reduced to one of priorities in setting up the interrelated studies needed to "wrap up" the issue.

Factorial Design of the MPT

Another option already mentioned to estimate the relative contribution of individual treatments and their interaction in

MPT is the use of "factorial design," in which relevant combinations of risk factors are managed within subgroups. The factorial design requires that each subject or unit have the same or predetermined probability of assignment to each treatment group. However, it is not possible to advise a thin man to lose weight or to treat a normotensive with antihypertensive drugs. Therefore, factorial design requires subgroups of subjects or randomized units having levels of risk factors sufficiently elevated to merit treatment by each of the methods under study; for example, "fat, hypertensive, hyperlipidemic cigarette smokers."

The National Cooperative Trial group[9] proposed a MPT design to obtain a maximum amount of precise information on the contribution of any and all treatments while intervening on groups contributing a substantial part of the total CHD incidence. Stratification of high-risk subjects into four cells was suggested as follows, each of which would then be randomized into treatment and control groups:

1. Hypercholesterolemia as the only risk factor.
2. Hypercholesterolemia plus hypertension.
3. Hypercholesterolemia plus cigarette smoking.
4. Hypercholesterolemia plus hypertension plus cigarette smoking.

Experimental subgroup 1 would be advised only in regard to diet and exercise, because recommendations on blood pressure and smoking control are not indicated for them. The sample size would be kept "reasonable" by the use of more frequently occurring endpoints of CHD morbidity rather than the rate of total mortality alone. Comparisons would be made to the randomly assigned control group having hypercholesterolemia as the only risk factor. Information on the individual contribution of each intervention would be obtained by providing the treatment appropriate to each subgroup. The definitive aspect of the MPT would be maintained by comparison of total mortality among *all* experimental and *all* control subgroups combined. The design would resolve the key question about the effect on the total mortality rate.

A subsequent conceptual development in this question of the

individual contribution of diet therapy is summarized here from the report to the National Heart and Lung Institute Task Force on Atherosclerosis:[14] The MPT is essential to determine whether application of the general body of knowledge on CHD risk factors can lead to significant reduction of CHD and death. There is a need to obtain a specific answer to the diet aspect of this question. The need for definitive answers on the benefit of treating hypertension and reducing cigarette smoking is less compelling because of the general acceptance of the desirability of their control. However, it is important to minimize the effect of change in confounding variables in any nondouble-blind study, including the MPT. Therefore, a design is proposed in which high-risk candidates are men with hypercholesterolemia who smoke cigarettes. Randomization into four groups would be performed:

1. Control (no intervention on diet or smoking).
2. Smoking intervention only.
3. Diet intervention only.
4. Diet plus smoking intervention.

Maximum similarity of design, measurement, and endpoints is recommended in all proposed programs, including double-blind studies among closed populations and nonblinded studies among the free-living population.

THE W.H.O. WORKING GROUP ON MPT

In November 1970 a group of cardiologists and epidemiologists were convened in Rome by the European Office of W.H.O. to discuss the concepts, problems, and detailed protocols for multifactor preventive trials in coronary heart disease. The two current European programs were reviewed in detail, one designed by Geoffrey Rose of London with randomly allocated industries, and another by Gosta Tibblin of Gothenburg with individual randomization from a community sample. Plans were made for extending these studies to other countries.

The arguments for MPT are succinctly summarized in the report of this working group:[13]

> 1) At some stage, multifactor trials will certainly be necessary,

since without them there can be no indication of the total effectiveness of applying current beliefs on IHD prevention. The urgency of the situation is such that they should not be postponed until the completion of single-factor trials.

2) Single-factor trials fail to measure the extent of any interaction (positive or negative) between the various factors. For example, the results of stopping cigarette smoking and at the same time lowering the serum cholesterol level may be greater or less than the sum of their two separate effects.

3) In trials of health advice it is impossible to prevent (or measure) a form of contamination within the intervention group: namely, when subjects are told to do one thing, they do other things as well. In other words, where the "treatment" consists of advice, a pure single-factor trial is impossible anyway.

4) The total effectiveness of a multifactor approach may well be greater than that of any single-factor treatment. This implies that there is a better chance that the trial with a multifactor design will provide a positive conclusion. In the present state of our knowledge, it would be helpful to provide *any* objective evidence that IHD can be prevented.

5) In the event of a negative outcome from a multifactor trial it could reasonably be inferred (subject to sufficient numbers) that each of the individual treatments, as well as the combinations, was probably ineffective. Thus a multifactor trial provides a means for more rapid, simultaneous evaluation of each of several different factors.

6) However, the strongest argument for multifactor trials in practice is their appropriateness to the real-life situation in which health policy must be determined. The medical approach to the management of high-risk individuals and groups is commonly multifactorial: a doctor offers more than one item of advice or treatment if this seems appropriate, selecting those particular items that seem suitable in the particular situation. The task of the public health researcher is if possible to estimate the efficacy of the policy which the majority of clinicians believe to be the most helpful, that is a multifactorial approach.

SUMMARY

The MPT in cardiovascular epidemiology marks a trend in epidemiology which merits critical attention.

The MPT concept is highly appropriate to chronic diseases associated with multiple risk factors.

The MPT allows tailoring of the treatment to the need, thereby following precepts widely acceptable in medicine.

The MPT tests the most fundamental and urgent hypothesis, whether primary prevention of CHD, with an associated reduction in total mortality, is indeed possible.

The MPT probably provides the best likelihood of demonstrating soon and with greatest efficiency any possibility of a major reduction in the incidence of CHD.

"Pure" preventive trials on single-risk factors are not possible when the treatment involves health advice in the open population; other changes occur which confound the conclusions.

MPT design, organization, and execution are more complex than in a single-factor trial and require greater staff experience.

More precise information on the contribution of individual treatments to prevention can be determined by parallel single-factor trials and multifactor trials with factorial design.

The knowledge obtained and the conclusions allowed from single-factor and multifactor trials are complementary.

ACKNOWLEDGMENTS

Many have made contributions to the concepts and design of multifactor preventive trials in vascular diseases. Among them are the following.

The U. S. National Cooperative Gorup. Participants: E. Benson, H. Blackburn, A. Keys, R. B. McGandy, M. Z. Nichaman, R. D. Remington, L. T. Sheffield, W. M. Smith, J. Stamler, F. J. Stare, S. L. Syme, H. L. Taylor.

The Makarska Conference on Mass Field Trials In Prevention of Coronary Disease. Participants: H. Blackburn, T. Chalmers, F. Epstein, S. M. Fox, III, I. Glasunov, J. G. Green, J. A. Heady, M. J. Karvonen, A. Keys, J. Morris, R. D. Remington, G. Rose, J. Stamler, H. L. Taylor, G. Tibblin, H. M. Whyte.

The Rome WHO Working Group on Multifactor Preventive Trials In Ischemic Heart Disease. Participants: A. Baubinene, H. Blackburn, D. Brunner, A. V. Caklin, D. G. S. Christie, Z. Fejfar, W. F. van Ganse, I. Glasunov, J. H. de Haas, I. Jhermann, Z. Jaksic, A. Jouve, V. Kallio, H. Kesteloot, M. D. Kornitzer, E. F. Krohn, F. Loogen, A. Menotti, C. L. C. van Nieuwenhuizen, Z. Pisa, M. Postiglione, V. Puddu, K. Pyorala, J. L.

Richard, G. Rose, S. L. Rywik, J. Simon, G. Tibblin, R. Vlaicu, L. Werko, L. Wilhelmsen.

REFERENCES

1. The Pooling Project Report. Current developments in North America. In Jones, R.J. (Ed.) *Atherosclerosis: Proceedings of the Second International Symposium.* Springer Verleg, New York, 1970. Council on Epidemiology, American Heart Association.
2. Report of the Inter-Society Commission for Heart Disease Resources. Primary prevention of atherosclerotic diseases. *Circulation, 42:*A55, 1970.
3. Truett, J., Cornfield, J., and Kannel, W. A multivariate analysis of the risk of coronary heart disease in Framingham. *J. Chronic Dis., 20:*511-524, 1967.
4. Schwartz, D., and Lellouch, J. Explanatory and pragmatic attitudes in therapeutic trials. *J. Chronic Dis., 20:*637, 1967.
5. National Diet-Heart Study Research Group. The national diet-heart study final report. *Circulation, 37* (Suppl. 1), 1968.
6. Taylor, H.L., Balke, B., Blackburn, H., Buskirk, E., Hamrell, B., and Remington, R. Studies of methodology and feasibility of physical activity in trials of prevention of coronary heart disease. *Medicine and Science in Sports,* in press.
7. Stamler, J. *Lectures on Preventive Cardiology.* New York, Grune & Stratton, 1967.
8. Report of the Coronary Drug Project Research Group. The coronary drug project. *J.A.M.A., 214:*1303-1313, 1970.
9. National Cooperative Trial on Multifactorial Prevention of First Heart Attacks and Coronary Mortality in Free-Living, High-Risk, Middle-Aged American Men. Submitted to the National Heart and Lung Institute, 1969.
10. Makarska Report on Clinical Trials in Ischemic Heart Disease. Council on Epidemiology and Prevention, International Society of Cardiology, 1968.
11. Rose, G. A proposed trial of heart disease prevention in industry. *Trans. Soc. Occup. Med., 20:*109-111, 1970.
12. Tibblin, G. Preventive cardiology in Gothenburg. *Pehr Dubb Journalen, 3,* 1969.
13. Report of a W.H.O. Working Group. Methodology of multifactor preventive trials in ischemic heart disease. Rome, Nov. 1970. Euro 5011 (3) Regional Office for Europe. W.H.O. Copenhagen, 1971.
14. Stamler, J. Position paper on the diet-heart issue for the National Heart and Lung Institute Task Force on Atherosclerosis. Aug. 19, 1970.
15. Keys, A. (Ed.) Coronary heart disease in seven countries. *Circulation, 41* (suppl. 1), 1970.

16. Stamler, J., Berkson, David M., and Lindberg, Howard A. Risk factors: Their significance for the etiopathogenesis and prevention of the atherosclerotic diseases. In Geer, J.C., and Wissler, R.W. (Eds.) *Proceedings of a Symposium of the American Society of Bacteriologists and Pathologists.* Montreal, Mar. 9, 1971. In press.
17. Cornfield, J., and Mitchell, S. Selected risk factors in coronary disease. Possible intervention effects. *Arch. Environ. Health, 19*:382-391, 1969.
18. Report of the Diet-Heart Review Panel of the National Heart Institute. *Mass Field Trials of the Diet-Heart Question.* American Heart Association Monograph No. 28, 1969.
19. Schork, M.A., and Remington, R.D. The determination of sample size in treatment-control comparisons for chronic disease studies in which dropout or non-adherence is a problem. *J. Chronic Dis., 20*:233, 1967.
20. Dayton, S., Pearce, M.L., Hashimoto, S., *et al.* A controlled clinical trial of a diet high in unsaturated fat in preventing complications of atherosclerosis. *Circulation, 39-40* (suppl. 2), 1969.

Chapter 8

THE BIRMINGHAM STROKE, EPIDEMIOLOGY AND REHABILITATION STUDY

PETER B. PEACOCK, CHARLES P. RILEY, THEODORE D. LAMPTON, SHERMAN S. RAFFEL, *and* JOHN S. WALKER

THE EPIDEMIOLOGY AND NATURAL HISTORY OF STROKE: A REVIEW OF THE LITERATURE: THE OBJECTIVES OF THE BIRMINGHAM STUDY

A STROKE HAS BEEN DEFINED as "a spontaneous more-or-less abrupt neurologic catastrophe of vascular origin—generally causing some combination of altered consciousness, blunting of intellect, alterations of personality, and specific neurologic deficits, such as motor and sensory paralysis, disturbances of speech and communication, and sometimes impairment of vision."[1] Lee and Hodes[2] point out that although the adult brain represents only 2 percent of the total body weight, it consumes more than 20 percent of the oxygen and 17 percent of the glucose used by the entire body and is completely dependent on an uninterrupted blood supply. Thus, while classifications exist[3] for use on the living patient, based on etiology, assumed pathology, the clinical picture and course, the assumed anatomical location or name of the vessel involved, or the existence of associated disease, most classifications are based on assumed changes in the cerebral vasculature.[4] The usual broad classification divides strokes into occlusive strokes (mostly thrombotic or embolic) and hemorrhagic strokes (intracerebral or subarachnoid).

Clinically, intracranial ischemic lesions may be asymptomatic, may be associated with nonlocalized manifestations such as syncope or confusion, may be associated with short-lived episodes of focal neurological dysfunction[5] leaving no or very little persistent neurological deficit (known as transient ischemic attacks), or may be associated with a persistent neurological deficit (a "completed" stroke). Because of the difficulty involved in identifying the lesser grades of stroke with any certainty, most epidemiological studies when discussing strokes are discussing "completed" strokes.

While careful retrospective and prospective studies[6] in limited localities of the U.S.A. have shown cerebral thrombosis and embolism making up 80 percent or more of the cerebral thrombosis-cerebral embolism-intracerebral hemorrhage complex (excluding subarachnoid hemorrhage and "other" strokes), the Vital Statistics of the United States in 1963 and again in 1967 show cerebral thrombosis and embolism making up only 36.5 percent of this complex. Some of this difference is accounted for by the higher case-fatality rate associated with cerebral hemorrhage[7] and some may be accounted for by deaths from cerebral thrombosis and embolism being certified incorrectly as deaths from cerebral hemorrhage. Thus Kuller[8] considered 43 of 168 deaths which had been attributed to cerebral hemorrhage among persons aged 40 to 64 years in Baltimore to have been incorrectly assigned. Of real interest, though of limited statistical value, was a study done by the editors of *Modern Medicine*[9] with 2662 physicians reporting having treated 12,390 stroke patients within the previous ninety days. Of these, 64 percent were thrombosis, 19 percent hemorrhage, and 7 percent embolism. Among the physicians aged younger than 35 years, 67 percent of their patients were called thromboses, while among the physicians aged 65 years or older, 48 percent of their patients were called thromboses.

Estimates of the immediate mortality from stroke vary from under 20 percent[7] to some 40 percent.[10] Of those who survive to enter hospital, Loewenson[11] found a five-year survival rate of 67 percent (77% for persons aged less than 60 years), while in a more extensive study of 843 cases, Robinson *et al.*[12] found a five-year survival rate of only 40 percent (62% for persons in their sixth decade).

Of the many papers which have been written concerning the natural history of stroke patients from the point of view of rehabilitation, three, spread over a period of fifteen years, might be selected for particular attention. Mahoney and Barthel[13] found that patients whose physical medicine rehabilitation therapy began within two weeks after the stroke did better than did those admitted to treatment later. Of the total group of 122 hemiplegic patients, 81 percent were able to get along independently at discharge. Boyle and Scalzitti[14] discussed 478 patients (out of 669) referred to the Department of Physical Medicine and Rehabilitation from the Milwaukee County Hospital and painted a much blacker picture. Of this group of patients, 224 died in hospital (170 on their first admission), 31 died out of hospital, 46 were lost to observation and 169 were traced one to three years later. Of these 169 living patients, only 63 had no disabling residual, 34 were little limited, 65 were moderately limited and 7 were bedridden. While age, sex, and the severity of the cerebrovascular accident had an important influence on rehabilitation potential, the number of physical and occupational therapy treatments and when these treatments were instituted had no measurable beneficial effects.

In addition to a good review, Marquardsen[10] reported 769 patients with acute cerebrovascular disease who were admitted to the Frederiksburg Hospital, Denmark, during the years 1940-52 with follow-up observation periods (for those who survived) ranging from 10 to 23 years. Of the 407 patients who survived the first three weeks, 52 percent were restored to independence in self-care and a further 15 percent achieved some measure of independence. Of those who had been in employment before the stroke, little over one-third went back to work. Of the adverse factors present at the time of admission, the most important were age over 70, severe motor deficit, impairment of consciousness of more than a few hours' duration, conjugate ocular deviation, and conceptual disorders. Of the survivors, 37 percent had further cerebrovascular accidents.

Most of the earlier estimates of stroke incidence are based on mortality figures. Some of these (taken from Stallones[15] and Kurtzke[5] and other sources) are reviewed later and have considerable value. The defects of death certificate data should, however, be remembered. Kuller[8] found that in only 256 out of 602 death certificates in Baltimore in which cerebrovascular disease was reported was cerebrovascular disease listed as the underlying cause. The relationship was particularly bad for cerebral thrombosis.

Only a limited number of morbidity studies have been reported from the U.S.A. and England. These may be divided into prevalence studies, registry studies, and incidence studies.

The prevalence of cerebral infarction in Evans County, Georgia, was reported as being as follows in cases per 1000.[16] The number of cases on which these rates have been based is given in parentheses and will indicate the instability of these figures.

Age	*White Males*	*White Females*	*N/White Males*	*N/White Females*
50-59	35.7 (8)	12.6 (3)	48.8 (6)	12.2 (2)
60-69	39.0 (6)	23.3 (4)	47.6 (4)	58.8 (7)

Several major registry studies are under way at the present time. A typical study in this group is that being conducted in Jefferson County, Alabama (see Table 8.1), but none of these has been reported as yet. Of the older registries in the U.S.A., the best known was that conducted in Middlesex, Connecticut,[17] from April 1, 1967, to March 31, 1968. Unfortunately, the 191 cases reported in this study included recurrent as well as first strokes, but using these data, the incidence in men aged 45 to 64 is found to be approximately 2.6 per 1000. The Oxford Record Linkage Study for 1963, reported on by Acheson and Fairbairn,[18] covered considerably more cases (630) and their reported incidence per 1000 population for cerebrovascular disease was as follows:

Age in Years	*I.C.D. Classification (7th)*									
	Male					*Female*				
	330	*331*	*332*	*334*	*All*	*330*	*331*	*332*	*334*	*All*
45-54	.13	.18	.22	.22	.76	.44	.22	.18	.13	.98
55-64	.41	.82	1.35	.88	3.47	.55	1.43	.71	.38	3.07

Note. 330 is subarachnoid hemorrhage, 331 is cerebral hemorrhage, 332 is cerebral infarct, and 334 is nonspecific.

Another study in Rochester, Minnesota,[19] based on 157 cases gave for the age group 45 to 54 years an incidence rate per 1000 of two for cerebral infarction and one for cerebral hemorrhage.

TABLE 8-1

CEREBROVASCULAR ACCIDENTS BY AGE, RACE AND SEX, SPECIFIC NUMBERS AND RATES PER 100,000 POPULATION, JEFFERSON COUNTY, ALABAMA, 1969

Race and	Age-Groups								
Sex	–40	40–44	45–49	50–54	55–59	60–64	65–69	70–74	75+	All Ages
White	2	5	9	24	25	37	47	57	109	315
Male	(1.4)	(36.6)	(69.0)	(202.8)	(238.4)	(485.6)	(804.1)	(1233.9)	(1985.8)	(152.4)
White	5	3	7	12	20	22	30	44	196	339
Female	(3.6)	(21.0)	(48.7)	(91.2)	(192.9)	(231.6)	(363.3)	(652.9)	(2288.4)	(150.5)
Nonwhite	1	10	8	13	28	31	41	36	66	234
Male	(1.6)	(266.3)	(172.2)	(290.7)	(496.4)	(742.6)	(1089.6)	(1406.9)	(2784.4)	(240.3)
Nonwhite	8	8	9	26	34	24	46	39	91	285
Female	(11.3)	(149.2)	(148.9)	(431.5)	(529.1)	(484.2)	(1112.5)	(1292.3)	(2683.6)	(258.9)
TOTAL	16	26	33	75	107	114	164	176	462	1173
	(3.9)	(70.1)	(85.6)	(211.3)	(313.6)	(434.3)	(756.3)	(1039.3)	(2331.6)	(183.5)

Note. Rates based on the 1970 census are given in parentheses.

The Chicago Stroke Study[20] was based on a large group of federal old-age-assistance applicants aged 65 to 69 years at the start of the study. The point prevalence of stroke in this group was 78 per 1000 and the three-year rate per 1000 was as follows (the number of strokes on which the rates are based are given in parentheses):

Category	*White Men*		*White Women*		*N/White Men*		*N/White Women*	
No TIA	35	(11)	54	(17)	63	(19)	41	(16)
Questionable TIA	61	(2)	57	(4)	116	(8)	153	(15)
Probably TIA	54	(1)	28	(1)	153	(6)	194	(11)

The twelve-year Framingham report[6] gave the following figures (note that the incidence is over a twelve-year period):

Age Group	*Men:*	*Cases*	*Incidence per 1000*	*Women:*	*Cases*	*Incidence per 1000*
40-49		9	11.7		7	7.4
50-59		15	24.6		21	26.7

Changes over time in the total incidence of cerebrovascular disease have not been remarkable. Stallones[15] noted a 25 percent reduction in the age-adjusted stroke death rates for the United States between 1940 and 1960, while Yates[21] found little change in total for England and Wales though there was a relative increase in occlusive stroke (broken by a dip during the 1940-45 war years) and a relative decrease in hemorrhagic stroke. Krueger and Paffenbarger[22] obtained results very similar to those of Yates when they looked at age-adjusted death rates from cerebrovascular disease in Memphis, Tennessee, for the period 1920-60.

Of particular interest in the epidemiological study of any disease is the consideration of risk factors. The geographical distribution of stroke shows most countries, including the U.S.A. (whites), with age-adjusted death rates from cerebrovascular disease, clustered closely round 100 per 100,000 persons per year.[15] Exceptions are Japan, with a rate of 209 (mostly hemorrhagic strokes), and Belgium, with a rate of 48 (mostly thrombotic strokes). Variations within countries are often as great as those between countries. For the U.S.A., Borhani[23] reported for the period 1959-61, for white males aged 35 to 65 years, that the age-standardized death rates from cerebrovascular disease were 90.3 in South Carolina, 66.6 in Alabama (only four states had higher rates than Alabama), and 34.3 in Wyoming (all rates were per 100,000 per year). In Japan, Takahashi[24] showed a similar variation, with rates in the north and some two and a half times those in the south.

Sex differences are not marked in cerebrovascular disease. Most studies show a small male excess in the age group 40 to 74 years, and a female excess thereafter.[12] Totals generally show a slight female excess, and thus in the Tecumseh study[25] the female death rate from stroke was 3.7 per 1000 per year and the male rate 3.4. The relationship to age is very obvious (see Table 8.1).

In the North American literature, discussions on the effect of race have dealt mostly with Caucasian-Negro and Caucasian-Japanese differences. Almost every investigator who has looked at Caucasian-Negro comparisons has found an excess of cerebrovascular disease among Negroes. It has been rare, however, for the two racial groups to be even approximately equivalent in their socioeconomic-physical environment. The Veteran Study[26] found in Georgia a Negro excess in every five-year age group from 25 to 74 years. (This study covered 426 deaths from stroke among whites and 180 deaths from stroke among Negroes.) In South Africa, however, Meyer[27] could find no difference. In Israel, Yablonski[28] found a two-times-higher rate (almost entirely due to hemorrhage) among Jews of Afro-Asian origin compared with Jews of European origin. Many authors have documented an excess of cerebrovascular disease among Japanese in Japan compared with white North Americans. One of the best-standardized of these studies was that by Resch *et al.*[29] Of interest was an earlier paper by Gordon[30] which reported that the cerebrovascular death rate for Japanese decreased progressively from Japan to Hawaii to the United States.

We have already noted the increased likelihood of persons who have had one stroke to develop another. There is also reasonably good evidence that persons who have had a TIA (transient ischemic attack as defined by Kurtzke[5]) are unduly liable to develop a "completed" stroke. As part of the Seal Beach study,

Friedman *et al.*[31] found that 8 of 44 patients with TIA followed for two years developed a thrombotic stroke.

Study after study has demonstrated a clear-cut relationship between hypertension and cerebrovascular disease. Robinson[12] found that 70 percent of his 843 cases of cerebral thrombosis had a blood pressure above 160/90 as their highest recorded blood pressure. Paffenbarger and Wing[32] found that 171 Harvard students who died of stroke ten to fifty years after their Harvard medical examination had a mean systolic blood pressure of 126 as students, compared with a mean of 122 for 684 paired controls (four controls for each stroke death) who did not die of a stroke. The Framingham study[6] reported a morbidity ratio of 2.32 for their hypertensives (systolic 160 plus and/or diastolic 95 plus) using brain infarction over a twelve-year follow-up period as their dependent variable. The Tecumseh study[25] recorded 33 percent of their male strokes and 62 percent of their female strokes as giving a history of hypertension compared with expected values of 20 percent and 40 percent respectively. A careful pathological study by Baker *et al.*[33] based on autopsies on 5033 persons showed Circle of Willis scores to be directly correlated with heart weight (by age and sex), with a history of hypertension, and to a lesser extent, with the recorded blood pressure.

Several authors have found a relationship between diabetes and cerebrovascular disease (especially thrombotic strokes). The Seal Beach study[34] found an incidence of 10.5 per 1000 for males and 14.5 per 1000 for females of thrombotic stroke among persons with a history of diabetes compared with 6.4 per 1000 for males and 4.8 per 1000 for females when there was no history of diabetes. The Chicago study[20] among patients with no history suggestive of TIA reported three-year incidence rates per 1000 for stroke among persons with or without diabetes mellitus to be for white males 81 and 31, respectively, for white females 86 and 45, for Negro males 105 and 57, and for Negro females 73 and 32.

Less truly definitive work has been done in investigating the relationship between ischemic heart disease and cerebral thrombosis than might be expected. Defining an abnormal ECG as one showing left ventricular hypertrophy and/or intraventricular block and/or nonspecific S-T and T-wave abnormality, the twelve-year Framingham report[6] gave the morbidity ratio for brain infarction among those without an abnormal ECG as 75 (based on 38 strokes) and among those with an abnormal ECG as 408 (based on 17 strokes). It might be noted that this latter morbidity ratio of 408 was higher than that found for myocardial infarction (161 based on 20 infarcts) among persons with an abnormal ECG. The Tecumseh study (1959-69) group, as reported by Johnson,[25] observed 25 stroke deaths among males with ECG abnormalities, which represented a mortality ratio of 186 percent. In Hiroshima, Japan, Johnson[35] reported a morbidity ratio of 141 (based on 9 strokes and 652 person-years of follow-up) among males with ST-T changes on their ECG. Among reported retrospective studies, Friedman[36] found coronary or arteriosclerotic heart disease in 42 percent (49 persons) of his stroke cases and in 24 percent (57 persons) of his controls. Despite the above findings, the statistical association between coronary disease and cerebrovascular disease reported by Aronson[37] was not impressive.

While Nefzger *et al.*[26] found no differences between the mean serum cholesterol levels of 369 cases of myocardial infarction and 414 cases of cerebral infarction (the study was limited to patients surviving at least one month), and while the close relationship between serum cholesterol and myocardial infarction is well known, a similarly clear relationship between serum cholesterol and cerebral infarction has not been shown. Chapman,[38] among white males aged 40 to 69 years, found a cerebral thrombosis incidence of 13 per 1000 (based on 3 strokes) where the serum cholesterol was 225-274 mg%, and an incidence of 19 per 1000 (based on 13 strokes) where the serum cholesterol was 275 or greater. The Seal Beach study[34] reported a cerebral thrombosis incidence among males of 5 per 1000 where the serum cholesterol was 220-249, 7 per 1000 where the serum cholesterol was 280-309, and 11 per 1000 where the serum cholesterol was over 340 mg%. Based on small numbers, the twelve-year Framingham study[6] showed morbidity ratios of 49, 112, and 217 for the three cholesterol levels <220, 220-259, and 260+ for the age group 30 to 49 years, but no relationship emerged for the age group 50 to 59 years.

In a retrospective study, Pearce and Aziz[39] found 25 percent of 60 patients with an acute stroke to have hyperuricemia (levels in excess of 7 mg/100 ml for males and 6 mg/100 ml for females), confirming technically less reliable studies reported by other investigators.

Ettinger *et al.*[40] have reported on coagulation studies comparing stroke patients and normal controls done in Minnesota (195 strokes and 55 normals in older age groups) and Japan (95 strokes and 26 normals in older age groups). The four tests used were the retarded thromboplastin generation test, prothrombin time, fibrinogen, and the recalcification clotting time. The authors state that "some identifiable coagulation changes do occur following an acute nonhemorrhagic stroke [but] we cannot conclude that these coagulation abnormalities. . .in any measure contributed to the development of the stroke." Stoica *et al.*,[41] in an unusual experiment, compared 24 patients with cerebral thrombosis (confirmed on angiography) with 12 controls by taking a base line and then exposing both groups to emotional strain (breathing through a narcosis mask). The thrombotic group showed a significantly reduced clotting time (heparin and recalcified plasma tests) and significantly decreased fibrinolysis.

The recent literature has included numerous papers on the relationship between oral contraceptives and cerebrovascular accidents. A typical early report was that of Cole,[42] who noted that five cerebrovascular accidents in young women (under the age of 40 years) had been seen at the North Carolina Baptist Hospital, Winston-Salem, in 1966-67, compared with seven (three associated with pregnancy) in the whole period 1959-66. All the cases seen in 1966-67 had been using oral contraceptives. Sartwell *et al.*,[43] in a retrospective study done in the U.S.A. with forty-eight hospitals, suggested that sequential products had the greater risk of causing thromboembolism; but Grant,[44] in clinical trials on 797 women, found most thromboembolism in combined preparations containing a relatively high dose of estrogen. The most authoritative paper in this area is that of Inman *et al.*[45] reporting the findings of the British Committee on Safety of Drugs. Based on 1305 cases of thromboembolism (including 83 strokes) among women on oral contraceptives, they found a positive correlation, statistically significant at $p < 0.001$, between the dose of estrogen and the (admittedly very small) risk of cerebral thrombosis.

Other variables (or risk factors) which have been looked at from the point of view of a possible relationship with cerebrovascular disease include smoking habits, the ponderal index, the vital capacity, parental mortality, the ingestion of alcohol, hemoglobin levels, and personality traits. For all of these the evidence is either conflicting (e.g. ponderal index and vital capacity) or else the results reported have been based on too small numbers to have any statistical significance.

Despite the recent small flurry of interest in the epidemiology of cerebrovascular disease which is reflected above, the study of stroke has tended to remain a stepchild. In 1964, the President's Commission on Heart Disease, Cancer and Stroke[46] reported through its subcommittee on stroke:

> In contrast to their concern with many less common diseases, the public and the professions have shown slight interest in the prevention, treatment, and recognition of basic problems of the victims of stroke. One indication of this apathy is that accurate information regarding the frequency of stroke is not available, though estimates state that at least two million people living in the United States show clinical evidence of this illness.

This stroke prevalence estimate of two million was based on the approximately 200,000 cerebrovascular deaths recorded for the United States (201,166 in 1963). The report of the Second National Conference on Cardiovascular Diseases (1964) indicated that increased longevity in the United States had resulted in an ever-increasing number of potential stroke patients, causing cerebrovascular disease to become a major medical and economic problem to the nation. This publication pointed out forcefully that even though there had been some increase of interest and investigation of cerebrovascular disease, "its epidemiology is still ill defined." The report told that most currently available data were derived from death certificates and other retrospective studies and noted that "the true incidence and prevalence of cerebrovascular disease is not known; it is obviously greater than death certificates indicate." Criticism of existing methods and the usefulness and validity of data obtained in this way was well documented.

The Birmingham stroke study was proposed in 1964 and funded in 1965 as a five-year study of (a) the natural history of stroke in an unbiased ambulant population and the evaluation of those personal and environmental factors which predisposed to the initiation or further progress of the disease and which might be susceptible to preventive measures, and (b) the effectiveness of intensive rehabilitation procedures applied to the stroke patient. A secondary objective of the epidemiological study was to determine whether information collected relatively inexpensively by lay interviewers using a standardized questionnaire would be as useful in predicting stroke as would a detailed medical history and examination.

The epidemiological study was the first large prospective study of stroke to be launched in the United States which covered a random sample of a total nonselected (except for age) ambulant population (in this study, that of Birmingham, Alabama) with a substantial proportion (about one-third) of nonwhites and located in a high-incidence geographical area.

The rehabilitation study was relevant because very poor results in the rehabilitation of stroke victims and very limited acceptance of them as candidates for vocational rehabilitation had been reported, and there was a dearth of properly randomized, controlled studies from which any firm conclusions could be drawn.

STUDY DESIGN AND METHODOLOGY

The Basic Design

It was estimated that a minimum of 50 strokes (of which 30 to 40 might be thrombotic strokes) would be needed in a prospective study before any statistically significant meaning could be attached to any but the most obvious of the variables (risk factors) being studied. Ideally the number of strokes studied should be at least twice this. It was known from existing stroke registries that first strokes were relatively uncommon under the age of 50 years (an incidence of less than 0.5 per 1000 persons per year for persons aged 40 to 49 years), which would make a prospective study on this age group impractical. For persons over the age of 70 years the expected annual stroke incidence was much higher (more than 10 per 1000), but this age group no longer represented a working population and the analysis would be confused by multiple pathology and interfering causes of death and disability. Also, the epidemiology of stroke in this population might be different from that found in younger working populations. This left the age group 50 to 69 years for study. While existing data suggested an annual incidence in this age group for new strokes of about 3 per 1000, it was felt that a study in the southeastern United States with improved notification might well increase this figure to 5. At this rate, a minimum of 10,000 completed person-years of follow-up would be needed.

The study was planned so that the minimum number of person interviews, examinations, and reinterviews required would be reached within five years. Allowing one year for a pretest, this left four years for the main study. Largely because of limitations in medical manpower and partly because it was considered necessary to gain experience as the study progressed, the decision was reached to partition the sample into four approximately equal parts (each quarter being, of itself, a random stratified sample of the total population aged 50 to 69 years) and to bring one new quarter into the study each year, with short reinterviews each year on all those who had been seen the previous year. This meant that that quarter of the sample seen the first year would be reinterviewed three times at yearly intervals, that quarter seen for the first time during the second year would be reinterviewed twice, and so on (see Table 8.3). The number of lengthy first interviews (which involved gaining the confidence of the respondent) and of medical examinations would thus be held constant from year to year, thought the number of reinterviews would increase. To obtain the required number of person-years of follow-up, it was originally estimated that about 2500 persons per year would be an appropriate quarter-sample, with about 2200 of these actually entering the study (giving all the questionnaire information that was required). A 30 percent systematic stratified random sample of these 2200 would be drawn in turn for the medical examination, yielding an estimated (allowing for refusals and so forth) 500 medical examinations each year. Information obtained by the lay interviewer on his questionnaire would not be made available to the medical examiners so that comparable items in the history obtained by both could later be compared without bias.

To check the quality of the medical examinations, with particular reference to neurological features, it was decided that 10 percent of those given a medical examination would be reexamined by one of a panel of neurologists. A decision was reached on what would constitute a "completed stroke" (simply called a "stroke" elsewhere in this report) for the purpose of this study and arrangements were made for an ongoing medical review of the information being collected.

Provision was made for appropriate reproducibility testing on the laboratory reports, for the standardized collection, recording, and preparation-for-analysis of data, and for a detailed cross-check to see that strokes were not missed, to ensure that strokes which were reported were in fact strokes, and to establish the type of strokes concerned. These matters are discussed further later in this report.

A publicity program was developed which would assist the interviewers in their work and which (at a different level) would bring us the support of the physicians and hospitals in the area.

The questionnaire construction involved problems in translating medical concepts into appropriate and easily understood questions. After specific cerebrovascular disease risk factors were designated and selected for exploration, conferences were held to determine which questions seemed appropriate and in what manner they should be asked. When the final questions for the pilot study were selected, the wording was checked against Dale and Chells' *Formula for Predicting Readability* in an effort to use words which could be comprehended by persons with a grade-school education. Four drafts were submitted to the investigators for revisions and suggestions. The questionnaire was given preliminary use on randomly selected "healthy" people and some persons who had suffered a stroke. Conferences were held with USPHS consultants of the Chronic Disease Program, who contributed freely in suggesting ways of improving the questionnaire.

The basic data for the epidemiology part of the study were gathered by the lay interviewers. These employees were recruited from persons in the community who had had experience in making household surveys in prior occupations. They did not necessarily have prior experience in the field of healthy surveying and therefore had to be specially trained with respect to this rather sensitive and personal area of interviewing. Based on the questionnaire that was developed and upon techniques of home interviewing that were culled from the literature, a handbook was prepared which outlined in detail the hows and whys of the techniques that were to be performed by the interviewer. In the first year of the project, the group of interviewers that were selected underwent a two-week period of daily training sessions in administering the health questionnaire and were given experience in doing so through the pilot study that was performed in a nearby community. Consultants on interview techniques from other health-survey-questionnarie studies were brought in and asked for their suggestions and advice concerning this particular study. In addition, the survey supervisor and the project coordinator had an opportunity to visit and consult with ongoing large-scale health studies in Tecumseh, Michigan, and Framingham Massachusetts. The interviewers were also instructed in the significance of certain of the medical implications of the responses to the health questionnaire by members of the investigator team and by physicians on the staff of the project. Throughout the project, there was regular and constant review of questionnaire techniques and interviewing problems and an opportunity to discuss any special issues which arose as a result of their field work. Since all raw data were to be coded for punch card processing, the interviewers also had to be familiar with this procedure and be able to translate the responses to the appropriate indicated punch card category.

In addition to the basic health questionnaire, the physical examination results were to be as uniform as possible with respect to the questions and the results of the physical examination by the various physicians who participated in the project. The physicians, the project coordinator, and the survey supervisor assisted one another in a cooperative effort to complete a form for recording all the physical examination and laboratory measurement data. Each physician was carefully instructed in its use and preparation for translating the raw data to the necessary computer-coded indices. The technicians that assisted the physicians were also instructed to do their data recording in a similar manner.

Key vital statistics (code number, name, age, race, sex, latest known address, telephone number, name and address of a relative or friend, whether in the physician-examination group, dates when interviewed, examined, and reinterviewed, whether a known stroke, whether died) were kept in a ledger (for the office staff) and on file cards (for the field staff) and were used in arranging each annual reinterview schedule. Each week, each member of the field staff was given an appropriate number of cards identifying the persons to be reinterviewed or brought in for medical examination. (This was in addition to first interviews.) All failures were discussed weekly and a decision made whether to have another try with the same interviewer, to change interviewers (we had both white and Negro interviewers to allow for racial prejudices), to follow up in some other way (e.g. by letter), or to record a nonresponse. It was found possible from the third year on, for reasons of economy and to save manpower, to conduct many of the reinterviews on the telephone.

The investigator team consisted of an epidemiologist (Dr. P. Peacock), who was project director, a psychologist (Dr. S. Raffel), who was project coordinator, a neurologist (Dr. S. Little), a neurosurgeon (Dr. G. Galbraith), a physiatrist (Dr. W. Fleming), and a statistician (Dr. D. Hurst). During the first four years of the project, two full-time physicians (reduced to one in the fourth year) were assigned by the United States Public Health Service to assist in the conduct of the research activities and to perform the necessary physical and laboratory examinations. This was done because of the interest that the Public Health Service had in the epidemiology of cerebrovascular disease. Two full-time physician equivalents were needed and used throughout the course of the project. In addition, the project employed radiology and laboratory consultation and worked closely with the Jefferson County Department of Health and the National Communicable Disease Center in their providing support through additional laboratory studies, especially serology.

All of the data obtained were coded for automatic data-processing devices, and much computer service plus program analysis was provided by members of the staff and statistical consultants to the project. One programmer-analyst equivalent and two assistants gave their full time to the study.

A survey supervisor was employed at the inception of the project, who was chiefly responsible for the training of interviewers, for keeping the response rate as high as possible, and for seeing that the data that were collected were properly transferred from their raw form into the coded materials. This person, together with the project coordinator and in consultation with the investigator team, devised the questionnaire and the medical examination and laboratory forms that were to be used in the data collection process. As the study developed, the services of from four to eight interviewers were required.

The protocol of the rehabilitation study called for a comparison of the progress under treatment of two groups of stroke patients. The total group was to include sixty patients, with the total group evenly divided on a random basis between the experimental group and controls. The experimental group (Group I) would receive treatment and care defined as intensive rehabilitative, while the control group (Group II) would receive care defined as conventional by criteria obtained from the records of treatment prescribed at University Hospital during the year 1964.

More specifically, conventional care for the purpose of this study would include the following procedures limited to application at the bedside of the patient:

1. Medical and surgical procedures listed as being routinely performed during a study of 71 conventional-care patients seen in University Hospital (July 1963 to June 1964).

2. Referral for appropriate surgical procedures associated with cerebrovascular disease.

3. Bedside physical therapy—passive and active exercises.

4. Use of braces, splints, arm slings, and walking frame.

5. Change of position.

6. Brief contact by social service worker either with patient or family during hospital period only.

7. Psychological and/or psychiatric evaluation and consultation involving temporary care for the disturbed, depressed, agitated, or psychotic patient.

Conventional care specifically excluded the following:

1. Speech therapy.

2. Long-term psychological therapy.

3. Application of long-term and intensive physical medicine and rehabilitation techniques, such as (a) physical therapy, (b) occupational therapy, (c) gait training, (d) muscle reeducation, and (e) activities of daily living.

4. Long-term and continuous social caseworker activities with patient or family of patient.

5. Vocational counseling.

The exclusions listed above formed a definition of an intensive and continuous physical-medicine rehabilitation effort.

All subjects would be admitted initially to University Hospital, and those selected for rehabilitation would be transferred at the appropriate time to Spain Rehabilitation Center by the attending physician. Patients in Group I hospitalized at the Spain Rehabilitation Center would be under the supervision of Dr. William Fleming, while those in Group II would be hospitalized at University Hospital under the supervision of either their own physician or a staff physician of the Departments of Medicine, Neurology, or Surgery.

Any resident of the city of Birmingham who had reached his 50th birthday and not yet reached his 70th and who could be diagnosed as having his first cerebrovascular accident not earlier than fourteen days prior to admission was eligible for inclusion. The patient would be admitted to the study after a seventy-two-hour waiting period, with financial assistance applied retroactively to the first day of admission. Because of the high mortality rate associated with hemorrhagic stroke, the admitting physician would select, if possible, persons believed to be having a thrombotic or ischemic stroke, but hemorrhagic accidents would not be excluded.

Every subject in both groups would be followed for as long as necessary to that level of physical, vocational, psychological, and social adjustment from which further improvement did not appear to be occurring. Criteria of physical recovery would be taken from available standard physical measurements. Other areas of adjustment would be evaluated by professional experts in the fields of psychology, social work, and vocational rehabilitation. Follow-up intervals for all subjects in both groups would be once per month for the first three months and every three months thereafter.

The Pilot Study

To test the operating assumptions that had been made and to assist in the construction of a suitable instrument (questionnaire), it was decided that the epidemiological survey should first proceed as a pilot study of an area geographically adjacent to Birmingham and having similar population characteristics. The area chosen was Fairfield, Alabama, a city of 18,000 contiguous with the boundaries of Birmingham. The statistical consultants drew a random sample from the city blocks which would provide approximately 300 respondents in the desired age group (50 to 69 years). The sampling unit was a dwelling with all persons in the selected dwelling being in the sample.

The actual operations consisted of block mapping, publicity and literature distribution, a household listing and dwelling unit survey, and administration of the health questionnaire. The protocol of the study directed that a 30 percent sample of those interviewed receive a physical examination. These were drawn as a stratified random sample of those interviewed. Once selected, the person was notified by the interviewer at home and an appointment was set. As can be expected, there were some minor difficulties, but the cooperation received was usually excellent. It was necessary to have night and Saturday appointments to accommodate the employed population, and help with transport was provided.

To classify the population, each person, based on his replies and the prepared criteria, was placed in one of four groups:

1. Complete stroke.
2. Transient ischemic attack.
3. Stroke prone, Group A.
4. Stroke prone, Group B.

The first group gave a history of a localizing neurological deficit which persisted more than twenty-four hours, while the second gave a history strongly suggestive of transient localizing neurological deficits not accountable for by any other cause. The third group gave a positive history for one or more of diabetes, cardiovascular disease (arteriosclerotic or hypertensive), or a family history of stroke. Stroke prone, Group B, formed a relatively pathology-free group (insofar as cardiocerebrovascular disease was concerned) in a susceptible age group. At the close of the pilot study, 268 respondents out of the 278 in the correct age group and in the dwelling drawn for the sample had been interviewed. This was considered a satisfactorily high response rate (96.4%).

The respondents were classified as follows:

	Number	*Percent*
Complete stroke	15	8
Transient ischemic attack	45	17
Stroke prone, Group A	90	33
Stroke prone, Group B	118	42
	268	100

Of the 80 persons in the questionnaire group (30%) who were called in for examination, examinations were obtained on 64 for an 80 percent response rate.

Each question in the pilot questionnaire was submitted to an exhaustive review to check whether the format was too complicated and the interviewers were missing questions that should have been asked (key positive answers in the main questionnaire led the interviewer into supplementary questionnaires), to check whether the questions asked were understood and the answers were reproducible (45% of the respondents were reinterviewed using another interviewer), and to check (using the physician-examined subsample as a yardstick) whether meaningful and analyzable responses were being obtained.

As a result of the pilot study, extensive changes were made in the questionnaire, which in its final form had 84 questions (mostly with subquestions) in the main questionnaire. The sequence was changed in several places and thus all the questions dealing with visual problems were brought together. For 29 questions the wording was changed. Thus No. 48 "Do you ever strangle or seem to strangle on what you eat or drink?" became No. 44 "Do you ever choke on what you eat or drink?" Similarly, No. 17 "Do you ever get pain in either leg which comes on while walking?" became No. 15 "Do you always get pain in your legs which comes on when walking and then goes away in a few minutes after you stop walking?" Nine questions, such as those asking if the patient had ever been told by a doctor that he had Parkinson's disease or multiple sclerosis, were deleted. Twelve questions were added, such as one asking, "How tall are you now?" (so that the ponderal index could be calculated) and others asking about thyroid disease and gout (not in the original questionnaire). An additional five questions, asking in slightly different words questions which had been asked previously in the questionnaire, were introduced as an internal check on replicability. Color coding was introduced for the various forms in use and all the questions were precoded to speed up and simplify the work of the key punch operator.

As a check on what the physicians were doing, with particular regard to their partly subjective assessment on what constituted a completed stroke, a TIA, or a stroke-prone (Group A or B) individual, forty charts (ten from each of the four physicians) from patients who had been medically examined were drawn at random, the "conclusion" sections were removed, and the four physicians were asked individually to record their evaluations. On each patient there were thus five evaluations: two from whichever physician first examined the patient (including the original record) and three others. The results may be summarized as follows:

Original Physician Evaluation	*Complete Stroke*	*TIA*	*Stroke Prone (A)*	*Stroke Prone (B)*
Number of persons in group	2	5	16	17
Physician agreed with himself	2	4	7	12
Of the other physicians				
None agreed	—	—	1	—
One agreed	1	2	6	4
Two agreed	—	1	6	5
Three agreed	1	2	3	8

As a result of this, the physician history-taking and examination form was substantially rewritten, an attempt was made to define previously undefined terms (such as what constituted "hypertension"), and the examining physicians made a daily habit of reviewing with their colleagues the patients they were seeing. In addition, the services of part-time physicians were largely discontinued.

Originally a letter was sent to a patient's private physician outlining what had been found on the medical examination only if the patient specifically requested and authorized this. As a result of discussions with private physicians during the pilot study, it became routine to send a letter to the private physician (if one was named) in respect to every patient seen.

The laboratory procedures used during the pilot study (glucose tolerance test, hematocrit, urinalysis, chest x-ray, serological test [for syphilis], and ECG) proved to be inadequately comprehensive by existing research standards. Tests for PBI, for serum cholesterol, for serum triglycerides, and for uric acid, together with thermography, pulmonary function testing, further x-rays, and submaximal exercise electrocardiography were added.

The Population Studied, Sampling Procedures, and Analysis

Birmingham, founded in 1870 on the site previously named Elyton, was named after the famous manufacturing city in England. It is the county seat of Jefferson County, Alabama, has an altitude of 600 feet and is located 98 miles north of the capital city of Montgomery, Alabama. Birmingham is the largest industrial city in the South between Atlanta and New Orleans and is serviced by a network of railroads, major airlines, state and federal highways, and a ready water access to the Gulf of Mexico. Its prime industries are the extraction of iron ore and steel refining together with the manufacture of heavy machinery. The city, located in Jones Valley, is surrounded by the most southerly ranges of the Appalchian Mountain system and has extensive deposits of coal, iron ore, limestone, bauxite, graphite, sand, gravel, and hard stone. Its educational facilities range from kindergarten through the doctoral level in almost any field of endeavor. Its medical school is one of the largest in the Southeast and contributes heavily to the city's overall economy.

The city of Birmingham had a population in 1950 of 326,037, in 1960 of 340,887, and in 1970 of 300,910 (decennial census figures). This last reduction largely represents the drift to residential townships within the metropolitan area (Jefferson County) but outside the city limits.

The 1960 census population was used in developing this survey and showed 39.7 percent of the population to be nonwhite compared with 28.7 percent of 293,977 persons for the rest of the county. For the whole county it is noted that nonwhites (99.89% Negro) made up 39 percent of the 1940 population, 37 percent of the 1950 population, and 35 percent of the 1960 population, with a clear downward trend. The median age for the nonwhite population resident in Birmingham in 1960 was 25.0 years compared with 31.6 years for the white population, and both these figures were some four years higher than the figures for the rest of the county. Within the city, the population aged 50 to 69 years was constituted as follows:

	White		*Nonwhites*		
	Male	*Female*	*Male*	*Female*	*Total*
Number aged 50-59 yrs.	10,225	12,172	6,367	7,379	36,143
60-69 yrs.	6,931	9,191	4,243	4,995	25,360
Total	17,156	21,363	10,610	12,374	61,503
Percentage of race-sex group	17.8	19.6	16.7	17.2	18.0

The percentage nonwhite in this age group was 37.4.

In the city of Birmingham in 1960, there were 101,855 households, of which 66,463 were white (average population per household 3.05) and 35,392 were nonwhite (average population per household 3.78). Only 1.4 percent of the total population lived in group quarters (i.e. in institutions and such) and not in one of these households.

The city is divided into 61 census tracts, and in stratifying the population these tracts were divided into seven main strata with one census tract (No. 27), which did not fit into any of these strata, classified separately. Within each stratum, the individual census tracts making up that stratum differed only narrowly from each other and from the following mean (or median) stratum values.

	Stratum							*Census Tract*
Number of census tracts	I	II	III	IV	V	VI	VII	*No. 27*
in stratum	9	11	6	8	10	8	8	1
Percent of population nonwhite	5.3	7.7	5.4	35.1	57.1	92.2	93.5	5.0
Median schooling (head of household)	12.2	11.1	12.0	9.2	8.5	8.6	7.6	9.0
Median household income	6932	5331	4517	4192	3159	3174	1842	1704
Median age (male)	32.1	30.4	35.0	27.0	24.6	23.8	25.3	41.3
Median age (female)	33.4	32.7	41.3	29.4	28.3	27.2	28.7	50.2
Population per household	3.25	3.18	2.68	3.48	3.65	3.90	3.31	1.54
Percent of males in labor force	84.2	80.2	79.4	77.0	73.2	69.5	74.1	50.2
Percent of males unemployed	2.6	4.1	6.0	7.3	9.4	11.4	9.4	8.9
Percent of females in labor force	33.6	36.1	46.2	34.9	34.6	37.8	45.1	42.0
Percent of females unemployed	3.5	4.4	3.7	7.5	7.9	7.1	8.6	8.2
Population in stratum aged 50-69 years	7825	11,956	9560	8786	8188	8243	6143	804

Each year within each stratum, a census tract (the primary sampling unit, or P.S.U.) was drawn on a probability proportional to size and without replacement. Additional census tracts were then chosen (again at random with a probability proportional to size) from whichever stratum happened to have the largest residual population in the age group 50 to 69 years (after subtracting the populations of those census tracts which had already been drawn as P.S.U's) until the total potential population drawn exceeded 10,000. Census tract number 27 was included in the first year's draw. It will be appreciated that over four years, at least two-thirds of all census tracts could be expected to have been drawn as P.S.U.'s, while any one year's sample would be comparable with that from any other year.

Once a census tract had been drawn as a P.S.U., a detailed block map was obtained and each block in the P.S.U. was counted and numbered. One-quarter of the blocks in each P.S.U. were then drawn as a simple random sample, and every person in the desired age group (50 to 69 years) resident in those blocks which had been drawn constituted the sample to be interviewed. It was expected that this would yield 2500 (or slightly more) persons each year with whom an interview would be attempted. The actual number of persons aged 50 to 69 years who were resident in the blocks drawn by this statistical method over the four years of the main study was 9334 (an average of 2341 per year). Fortunately a better-than-expected interview response rate was obtained and the required 8800 persons were actually interviewed (see Table 8.2). It appears that the reason for this difficulty was the decrease in the population of the city over the decade 1960-70 (see earlier in this section of the report), which had not been anticipated in the planning.

The other samplings used in this study were a 30 percent draw from the questionnaire-interviewed group for physician examination, a 10 percent draw from the physician-examined group for neurological examination, and a 50 percent draw of those considered suitable for the rehabilitation experiment for inclusion in the intensive rehabilitation group. For each of the strata within these samplings, an appropriate number of sealed envelopes were prepared ahead of time (with the desired percentage of "to-be-included-in-the-study" instructions) and for each person under consideration an envelope was allocated at random. The questionnaire-interviewed group was stratified for the pilot study into apparent clinical groupings (see under "Pilot Study" for details) and for the main study into age-race-sex groups. The physician-examined group was divided into "suspect strokes" (completed stroke or TIA) and "others," and after the first year of the study the sample for neurological examination included all the suspect strokes and a sufficient sample from the "others" to bring the proportion up to 10 percent. The "suitable-for-rehabilitation" group was stratified into staff patients and private patients.

Once collected, the data were checked and punched (the forms were all precoded) onto IBM cards. One or two summary cards were then prepared per respondent (one for the interviewer data and one for the physician and laboratory data) with provision on each for the entry of relevant reinterview, hospital, or death data. These summary cards could then be handled much easier on the computer (most of the analysis was done on an IBM 1740) than could the variable number of basic cards (up to twenty per respondent) held in the main deck. For each of the variables which have been analyzed, an edit program has been run to exclude "impossible" results, and several printouts of selected variables have been made, which could be checked against the data on the original record forms.

For the rehabilitation study, all the forms used were developed locally, using consultants as necessary, and were pretested. Each form was precoded for computer analysis. The numbers involved in this study have, however, been so small (*q.v.*) that all the analyses performed on these data have been hand-tabulated.

Throughout the "Results" and "Discussion" sections of this report, the various risk factors (independent variables) are discussed in terms of relative risk (*R.R.*).

		Disease (dependent variable) Present	Absent
Risk factor (independent variable)	*Present*	a	b
	Absent	c	d

By definition, the relative risk associated with a risk factor is the ratio of the incidence of some given disease (outcome) among those exposed to the factor to the incidence of the disease among those not exposed to the factor. For the above 2 × 2 table,

$$R.R. = \frac{a}{a+b} \cdot \frac{c+d}{c}$$

In terms of the definition, a relative risk can be obtained in a prospective study but cannot be obtained in a case-control retrospective study, since such a study does not yield incidence figures. A prevalence study (a retrospective or cross-sectional study of a total population sample which has been appropriately weighted if different sampling fractions were used for various strata) will give an approximation to a relative risk provided the prevalence-incidence ratios in the exposed (to the risk factor) and nonexposed groups are approximately the same. Thus, if a risk factor increases the case fatality rate or shortens the life expectancy of persons who experience the disease (outcome) being used as a dependent variable vis-à-vis those persons who do not have the risk factor, then the relative risk obtained will be in error. Usually the assumption has been made that the presence or absence of a risk factor does not alter the prevalence-incidence ratio.

It can be shown[47] that the size of a relative risk associated with one risk factor is directly influenced by the prevalence of other risk factors in the same population, and with independent risk factors with independent pure risks this relationship can be expressed by the equation

$$R.R._{A(B'C'...N')} = \frac{1-a\Omega_{B'C'...N'}}{1-\bar{a}\Omega_{B'C'...N'}}$$

(the relative risk of risk factor *A* in the presence of risk factor *B*, *C*, etc.)

where $\Omega_{B'C'...N'} = \Omega_{B'}\Omega_{C'}...\Omega_{N'}$

and $\Omega_{B'} = [\bar{b}-p_B(\bar{b}-b)]$

and p_B is the proportion of the population with risk factor *B*

and $(1-b)$ is the pure risk (the risk in the absence of other risk factors) of developing disease associated with risk factor *B*

and $(1-\bar{b})$ is the pure risk of developing disease among persons who do not have risk factor *B*

It is noted that (modified from Cornfield[48])

$$R.R. = \frac{a}{c} \cdot \frac{c+d}{a+b} = \frac{ad}{bc}$$

where c is "small" compared with d and a is "small" compared with b (i.e. the incidence of the disease in both exposed and nonexposed groups is "small"). Under these circumstances, the relative risk can be approximated by the odds ratio (cross ratio) or $\frac{ad}{bc}$. This is the situation in the prospective part of this study. In the retrospective part of the study, the differences betwen the relative risk and the odds ratio [actually an amended form of it

$$\frac{(2a+1)\ (2d+1)}{(2b+1)\ (2c+1)}$$

suggested by Haldane[49]] are larger but fortunately of little practical importance. Thus for the 26 relative risks in Table 8.5a which are greater than 1, the odds ratios are on the average 5.7 percent bigger than their corresponding relative risks, but for those relative risks of less than 3 (and these are the ones for which statistical significance becomes questionable) the average difference is only 3.6.

Whether a relative risk is significantly greater than 1 can be established using the standard 2 × 2 equation for χ^2 (calculated, but not shown in the tables to save space), but this does not enable us to compare two relative risks or to compare the relative risk we have obtained with some arbitrary standard. To obtain a variance (this is only applicable when the relative risk can be approximated by the odds ratio, as was the situation in this study), the best technique appears to be that of Woolf[50] as modified by Haldane[49] and later by Sheehe,[51] whereby we make the transformation

$$y = \ln \frac{(2a+1)\ (2d+1)}{(2c+1)\ (2b+1)}$$

$$\text{and } V(y) = \frac{1}{a+1} + \frac{1}{b+1} + \frac{1}{c+1} + \frac{1}{d+1}$$

(Haldane's own equation does not allow for two cells being zero.) This approach has been used for the tables given in this study.

When dealing with small numbers, even a large relative risk may not be significantly greater than 1 and, rather than looking at the relative risk per se, one looks for a $y/S.E.(y)$ value that is greater than t for $n - 2$ degrees of freedom (n here is the number of stroke). Consider white males aged 50 to 59 years (Table 8.7b) for an example. Here $n - 2 = 4$. The largest relative risk in this category is for hardened arteries (14.89) based on $a=2$ and $y/S.E.(y) = 3.79$. The tabulated t values for 4 degrees of freedom are 2.78 for $p < 0.05$ and 4.60 for $p < 0.01$. With small numbers like this it is not difficult to work out the exact probability, and we find (on the assumption that hardened arteries and strokes are independent) that the probability of getting 2 or more strokes among the 38 persons (out of 1170) with hardened arteries is

0.014, or $0.01 < p < 0.05$. Unfortunately when the *a* cells in this study have a value of 1, the modification of the odds ratio (q.v.) introduced by Haldane[49] and used in the tabulations for this study grossly overestimates the true odds ratio $\frac{ad}{bc}$ and the relative risk. Conversely in those (isolated) examples where the *c* cells have a value of 1, the modified odds ratio grossly underestimates the true odds ratio. Thus we will, when considering statistical significance for examples when *a* or *c* equals 1, use $y = \ln \left(\frac{ad}{bc}\right)$ rather than the *y* value given in the tables. In addition, when $a =$ 1, 2, or 3, we will use

$$V(y) = \frac{1}{a} + \frac{1}{b} + \frac{1}{c} + \frac{1}{d}$$ [50]

rather than the tabulated value since, under these circumstances, Sheehe's modification underestimates the variance (in the "hardened arteries" example given above this would reduce $y/S.E.(y)$ to 3.23).

Considerable thought was given to whether the results should be given in the form of morbidity ratios (rather than relative risks) as has been done for the Framingham study (*q.v.*). The equation for the morbidity ratio (M.R.), using our 2×2 table, is

$$M.R. = \frac{a(a+b+c+d)}{(a+b)(a+c)}$$

and it is noted that

$$\frac{M.R.}{R.R.} = \frac{ac+bc+cd+c^2}{ac+ad+cd+c^2}$$

so that the *M.R.* will equal the *R.R.* if and only if $bc = ad$ (i.e. the odds ratio = 1) and for an odds ratio greater than 1, then $R.R. > M.R.$ It was decided that the relative risk gave a more direct picture of the situation, but for the benefit of other investigators who may wish to use other measures of excess risk, the values for *a, b, c,* and *d* have been given in the tables.

Standard tests of significance must be applied with great caution when looking at 62 variables simultaneously, as in this study. We were not aware of any established method. While not entirely comparable (because we were using varying though overlapping controls in this study), the tables prepared by Dunnett[52] for comparing several treatments with a control appeared to be usable, but unfortunately the tables extended to only nine treatments. Based on these tables, however, a t for a two-sided comparison between the 62 relative risks and the control value of 1 for a joint confidence coefficient of $P = 95$ percent can safely be assumed to be not greater than 4.76 ($d.f. = 120$), and for $P = 99$ percent, not greater than 5.29 (d.f. = 120).

The Variables Being Studied

The dependent variable in the epidemiological study (both retrospective and prospective) was a stroke, divided for the purpose of the prospective study into thrombotic stroke, embolic stroke, cerebral hemorrhage, and subarachnoid hemorrhage. A localizing neurological deficit which persisted for longer than twenty-four hours, for which no other cause was detected, and which was confirmed by a physician constituted a completed stroke. Every attempt was made to ensure that all suspect strokes were recorded and all the relevant information collected about them. This was done as follows:

1. All persons in the questionnaire interview group were asked to notify of anything resembling a stroke. Preaddressed, prestamped postcards, which only needed to be dropped into the mail, were given to each person. As an extra encouragement, anyone notifying of a stroke was offered inclusion in the rehabilitation study, which would pick up the cost of rehabilitative care. Suspect strokes were investigated in detail.

2. The annual reinterview probed extensively for any history which might suggest a stroke. If they would accept and there was any doubt, anyone with such a history was brought in for a neurological examination.

3. All the physicians in the community were asked to notify regarding strokes and provide relevant information on each case they saw.

4. The records of the stroke registry (conducted by a separate staff), which investigated every hospital record in which "stroke" (or an equivalent term) was mentioned for every hospital in the

three-county area surrounding Birmingham, were cross-checked and the relevant hospital extracts taken.

5. The county death records were reviewed. For all deaths (including strokes) within the study population, death certificates and autopsy records (if any autopsy had been done) were obtained.

The independent variables from the questionnaire-interviewer study (retrospective and prospective) which have been developed and analyzed in this report are all history items and are as follows: In the retrospective part of the study, where a history of a previous (old) stroke was obtained, the rest of the interview was restructured by adding the words "Before your stroke did you. . .?" to each question. This was to exclude, as far as possible, complaints which occurred as a result of the stroke.

1. *High blood pressure.* A respondent was classified as giving a history of high blood pressure if he answered "Yes" to all three of the sequential questions "Have you ever had your blood pressure checked?", "Did he say your blood pressure was high?", and "Did the doctor give you any medicine for your blood pressure at that time?" The reason for including this third requirement was the very high proportion (39% of the first 3000 patients seen) of respondents answered "Yes" to the first two questions and the clinical feeling that if the doctor had taken his findings seriously he would have initiated some treatment. Twenty-five percent of the 3802 respondents in this study met all three requirements.

2. *Diabetes.* A respondent was classified as giving a history of diabetes if he answered "Yes" to "Has a doctor ever told you that you had diabetes, or sugar diabetes?" and in reply to the question "What kinds of treatment have you had for diabetes?" answered "Yes" to one or more of "Detailed diet instructions," "Oral medication," or "Insulin injections." The addition of this second requirement led to a reduction in the proportion of respondents recorded as giving a history of diabetes from 7.1 percent to 5.9 percent.

3. *Heart attack.* A respondent was classified as giving a history of a heart attack if he answered "Yes" to the question "Have you ever had a heart attack?" The additional questions which

were asked about the when, where, and nature of the heart attack and how it was treated (see, however, under "Chest pain") did not add to the discriminant value of this single question. Five percent of the study population gave this history.

4. *Chest pain.* A respondent was classified as giving a history of chest pain if he answered "Yes" to the question "Have you ever had a severe pain across the front of your chest lasting for half an hour or more?" or, having given a history of a heart attack (see above), answered "Yes" to "Did you have any pain in your chest with these attacks?" Eight percent of the study population gave this history.

5. *Intermittent claudication.* A positive history was a "Yes" response to "Do you always get pain in your legs which comes on while walking and then goes away in a few minutes after you stop walking?" Four and nine-tenths percent of the study population gave this history.

6. *Hardening of arteries.* A positive history was a "Yes" response to "Have you ever been told by a doctor that you had hardening of the arteries?" Three and five-tenths percent of the study population gave this history.

7. *Pounding in head.* A positive history was a "Yes" response to "Do you ever hear or seem to feel a pounding or beating in your head?" Five and nine-tenths percent of the study population gave this history.

8. *Weight increase of more than twenty pounds.* This history was obtained by subtracting the answer to "How much did you weigh when you were 30 years of age? from the answer to "How much do you weigh now?" Thirty-three percent of the study population gave this history.

9. *Ponderal index of less than twelve.* The height in inches (obtained from the question "How tall are you now?") was divided by the cube root of the present weight in pounds (see above). Thirty-three percent of the study population fell into this category.

10. *Shortness of breath.* A positive history was a "Yes" response to "Have you ever been troubled with shortness of breath

before you expected to be, or for no good reason?" Seven and nine-tenths percent of the study population gave this history.

11. *Gout.* A positive history was a "Yes" to either "Have you ever had gout?" or "Have you ever had joint pain of the big toe?" Six and two-tenths percent of the study population gave this history.

12. *Cigarette smoker.* A cigarette smoker was defined as a person who had smoked more than ten cigarettes a day in the last two years or (for the retrospective study) in the two years preceding the stroke. This information was obtained from the conditional questions "Have you ever smoked?", "Do you smoke now? Cigarettes?", "About how many do/did you smoke a day, on the average?", "How many years have/did you smoke(d) this amount per day?", and "When did you quit smoking?" coupled with (if relevant) the recorded date of the first stroke. Using this definition, 21 percent of the study population were classified as cigarette smokers.

13. *Alcohol drinker.* An alcohol drinker was defined as a person who answered "Yes" to either "Do you drink any alcoholic beverage, such as beer, wine or whiskey?" or "Did you ever drink any alcoholic beverages?", and whose answer to the question "About how often do (did) you have a drink?" fell into the once-a-month-or-more-frequently category. Using this definition, 24 percent of the study population were classified as alcohol drinkers.

14. *Family history.* A positive history was a "Yes" response to "Do you know if anyone in your family has ever had a stroke?" The strict logic of this question might be queried, but it seemed to be understood in the form that was intended. Further information was obtained on which family members had been affected, but attempts to quantify this were not successful. Thirty-six percent of the study population gave a family history as defined.

15. *Temporary weakness of arm or leg.* A positive history was a "Yes" response to "Have you ever had an unexplained weakness or loss of strength of an arm or leg which lasted only a short while? Three and eight-tenths percent of the study population gave this history.

16. *Temporary weakness of face.* A positive history was a

"Yes" response to "Have you ever had such a weakness (referring to the above question) of either side of your face?" One and four-tenths percent of the study population gave this history.

17. *Sensory loss involving arm or leg.* A positive history was a "Yes" response to either "Have you ever had a loss of feeling or numbness of an arm or leg about which you became worried?" or "Have you ever burned your hands or feet and not felt the pain?" Six and six-tenths percent of the study population gave this history.

18. *Loss of eyesight.* An attempt was made to distinguish between a chronic condition as asked for by "Do you have any trouble with your eyesight that glasses do not take care of?" and a short-term loss as asked for by "Have you ever had any trouble with your eyes, such as spells of blindness in one or both eyes, with the sight returning in a few minutes or a few hours?", "Have you ever had spells of half-blindness in one or both eyes so that you only see half of things when you look right at them?" and "Have you ever had dimness or loss of eyesight which lasted a few minutes or more?" The questions were, however, poorly understood, and for our purposes here a "Yes" answer to any of these questions has been taken as a positive history. Using these criteria, 20 percent of the study population gave a history of loss of eyesight.

19. *Double vision.* A positive history was a "Yes" response to "Have you ever had spells when you see two things where there should be only one?" Six and six-tenths percent of the study population gave this history.

20. *Incoordination.* A positive history was a "Yes" response to either "Do you often drop things out of your hand without being able to stop it? or "Do you ever have a shaking or jerking of your arms or legs that you cannot control?" Nine and eight-tenths percent of the study population gave this history.

21. *Fainting or blackouts.* A positive history was a "Yes" response to any of the questions "In the past 10 years have you ever had fainting or falling-out spells?", "Do you ever have spells when you suddenly get weak in the knees and fall?", or "Have you ever had blackout spells?" Eight and four-tenths percent of the study population gave this history.

22. *Headaches.* A positive history was an answer to the question "About how often do you get a headache?" indicating that headaches were occurring at monthly or shorter intervals. Twenty-three percent of the study population gave this history.

23. *Deafness.* A positive history was a "Yes" response to "Do you think you are getting deaf?" Eleven percent of the study population gave this history.

24. *Speech disturbances.* A positive history was a "Yes" response to any of the questions "Do you ever have trouble finding the right words in trying to say things just as clearly as they seem in your mind?", "Do you ever have spells where what you say is not what you wanted to say?", or "Are there ever times when your speech becomes thick like having a mouth full of mush?" Ten percent of the study population gave this history.

25. *Confusion.* A positive history was a "Yes" response to "Are there ever times when you just get mixed up and confused which last a few minutes or hours?" Three and seven-tenths percent of the study population gave this history.

26. *Choking.* A positive history was a "Yes" response to "Are there times when you have choking spells, or difficulty in swallowing?" Six and three-tenths percent of the study population gave this history.

27. *Dizziness.* A positive history was a "Yes" response to any of the questions "Do you ever get dizzy spells?", "Do you ever get dizzy enough to have trouble with your balance when you stand or sit up suddenly?", "Do you often, for no known reason, lose your balance or stagger while walking?", or "Does looking up and twisting your head to one side ever bring on a dizzy spell?" Twenty-four percent of the study population gave this history.

28. *Memory loss.* A respondent was classified (for the prospective study only) as giving a history of memory loss if he answered "Yes" to the question "Have you had enough trouble with your memory to interfere with your work or getting along with people?" Two percent of the study population gave this history.

29. *Transient ischemic attacks (TIA).* To define a TIA from the interviewer study, the decision was reached to take all the questions relating to possible temporary cerebral dysfunction and form a composite. The diagnosis of TIA was thus recorded if

"Yes" answers were received to three or more of the following questions:

1. Have you ever had an unexplained weakness or loss of strength of an arm or leg which lasted only a short while?
2. Have you ever had such a weakness of either side of your face?
3. Have you ever had a loss of feeling or numbness of an arm or leg about which you became worried?
4. Have you ever had a loss of feeling over most of your body?
5. Have you ever had a weakness or loss of strength over most of one side of your body?
6. Have you ever burned your hands or feet and not felt the pain?
7. Have you ever had any trouble with your eyes, such as spells of blindness in one or both eyes, with the sight returning in a few minutes or a few hours?
8. Have you ever had spells of half-blindness in one or both eyes so that you only see half of things when you look right at them?
9. Have you ever had dimness or loss of your eyesight which lasted a few minutes or more?
10. Have there ever been times when you were looking at objects and they seemed to be floating around in the air?
11. Have you ever had spells when you see two things where there should be only one?
12. In the past 10 years have you ever had fainting or falling-out spells?
13. Do you ever have spells when you suddenly get weak in the knees and fall?
14. Have you ever had blackout spells?
15. Do you ever have trouble finding the right word in trying to say things just as clearly as they seem in your mind?
16. Do you ever have spells where what you say is not what you wanted to say?
17. Are there ever times you just get mixed up and confused which last a few minutes or hours?
18. Are there ever times when your speech becomes thick, like having a mouth full of mush?
19. Are there times when you have choking spells, or difficulty in swallowing?
20. Do you ever choke on what you eat or drink?

During the course of the questionnaire-interviewer study, information was also collected with regard to occupational history, head injuries, the occurrence of fits, poliomyelitis, getting along with people, nervous or mental trouble, memory defects, thyroid disease, and tinnitus. On investigation, it appeared that this information was either unreliable or could not be classified and we have not proceeded further with the analysis thereof.

The independent variables about which information was obtained from the physician-examined group of respondents may be considered in four categories. In the first category are items from the medical history (structured but not given a formed phraseology), in the second are items from the medical examination, in the third are testing procedures conducted at the time of the respondent's visit, and in the fourth category are laboratory procedures done elsewhere on specimens which were collected during the examination. The variables which have been developed and analyzed in this report are as follows: For each of the history and examination variables, the physician was asked to grade his patient on a scale running through Code 0 (no data), 1 (absent), 2 (questionable), 3 (mild, a few, a little), 4 (moderate), to 5 (severe, very many). When these variables have been dichotomized in the analysis into "variable present," "variable absent," a code value of three or more has been taken (unless otherwise specified) as indicating that the variable concerned was present.

Physician history items were as follows:

1. *Hypertension.* Any history of hypertension was recorded (Code 3). Code 4 indicated that treatment was required and Code 5 that some target organ was involved.

2. *Diabetes.* Code 3 indicated adult-onset type controlled by diet or medication, Code 4 indicated that insulin was required, and Code 5 indicated definite target organ involvement including retinopathy.

3. *Ischemic heart disease.* This covered a history of angina pectoris (Code 3 being probable, Code 4 definite, and Code 5 angina at rest) and/or a history of myocardial infarction (Code 3 being associated with intense, prolonged anginal pain, Code 4 with clear-cut ECG changes, and Code 5 with two or more infarctions).

4. *Valvular heart disease.* Code 3 covered a history of heart murmur, Code 4 definite asymptomatic valvular disease, and Code 5 symptomatic valvular disease.

5. *Cardiac dysrhythmias.* Code 3 covered a history of fre-

quent palpitations, Code 4 atrial fibrillation, and Code 5 problem symptomatology and a history of treatment.

6. *Congestive heart failure.* Code 3 covered a history of probable failure, Code 4 paroxysmal nocturnal dyspnea and orthopnea, and Code 5 intractable failure.

7. *Intermittent claudication.* Code 3 covered a history of calf pain which spontaneously disappeared so that walking could be continued, Code 4 calf pain which stabilized at a variable level of intensity, and Code 5 pain which became worse and forced the patient to stop walking.

8. *Decreased monocular vision.* As per the general coding, but excluding refractive errors.

9. *Decreased binocular vision.* As per the general coding, but excluding refractive errors.

10. *Diplopia.* As per the general coding.

11. *Vertigo.* As per the general coding, looking for a true rotary whirling and excluding simple giddiness and nausea.

12. *Deafness.* Code 3 covered a history of nonhandicapping impairment, Code 4 a mild handicap, and Code 5 near-total to total deafness.

13. *Memory deterioration.* As per the general coding, using the response to the general question "Do you think your memory has decreased in the last few years?".

14. *Hypothyroidism.* As per the general coding.

In addition to the above items, the physician's history also covered a family history, a record of parental death ages (this information duplicating on a subsample that already obtained by the lay interviewers), and a history of embolic, thrombotic, and hemorrhagic disorders, together with the use of anticoagulants (not used as independent variables but as aids in determining whether a possible TIA or completed stroke had occurred or not). Other conditions asked about were syphilis, polycythemia, hypoglycemia, gout, the menopausal syndrome, seizures, syncope, hemiplegia, monoplegia, facial paresis, extrapyramidal disorders, cerebellar disorders, tinnitus, dysarthria, dysphagia, and dysphasia together with the use (or misuse) of alcohol and tobacco. Except for the last two items mentioned (which duplicated what had already been obtained by the lay interviewers), the number giving a positive history for any one item were too small to use them as independent variables and their chief use has been in developing a total diagnostic patient profile.

Physician examination items were as follows:

15. *Arcus senilis*. An incomplete light ring was given Code 3, a complete ring was given Code 4, and a complete heavy ring was given Code 5.

16. *Arteriosclerotic optic fundi*. Early compression of the vein at an arterial crossing with beginning copper-wire arterial light streak was given Code 3. Tapering of the veins with some sheathing of the arteries and a marked copper-wire appearance was Code 4. A silver-wire appearance of the light streak and marked perivascular sheathing were Code 5.

17. *Optic fundi (Keith Wagner Scale)*. Code 3 (K.W. grade 2) covered arteriolar narrowing to half (or less) of the corresponding veins, Code 4 (K.W. grade 3) flame-shaped hemorrhages and/or cotton wool patches, and Code 5 (K.W. grade 4) edema and blurring of the optic disk.

18. *Congestive heart failure (examination)*. Cardiomegaly, an S-3 Gallop and/or peripheral edema and venous distension was given Code 3; orthopnea, rales, tachycardia, Code 4; and pulmonary edema and/or anasarca, Code 5.

19. *Valvular heart disease (examination)*. Code 3 covered a single valve murmur without cardiomegaly, Code 4 a single valve murmur with some functional impairment, and Code 5 multiple valve involvement or a single valve murmur with severe impairment.

20. *Dysrhythmia (examination)*. Code 3 covered premature contractions, Code 4 atrial fibrillation, and Code 5 any other arrhythmia.

21. *Cervical bruits*. A Code 3 bruit was loud and filled systole while a Code 4 had an additional short diastolic component and a Code 5 a long diastolic component.

22. *Supraclavicular bruits.* As for cervical bruits.

Additional examination items which were recorded but have not been analyzed in detail because of the small numbers involved were a check for hypothyroidism and gout. A complete neurological examination was done looking for evidence of TIA or stroke (the dependent variable). Cardiomegaly was recorded but it was felt that the chest x-ray gave a better objective measure of this parameter. Peripheral pulses (the dorsalis pedis and posterior tibial arteries) were felt for and recorded, but the interexaminer reproducibility of these estimates of peripheral vascular disease was so bad that further analysis was not done.

Testing procedures recorded at the time of the patients' visits and subsequently analyzed as independent variables were the following:

23. *Blood pressure.* Arterial blood pressures were measured using a mercury-columnated sphygmomanometer with a 13-cm cuff. All measurements were made (after the physician completed his history and physical examination) by trained technicians who were periodically checked for accuracy and method. The brachial blood pressures were recorded in both arms after five minutes' delay with the patient sitting, with the patient recumbent for five minutes, and immediately upon standing from recumbency. The blood pressures used for the main analysis in this report are those from the right arm (unless there was some physical difficulty in taking from the right arm) in the sitting position. Systolic pressures were recorded from the appearance of sound (first phase) and diastolic pressures as the cessation of sound (fifth phase). Where the fifth phase was absent, the fourth phase was recorded.

For the analysis of the blood pressures (systolic and diastolic), they have been trichotomized since it seemed possible that the relationship between blood pressure and stroke might not be linear. The cutting points which were chosen (134 and 156 for systolic and 82 and 90 for diastolic) were based on the following table for systolic pressures and a similar one for diastolic pressures obtained at the end of the second year of the study and represented the thirtieth and seventieth percentiles for the total population.

	Total	*White males*		*White females*		*N/White males*		*N/White females*	
Percentile	*population*	*50-59*	*60-69*	*50-59*	*60-69*	*50-59*	*60-69*	*50-59*	*60-96*
90	182	170	176	168	180	186	195	220	216
80	166	155	162	152	164	178	180	200	190
70	156	150	158	142	158	168	172	170	180
60	150	142	150	140	150	160	162	158	170
50	140	138	142	136	140	142	154	148	160
40	138	132	140	130	136	140	150	142	150
30	134	130	134	125	130	136	140	136	140
20	124	122	130	120	120	130	134	130	140
10	116	116	120	112	112	120	130	130	130
N	967	141	142	184	227	51	60	69	93

24. *Resting electrocardiogram.* Standard twelve-lead electrocardiograms were taken and coded according to the Minnesota code by a single observer. The three indices of electrocardiographic abnormality which have been in our analysis for this report were abnormal Q-waves (code items 111-117, 121-128), abnormal R-waves (code items 31, 33) and abnormal ST-T segments (code items 41-43 read in conjunction with code items 51-53).

25. *Thermography.* Supraorbital skin temperatures were recorded on both sides using a thermocouple accurate to within 0.4 degree Fahrenheit. A difference of one degree Fahrenheit or greater between the two sides of the head was treated as an independent variable for purposes of analysis.

26. *Ponderal index (physician group).* Height and weight were recorded and a ponderal index (height in inches divided by the cube root of the weight in pounds) calculated for the physician-examined group.

27. *Chest x-rays.* Chest x-rays were obtained using a special cassette and grid which made possible accurate measurements of heart size.

28. *Submaximal exercise electrocardiography.* A subgroup of the physician-examined group who were free of handicapping dyspnea on exercise, physical deformities, or acute illness and who did not have second- or third-degree heart block, LBBB, or ST-T changes (code 41-43, 51-53) on a standard resting ECG were given a submaximal exercise electrocardiogram. Recordings of V5 were obtained continuously as the patient built up to 90 percent of his predicted maximal heart rate and maintained this level

for two minutes. The target heart rate was attained as quickly as was reasonable by gradually increasing both treadmill grade (starting at 10%) and speed (starting at 1.7 mph). The signal was under continuous observation on the oscilloscope and the test was terminated if necessary. A positive test was an ST segment depression of 0.1 millivolts or greater beginning with J-point depression and continuing flat or downsloping for a duration at least equivalent to the QRS duration before returning to the isoelectric line.

29. *Vital capacity.* This was recorded using the best of three readings obtained on the Pulmonor. The reproducibility of this test in this age group was found to be poor, and the introduction of corrections for age, sex, and body build tended to confuse rather than clarify the issue.

30. *Transient ischemic attacks (TIA).* The physicians doing the examinations made a clinical decision on each patient, based on the total history and examination, as to whether that patient had suffered a TIA, and this decision was recorded. There was some question whether TIA (diagnosed in this fashion) was to be regarded as an independent variable or as a part of the stroke complex (i.e. part of the dependent variable, which would have meant excluding individuals with this diagnosis from the prospective study). Because of the subjective nature of this diagnosis, it was eventually decided to use TIA as an independent variable for the prospective study.

Laboratory procedures which were done and which have been analyzed as independent variables were the following:

31. *Blood glucose.* This was measured two hours after an oral load of 75 gm of carbohydrate (Galaxy GTT 75 Dextrose cola beverage). This determination was done on an autoanalyzer.

32. *Serum cholesterol.* This was obtained by solvent distribution of the saponified lipid fraction fractionated between petroleum ethers and aqueous alcohol (the ALBK method).

33. *Serum triglycerides.* This was obtained by the direct assay of lipid glycerol from which the phospholipid glycerol (together with most of the mono-and diglycerides) was physically removed.

These variables can be considered together. In the analysis, each has been trichotomized since it seemed possible that their relationship with stroke incidence might not be linear. The cutting points used were the seventieth percentile for the upper cut (established at the end of the second year of the study) on all three, the thirtieth percentile for the lower cut on serum cholesterol, and the tenth percentile for the lower cut on blood glucose and triglycerides. Thus, the upper and lower cutting points were as follows:

	Upper	*Lower*
Blood glucose	150 mg/100 ml	90 mg/100 ml
Serum cholesterol	277 mg/100 ml	227 mg/100 ml
Serum triglycerides	4 mEq/liter	2 mEq/liter

For the first two years of the main study, the laboratory determinations were done by the Medical Laboratory Section of the National Communicable Disease Center, Atlanta. It then became necessary to transfer the laboratory work to the State Public Health Laboratory in Birmingham, which had not previously done this kind of work. During the transition period, the Communicable Disease Center laboratory (CDC) was too swamped with work (from the large Cooperative Coronary Disease Diet Project) for a replication study (with a quick response) with them to be possible. However, twenty-six serum samples were divided into four equal parts and each part was given a different (false) name. Then, without the two laboratories knowing that a test was being conducted, two of the parts were sent to the local laboratory (PHL) and the other two parts to a large reputable laboratory (UML) on the West Coast. The results, insofar as serum cholesterol is concerned, may be summarized as follows. Note that the CDC values are not directly comparable with the other two since they are based on a different (larger) population. The PHL and UML values used for the percentile figures are each a mean of separate values.

Steps were taken to correct this, and subsequent CDC report graded PHL as "A Satisfactory" though one noted that the PHL values were still some 4 percent higher than the CDC median reference laboratory values. The small increase in the proportion of serum cholesterol values in excess of 277 mg% found in the last two years of the study (34.2% compared with 30% in the first two years of the study) is probably accounted for by this.

SERUM CHOLESTEROL VALUES IN MG%

Percentile	*CDC (values from years 1 and 2)*	*PHL (trial group)*	*UML (trial group)*
10	192	198	192
20	208	227	211
30	227	254	220
40	238	265	225
50	250	270	233
60	261	298	240
70	277	306	248
80	297	334	250
90	324	390	289
Mean difference between the two values on each patient done in one laboratory		17.8	11.1
Standard deviation of above		17.1	10.7
Mean difference between the two mean values obtained for each patient, comparing labs		52.2	(for 23 of the 26 means, the PHL value was the higher)
Standard deviation of above		32.1	

Additional laboratory procedures which were done but which are not analyzed as independent variables in this report were estimates of uric acid and protein-bound iodine (PBI) and a packed cell volume (hematocrit). Preliminary analyses showed no relationship between these parameters and the incidence of stroke. The analysis for the epidemiological study thus deals with sixty-two independent variables.

For the rehabilitation study, the patients admitted to the randomized group were assessed on entry to the study and this assessment compared with a final assessment done when no further improvement seemed likely. Each assessment was from a composite picture compiled using standardized reports from a psychiatrist, a neurologist, an occupational therapist, a nurse, a psychologist, a speech therapist, a physiotherapist, a social worker, and a vocational therapist. The standard forms used were developed locally and are available on request. This assessment was in terms of personal-care status and vocational status.

Personal Care

The levels and criteria used were as follows:

1. *Bed patient.* Completely dependent in bed.

2. *Requires custodial care.* An individual who may be able to sit in a wheelchair or stand with support but who is essentially dependent upon attendant care for help in necessary personal care or daily activities such as eating, dressing, and toilet.

3. *Requires assistance at home.* An individual who is capable of functioning at home with minimal attendant care.

4. *Completely independent at home.* An individual who is able to care for himself during the day without requiring assistance, thus releasing someone else from the home.

5. *Requires limited assistance outside the home.* An individual who is capable of performing the essential activities independently within the home but who requires assistance occasionally or under special circumstances for elevation, travel, and toilet activities or else needs special arrangements, such as ramps, hand rails, toilet equipment, and so forth.

6. *Completely independent outside the home.* An individual who is completely independent with or without apparatus (braces, prostheses, crutches, wheelchair) in all essential daily activities, including elevation and public travel.

Vocational

The levels and criteria of vocational status were the following:

1. *Not employable.*

2. *Home employment with assistance.* An individual who is able to carry on some functions of the business with assistance or who is able to help others in a business conducted at home; also, a housewife who can assist others in household duties or who would require help in performing daily household duties.

3. *Sheltered workshop or home employment.* An individual who is capable of productive work in a sheltered workshop or at home or a housewife who can manage some household and child-care activities, exclusive of shopping and heavy lifting.

4. *Part-time employment.* An individual who is capable of part-time employment in open industry under special conditions or a housewife who can manage most household and child-care activities, exclusive of shopping and heavy lifting.

5. *Full-time employment with special arrangements.* An in-

dividual who is capable of full-time employment under special working conditions, such as a standing device, adaptive equipment, messenger service, and so on; also, a housewife who can do household and childcare activities but cannot carry packages, manage a child in the carriage, or perform heavy household duties not essential for the day-to-day management of the house.

6. *Full-time independent employment.* An individual who is capable of full-time competitve employment or a housewife who is able to perform all household and child-care activities, including shopping.

RESULTS AND DISCUSSION

Response Rates

In the main study, interviews were successfully completed on 8802 (or 94%) of the persons drawn for the sample, which was a stratified, unweighted, random sample of the total population of Birmingham aged 50 to 69 years. Of these, 1991, or 75 of those chosen for examination, have been examined by a physician (see Table, 8.2).

Over the four years of the main study, interviewer response rates were 97 percent, 94 percent, 90 percent, and 95 percent, respectively, with a drop-off in the third year which was corrected in the fourth year when what was happening was appreciated.

The disadvantages of using the 1960 census as a basis for population samples drawn in 1965-70 became obvious as the study

TABLE 8.2
RACE, SEX, AND AGE DISTRIBUTION OF SUBJECTS INTERVIEWED AND EXAMINED

Race and Sex	*Age in Years*	*Numbers Interviewed*	*Percent of Number Chosen for Interview*	*Numbers Examined*	*Percent of Number Chosen for Exam*
White male	50-59	1204	93	281	78
	60-69	1122	94	262	78
White female	50-59	1689	95	399	79
	60-69	1645	95	429	87
N/White male	50-59	664	94	121	61
	60-69	626	94	128	68
N/W female	50-59	898	94	168	62
	60-69	954	95	203	71
Total		8802	94	1991	75

progressed, though fortunately this did not disturb the random nature of the sample. A comparison between the number of persons found and listed (though not necessarily interviewed) in the households drawn for the sample and the theoretical numbers (16.26% of the numbers in the race-sex-age groups provided by the 1960 census) gave the following result:

Race	*Sex*	*Age (in years)*	*Number in* Household Listing	*Number in* Theoretical Sample
White	Male	50-59	1295	1663
		60-69	1194	1127
	Female	50-59	1778	1979
		60-69	1732	1494
Nonwhite	Male	50-59	710	1035
		60-69	666	690
	Female	50-59	955	1200
		60-69	1004	812
Total			9334	10,000

It appears that most of the differences found were due to selective out-migration of the younger age group. We have no reason to believe that the household listings (which were rechecked) were not accurate.

The response rate to the invitations to come in for a physical examination was much lower (75% overall) though comparable to that reported in major studies elsewhere. Thus the Framingham study[53] had an examination response rate of 69 percent. There was considerable variation by age, race, and sex (see Table 8.2), with a four-year response rate for white females aged 60 to 69 years of 87 percent compared with 61 percent for nonwhite males aged 50 to 59 years. In a review of the first-year nonrespondents (166 in number), the reasons for nonresponse that were given were as follows:

Not enough time, other commitments, too busy	48 percent
In good health, will go to own doctor if needed	18 percent
Scared of doctors, in poor health, scared something is wrong	18 percent
Others	15 percent

One notes that the total examination took more than two hours to complete, and thus working (aged 50 to 59) nonwhites would find it harder to get away. Over the four years of the study, the overall response rates were 76 percent, 77 percent, 77 percent, and 66 percent, respectively. The drop in the last year of the study was attributable to having no Public Health Service medical officers that year, with the result that medical appointments (especially in the evening and on Saturdays) were more difficult to arrange.

Tables 8.3a and b record the number of interviews (or examinations) and reinterviews obtained on the interview and examination groups, excluding from each reinterview figure those persons who had a stroke recorded at any previous examination or interview. For the prospective study, we thus have information on 10,876 patient-years under observations for the interview group,

TABLE 8.3a

NUMBER OF INTERVIEWS AND REINTERVIEWS (AT YEARLY INTERVALS) OBTAINED ON QUESTIONNAIRE RESPONDENTS, EXCLUDING FROM EACH REINTERVIEW FIGURE THOSE WHO HAD A STROKE RECORDED AT ANY PREVIOUS INTERVIEW

Year of entry to study	*Number of interviews obtained and first strokes recorded*			
	1st interview	*1st reinterview*	*2nd reinterview*	*3rd reinterview*
1966-67	2261	2016	1835	1646
1967-68	1982	1774	1568	
1968-69	2302	2019		
1969-70	2257			
Total	8802	5809	3421	1646
Number of first strokes	283	50	27	10

TABLE 8.3b

NUMBER OF PERSONS EXAMINED AND REINTERVIEWS (AT YEARLY INTERVALS) OBTAINED ON THESE PERSONS, EXCLUDING FROM EACH REINTERVIEW FIGURE THOSE WHO HAD A STROKE RECORDED AT ANY PREVIOUS EXAMINATION OR INTERVIEW

Year of entry to study	*Number of persons examined and reinterviewed and first strokes recorded*			
	Examined	*1st reinterview*	*2nd reinterview*	*3rd reinterview*
1966-67	565	514	465	414
1967-68	484	437	402	
1968-69	495	442		
1969-70	447			
Total	1991	1393	867	414
Number of first strokes	75	9	5	4

and 2674 patient-years under observation for the examination subgroup.

By taking the sum of patient losses over all completed time intervals [i.e. (2261 – 2016) + (2016 – 1835) + . . . + (2302 – 2019)] and subtracting from this the persons first recorded as having a stroke at the start of the interval (247) and persons who died of causes other than stroke during the interval (181), we find that the average percentage of patients who moved out of Birmingham or who could not be traced was 864 out of 12,170, or 7.1 percent per year.

Prevalence Rates: Recurrence Rates and Death Rates Among Persons with a Previous History of Stroke

An acceptable history of a completed stroke was obtained from 283 (3.2%) of those interviewed for the first time (see Table 8.3a) and from 75 (3.8%) of the subsample of those interviewed (i.e. the 75 are included in the 283 interviewer strokes) who were brought in for a medical examination (see Table 8.3b). Findings based on these strokes constitute the less important retrospective part of our study. These retrospectively diagnosed strokes came in as follows over the four years of the study:

Year	*Interview Group*	*Examination Group*
1966-67	81	26
1967-68	61	14
1968-69	71	17
1969-70	70	18

Prevalence rates are given in Table 8.4 and for every subcategory show an excess in older persons among males and among nonwhites.

TABLE 8.4
PREVALENCE AND INCIDENCE RATES OF STROKE IN THE INTERVIEWER GROUP BY AGE, RACE, AND SEX

Race and Sex	*Age in Years*	*Prevalence Rates (old strokes) per 1000 Persons*	*Incidence Rates per 1000 Persons per Year* All strokes	*Cerebral thrombosis*	*Cerebral hemorrhage*
White	50-59	28 (34)	4 (6)	2 (3)	2 (3)
male	60-69	41 (46)	12 (17)	9 (12)	3 (4)
White	50-59	14 (24)	3 (6)	2 (4)	0 (0)
female	60-69	25 (41)	7 (15)	5 (10)	1 (2)
N/White	50-59	30 (20)	16 (13)	10 (8)	4 (3)
male	60-69	73 (46)	16 (12)	8 (6)	5 (4)
N/White	50-59	31 (28)	5 (5)	2 (2)	3 (3)
female	60-69	46 (44)	11 (13)	9 (10)	3 (3)
Total		32.2 (283)	8.0 (87)	5.1 (55)	2.0 (22)

Note. 1. The number of strokes is shown in parentheses. 2. The stroke due to cerebral embolism was in a nonwhite male aged 63 years, and the two strokes due to subarachnoid hemorrhage were in nonwhite males aged 54 and 59 years, respectively. The distribution of the unclassified strokes can be obtained by subtraction.

An attempt was made to see how good the lay reinterview record was by itself in diagnosing the type of stroke, and a computer program was developed for this purpose. Based on the 50 living cases from the prospective study on whom the final diagnosis was most firmly established, the final comparison was as follows:

Type of Stroke	*Original (Computer) Count*	*Final (Confirmed) Count*	*Changes* Removed from Original List	*Changes* Added to Final List
Cerebral thrombosis	32	33	6	7
Cerebral embolism	0	1	0	1
Cerebral hemorrhage	14	10	10	6
Subarachnoid hemorrhage	0	1	0	1
Unknown	4	5	3	4

While the situation with regard to cerebral thrombosis was not too bad, that with regard to cerebral hemorrhage was impossible. Of 14 patients diagnosed from the reinterview record as having cerebral hemorrhage, only 4 could be confirmed! For this reason, no attempt has been made in this report to classify the strokes diagnosed retrospectively (i.e. at the time of their admission to the study) according to type, though the much higher mortality in the prospective study of the hemorrhagic strokes (11 out of 24, or 46%) compared with the occlusive strokes (13 out of 56, or 23%) coupled with the higher incidence of occlusive stroke would suggest that most of the survivors coming into a retrospective study would have had an occlusive stroke.

There still remains some doubt whether a physician taking an independent history for stroke and doing a complete physical examination would have agreed with the interviewer records (based on a statement by the respondent that he had had a stroke which had been diagnosed by a physician) that these 283 strokes found retrospectively were actually "completed" strokes. When the records for those respondents who had both been interviewed and had had a medical examination were compared, the following was found (note that the interviewer record was not available to the examining physician):

		Physician Rating: Completed Stroke	*Physician Rating:* Not a Completed Stroke	*Total*
Interviewer Rating:	Complete stroke	49	26 (12)	75
	Not a complete stroke	21 (9)	1895	1916
	Total	70	1921	1991

The four inner cells of this 2 × 2 table differ remarkably according to the year concerned:

1966-67		*1967-68*		*1968-69*		*1969-70*	
21	5 (1)	7	7 (3)	10	7 (4)	11	7 (4)
1 (1)	538	7 (4)	463	9 (3)	469	4 (1)	425

Regarding the interviewer's history-taking as a screening test and the medical examiner's finding as definitive (though we cannot be sure of this, for the retrospective diagnosis of a stroke by a physician also has a large subjective component), the sensitivity of the screening test was 70 percent overall and varied from a high of 95 percent to a low of 50 percent over the four years of the study! The specificity never fell below 98.3 percent. While the questionnaire and the interviewers were unchanged during the study, the physician staff did change, and the above change over time is probably largely due to this. The question arises whether the "false positives" (26) and "false negatives" (21) were nearmisses or not. The figures in parentheses give the number of patients who were diagnosed as TIA (i.e. a nearmiss). Thus, of the 26 "false positives," 12 were diagnosed by the physician as TIA, while of the 21 "false negatives," 9 were classified from the questionnaire as being TIA. Basically, this comparison highlights the difficulty of making a retrospective diagnosis of a completed stroke and makes the prospective study more important.

Let us consider the 283 strokes which were found retrospectively (by the interviewer questionnaire) in more detail. We have 343 patient-years of follow-up on this group. There were 11 who had recurrent strokes recorded, for an incidence rate of 32 per 1000 per year or four times the incidence rate for new strokes. Six of the 11 (56%) recurrent-strokes victims died from this stroke compared with a death rate of 24 out of 87 (28%) for first strokes. Deaths from other causes in this group of old strokes amounted to 21 (7 heart disease, 4 cancer, 2 influenza-pneumonia, 2 accidental, 6 others), for a nonstroke death rate of 61 per 1000 per year. This can be compared with the deaths from other causes in the initially stroke-free main prospective study group, amounting to 181 (57 heart disease, 42 cancer, 12 influenza-pneumonia, 7 accidents, 63 others), for a nonstroke death rate of 19 per 1000 per year.

Findings from the Retrospective Studies

For the retrospective study, the relative risks of a stroke (all types combined) associated with 56 of the variables treated within this report are given in Tables 8.5a (interviewer findings) and 8.5b (medical examination findings). From these tables it is also possible to obtain (by adding columns *a* and *b*) the prevalence in the population of the variable concerned. A logarithmic (natural logs) conversion *y* of the relative risk (actually of a slightly changed version of the odds ratio) is given along with the square root of the variance of *y*; $y/S.E.(y)$ can be approximately equated to a *t* value to calculate whether any given relative risk (considered singly) is significantly different from 1.

With the large sample size used for Table 8.5a (interviewer

TABLE 8.5a

THE RETROSPECTIVE INTERVIEWER STUDY: THE RELATIVE RISKS OF A STROKE (ALL TYPES COMBINED) ASSOCIATED WITH SELECTED VARIABLES FROM THE HISTORIES GIVEN BY 8802 RESPONDENTS

History of:	*Number of respondents*						
	Exposed to risk factor		*Not exposed*		*Rel. Risk*	*y*	*S.E.(y)*
	Stroke (a)	*No stroke (b)*	*Stroke (c)*	*No stroke (d)*			
Treated hypertension	159	2055	124	6464	3.82	1.39	0.12
Treated diabetes	43	481	240	8038	2.83	1.10	0.17
Heart attack	46	398	237	8121	3.65	1.38	0.17
Chest pain	54	654	229	7865	2.70	1.05	0.16
Inter. claudication	60	371	223	8148	5.23	1.78	0.15
Hardened arteries	32	279	251	8240	3.48	1.34	0.19
Pounding in head	51	474	232	8045	3.47	1.32	0.16
Weight increase > 20 pounds	77	2874	206	5645	0.74	—0.31	0.13
Ponderal index < 12	97	2798	186	5721	1.06	0.06	0.13
Shortness of breath	52	644	231	7875	2.62	1.02	0.16
Gout	30	513	253	8006	1.80	0.63	0.20
Cigarette smoking	66	1823	217	6696	1.11	0.11	0.14
Use of alcohol	92	2060	191	6459	1.49	0.41	0.13
Family history of stroke	123	3018	160	5501	1.39	0.34	0.12
Temp. weakness arm or leg	44	292	239	8227	4.64	1.65	0.17
Temp. weakness face	20	103	263	8416	5.37	1.84	0.25
Sensory loss arm or leg	50	531	233	7988	3.04	1.18	0.16
Loss of eyesight	77	1643	206	6876	1.54	0.45	0.14
Double vision	51	535	232	7984	3.08	1.19	0.16
Incoordination	62	799	221	7720	2.59	1.00	0.15
Fainting	52	694	231	7825	2.43	0.94	0.16
Headaches	113	1912	170	6607	2.22	0.83	0.12
Deafness	40	900	243	7619	1.38	0.34	0.17
Speech disturbances	65	820	218	7699	2.67	1.03	0.15
Confusion	6	316	277	8203	0.57	—0.49	0.39
Choking	32	520	251	7999	1.91	0.68	0.19
Dizziness	104	1978	179	6541	1.88	0.65	0.13

Note. 1. $y = \ln \frac{(2a+1)\ (2d+1)}{(2b+1)\ (2c+1)}$ (Haldane 1956)

2. $V(y) = \frac{1}{a+1} + \frac{1}{b+1} + \frac{1}{c+1} + \frac{1}{d+1}$ (Sheehe 1965)

findings), only a weight increase of more than twenty pounds, the ponderal index, a history of cigarette smoking, deafness, and confusion have relative risks which are not significantly ($p < 0.05$) greater than 1. A history of gout, of drinking alcohol, of loss of eyesight, and of family members who have had a stroke are significantly greater than 1 at $p < 0.01$, and all the other variables are significant at $p < 0.001$ (considering each as a single comparison). Much the most important variable is obviously a history of treated hypertension [$y/S.E.(y) = 11.5$] though many other history items suggestive of other preexistent cardiovascular disease (heart attack, chest pain, intermittent claudication, hardened arteries), of diabetes, and of neurological disease (temporary muscular weaknesses, sensory loss, double vision, incoordination) occur much more frequently in the past record of stroke patients than can be expected by chance. General items such as a family history of stroke, cigarette smoking, weight changes, and the use of alcohol appear to be of much less importance.

The history items from the physicians' records (Table 8.5b) give results very similar to those obtained by the lay interviewers (Table 8.5a) for those questions which were common (in general terms) to both. Table 8.5c records the prevalence of those variables which were asked about by both. A history suggestive of intermittent claudication and of loss of eyesight was more often obtained by the lay interviewers, and a history of deafness was less often obtained. The difference with regard to hypertension (*q.v.*) was because "treated" hypertension was the independent variable used for the interviewer study and the physicians did not operate under this restriction.

From the histories obtained by the physicians, hypertension again stands out as the most important variable; but congestive heart failure, diabetes, diplopia, decreased binocular vision, vertigo, intermittent claudication, and memory deterioration all have relative risks significantly ($p < 0.01$) greater than 1. Among the examination variables which were looked at, changes in the optic fundi, congestive heart failure, abnormal Q waves and abnormal ST segments on the ECG, and a positive thermography test all occur significantly ($p < 0.01$) more frequently in patients with

TABLE 8.5b

THE RETROSPECTIVE EXAMINATION STUDY: THE RELATIVE RISKS OF A STROKE (ALL TYPES COMBINED) ASSOCIATED WITH SELECTED VARIABLES FROM THE MEDICAL HISTORY EXAMINATION AND LABORATORY FINDINGS ON 1991 RESPONDENTS

Variable	*Number of respondents*				*Rel.*		
	Exposed to risk factor		*Not exposed*		*Risk*	*y*	*S.E.(y)*
	Stroke (c)	*No stroke (d)*	*Stroke (a)*	*No stroke (b)*			
History of:							
Hyptertension	53	600	22	1316	4.94	1.65	0.25
Diabetes	14	131	61	1785	2.92	1.16	0.30
Ischemic heart disease	9	130	66	1786	1.82	0.67	0.35
Valvular heart disease	2	28	73	1888	1.79	0.81	0.62
Cardiac dysrhythmia	6	143	69	1773	1.07	0.14	0.40
Congestive heart failure	11	69	64	1847	4.10	1.55	0.34
Inter. claudication	6	43	69	1873	3.45	1.39	0.42
Decr. monocular vision	6	124	69	1792	1.24	0.29	0.41
Decr. binocular vision	20	222	55	1694	2.63	1.03	0.26
Diplopia	8	62	67	1854	3.28	1.32	0.38
Vertigo	16	171	59	1745	2.62	1.03	0.29
Deafness	17	297	58	1619	1.56	0.48	0.28
Memory deteriation	23	168	52	1748	4.17	1.53	0.26
Hypothyroidism	1	32	74	1884	0.80	0.15	0.74
Exam findings of:							
Arcus senilis	20	353	29	1924	1.95	0.70	0.29
A.S. fundi	21	171	28	1206	4.82	1.67	0.29
K.W. fundi > gr. 2	26	332	49	1584	2.42	0.93	0.25
Congestive heart failure	9	30	66	1886	6.82	2.18	0.38
Valvular heart disease	10	151	65	1765	1.75	0.62	0.34
Dysrhythmia	7	84	68	1832	2.15	0.86	0.39
Cervical bruits	4	110	71	1806	0.93	0.02	0.47
Supraclavicular bruits	1	65	74	1851	0.39	—0.56	0.73
Systolic B.P. < 134	18	685	57	1231	0.58	—0.55	0.27
Systolic B.P. 134-156	29	658	46	1258	1.20	0.19	0.24
Systolic B.P. > 156	28	573	47	1343	1.38	0.34	0.24
Diastolic B.P. < 82	24	860	51	1056	0.59	—0.54	0.25
Diastolic B.P. 82-90	20	536	55	1380	0.94	—0.05	0.26
Diastolic B.P. > 90	31	520	44	1396	1.84	0.64	0.24
Abn. Q on ECG	6	51	69	1865	2.95	1.21	0.42

TABLE 8.5b (con't.)

Variable	*Number of respondents*				*Rel. Risk*	*y*	*S.E.(y)*
	Exposed to risk factor		*Not exposed*				
	Stroke (c)	*No stroke (d)*	*Stroke (a)*	*No stroke(b)*			
Abn. R on ECG	9	186	66	1730	1.26	0.28	0.35
Abn. ST on ECG	25	377	50	1549	1.99	0.73	0.24
Therm. dif. > 1° F	12	87	63	1829	3.64	1.41	0.32
Ponderal index < 12	39	659	36	1257	2.01	0.72	0.23
2-hr. blood glucose < 90	12	215	60	1619	1.48	0.44	0.31
2-hr. blood glucose 90-150	33	866	39	968	0.95	—0.06	0.24
2-hr. blood glucose > 150	27	753	45	1981	0.87	—0.14	0.24
Cholesterol < 227	19	498	51	1294	0.97	—0.02	0.27
Cholesterol 227-277	31	716	39	1076	1.19	0.18	0.24
Cholesterol > 277	20	578	50	1214	0.85	—0.16	0.26
Triglycerides < 2	2	142	65	1561	0.35	—0.87	0.60
Triglycerides 2-4	34	961	33	742	0.80	—0.23	0.25
Triglycerides > 4	31	600	36	1103	1.55	0.46	0.25

Note. 1. *y and V(y)* are as for Table 8.5a.
2. Arcus senilis and A.S. fundi were not recorded in the first year (565 patients).
3. Laboratory data (due to spoiled specimens etc.) were not available on all patients.

a past history of a completed stroke. In this retrospective examination study, systolic blood pressure, bruits, and the laboratory variables which were looked at (blood glucose, cholesterol, triglycerides) are not associated with any significant change in relative risk. The contrast between the history findings and the examination-laboratory findings with regard to systolic hypertension and diabetes is of particular interest.

Incidence Rates: Findings from the Stroke Registry

The characteristics, with regard to the interviewer variables under consideration, of the population (8519 individuals) admitted to the prospective study is given, broken down by race, sex, and age, in Table 8.6 Amongst these variables, a history of a heart attack, of chest pain, of hardened arteries, and of cigarette smoking were found much more frequently (Obs/Exp > 1.4) among white males. For white females, a family history of stroke and a history of pounding in the head were found to excess. For nonwhite males, the use of alcohol stands out, and for nonwhite

TABLE 8.5c

PREVALENCE OF SELECTED VARIABLES FROM THE RETROSPECTIVE STUDY, COMPARING THE FIRST AND SECOND HALVES OF THE EXAMINATION GROUP (PHYSICIAN FINDINGS) WITH EACH OTHER AND WITH THE TOTAL INTERVIEWER GROUP FOR COMPARABLE VARIABLES

Variable	*Percentage of population with variable from:* Physician exam, Year 1 and 2,	Physician exam, Year 3 and 4	Interviewer Record
History of:	($n = 1049$)	($n = 942$)	($n = 8802$)
Hypertension	30 (all)	36 (all)	25 (treated)
Diabetes (treated)	6	8	6
Ischemic heart disease (angina)	7	7	8 (chest pain
Intermittent claudication	3	2	5
Loss of eyesight	12	13	20
Deafness	16	15	1
Finding of:			
K. W. fundi > gr. 2	17	18	—
Valvular heart disease	6	10	—
Supraclavicular bruits	3	4	—
Systolic B.P. > 156	30	29	—
Diastolic B.P. > 90	29	26	—
Abn. ST on ECG	21	20	—
2-hr. blood glucose > 150	35	45	—
Cholesterol > 277	31	33	—
Triglycerides > 4	4	3	—
Therm. dif. > 1° F	4	5	—
Ponderal index < 12	33	38	33
Vital capacity < 3.5 (male), or 2.5 (female)	20	34	—

females, a history of treated hypertension, of treated diabetes, and of confusion together with a low ponderal index (i.e. overweight) were found to excess.

The 87 accepted first strokes ("completed" strokes) recorded during the four years of the main prospective study were classified on the basis of the following information:

NUMBER OF PERSONS WITH FIRST STROKES WHO

	Died	*Did Not Die*
Number of accepted strokes	24 (all with death certificates)	63
With adequate hospital records	12	30
Lumbar puncture performed	5	18
Autopsy performed	5	—
Cerebral angiogram performed	1	8
Physicians's diagnosis (patients not treated in hospital) checked by staff neurologist	—	30

TABLE 8.6
THE PROSPECTIVE INTERVIEWER STUDY: NUMBERS OF RESPONDENTS IN EACH RACE-SEX-AGE CATEGORY AND THE NUMBERS EXPOSED TO SELECTED RISK FACTORS DERIVED FROM THEIR HISTORIES

Race:	*White*				*Nonwhite*			
Sex:	*Male*		*Female*		*Male*		*Female*	
Age group:	*50-59*	*60-69*	*50-59*	*60-69*	*50-59*	*60-69*	*50-59*	*60-69*
No. in category:	1170	1076	1665	1604	644	580	870	910
No. with a history of:								
Treated hypertension	157	221	322	455	119	154	274	353
Treated diabetes	44	66	62	97	28	36	62	86
Heart attack	90	94	60	69	11	13	33	28
Chest pain	117	140	112	132	18	31	59	45
Inter. claudication	47	56	62	66	20	33	45	42
Hardened arteries	38	73	34	90	7	5	11	21
Pounding in head	45	45	136	118	24	26	39	41
Weight increase > 20 lbs.	341	380	457	530	178	162	421	405
Ponderal index < 12	185	186	446	541	182	171	532	555
Shortness of breath	87	97	116	138	27	54	56	69
Gout	54	50	99	95	25	49	73	68
Cigarette smoking	462	316	333	222	185	123	104	78
Use of alcohol	375	321	189	170	296	283	228	198
Family history of stroke	364	411	665	709	155	154	280	280
Temp. weakness arm or leg	39	27	56	46	14	27	41	42
Temp. weakness face	14	12	32	28	3	3	5	6
Sensory loss arm or leg	81	67	95	84	27	40	73	64
Loss of eyesight	155	207	227	329	112	143	221	249
Double vision	52	67	63	76	47	44	87	99
Incoordination	73	105	114	190	40	63	101	113
Fainting	78	80	144	141	44	54	71	82
Headaches	242	187	473	351	117	107	236	199
Deafness	104	197	130	182	51	84	67	85
Speech disturbances	75	84	146	150	57	62	115	131
Confusion	29	30	46	39	16	38	53	65
Choking	59	79	119	166	9	12	46	30
Dizziness	17	19	30	27	12	10	18	44
Memory loss	204	248	383	443	108	119	224	249

With the available information, out of the 87 strokes, only 7 had to be classified as "type unknown." It will be noticed that 12 of the 24 deaths occurred before the patient was admitted to the hospital (or admitted long enough to have an adequate hospital record). Also, 33 of the 63 who did not die (38% of all prospective strokes) were not admitted to the hospital but were diagnosed and treated by their physicians at home. The diagnosis on the 12 early deaths is based on death certificate data and on supplementary data from the families and attending physicians (only one autopsy was obtained on this group). The hospital data on the 42 who were hospitalized was standardized and reasonably adequate. Of the 33 who were treated at home, 30 were brought into our clinic and had the diagnosis confirmed by a staff neurologist. Three for whom suitable appointments could not be made appeared to be clear-cut cases confirmed by their attending physicians. Two further patients diagnosed as "completed stroke treated at home" were not accepted by our staff neurologists (one was diagnosed as a Bell's palsy and the other as a TIA consequently on general arteriosclerosis) and are not included in the list of accepted strokes.

Incidence rates by age, race, and sex are given in Table 8.4 and show (as with the prevalence rates) an excess among older persons, among nonwhites, and among males. The overall (8.0 new strokes per 1000 persons per year) and categorical incidence rates may overestimate the true rates (such an overestimate is inherent in this type of prospective study where the numerator is obtained from interview and extraneous information and the demoninator from interview information only) by not more than 5 percent (i.e. giving a true rate of about 7.6 per 1000 per year).

The distribution of deaths, hospitalized cases (nondeaths), and home-treated cases varied by age, race, and sex.

Race, Sex and Age		*Died*	*Hospital: Did Not Die*	*At Home: Did Not Die*
White males	50-59	2	3	1
	60-69	2	2	13
White females	50-59	0	1	5
	60-69	2	7	6
N/White males	50-59	5	7	1
	60-69	4	6	2
N/White females	50-59	2	1	2
	60-69	7	3	3
Total		24	30	33

For comparison with the incidence rates obtained in the prospective study, figures obtained by the Birmingham Stroke Registry for Jefferson County (which includes the city of Birmingham) for 1969 are given in Table 8.1. The registry also is conducted by the Department of Public Health and Epidemiology of the University of Alabama in Birmingham, but is funded under different auspices (contract No. PH 86-68-165 with the Heart Disease and Stroke Control Program, Division of Chronic Disease Programs, Regional Medical Programs Service) and staffed separately from the stroke study discussed in this report. These figures give an idea of the dimensions of the problem spread over all age brackets and over a total community. It will be noticed that the registry incidence starting at about 0.7 per 1000 in the age bracket 40 to 44 years increases by approximately 60 percent (compounded) for each five-year age group thereafter and is in excess of 10 per 1000 in the age bracket 70 to 74 years. For all age groups, the nonwhite rates are considerably higher than the white rates. Except in the very youngest (under 40) and very oldest (over 75) age groups, the white male rate is considerably higher than the white female rate, but among nonwhites there are no marked differences by sex.

The death rates recorded by the stroke registry were, for persons aged 50 to 54 years, 35 out of 75 (47%); for persons aged 55 to 59 years, 49 out of 107 (46%); for persons aged 60 to 64 years, 56 out of 114 (49%); and for persons aged 65 to 69 years, 82 out of 164 (50%).

If only cases of stroke who died before admission to the hospital or who were admitted to hospital are taken into account in the prospective study, the incidence figures obtained in the prospective study are similar to these given by the registry study:

Group	*Incidence Rates per 1000 per Year*		
	Registry	*Prospective Study (Deaths and Hospital)*	*Prospective Study (Home)*
Aged 50-59	2.6	3.8	1.6
Aged 60-69	5.7	6.2	4.5
White	2.8	2.7	3.5
Nonwhite	6.3	9.2	2.1
Male	4.7	7.0	3.8
Female	3.4	3.6	2.4

The higher incidence of strokes in older persons, among nonwhites, and among males (perhaps white males only) is confirmed. Case fatality rates are similar, with 48 percent of the registry cases and 44 percent of the early death and hospital admission prospective study cases dying during the acute episode. It appears that a registry study can reasonably reflect certain features of this latter component of a prospective study.

A different picture emerges when cases of stroke that are not admitted to hospital and do not die are taken into account. This may not be generally true across the United States, but at least in the Birmingham area (where there is no shortage of hospital beds though financial barriers to hospital admission do exist) about one-third of our stroke cases were not admitted to hospital. These cases treated at home were typically older, white, and male with a relatively mild thrombotic stroke, who regained full or near-full function with little or no assistance from an organized rehabilitation program.

Of the 87 strokes found in the prospective study, 22 (10 deaths) were due to cerebral hemorrhage, 2 (1 death) were due to a subarachnoid hemorrhage, 55 (13 deaths) were due to cerebral thrombosis, 1 was due to cerebral embolism, and for 7 the type of stroke could not be determined. For the physician-examined subgroup there were 18 new strokes in the prospective study, giving a rate of 6.6 per 1000 per year. Thirteen of these strokes were cerebral thrombosis, 3 were cerebral hemorrhage, and 2 were unclassified.

The distribution of cases between thrombotic and hemorrhagic strokes confirmed other reports. For those stroke cases that died, the cerebral thrombosis-cerebral hemorrhage ratio was 1.3, while for those that survived, the ratio was 3.5. If the figures for whites only are considered, these two ratios become 0.5 and 5.4, respectively, while for nonwhites they were 1.8 and 2.1, respectively. Another large difference between whites and nonwhites emerges when we look at death rates. For cerebral hemorrhage the rates were essentially similar (44% for whites and 46% for nonwhites), but for cerebral thrombosis the white rate was 6 percent and the nonwhite rate 46 percent, reflecting the large number of relatively benign, mild thrombotic strokes found among older whites.

In general, relatively more of the thrombotic strokes were admitted to hospital than were strokes due to cerebral hemorrhage, and the surviving hospital population, in particular, included a relatively high proportion of thrombotic strokes.

	Died Before Admission to Hospital	*Admitted to Hospital:*		*At Home:*
		Died	*Did Not Die*	*Did Not Die*
Cerebral thrombosis	6	7	20	22
Cerebral hemorrhage	5	5	4	8
Other	1	0	6	3

Findings from the Prospective Studies

Using all 87 strokes (including cerebral thrombosis, cerebral hemorrhage, other and unclassified) as the dependent variable, Table 8.7a gives the relative risks associated with the variables under investigation in the interviewer study. Tables 8.7b,c,d, and e give this same information for each of the eight major race-sex-age groups. In relating Table 8.7a to Table 8.5a (that dealing with the retrospective interviewer study) it will be appreciated that for each variable, the persons in column *b* (exposed, no stroke) of Table 8.5a are distributed between colunm *a* (exposed, stroke) and column *b* of Table 8.7a, while the persons in column *d* (not exposed, no stroke) of Table 8.5a are distributed between columns *c* (not exposed, stroke) and *d* of Table 8.7a. To save space, only the column *a* (exposed, stroke) values are given in Table 8.7b,c,d, and e. However, the *b*, *c*, and *d* values can be readily derived. Consider, as an example, the figures for "Treated hypertension" among white males aged 50 to 59 years. Table 8.7b gives the values for *a* as 1, and for $a + c$ (all strokes in this race-sex-age group) as 6. Thus *c* is $6 - 1 = 5$. Also, (from Table 8.6) $a + b$ (all exposed persons) $= 157$. Thus *b* is $157 - 1 = 156$. Finally $a + b + c + d$ (all white males aged 50 to 59 years) is (from Table 8.7b) 1170, and thus $d = 1170 - 1 - 156 - 5 = 1008$.

In striking contrast to the retrospective study, relatively few of the variables considered in the prospective study have a relative risk which is significantly greater than 1 when each variable is considered independently. Those variables which do fall into this category are a history of treated hypertension, treated dia-

TABLE 8.7a

THE PROSPECTIVE INTERVIEWER STUDY: THE RELATIVE RISKS OF A FIRST STROKE (ALL TYPES COMBINED) ASSOCIATED WITH SELECTED VARIABLES FROM THE HISTORIES GIVEN BY 8519 RESPONDENTS

History of:	*Number of respondents* *Exposed to risk factor* *Stroke (a)*	*No stroke (b)*	*Not exposed* *Stroke (c)*	*No stroke (d)*	*Rel. Risk*	*y*	*S.E.(y)*
Treated hypertension	44	2011	43	6421	3.22	1.18	0.21
Treated diabetes	15	466	72	7966	3.48	1.29	0.28
Heart attack	11	387	76	8045	2.95	1.14	0.31
Chest pain	14	640	73	7792	2.31	0.87	0.29
Inter. claudication	4	367	83	8065	1.06	016	0.46
Hardened arteries	6	273	81	8159	2.19	0.86	0.40
Pounding in head	6	468	81	7964	1.26	0.30	0.40
Weight increase > 20 pounds	32	2842	55	5590	1.14	0.14	0.22
Ponderal index < 12	36	2762	51	5670	1.44	0.37	0.22
Shortness of breath	11	633	76	7799	1.77	0.61	0.31
Gout	7	506	80	7926	1.36	0.37	0.37
Cigarette smoking	17	1806	70	6626	0.89	—0.09	0.26
Use of alcohol	31	2029	56	6403	1.74	0.56	0.22
Family history of stroke	26	2992	61	5440	0.78	—0.24	0.23
Temp. weakness arm or leg	6	286	81	8146	2.09	0.82	0.40
Temp. weakness face	1	102	86	8330	0.95	0.34	0.72
Sensory loss arm or leg	7	524	80	7908	1.32	0.34	0.37
Loss of eyesight	28	1615	59	6817	1.99	0.70	0.23
Double vision	10	525	77	7907	1.94	0.71	0.32
Incoordination	11	788	76	7644	1.40	0.37	0.31
Fainting	11	683	76	7749	1.63	0.53	0.31
Headaches	27	1885	60	6547	1.55	0.45	0.23
Deafness	15	885	72	7547	1.76	0.60	0.28
Speech disturbances	13	807	74	7625	1.65	0.53	0.29
Confusion	6	310	81	8122	1.92	0.73	0.40
Choking	7	513	80	7919	1.34	0.36	0.37
Dizziness	35	1943	52	6489	2.22	0.81	0.22
Memory loss	5	172	82	8260	2.87	1.16	0.43

TABLE 8.7b

THE PROSPECTIVE INTERVIEWER STUDY: THE RELATIVE RISKS OF A FIRST STROKE (ALL TYPES COMBINED) ASSOCIATED WITH SELECTED VARIABLES FROM THE HISTORIES GIVEN BY 1170 WHITE MALES AGED 50-59 YEARS AND 1076 WHITE MALES AGED 60-69 YEARS

History of:	*White males aged 50-59 yrs.* *R.R.*	*y*	*S.E.(y)*	*White males aged 60-69 yrs.* *R.R.*	*y*	*S.E.(y)*
Treated hypertension	1.29 (1)	0.56	0.82	7.09 (11)	1.96	0.48
Treated diabetes	5.12 (1)	1.95	0.83	3.28 (3)	1.33	0.58
Heart attack	2.40 (1)	1.19	0.82	4.35 (5)	1.56	0.51
Chest pain	1.80 (1)	0.89	0.82	5.94 (8)	1.83	0.47
Inter. claudication	0 (0)	0.59	1.08	0 (0)	—0.68	1.04
Hardened arteries	14.89 (2)	2.84	0.75	2.94 (3)	1.22	0.58
Pounding in head	0 (0)	0.63	1.08	1.43 (1)	0.73	0.76
Weight increase > 20 lbs.	1.22 (2)	0.30	0.73	1.28 (7)	0.27	0.47
Ponderal index < 12	2.66 (2)	0.73	1.09	1.47 (4)	0.47	0.53
Shortness of breath	2.49 (1)	1.22	0.82	1.35 (2)	0.49	0.64
Gout	0 (0)	0.45	1.08	1.28 (1)	0.62	0.76
Cigarette smoking	1.53 (3)	0.43	0.71	1.00 (5)	0.05	0.50
Use of alcohol	10.60 (5)	2.06	0.82	1.65 (7)	0.52	0.47
Family history of stroke	2.21 (3)	0.80	0.71	1.13 (7)	0.14	0.47
Temp. weakness of arm or leg	5.80 (1)	2.07	0.83	0 (0)	0.07	1.05
Temp. weakness of face	0 (0)	1.81	1.10	0 (0)	0.87	1.06
Sensory loss arm or leg	0 (0)	0.02	1.08	3.23 (3)	1.31	0.58
Loss of eyesight	1.31 (1)	0.58	0.82	2.29 (6)	0.88	0.48
Double vision	0 (0)	0.49	1.08	0.94 (1)	0.30	0.76
Incoordination	3.01 (1)	1.41	0.83	1.49 (2)	0.59	0.64
Fainting	0 (0)	0.06	1.08	1.66 (2)	0.70	0.64
Headaches	3.83 (3)	1.35	0.71	1.45 (4)	0.46	0.53
Deafness	2.05 (1)	1.03	0.82	1.86 (5)	0.68	0.50
Speech disturbances	2.92 (1)	1.38	0.83	0.74 (1)	0.06	0.76
Confusion	0 (0)	1.08	1.08	2.18 (1)	1.15	0.77
Choking	0 (0)	0.35	1.08	0.79 (1)	0.12	0.76
Dizziness	9.47 (4)	2.16	0.73	1.82 (6)	0.64	0.48
Memory loss	33.91 (2)	3.72	0.77	0 (0)	0.42	1.05

Note. 1. y and $V(y)$ are as for Table 8.5a.

2. The number of strokes in exposed persons (a) is given after the R.R. in parentheses. There were 6 strokes in white males aged 50-59 and 17 strokes in white males aged 60-69. Read in conjunction with Table 8.6, cells b, c, and d of the 2×2 table can be obtained by subtraction.

TABLE 8.7c

THE PROSPECTIVE INTERVIEWER STUDY: THE RELATIVE RISKS OF A FIRST STROKE (ALL TYPES COMBINED) ASSOCIATED WITH SELECTED VARIABLES FROM THE HISTORIES GIVEN BY 1665 WHITE FEMALES AGED 50-59 YEARS AND 1604 WHITE FEMALES AGED 60-69 YEARS

History of:	*White females aged 50-59 yrs.* R.R.	*y*	*S.E.(y)*	*White females aged 60-69 yrs.* R.R.	*y*	*S.E.(y)*
Treated hypertension	4.17 (3)	1.43	0.71	5.05 (10)	1.59	0.51
Treated diabetes	12.93 (2)	2.68	0.74	5.65 (4)	1.83	0.54
Heart attack	0 (0)	0.71	1.08	3.42 (2)	1.42	0.65
Chest pain	0 (0)	0.05	1.07	2.79 (3)	1.15	0.58
Inter. claudication	5.17 (1)	1.96	0.83	0 (0)	—0.30	1.04
Hardened arteries	9.59 (1)	2.58	0.83	0 (0)	—0.63	1.03
Pounding in head	0 (0)	—0.15	1.07	3.15 (3)	1.27	0.58
Weight increase > 20 lbs.	0 (0)	—1.60	1.07	1.01 (5)	0.06	0.51
Ponderal index < 12	2.73 (3)	1.00	0.71	0.71 (4)	—0.27	0.53
Shortness of breath	0 (0)	0.02	1.07	2.66 (3)	1.10	0.58
Gout	0 (0)	0.18	1.07	1.13 (1)	0.49	0.76
Cigarette smoking	0 (0)	—1.18	1.07	0.96 (2)	0.14	0.64
Use of alcohol	0 (0)	—0.52	1.07	0 (0)	—1.31	1.03
Family history of stroke	0.75 (2)	—0.18	0.73	1.44 (8)	0.36	0.49
Temp. weakness of arm or leg	5.75 (1)	2.06	0.83	2.42 (1)	1.25	0.77
Temp. weakness face	0 (0)	1.35	1.08	4.02 (1)	1.77	0.78
Sensory loss arm or leg	3.31 (1)	1.51	0.82	1.29 (1)	0.62	0.76
Loss of eyesight	1.27 (1)	0.54	0.82	3.39 (7)	1.24	0.49
Double vision	5.09 (1)	1.93	0.82	7.31 (4)	2.10	0.55
Incoordination	0 (0)	0.03	1.07	3.72 (5)	1.38	0.51
Fainting	2.11 (1)	1.06	0.82	0.74 (1)	0.06	0.76
Headaches	5.04 (4)	1.52	0.73	2.38 (6)	0.90	0.50
Deafness	5.90 (2)	1.89	0.74	1.95 (3)	0.79	0.58
Speech disturbances	2.08 (1)	1.04	0.82	1.49 (2)	0.58	0.64
Confusion	7.04 (1)	2.27	0.83	2.87 (1)	1.43	0.77
Choking	6.50 (2)	1.98	0.74	2.17 (3)	0.89	0.58
Dizziness	1.67 (2)	0.62	0.73	2.29 (7)	0.84	0.49
Memory loss	10.90 (1)	2.71	0.84	4.17 (1)	1.81	0.78

Note. 1. y and V (y) are as for Table 8.5a.

2. The number of strokes in exposed persons (a) is given after the R.R. in parentheses. There were 6 strokes in white females aged 50-59 and 15 strokes in white females aged 60-69. Read in conjunction with Table 8.6, cells b, c, and d of the 2×2 table can be obtained by subtraction.

TABLE 8.7d

THE PROSPECTIVE INTERVIEWER STUDY: THE RELATIVE RISKS OF A FIRST STROKE (ALL TYPES COMBINED) ASSOCIATED WITH SELECTED VARIABLES FROM THE HISTORIES GIVEN BY 644 NONWHITE MALES AGED 50-59 YEARS AND 580 NONWHITE MALES AGED 60-69 YEARS

History of:	*Nonwhite males aged 50-59 yrs.*			*Nonwhite males aged 60-69 yrs.*		
	R.R.	*y*	*S.E.(y)*	*R.R.*	*y*	*S.E.(y)*
Treated hypertension	3.78 (6)	1.37	0.53	0.92 (3)	0.01	0.60
Treated diabetes	4.00 (2)	1.60	0.67	0 (0)	—0.54	1.05
Heart attack	4.80 (1)	1.96	0.82	8.72 (2)	2.45	0.71
Chest pain	2.90 (1)	1.44	0.80	1.61 (1)	0.83	0.78
Inter. claudication	0 (0)	0.10	1.05	3.32 (2)	1.40	0.68
Hardened arteries	0 (0)	1.12	1.09	0 (0)	1.41	1.12
Pounding in head	0 (0)	—0.08	1.05	0 (0)	—0.20	1.06
Weight increase > 20 lbs.	1.16 (4)	0.21	0.55	1.84 (5)	0.65	0.55
Ponderal index < 12	2.96 (7)	1.10	0.53	1.71 (5)	0.57	0.55
Shortness of breath	6.86 (3)	2.11	0.62	0 (0)	—0.97	1.05
Gout	0 (0)	—0.13	1.05	0.98 (1)	0.33	0.78
Cigarette smoking	1.10 (4)	0.16	0.55	1.24 (3)	0.31	0.60
Use of alcohol	1.88 (8)	0.61	0.53	1.05 (6)	0.05	0.54
Family history of stroke	0.95 (3)	0.04	0.59	0 (0)	—2.23	1.04
Temp. weakness of arm or leg	3.75 (1)	1.70	0.81	0 (0)	—0.24	1.06
Temp. weakness face	0 (0)	1.89	1.15	0 (0)	1.86	1.52
Sensory loss arm or leg	0 (0)	—0.21	1.05	1.23 (1)	0.56	0.78
Loss of eyesight	1.43 (3)	0.46	0.59	2.18 (5)	0.82	0.55
Double vision	1.06 (1)	0.41	0.77	1.11 (1)	0.45	0.78
Incoordination	2.75 (2)	1.21	0.67	0.75 (1)	0.05	0.78
Fainting	2.48 (2)	1.10	0.66	1.95 (2)	0.85	0.67
Headaches	2.82 (5)	1.09	0.54	0.88 (2)	0.04	0.66
Deafness	3.49 (3)	1.39	0.60	0.54 (1)	—0.28	0.77
Speech disturbances	4.58 (4)	1.63	0.57	0.76 (1)	0.07	0.78
Confusion	3.27 (1)	1.56	0.80	1.30 (1)	0.61	0.78
Choking	0 (0)	0.88	1.08	0 (0)	0.58	1.07
Dizziness	4.25 (6)	1.50	0.53	3.37 (5)	1.27	0.55
Memory loss	0 (0)	0.60	1.07	0 (0)	0.75	1.08

Note. 1. *y* and *V* (*y*) are as for Table 8.5a.

2. The number of strokes in exposed persons (a) is given after R.R. in parentheses. There were 13 strokes in nonwhite males aged 50-59 and 12 strokes in nonwhite males aged 60-69. Read in conjunction with Table 8.6, cells b, c, and d of the 2×2 table can be obtained by subtraction.

TABLE 8.7e

THE PROSPECTIVE INTERVIEWER STUDY: THE RELATIVE RISKS OF A FIRST STROKE (ALL TYPES COMBINED ASSOCIATED WITH SELECTED VARIABLES FROM THE HISTORIES GIVEN BY 870 NONWHITE FEMALES AGED 50-59 YEARS AND 910 NONWHITE FEMALES AGED 60-69 YEARS

History of:	*Nonwhite females aged 50-59 yrs.*			*Nonwhite females aged 60-69 yrs.*		
	R.R.	*y*	*S.E.(y)*	*R.R.*	*y*	*S.E.(y)*
Treated hypertension	1.45 (2)	0.44	0.77	2.52 (8)	0.90	0.53
Treated diabetes	3.26 (1)	1.47	0.85	1.74 (2)	0.74	0.66
Heart attack	0 (0)	0.81	1.09	0 (0)	0.12	1.05
Chest pain	0 (0)	0.21	1.09	0 (0)	—0.37	1.05
Inter. claudication	0 (0)	0.49	1.09	1.72 (1)	0.90	0.78
Hardened arteries	0 (0)	1.91	1.12	0 (0)	0.41	1.06
Pounding in head	0 (0)	0.64	1.09	3.85 (2)	1.55	0.66
Weight increase > 20 lbs.	0.27 (1)	—1.04	0.84	1.96 (8)	0.66	0.53
Ponderal index < 12	0.95 (3)	—0.12	0.77	1.02 (8)	—0.01	0.53
Shortness of breath	3.63 (1)	1.58	0.85	1.02 (1)	0.37	0.77
Gout	0 (0)	—0.02	1.09	5.50 (4)	1.81	0.56
Cigarette smoking	0 (0)	—0.41	1.08	0 (0)	—0.95	1.04
Use of alcohol	1.88 (2)	0.70	0.77	1.08 (3)	0.18	0.59
Family history of stroke	0 (0)	0.01	1.09	0.68 (3)	0.29	0.59
Temp. weakness of arm or leg	5.05 (1)	1.91	0.85	1.72 (1)	0.90	0.78
Temp. weakness face	0 (0)	2.22	1.16	0 (0)	1.62	1.10
Sensory loss arm or leg	0 (0)	—0.02	1.09	1.10 (1)	0.45	0.77
Loss of eyesight	1.96 (2)	0.74	0.77	0.80 (3)	—0.13	0.59
Double vision	0 (0)	—0.21	1.08	1.49 (2)	0.58	0.65
Incoordination	0 (0)	—0.38	1.08	0 (0)	—1.36	1.04
Fainting	0 (0)	—1.66	1.08	3.03 (3)	1.23	0.60
Headaches	0 (0)	—1.42	1.08	1.07 (3)	0.17	0.59
Deafness	0 (0)	0.07	1.09	0 (0)	—1.04	1.04
Speech disturbances	0 (0)	—0.53	1.08	1.78 (3)	0.69	0.59
Confusion	0 (0)	0.32	1.09	1.08 (1)	0.44	0.77
Choking	4.48 (1)	1.79	0.85	0 (0)	0.05	1.05
Dizziness	0.72 (1)	—0.04	0.84	1.18 (4)	0.23	0.55
Memory loss	11.83 (1)	2.78	0.87	0 (0)	0.56	1.06

Note. 1. y and V (y) are as for Table 8.5a.

2. The number of strokes in exposed persons (a) is given after the R.R. in parentheses. There were 5 strokes in nonwhite females aged 50-59 and 13 strokes in nonwhite females aged 60-69. Read in conjunction with Table 8.6, cells b, c, and d of the 2×2 table can be obtained by subtraction.

betes, a heart attack, loss of eyesight, and dizziness (all $p < 0.01$) together with a history of chest pain, hardened arteries, the use of alcohol, a temporary weakness of an arm or leg, double vision, deafness, and memory loss (all $p < 0.05$). Much the most important of these is a history of treated hypertension, both from the approximate *t value* [$y/S.E.(y) = 5.6$] obtained and from the relatively good sensitivity (51%) and specificity (99.3%) found when a history of treated hypertension is used as a screening test. While not reaching statistical significance, it is noted, however, that all the risk factors considered, with the exception of cigarette smoking, a family history of stroke, and temporary weakness of the face (the numbers in this last group were very small) did have a relative risk of greater than 1.

When one looks next at the figures for the eight race-sex-age subgroups, it is important to appreciate that one is dealing with very small numbers. With this in mind, we find that those variables for which there was a significantly increased relative risk ($p < 0.05$) were as follows:

Category	*A History of*
White males aged 50-59	hardened arteries use of alcohol (exact probability 0.015) memory loss
White males aged 60-69	treated hypertension heart attack chest pain
White females aged 50-59	treated diabetes
White females aged 60-69	treated hypertension treated diabetes loss of eyesight double vision incoordination
Nonwhite males aged 50-59	treated hypertension speech disturbances dizziness
Nonwhite males aged 60-69	heart attack dizziness
Nonwhite females aged 50-59	(none)
Nonwhite females aged 60-69	gout

We note again that large relative risks by themselves need not be meaningful. For white females aged 60 to 69 years, the relative risk associated with hardened arteries (9.59) and choking (6.50) were substantial, yet the exact probabilities were 0.12 and 0.06, respectively.

The relative risks for a first attack of thrombotic stroke associated with the variables looked at in the prospective interviewer study are given in Table 8.8a. In Table 8.8b, persons aged 50 to

TABLE 8.8a

THE PROSPECTIVE INTERVIEWER STUDY: THE RELATIVE RISKS OF A FIRST STROKE (DUE TO CEREBRAL THROMBOSIS) ASSOCIATED WITH SELECTED VARIABLES FROM THE HISTORIES GIVEN BY 8519 RESPONDENTS

History of:	*Number of respondents.* *Exposed to risk factor* *Stroke (a)*	*No stroke (b)*	*Not exposed* *Stroke (c)*	*No stroke (d)*	*Rel. Risk*	*y*	*S.E.(y)*
Treated hypertension	30	2025	25	6439	3.77	1.33	0.27
Treated diabetes	8	473	47	7991	2.84	1.10	0.37
Heart attack	10	388	45	8076	4.34	1.56	0.34
Chest pain	10	644	45	7820	2.67	1.03	0.34
Inter. claudication	2	369	53	8095	0.83	0.02	0.60
Hardened arteries	6	273	49	8191	3.62	1.37	0.41
Pounding in head	5	469	50	7995	1.70	0.61	0.43
Weight increase > 20 pounds	23	2851	32	5613	1.41	0.35	0.27
Ponderal index < 12	23	2775	32	5689	1.47	0.39	0.27
Shortness of breath	7	637	48	7827	1.78	0.64	0.38
Gout	4	509	51	7955	1.22	0.31	0.47
Cigarette smoking	14	1809	41	6655	1.25	0.25	0.30
Use of alcohol	18	2042	37	6422	1.52	0.44	0.28
Family history of stroke	19	2999	36	5465	0.96	—0.03	0.28
Temp. weakness arm or leg	4	288	51	8176	2.21	0.90	0.47
Teamp. weakness face	1	102	54	8362	1.51	0.81	0.72
Sensory loss arm or leg	5	526	50	7938	1.50	0.49	0.43
Loss of eyesight	17	1626	38	6838	1.87	0.64	0.29
Double vision	6	529	49	7935	1.83	0.67	0.41
Incoordination	7	792	48	7672	1.41	0.40	0.38
Fainting	6	688	49	7776	1.38	0.39	0.40
Headaches	17	1895	38	6569	1.54	0.45	0.29
Deafness	10	890	45	7574	1.88	0.67	0.34
Speech disturbances	7	813	48	7651	1.37	0.37	0.38
Confusion	4	312	51	8152	2.04	0.82	0.47
Choking	3	517	52	7947	0.89	0.02	0.52
Dizziness	20	1958	35	6506	1.89	0.65	0.28
Memory loss	3	174	52	8290	2.72	1.15	0.52

Note. y and V (y) are as for Table 8.5a.

TABLE 8.8b

THE PROSPECTIVE INTERVIEWER STUDY: THE RELATIVE RISKS OF A FIRST STROKE (DUE TO CEREBRAL THROMBOSIS) ASSOCIATED WITH SELECTED VARIABLES FROM THE HISTORIES OF 4170 RESPONDENTS AGED 60-69 AND 4349 RESPONDENTS AGED 50-59

History of:	*Aged 60-69*			*Aged 50-59*		
	R.R.	*y*	*S.E.(y)*	*R.R.*	*y*	*S.E.(y)*
Treated hypertension	3.47 (22)	1.25	0.32	3.54 (8)	1.28	0.46
Treated diabetes	2.56 (6)	1.01	0.42	2.82 (2)	1.23	0.63
Heart attacks	5.18 (8)	1.72	0.38	2.86 (2)	1.24	0.63
Chest pain	2.93 (8)	1.13	0.38	1.76 (2)	0.76	0.63
Inter. claudication	0.55 (1)	—0.22	0.73	1.50 (1)	0.78	0.75
Hardened arteries	1.80 (3)	0.73	0.53	10.14 (3)	2.46	0.57
Pounding in head	2.60 (5)	1.04	0.49	0 (0)	—0.74	1.03
Weight increase > 20 lbs.	1.64 (18)	0.50	0.32	0.88 (5)	—0.07	0.49
Ponderal index < 12	1.09 (14)	0.10	0.33	2.51 (9)	0.92	0.46
Shortness of breath	1.25 (4)	0.33	0.48	3.04 (3)	1.24	0.57
Gout	1.75 (4)	0.67	0.48	0 (0)	—0.77	1.03
Cigarette smoking	1.44 (9)	0.40	0.37	1.25 (5)	0.28	0.49
Use of alcohol	1.18 (10)	0.19	0.36	2.66 (8)	0.99	0.46
Family history of stroke	0.98 (14)	— 0	0.33	0.82 (5)	—0.14	0.49
Temp. weakness of arm or leg	1.58 (2)	0.66	0.61	3.73 (2)	1.51	0.63
Temp. weakness face	2.27 (1)	1.21	0.74	0 (0)	0.80	1.04
Sensory loss arm or leg	2.33 (5)	0.93	0.45	0 (0)	—0.87	1.03
Loss of eyesight	2.04 (14)	0.73	0.33	1.09 (3)	0.20	0.56
Double vision	2.06 (5)	0.81	0.45	1.03 (1)	0.40	0.75
Incoordination	1.19 (5)	0.25	0.44	1.63 (2)	0.68	0.63
Fainting	1.26 (4)	0.33	0.48	1.59 (2)	0.65	0.63
Headaches	1.05 (8)	0.09	0.38	3.46 (9)	1.24	0.46
Deafness	1.49 (7)	0.45	0.38	2.43 (3)	1.01	0.56
Speech disturbances	1.03 (4)	0.13	0.48	2.16 (3)	0.89	0.56
Confusion	1.99 (3)	0.83	0.53	1.82 (1)	0.97	0.75
Choking	0.75 (2)	—0.08	0.60	1.10 (1)	0.47	0.75
Dizziness	1.53 (13)	0.44	0.33	2.61 (7)	0.98	0.47
Memory loss	1.10 (1)	0.48	0.73	7.40 (2)	2.20	0.64

Note. 1. *y* and *V* (*y*) are as for Table 8.5a.

2. The number of persons exposed to the factor who developed stroke (cell a) is given in parentheses after the R.R. Given that the number of persons aged 60-69 who developed stroke was 38 and the number of persons aged 50-59 who developed stroke was 17, read in conjunction with Table 8.6, one can readily obtain by substraction the other cells b, c, and d, of the usual 2×2 table for each variable.

TABLE 8.8c

THE PROSPECTIVE INTERVIEWER STUDY: THE RELATIVE RISKS OF A FIRST STROKE (DUE TO CEREBRAL THROMBOSIS) ASSOCIATED WITH SELECTED VARIABLES FROM THE HISTORIES OF 5049 FEMALE RESPONDENTS AND 3470 MALE RESPONDENTS

History of:	*Female*			*Male*		
	R.R.	*y*	*S.E.(y)*	*R.R.*	*y*	*S.E.(y)*
Treated hypertension	3.54 (15)	1.26	0.38	4.64 (15)	1.53	0.36
Treated diabetes	3.68 (5)	1.38	0.46	2.18 (3)	0.92	0.54
Heart attack	2.13 (2)	0.96	0.62	5.97 (8)	1.85	0.40
Chest pain	1.12 (2)	0.32	0.61	3.94 (8)	1.42	0.40
Inter. claudication	1.87 (2)	0.83	0.61	0 (0)	—1.03	1.02
Hardened arteries	1.25 (1)	0.61	0.74	5.67 (5)	1.84	0.46
Pounding in head	1.84 (3)	0.74	0.54	0.85 (1)	0.22	0.74
Weight increase > 20 lbs.	1.12 (10)	0.12	0.39	1.84 (13)	0.62	0.36
Ponderal index < 12	1.43 (13)	0.36	0.38	2.00 (10)	0.71	0.38
Shortness of breath	1.61 (3)	0.60	0.54	1.94 (4)	0.76	0.49
Gout	1.84 (3)	0.74	0.54	0.66 (1)	—0.03	0.74
Cigarette smoking	0.49 (2)	—0.52	0.61	1.55 (12)	0.45	0.36
Use of alcohol	0.45 (2)	—0.59	0.61	2.12 (16)	0.75	0.36
Family history of stroke	1.01 (10)	0.02	0.39	0.99 (9)	0.02	0.38
Temp. weakness of arm or leg	2.19 (2)	.99	0.62	2.33 (2)	1.05	0.62
Temp. weakness face	2.80 (1)	1.42	0.74	0 (0)	—0.13	1.02
Sensory loss arm or leg	1.25 (2)	0.42	0.61	1.75 (3)	0.69	0.54
Loss of eyesight	2.08 (9)	0.76	0.40	1.76 (8)	0.60	0.39
Double vision	1.90 (3)	0.77	0.54	1.79 (3)	0.72	0.54
Incoordination	1.59 (4)	0.56	0.50	1.31 (3)	0.40	0.54
Fainting	0.42 (1)	—0.48	0.74	2.63 (5)	1.05	0.46
Headaches	1.34 (8)	0.32	0.40	1.94 (9)	0.70	0.39
Deafness	1.80 (4)	0.68	0.50	1.80 (6)	0.65	0.43
Speech disturbances	1.08 (3)	0.21	0.54	1.84 (4)	0.71	0.49
Confusion	1.99 (2)	0.89	0.62	2.20 (2)	1.00	0.61
Choking	1.08 (2)	0.28	0.61	0.74 (1)	0.08	0.74
Dizziness	1.28 (8)	0.28	0.40	2.90 (12)	1.08	0.37
Memory loss	3.45 (2)	1.44	0.62	2.10 (1)	1.13	0.74

Note. 1. y and V (y) are as for Table 8.5a.

2. The number of persons exposed to the factor who developed stroke (cell a) is given in parentheses after the R.R. Given that the number of females who developed stroke was 26 and the number of males who developed stroke was 29, read in conjunction with Table 8.6, one can readily obtain by stubtraction the other cells b, c, and d, of the usual 2×2 table for each variable.

TABLE 8.8d

THE PROSPECTIVE INTERVIEWER STUDY: THE RELATIVE RISKS OF A FIRST STROKE (DUE TO CEREBRAL THROMBOSIS) ASSOCIATED WITH SELECTED VARIABLES FROM THE HISTORIES OF 3004 NONWHITE RESPONDENTS AND 5515 WHITE RESPONDENTS

History of:	*Nonwhite* *R.R.*	*y*	*S.E.(y)*	*White* *R.R.*	*y*	*S.E.(y)*
Treated hypertension	2.34 (13)	0.85	0.38	5.35 (17)	1.68	0.36
Treated diabetes	1.10 (2)	0.29	0.62	5.09 (6)	1.70	0.43
Heart attack	4.48 (3)	1.65	0.55	5.29 (7)	1.73	0.41
Chest pain	1.55 (2)	0.64	0.62	3.81 (8)	1.38	0.40
Inter. claudication	0.82 (1)	0.18	0.74	0.82 (1)	0.18	0.73
Hardened arteries	0 (0)	0.22	1.03	5.86 (6)	1.84	0.43
Pounding in head	0.88 (1)	0.27	0.74	2.40 (4)	0.98	0.49
Weight increase > 20 lbs.	1.35 (12)	0.31	0.38	1.36 (11)	0.32	0.37
Ponderal index < 12	1.48 (15)	0.38	0.38	1.17 (8)	0.19	0.40
Shortness of breath	1.77 (3)	0.71	0.54	1.85 (4)	0.72	0.49
Gout	1.08 (2)	0.28	0.62	1.30 (2)	0.46	0.61
Cigarette smoking	1.54 (6)	0.49	0.44	1.20 (8)	0.21	0.40
Use of alcohol	1.24 (10)	0.24	0.39	1.51 (8)	0.45	0.40
Family history of stroke	0.58 (5)	—0.47	0.46	1.46 (14)	0.38	0.36
Temp. weakness of arm or leg	1.94 (2)	0.86	0.62	2.36 (2)	1.06	0.61
Temp. weakness face	0 (0)	1.16	1.05	2.25 (1)	1.20	0.74
Sensory loss arm or leg	1.14 (2)	0.33	0.62	1.83 (3)	0.74	0.54
Loss of eyesight	1.40 (8)	0.37	0.41	2.25 (9)	0.84	0.38
Double vision	1.28 (3)	0.38	0.54	2.35 (3)	0.99	0.54
Incoordination	0.71 (2)	—0.15	0.61	2.18 (5)	0.85	0.46
Fainting	1.99 (4)	0.79	0.50	0.85 (2)	0.03	0.61
Headaches	1.58 (8)	0.49	0.41	1.53 (9)	0.45	0.38
Deafness	0.79 (2)	—0.04	0.61	3.05 (8)	1.16	0.40
Speech disturbances	1.31 (4)	0.37	0.50	1.28 (3)	0.38	0.54
Confusion	1.37 (2)	0.52	0.62	2.76 (2)	1.22	0.61
Choking	0 (0)	—0.58	1.02	1.39 (3)	0.46	0.54
Dizziness	1.74 (9)	0.58	0.40	2.03 (11)	0.72	0.37
Memory loss	1.39 (1)	0.71	0.74	4.32 (2)	1.62	0.62

Note. 1. y and $V(y)$ are as for Table 8.5a.

2. The number of persons exposed to the factor who developed stroke (cell a) is given in parentheses after the R.R. Given that the number of nonwhites who developed stroke was 26 and the number of whites who developed stroke was 29, read in conjunction with Table 8.6, one can readily obtain by subtraction the other cells b, c, and d, of the usual 2×2 table for each variable.

59 years and 60 to 69 years are compared; in Table 8.8c, males and females are compared; and in Table 8.8d, whites and non-whites are compared with respect to the relative risks for a thrombotic stroke. Table 8.9a,b,c, and d repeat this procedure for the 22 strokes due to cerebral hemorrhage. For comparative purposes it is better to look at Tables 8.7a (all strokes), 8.8a (all cerebral thrombosis), and 8.9a (all cerebral hemorrhage) together. Variables which do not have a relative risk significantly greater than 1 are not given in the following list.

Variable	*Relative Risk Significantly ($p < 0.05$) Greater than 1 for*		
A History of	*All Strokes*	*Cerebral Thrombosis*	*Cerebral Hemorrhage*
Treated hypertension	Yes	Yes	No
Treated diabetes	Yes	Yes	Yes
Heart attack	Yes	Yes	No
Chest pain	Yes	Yes	No
Hardened arteries	Yes	Yes	No
Use of alcohol	Yes	No	Yes
Temporary weakness arm or leg	Yes	No	No
Loss of eyesight	Yes	Yes	No
Double vision	Yes	No	No
Deafness	Yes	No	No
Dizziness	Yes	Yes	Yes
Memory loss	Yes	Yes	No

The results with regard to treated hypertension (significant for thrombosis only) and the use of alcohol (significant for hemorrhage only) are of particular interest.

TABLE 8.9a

THE PROSPECTIVE INTERVIEWER STUDY: THE RELATIVE RISKS OF A FIRST STROKE (DUE TO CEREBRAL HEMORRHAGE) ASSOCIATED WITH SELECTED VARIABLES FROM THE HISTORIES GIVEN BY 8519 RESPONDENTS

History of:	*Number of respondents* — *Exposed to risk factor* — *Stroke (a)*	*No stroke (b)*	*Not exposed* — *Stroke (c)*	*No stroke (d)*	*Rel. Risk*	*y*	*S.E.(y)*
Treated hypertension	9	2046	13	6451	2.18	0.79	0.41
Treated diabetes	4	477	18	8020	3.71	1.41	0.50
Heart attack	1	397	21	8100	0.97	0.35	0.74
Chest pain	3	651	19	7846	1.90	0.77	0.55
Inter. claudication	2	369	20	8128	2.20	0.98	0.62
Hardened arteries	0	279	22	8218	0.00	—0.42	1.02
Pounding in head	1	473	21	8024	0.81	0.16	0.74
Weight increase > 20 pounds	7	2867	15	5630	0.92	—0.05	0.43
Ponderal index < 12	10	2788	12	5709	1.70	0.54	0.41
Shortness of breath	3	641	19	7856	1.93	0.78	0.55
Gout	3	510	19	7987	2.46	1.03	0.55
Cigarette smoking	3	1820	19	6677	0.58	—0.42	0.55
Use of alcohol	11	2049	11	6448	3.14	1.14	0.41
Family history of stroke	5	3013	17	5484	0.54	—0.56	0.47
Temp. weakness arm or leg	1	291	21	8206	1.34	0.67	0.74
Temp. weakness face	0	103	22	8394	0.00	0.58	1.03
Sensory loss arm or leg	1	530	21	7967	0.72	0.04	0.74
Loss of eyesight	6	1637	16	6860	1.57	0.50	0.45
Double vision	2	533	20	7964	1.49	0.60	0.62
Incoordination	4	795	18	7702	2.15	0.85	0.50
Fainting	3	691	19	7806	1.78	0.70	0.55
Headaches	7	1905	15	6592	1.61	0.51	0.43
Deafness	4	896	18	7601	1.88	0.72	0.50
Speech disturbances	4	816	18	7681	2.09	0.82	0.50
Confusion	1	315	21	8182	1.24	0.59	0.74
Choking	2	518	20	7979	1.54	0.63	0.62
Dizziness	11	1967	11	6530	3.31	1.20	0.41
Memory loss	1	176	21	8321	2.24	1.19	0.74

Note. y and $V(y)$ are as for Table 8.5a.

TABLE 8.9b

THE PROSPECTIVE INTERVIEWER STUDY: THE RELATIVE RISKS OF A FIRST STROKE (DUE TO CEREBRAL HEMORRHAGE) ASSOCIATED WITH SELECTED VARIABLES FROM THE HISTORIES OF 4170 RESPONDENTS AGED 60-69 AND 4349 RESPONDENTS AGED 50-59

History of:	*Persons aged 60-69 yrs.*			*Persons aged 50-59 yrs.*		
	R.R.	*y*	*S.E.(y)*	*R.R.*	*y*	*S.E.(y)*
Treated hypertension	2.16 (6)	0.78	0.52	1.99 (3)	0.76	0.63
Treated diabetes	1.14 (1)	0.49	0.76	10.59 (3)	2.44	0.63
Heart attack	1.62 (1)	0.84	0.76	0 (0)	0.11	1.05
Chest pain	3.29 (3)	1.30	0.59	0 (0)	—0.37	1.05
Inter. claudication	3.67 (2)	1.48	0.65	0 (0)	0.22	1.05
Hardened arteries	0 (0)	—0.25	1.04	0 (0)	0.90	1.05
Pounding in head	1.43 (1)	0.71	0.76	0 (0)	—0.13	1.05
Weight increase > 20 lbs.	1.14 (5)	0.16	0.53	0.60 (2)	—0.35	0.68
Ponderal index < 12	1.60 (6)	0.48	0.52	1.79 (4)	0.60	0.61
Shortness of breath	0.89 (1)	0.24	0.76	4.06 (2)	1.56	0.68
Gout	4.47 (3)	1.61	0.59	0 (0)	—0.16	1.05
Cigarette smoking	0.39 (1)	—0.59	0.76	0.86 (2)	0	0.68
Use of alcohol	2.06 (5)	0.76	0.53	5.99 (6)	1.72	0.63
Family history of stroke	0.50 (3)	—0.58	0.58	0.56 (2)	—0.42	0.68
Temp. weakness of arm or leg	0 (0)	0.04	1.04	3.50 (1)	1.60	0.78
Temp. weakness face	0 (0)	1.12	1.04	0 (0)	1.42	1.06
Sensory loss arm or leg	1.28 (1)	0.61	0.76	0 (0)	—0.26	1.05
Loss of eyesight	1.55 (4)	0.50	0.55	1.45 (2)	0.52	0.68
Double vision	2.47 (2)	1.08	0.65	0 (0)	—0.15	1.05
Incoordination	2.36 (3)	0.96	0.58	1.53 (1)	0.77	0.78
Fainting	3.20 (3)	1.27	0.59	0 (0)	—0.47	1.05
Headaches	2.46 (5)	0.94	0.53	0.88 (2)	0.02	0.68
Deafness	1.20 (2)	0.36	0.65	3.24 (2)	1.33	0.68
Speech disturbances	1.59 (2)	0.64	0.65	2.88 (2)	1.21	0.68
Confusion	1.94 (1)	1.02	0.76	0 (0)	0.42	1.05
Choking	1.13 (1)	0.48	0.76	2.21 (1)	1.13	0.78
Dizziness	2.52 (6)	0.94	0.52	4.66 (5)	1.52	0.61
Memory loss	0 (0)	0.40	1.04	6.94 (1)	2.28	0.79

Note. 1. y and V (y) are as for Table 8.5a.

2. The number of persons exposed to the factor who developed stroke (cell a) is given in parentheses after the R.R. Given that the number of persons aged 60-69 who developed stroke was 13 and the number of persons aged 50-59 who devolped stroke was 9, read in conjunction with Table 8.6, one can readily obtain by subtraction the other cells b, c, and d, of the usual 2×2 table for each variable.

TABLE 8.9c

THE PROSPECTIVE INTERVIEWER STUDY: THE RELATIVE RISKS OF A FIRST STROKE (DUE TO CEREBRAL HEMORRHAGE) ASSOCIATED WITH SELECTED VARIABLES FROM THE HISTORIES OF 5049 FEMALE RESPONDENTS AND 3470 MALE RESPONDENTS

History of:	*Females* *R.R.*	*y*	*S.E.(y)*	*Males* *R.R.*	*y*	*S.E.(y)*
Treated hypertension	7.79 (6)	1.91	0.69	1.18 (3)	0.27	0.58
Treated diabetes	5.15 (2)	1.78	0.69	3.16 (2)	1.33	0.64
Heart attack	0 (0)	0.40	1.06	1.21 (1)	0.55	0.76
Chest pain	0 (0)	—0.23	1.06	2.82 (3)	1.15	0.58
Inter. claudication	0 (0)	0.27	1.06	3.54 (2)	1.45	0.64
Hardened arteries	0 (0)	0.61	1.06	0 (0)	—0.07	1.04
Pounding in head	2.02 (1)	1.04	0.79	0 (0)	—0.21	1.04
Weight increase > 20 lbs.	1.07 (3)	0.12	0.65	0.91 (4)	—0.02	0.54
Ponderal index < 12	1.43 (4)	0.36	0.63	2.84 (6)	1.07	0.50
Shortness of breath	1.76 (1)	0.90	0.79	2.02 (2)	0.88	0.64
Gout	4.70 (2)	1.69	0.69	1.42 (1)	0.72	0.76
Cigarette smoking	0 (0)	—1.07	1.05	0.85 (3)	—0.06	0.58
Use of alcohol	3.27 (3)	1.24	0.65	2.30 (8)	0.81	0.51
Family history of stroke	0.54 (2)	—0.48	0.69	0.60 (3)	—0.40	0.58
Temp. weakness of arm or leg	3.75 (1)	1.66	0.79	0 (0)	0.07	1.04
Temp. weakness face	0 (0)	1.40	1.06	0 (0)	1.29	1.05
Sensory loss arm or leg	0 (0)	—0.13	1.06	1.16 (1)	0.52	0.76
Loss of eyesight	2.35 (3)	0.91	0.65	1.26 (3)	0.34	0.58
Double vision	4.84 (2)	1.72	0.69	0 (0)	—0.63	1.04
Incoordination	1.25 (1)	0.56	0.79	3.10 (3)	1.24	0.58
Fainting	3.51 (2)	1.40	0.69	0.97 (1)	0.33	0.76
Headaches	1.81 (3)	0.65	0.65	1.73 (4)	0.61	0.54
Deafness	0 (0)	—0.54	1.06	2.76 (4)	1.09	0.54
Speech disturbances	2.77 (2)	1.16	0.69	1.91 (2)	0.83	0.64
Confusion	0 (0)	0.33	1.06	2.29 (1)	1.19	0.76
Choking	4.33 (2)	1.61	0.69	0 (0)	—0.34	1.04
Dizziness	2.89 (4)	1.06	0.63	4.11 (7)	1.42	0.50
Memory loss	0 (0)	0.88	1.06	4.53 (1)	1.88	0.77

Note. 1. y and $V(y)$ are as for Table 8.5a.

2. The number of persons exposed to the factor who developed stroke (cell a) is given in parentheses after the R.R. Given that the number of females who developed stroke was 8 and the number of males who developed stroke was 14, read in conjunction with Table 8.6, one can readily obtain by subtraction the other cells b, c, and d, of the usual 2×2 table for each variable.

TABLE 8.9d

THE PROSPECTIVE INTERVIEWER STUDY: THE RELATIVE RISKS OF A FIRST STROKE (DUE TO CEREBRAL HEMORRHAGE) ASSOCIATED WITH SELECTED VARIABLES FROM THE HISTORIES OF 3004 NONWHITE RESPONDENTS AND 5515 WHITE RESPONDENTS

History of:	*Nonwhites* R.R.	y	S.E.(y)	*Whites* R.R.	y	S.E.(y)
Treated hypertension	1.46 (5)	0.41	0.53	3.02 (4)	1.13	0.61
Treated diabetes	3.95 (3)	1.48	0.59	2.44 (1)	1.23	0.78
Heart attack	0 (0)	0.23	1.04	2.08 (1)	1.07	0.78
Chest pain	0 (0)	—0.37	1.04	5.00 (3)	1.68	0.63
Inter. claudication	3.72 (2)	1.50	0.65	0 (0)	0.18	1.05
Hardened arteries	0 (0)	0.89	1.05	0 (0)	0.16	1.05
Pounding in head	1.84 (1)	0.97	0.76	0 (0)	—0.24	1.05
Weight increase > 20 lbs.	0.99 (5)	0.02	0.53	0.64 (2)	—0.30	0.68
Ponderal index < 12	0.93 (6)	—0.06	0.52	2.45 (4)	0.92	0.61
Shortness of breath	2.47 (2)	1.08	0.65	1.45 (1)	0.71	0.78
Gout	3.89 (3)	1.47	0.59	0 (0)	—0.09	1.05
Cigarette smoking	0.43 (1)	—0.49	0.76	0.90 (2)	0.04	0.68
Use of alcohol	2.32 (7)	0.83	0.52	3.38 (4)	1.24	0.61
Family history of stroke	0 (0)	—2.40	1.04	1.96 (5)	0.65	0.61
Temp. weakness of arm or leg	1.94 (1)	1.02	0.77	0 (0)	0.51	1.05
Temp. weakness face	0 (0)	1.84	1.06	0 (0)	1.19	1.05
Sensory loss arm or leg	0 (0)	—0.68	1.04	1.98 (1)	1.03	0.78
Loss of eyesight	0.94 (3)	0.04	0.59	2.50 (3)	0.99	0.63
Double vision	0.82 (1)	0.16	0.76	2.55 (1)	1.28	0.78
Incoordination	0.71 (1)	0.02	0.76	5.22 (3)	1.73	0.63
Fainting	3.29 (3)	1.30	0.59	0 (0)	—0.51	1.05
Headaches	0.30 (1)	—0.86	0.76	6.80 (6)	1.84	0.63
Deafness	1.72 (2)	0.72	0.65	2.28 (2)	0.98	0.68
Speech disturbances	2.17 (3)	0.88	0.59	1.39 (1)	0.67	0.78
Confusion	1.37 (1)	0.68	0.76	0 (0)	0.67	1.05
Choking	2.50 (1)	1.28	0.77	1.50 (1)	0.75	0.78
Dizziness	2.06 (5)	0.76	0.53	6.63 (6)	1.82	0.63
Memory loss	0 (0)	0.20	1.04	7.29 (1)	2.33	0.79

Note. 1. y and $V(y)$ are as for Table 8.5a.

2. The number of persons exposed to the factor who developed stroke (cell a) is given in parentheses after the R.R. Given that the number of nonwhites who developed stroke was 13 and the number of whites who developed stroke was 9, read in conjunction with Table 8.6, one can readily obtain by subtraction the other cells b, c, and d, of the usual 2×2 table for each variable.

Our findings dealing with the age-sex-race comparisons can be displayed in a similar fashion. For the age comparison (see Tables 8.8b and 8.9b), we find the following:

	Relative Risk Significantly ($p < 0.05$) Greater than 1 for			
Variable	*Cerebral Thrombosis*		*Cerebral Hemorrhage*	
A History of	*Aged 50-59*	*Aged 60-69*	*Aged 50-59*	*Aged 60-69*
Treated hypertension	Yes	Yes	No	No
Treated diabetes	No	Yes	Yes	No
Heart attack	No	Yes	No	No
Chest pain	No	Yes	No	No
Hardened arteries	Yes	No	No	No
Pounding in head	No	Yes	No	No
Gout	No	No	No	Yes
Use of alcohol	Yes	No	Yes	No
Sensory loss arm or leg	No	Yes	No	No
Loss of eyesight	No	Yes	No	No
Headaches	Yes	No	No	No
Dizziness	No	No	Yes	No
Memory loss	Yes	No	No	No

The results for the age group 50 to 59 years are of special interest, with a history of hardened arteries (thrombosis only), use of alcohol (thrombosis and hemorrhage), headaches (thrombosis only), dizziness (hemorrhage only), and memory loss (thrombosis only) carrying a significant relative risk in this younger age group but not in the age group 60 to 69 years.

For the comparison by sex (see Tables 8.8c and 8.9c), we find the following:

Variable A History of	*Relative Risk Significantly ($p < 0.05$) Greater than 1 for* Cerebral Thrombosis *Male*	*Female*	*Cerebral Hemorrhage* *Male*	*Female*
Treated hypertension	Yes	Yes	No	Yes
Treated diabetes	No	Yes	No	No
Heart attack	Yes	No	No	No
Chest pain	Yes	No	No	No
Hardened arteries	Yes	No	No	No
Use of alcohol	Yes	No	No	No
Fainting	Yes	No	No	No
Dizziness	Yes	No	Yes	No

Of interest in this comparison is the very small number of risk factors which have emerged (hypertension and diabetes for thrombosis and hypertension alone for hemorrhage) as having a significant relative risk for females.

For the comparison by race (see Tables 8.8d and 8.9d), we find the following:

Variable A History of	*Relative Risk Significantly ($p < 005$) Greater than 1 for* Cerebral Thrombosis *White*	*Nonwhite*	*Cerebral Hemorrhage* *White*	*Nonwhite*
Treated hypertension	Yes	Yes	No	No
Treated diabetes	Yes	No	No	Yes
Heart attack	Yes	Yes	No	No
Chest pain	Yes	No	Yes	No
Hardened arteries	Yes	No	No	No
Gout	No	No	No	Yes
Loss of eyesight	Yes	No	No	No
Incoordination	No	No	Yes	No
Headaches	No	No	Yes	No
Deafness	Yes	No	No	No
Dizziness	No	No	Yes	No
Memory loss	Yes	No	No	No

Only a history of treated hypertension and a heart attack (for thrombosis) and a history of treated diabetes and gout (for hemorrhage) have emerged as significant risk factors for nonwhites.

The cardiovascular disease history is particularly relevant for cerebral thrombosis among whites.

Among the 1916 persons being followed for the prospective examination study, there were 18 strokes, of which 13 were ascribed to cerebral thrombosis and 3 to cerebral hemorrhage. Thirteen were white and 9 were male. Three of the 18 died from stroke (2 before they reached hospital), 5 were hospitalized and did not die from their stroke (and 10 were treated at home and survived their stroke, yielding a rather higher percentage of survivors (85%) and "treated-at-home" patients (56%) than was the situation with the prospective study strokes as a whole (72% and 38%).

The relative risks associated with the variables looked at in the examination study with regard to all strokes and thrombotic strokes are presented in Tables 8.10 and 8.11. There were too few hemorrhagic strokes in this physician-examined subgroup to make an analysis for hemorrhagic stroke worthwhile. A breakdown by age, race, and sex was not realistic.

TABLE 8.10

THE PROSPECTIVE EXAMINATION STUDY: THE RELATIVE RISKS OF A FIRST STROKE (ALL TYPES COMBINED) ASSOCIATED WITH SELECTED VARIABLES FROM THE MEDICAL HISTORY, EXAMINATION AND LABORATORY FINDINGS ON 1916 RESPONDENTS

Variable:	*Number of respondents*						
	Exposed to risk factor		*Not exposed*		*Rel.*		
History of:	*Stroke (a)*	*No stroke (b)*	*Stroke (c)*	*No stroke (d)*	*Risk*	*y*	*S.E.(y)*
Hypertension	12	588	6	1310	4.39	1.45	.47
Diabetes	6	125	12	1773	6.81	1.99	.48
Ischemic heart disease	8	122	10	1776	10.99	2.46	.46
Valvular heart disease	0	28	18	1870	0.00	0.57	1.04
Cardiac dysrhythmia	3	140	15	1758	2.48	1.04	.57
Cong. heart failure	4	65	14	1883	7.85	2.19	.53
Inter. claudication	2	41	16	1857	5.44	1.91	.65
Decr. monocular vision	4	120	14	1778	4.13	1.52	.52
Decr. binocular vision	1	221	17	1677	0.45	—0.43	.75
Diplopia	3	59	15	1839	5.98	1.94	.57
Vertigo	4	167	14	1731	2.92	1.16	.52
Deafness	4	293	14	1605	1.56	0.53	.52
Memory deterioration	1	167	17	1731	0.61	—0.12	.74
Hypothyroidism	0	32	18	1866	0.00	0.44	1.04

TABLE 8-10 (con't.)

Variable: History of:	*Number of respondents* — *Exposed to risk factor* — *Stroke (a)*	*No stroke (b)*	*Not exposed* — *Stroke (c)*	*No stroke (d)*	*Rel. Risk*	*y*	*S.E.(y)*
Exam findings of:							
Arcus senilis	2	351	6	1018	0.97	0.10	.69
A.S. fundi	3	168	5	1201	4.23	1.51	.65
K.W. fundi > gr. 2	10	322	8	1576	5.96	1.80	.45
Congestive heart failure	1	29	17	1869	3.70	1.69	.76
Valvular heart disease	2	149	16	1749	1.46	0.57	.63
Dysrhythmia	3	81	15	1817	4.36	1.61	.57
Cervical bruits	2	108	16	1790	2.05	0.91	.63
Supraclavicular bruits	4	61	14	1837	8.13	2.22	.53
Systolic B.P. < 134	2	683	16	1215	0.22	—1.31	.63
Systolic B.P. 134-156	4	654	14	1244	0.55	—0 52	.51
Systolic B.P. > 156	12	561	6	1337	4.68	1.52	.47
Diastolic B.P. < 82	2	858	16	1040	0.15	—1.70	.63
Diastolic B.P. 82-90	7	529	11	1369	1.64	0.52	.46
Diastolic B.P. > 90	9	511	9	1387	2.68	1 00	.45
Exam findings of:							
Abn. Q on ECG	3	47	15	1850	7.46	2.17	.58
Abn. R on ECG	4	182	14	1716	2.66	1.07	.52
Abn. ST on ECG	14	363	4	1545	14.38	2.62	.52
Therm. dif. > 1° F	3	84	15	1814	4.20	1.58	.57
Ponderal index < 12	9	723	9	1175	1.62	0.48	.45
2-hr. blood glucose < 90	3	212	14	1605	1.61	0.60	.57
2-hr. blood glucose 90-150	8	858	9	959	0.99	0.00	.46
2-hr. blood glucose > 150	6	747	11	1070	0.78	—0.21	.48
Cholesterol < 227	3	495	14	1280	0.57	—0.47	.57
Cholesterol 227-277	6	710	11	1065	0.82	—0.17	.48
Cholesterol > 277	8	570	9	1205	1.87	0.63	.46
Triglycerides < 2	2	140	14	1547	1.57	0.64	.64
Triglycerides 2-4	8	953	8	734	0.77	—0.26	.47
Triglycerides > 4	6	594	10	1093	1.10	0.13	.49

Note. 1. *y* and *V* (*y*) are as for Table 8.5a.
2. Arcus senilis and A.S. fundi were not recorded in the first year so these patients are not recorded in the follow-up.
3. Laboratory data was not available on all patients.

TABLE 8.11
THE PROSPECTIVE EXAMINATION STUDY: THE RELATIVE RISKS OF A FIRST STROKE (CEREBRAL THROMBOSIS) ASSOCIATED WITH SELECTED VARIABLES FROM THE MEDICAL HISTORY, EXAMINATION AND LABORATORY FINDINGS ON 1916 RESPONDENTS

Variables:	*Number of respondents*						
	Exposed to risk factor		*Not exposed*		*Rel.*		
History of:	*Stroke (a)*	*No stroke (b)*	*Stroke (c)*	*No stroke (d)*	*Risk*	*y*	*S.E.(y)*
Hypertension	9	591	4	1312	4.94	1.54	.55
Diabetes	4	127	9	1776	6.06	1.89	.55
Ischemic heart disease	8	128	5	1781	21.01	3.06	.54
Valvular heart disease	0	28	13	1875	0.00	0.88	1.05
Cardiac dysrhythmia	2	141	11	1762	2.25	0.99	.65
Cong. heart failure	3	66	10	1837	8.03	2.22	.60
Inter. claudication	2	41	11	1862	7.92	2.28	.66
Decr. monocular vision	2	122	11	1781	2.63	1.15	.65
Decr. binocular vision	1	221	12	1682	0.64	—0.09	.76
Diplopia	1	61	12	1842	2.49	1.28	.77
Vertigo	2	169	11	1734	1.86	0.80	.65
Deafness	4	293	9	1610	2.42	0.95	.55
Memory deterioration	1	167	12	1736	0.87	0.22	.76
Hypothyroidism	0	32	13	1871	0.00	0.75	1.05
Exam findings of:							
Arcus senilis	2	351	5	1019	1.15	.28	.71
A.S. fundi	2	169	5	1201	2.78	1.17	.71
K.W. fundi > gr. 2	7	325	6	1578	5.57	1.72	.52
Congestive heart failure	1	29	12	1894	5.29	2.04	.78
Valvular heart disease	2	149	11	1754	2.13	0.93	.65
Dysrhythmia	2	82	11	1821	3.97	1.57	.66
Cervical bruits	2	108	11	1795	2.99	1.28	.65
Supraclavicular bruits	3	62	10	1831	8.50	2.28	.60
Systolic B.P. < 134	1	684	12	1219	0.15	—1.54	.76
Systolic B.P. 134-156	3	655	10	1248	0.57	—0.45	.59
Systolic B.P. > 156	9	564	4	1339	5.27	1.61	.55
Diastolic B.P. < 82	2	858	11	1045	0.22	—1.33	.64
Diastolic B.P. 82-90	4	532	9	1371	1.14	0.20	.55
Diastolic B.P. > 90	7	513	6	1390	3.13	1.14	.52

Exam finding of:							
Abn. Q on ECG	3	47	10	1856	11.20	2.56	.61
Abn. R on ECG	3	183	10	1720	2.79	1.14	.59
Abn. ST on ECG	10	367	3	1536	13.61	2.53	.59
Therm. dif. > 1° F	2	85	11	1818	3.82	1.53	.65
Ponderal index < 12	5	727	8	1176	1.01	0.04	.53
2-hr. blood glucose < 90	2	213	9	1610	1.62	0.68	.66
2-hr. blood glucose 90-150	6	860	5	963	1.34	0.28	.56
2-hr. blood glucose > 150	3	750	8	1073	0.54	—0.53	.60
Cholsterol < 227	2	496	9	1285	0.58	—0.39	.66
Cholesterol 227-277	4	712	7	1069	0.86	—0.10	.57
Cholesterol < 277	5	573	6	1208	1.75	0.58	.56
Triglycerides < 2	1	141	9	1552	1.22	0.55	.78
Triglycerides 2-4	5	956	5	737	0.77	—0.26	.58
Triglycerides > 4	4	596	6	1097	1.23	0.24	.59

Note. 1. y and $V(y)$ are as for Table 8.5a.
2. Arcus senilis and A.S. fundi were not recorded in the first year so these patients are not recorded in the follow-up.
3. Laboratory data was not available on all patients.

Our findings can again be summarized in the form of a simple listing with only variables having a relative risk significantly ($p < 0.05$) greater than 1 being listed.

Variable	*Relative Risk Significantly (p < 0.05) greater than 1 for* All Strokes	Cerebral Thrombosis
History of		
Hypertension	Yes	Yes
Diabetes	Yes	Yes
Ischemic heart disease	Yes	Yes
Congestive heart failure	Yes	Yes
Intermittent claudication	Yes	Yes
Decreased monocular vision	Yes	No
Diplopia	Yes	No
Vertigo	Yes	Yes
Finding of		
K.W. fundi > gr. 2	Yes	Yes
Cardiac dysrhythmia	Yes	No
Supraclavicular bruits	Yes	Yes
Systolic B.P. > 156	Yes	Yes
Diastolic B.P. > 90	Yes	No
Abn. Q on ECG	Yes	Yes
Abn. ST on ECG	Yes	Yes
Therm. dif. > 1° F	Yes	No

Repeating what was found in the retrospective study, high levels of blood glucose, cholesterol, and triglycerides were not associated with relative risks significantly greater than 1. In fact, for blood glucose the highest relative risk (though not statistically significant) was found for those persons with the lowest two-hour level.

In terms of sensitivity, in addition to the relative risk and the $y/S.E.(y)$ ratio, the most important examination variables were an abnormal ST segment on the ECG (sensitivity 78%), a systolic blood pressure above 156 (sensitivity 67%), and K.W. fundi > grade 2 (sensitivity 56%). The most important history variable was a history of ischemic heart disease (sensitivity 44%), which defined in a more precise fashion the two variables "heart attack" and "chest pain" used in the interviewer study. Of particular interest is the relation with hypertension (on examination) which was found, since the retrospective examination study (see Table 8.5b) did not display this. The findings from the history items replicated closely those obtained in the prospective interviewer study where these items covered more or less the same ground.

There are four variables which we have not yet considered. The percentages of the examined population who were recorded as having an abnormally reduced vital capacity varied so much from year to year of the study (see Table 8.5c) that little reliance can be placed on the findings, which showed no significant difference between the normal and the abnormals.

	Number of Persons (All Strokes)		*Number of Persons (Thrombotic Strokes)*	
	Stroke	*No Stroke*	*Stroke*	*No Stroke*
Vital capacity abnormal	7	510	4	513
Vital capacity normal	11	1388	9	1390
χ^2	1.31		0.10	

Of the 1916 persons accepted for the prospective examination study, a selected healthy subgroup of 602 persons with normal resting electrocardiograms were tested using submaximal exercise electrocardiography (see under Section 8 of this report for details concerning the procedure). As anticipated, in view of how they were selected, this subgroup has shown fewer strokes than expected

(Observed 2, Expected 5.7). It is planned to follow this subgroup for an extended period but, in the meanwhile, the results on this subgroup are as follows:

		Occurred	*New Stroke Did Not Occur*	*Total*
GXT	Positive	1	94	95
	Negative	1	506	507
	Total	2	600	602

The incidence rate of stroke in the GXT-negative group is the lowest of any group that has been followed, and it is possible that this test may define an essentially stroke-free population in contrast to the other variables that have been considered.

During the first three years of the main study, heart volume was calculated on 1076 of the 1544 persons seen in the physician-examination study. This program was discontinued in the fourth year because of the high costs and difficulty in obtaining professional radiological services. That only 70 percent of the eligibles had this screening test is accounted for by difficulties in scheduling, with occasional long delays for the patients, and the need, especially with patients seen in the evening or on weekends, for many patients to pay an additional visit to the Medical Center.

Standard posterior-anterior and lateral end-inspiratory roentgenograms of the chest were employed using the ellipsoid approximation techniques of Rohrer and Kahlstorf.[54] The formula used for calculation of heart volume ($V = 0.41 \cdot L \cdot b \cdot d$) was most recently described by Evans and Carpenter.[55]

Thirteen new strokes (of which 11 were thrombotic) have occurred during the follow-up period among the 1076 individuals whose heart volume was measured. The distributions of the thrombotic strokes by heart volume were as follows:

Number of Persons							
Heart Volume Trichotomized				*Heart Volume Dichotomized*			
Volume	*Stroke*	*No Stroke*	*Total*	*Volume*	*Stroke*	*No Stroke*	*Total*
> 70th Percentile (767 ml)	5	318	323	> 50th percentile (665 ml)	8	530	538

Number of Persons (con't.)

Heart Volume Trichotomized				*Heart Volume Dichotobized*			
Volume	*Stroke*	*No Stroke*	*Total*	*Volume*	*Stroke*	*No Stroke*	*Total*
30th-70th percentile	5	425	430	$\bar{<}$ 50th percentile	3	535	538
< 30th percentile (584 ml)	1	322	323	Total	11	1065	1076
Total	11	1065	1076				

In both cases the χ^2 fails to achieve statistical significance ($p < 0.05$), but the direction is very suggestive.

Of considerable interest and importance is the question whether transient ischemic attacks (TIA) precede a completed stroke in a significantly high proportion of cases. Using the composite definition of TIA developed for the interviewer study, the following results were obtained:

		Number of Persons		
		Stroke	*No Stroke*	*Total*
TIA	Present	21	511	532
	Absent	66	7921	7987
	Total	87	8432	8519

The relative risk of stroke for the TIA present group is 4.97 and the $\chi^2 = 48.1$, indicating that this relative risk is significantly ($p < 0.001$) greater than 1. Since $y = 1.61$ and $V(y) = 0.0625$, the 95 percent confidence interval of this relative risk is approximately 3.04 to 8.25.

The examining physicians used the entire clinical profile of each patient (including a fairly extensive neurological examination) in forming their opinion whether the patient had suffered from a TIA, and this opinion was recorded on a five-notch scale (discussed earlier in this report). The results obtained in the prospective examination study, treating all patients given Code 2 or higher as "TIA present," were as follows:

		Number of Persons		
		Stroke	*No Stroke*	*Total*
TIA	Present	3	323	326
	Absent	15	1575	1590
	Total	18	1898	1916

The relative risk of stroke for the TIA-present group is 0.98, which is, of course, not significantly different from 1. The sensitivity (17%) is already low, and taking the cut-point for what constituted a TIA-present to be Code 3+ or even Code 4+ would reduce it still further.

The contrast between the success of the one method of classifying TIA and the apparent failure of the other method of classifying TIA when used as stroke predictors is striking. Note, however, that the variance of the relative risk associated with TIA in the examination study is such that a relative risk of 3.6 is within the 95 percent confidence limits.

Discussion of Risk Factors

The results which we have obtained can be presented in a different way and discussed in terms of group of risk factors. All strokes are being used as the dependent variable in the following listings.

Changes in Blood Pressure

Previously reported studies (*q.v.*) have consistently shown or suggested that hypertension predisposes to a stroke. Our overall results may be shown as follows:

Variable	*95 Percent Confidence Interval of R.R. (If Not Overlapping 1)*			
	Retrospective Interview	*Retrospective Examination*	*Prospective Interview*	*Prospective Examination*
History of hypertension	3.2 – 5.1	3.2 – 8.6	2.1 – 5.0	1.6 – 16
Systolic B.P. > 156		NS		1.8 – 12
Diastolic B.P. > 90		1.2 – 3.1		1.1 – 6.7
Abn. R. on ECG		NS		NS
Heart volume > 665				NS

Note NS means that the 95 percent confidence interval for the relative risk overlapped the value 1.

Within age-race-sex groups and for cerebral thrombosis and cerebral hemorrhage as well as all strokes, all of the analyses recorded on this group of risk factors yielded a relative risk of greater than 1, and a relative risk not significantly greater than 1 usually reflected small numbers in the subcategory concerned. With only three exceptions (including those categories shown as NS), the 95 percent confidence interval overlapped an estimated central relative risk of 4.0, and these exceptions merit special attention. All three (systolic B.P. > 156, diastolic B.P. > 90, abnormal R wave on ECG) occurred in the retrospective physician-examination study. Four possible explanations suggest themselves:

1. As a result of a stroke the blood pressure drops.
2. Persons with a high blood pressure who have a stroke die at time of stroke or shortly thereafter and do not appear in a retrospective study.
3. Persons who have a stroke have any hypertension they may have at that time diagnosed and treated.
4. A person who has had a stroke so changes his mode of life that his blood pressure, even if once raised, returns to near-normal limits.

These explanations are not mutually exclusive and, in our opinion, probably all play a role.

Reverting to the above list, we note that the inexpensive interviewer study was as good as the expensive physician examination in relating a history of hypertension to the subsequent occurrence of stroke. Fifty-one percent of all strokes (55% of thrombotic strokes and 38% of hemorrhagic strokes) occurred in persons who gave a history of treated hypertension. (These percentages are the "sensitivity" of this question.) This offers an obvious opportunity for preventing stroke since most hypertension is amenable to therapy.

Ischemic Heart Disease

Despite apparent similarities (there are also many differences) between the pathology of cerebral thrombosis and coronary thrombosis, the epidemiological relationships between these two important syndromes (respectively the third and first cause of all deaths in the U.S.A.) have not been as close as might be expected (*q.v.*). Our findings from the four main studies, with "all strokes" as the dependent variable, may be listed as follows:

Variable	*95 Percent Confidence Interval of R.R. (If Not Overlapping 1)*			
	Retrospective Interview	*Retrospective Examination*	*Prospective Interview*	*Prospective Examination*
History of heart attack	2.8 – 5.6		1.7 – 5.8	
History of chest pain	2.1 – 3.9		1.3 – 4.3	
History of ischemic heart disease		NS		4.6 – 30
ST changes on ECG		1.3 – 3.3		4.8 – 35
Abn. Q waves on ECG		1.4 – 7.8		2.7 – 27
Abn. exercise ECG				NS

The retrospective and prospective interviewer study gave results which were consistent with each other. The sensitivity in the prospective study of the heart attack and chest pain questions were only 13 percent and 16 percent respectively, which somewhat reduced their practical value. The only race-sex-age groups in which the relative risks associated with these variables were significantly greater than 1, were white males aged 60 to 69 (as expected, in this subgroup the sensitivity of the two questions were 29% and 47%) for both questions and nonwhite males aged 60 to 69 for the heart attack question. Again as expected, these two questions gave significant relative risks for thrombotic stroke (but not for hemorrhagic stroke), and within the thrombotic group for older white males only.

The variables dealing with possible ischemic heart disease in the physician-examination study were a history of ischemic heart disease (an infarct or angina), abnormal ST segments on the resting and submaximal exercise ECG, and abnormal Q waves on the ECG. The first two of these variables proved to have the highest relative risks of any variables tested in the prospective study (not in the retrospective study), with a high sensitivity for all strokes (44% and 78%, respectively) and particularly for thrombotic stroke (61% and 77%). As noted under "Results" a normal submaximal exercise ECG defined a population with a greatly reduced relative risk (0.16).

This result suggests the possible value of an initial screening using a resting ECG (for which a physician is not required) and looking for ST-segment changes. For those with a normal ECG and no history of other cardiac disease and where the patient's occupation is such that stroke proneness must be excluded, if possible, a submaximal exercise ECG might be considered.

Diabetes

Several investigators have found a positive relationship between diabetes and stroke (*q.v.*). Our findings may be reviewed as follows:

Variable	*95 Percent Confidence Limits of R.R. (If Not Overlapping 1)*			
	Retrospective Interview	*Retrospective Examination*	*Prospective Interview*	*Prospective Examination*
History of treated diabetes	2.1 – 4.2	1.7 – 5.8	2.0 – 6.3	2.8 – 18
Two-hr. blood glucose < 90		NS		NS
Two-hr. blood glucose > 150		NS		NS

A history of treated diabetes carried approximately the same (significant) relative risk retrospectively and prospectively, with lay interviewer and physician getting the same results. In the prospective study, this history had a sensitivity of 17 percent when asked for by a lay interviewer and 33 percent when asked for by a physician. By subcategory, this question picked out the older white female with cerebral thrombosis and the younger nonwhite with cerebral hemorrhage.

In contrast, the finding of a raised two-hour blood glucose (at a level usually regarded as being diagnostic of diabetes) was not associated with any increases of relative risk either retrospectively or prospectively. A low two-hour blood glucose (< 90) actually carried a higher (though not significant) relative risk.

A number of possible explanations for these apparently contradictory findings may be offered:

1. It may not be the diabetes but the therapeutic agents being used to treat the diabetes that are causing the increased relative risk associated with a history of treated diabetes.

2. It may be that the treated diabetics had normal or low two-hour blood glucose levels and it is this symptomatic and hence treated group of diabetics that go on to get a stroke, while a high two-hour blood glucose by itself is not diabetes at all.

3. It may be that it is largely only hypertensive diabetics who develop a stroke. This group, symptomatic because of the hypertension, came under treatment for their diabetes. It is of interest that an earlier analysis of our data (at the end of the third year) showed that all the diabetics who had a stroke (in the prospective study) were also hypertensives.

These explanations are not mutually exclusive, and it appears probable that they all play a role.

Other Heart Disease

Except in regard to cerebral embolism, and to a lesser extent, subarachnoid hemorrhage, very little acceptable data have been published relating other manifestations of heart disease to stroke. Our findings may be summarized as follows: Shortness of breath and vital capacity are for convenience, considered as variables in this group, since we do not have a separate cardiopulmonary group.

In this list, only a history of congestive heart failure and a finding of cardiac dysrhythmia stand out as having a significantly increased relative risk in the prospective study. For a history of congestive heart failure, this significantly increased relative risk persisted when thrombotic strokes alone were considered. Neither of these variables had a good sensitivity in the prospective study (22% and 17%, respectively). Except for a limited number of patients probably already under treatment from their family physician, this group of variables appears to be of minor importance.

Variable	*95 Percent Confidence Limits of R.R. (If Not Overlapping 1)* *Retrospective Interview*	*Retrospective Examination*	*Prospective Interview*	*Prospective Examination*
History of valvular heart disease		NS		NS
History of cardiac dysrhythmia		NS		NS
History of congestive heart failure		2.4 – 9.3		3.0 – 25
History of shortness of breath	2.0 – 3.8		NS	
Finding of valvular heart diesase		NS		NS
Finding of cardiac dysrhythmia		1.1 – 5.2		1.6 – 15
Finding of congestive heart failure		4.1 – 11		NS
Abnormally reduced vital capacity				NS

Extracardiac Vascular Disease

This area has received particular attention from the neurosurgeons and vascular surgeons because of the possibility of successful surgical intervention. The relationship between extracranial vascular disease and intracranial disease (other than that directly attributable to the thrombosis, stenosis, kinking or absence of an extracranial vessel) has, however, not been well documented. Our findings may be summarized as follows: Arcus senilis, a history of pounding in the head and memory loss, may be associated with the vague syndrome known as "generalized arteriosclerosis" and is included with this group of variables for convenience.

Variable	*95 Percent Confidence Limits of R.R. (If Not Overlapping 1)*			
	Retrospective Interview	*Retrospective Examination*	*Prospective Interview*	*Prospective Examination*
History of intermittent claudication	4.4 – 8.0	1.7 – 9.3	NS	1.3 – 7.5
History of pounding in the head	2.7 – 5.1		NS	
History of memory loss		2.7 – 7.7	1.3 – 7.5	NS
History of hardened arteries	2.6 – 5.6		1.1 – 5.2	
Finding of arcus senilis		1.1 – 3.6		NS
Finding of A.S. fundi		2.9 – 9.5		NS
Finding of K.W. fundi > gr. 2		1.5 – 4.2		2.4 – 15
Finding of cervical bruits		NS		NS
Finding of supraclavicular bruits		NS		3.2 – 25
Finding of thermographic difference > 1° F		2.1 – 7.8		1.5 – 15

In the prospective interviewer study, a history of memory loss and hardened arteries had a significantly increased relative risk for cerebral thrombosis only and for younger white males only. In the prospective examination study, the significantly increased relative risks associated with a history of intermittent claudication and the finding of K.W. fundi > grade 2 and supraclavicular bruits (not the thermography difference), were still found when thrombotic strokes only were considered.

It appears that these questions were selective to some extent for cerebral thrombosis. Looking at cerebral thrombosis only, the examination finding of K.W. fundi > grade 2 had a sensitivity of 62 percent but none of the other questions had a good sensitivity (supraclavicular bruits 23%, thermography and intermittent claudication 15%, hardened arteries 11%, memory loss 5%). From a practical viewpoint, it would seem worthwhile to ask younger white males about memory loss and hardened arteries, and for all groups in a clinical setting to examine their fundi and listen for supraclavicular bruits. The classification of optic fundi on the K.W. scale and the interpretation of supraclavicular bruits are not easy and it is unlikely that these diagnostic tools could be used effectively in mass surveys.

Excessive Weight and Changes in Serum Lipids

Published findings relating stroke incidence to body weight, to changes in weight, and to serum lipids have been equivocal (*q.v.*). The usually quoted belief is that high serum cholesterol levels in younger males (but not in older males or in females) are associated with an increased risk of developing a stroke. Our findings may be summarized as follows:

Variable	*95 Percent Confidence Limits of R.R. (If Not Overlapping 1)*			
	Retrospective Interview	*Retrospective Examination*	*Prospective Interview*	*Prospective Examination*
Weight increase > 20 lbs.		NS		NS
Ponderal index < 12	NS	1.3 – 3.2	NS	NS
Serum cholesterol > 277		NS		NS
Serum triglycerides > 4		NS		NS

The different findings with regard to the ponderal index in the two retrospective studies may relate to a poor estimate of height and weight obtained by the interviewer (on asking the respondent) compared with the measured findings obtained at examination. The increased ponderal index among stroke patients found retrospectively at examination may be an effect rather than a cause. The other findings were all nonsignificant though those for serum cholesterol were suggestive.

	All Strokes		*Cerebral Thrombosis*	
	Stroke	*No Stroke*	*Stroke*	*No Stroke*
Serum cholesterol > 277	8	570	5	573
≦ 277	9	1205	6	1208
Morbidity ratio	146		141	
χ^2	1.72		0.88	

It appears that this group of variables in this age group (50-69 years) add little, if anything, to our ability to assess the probability of a future stroke.

Neurological Dysfunction

Except for occasional studies relating TIA (as a syndrome) to stroke incidence, very little acceptable data have been published regarding the relationship, if any, between individual manifestations of neurological dysfunction and a subsequent completed stroke. In the planning of the epidemiological study reported on here, particular attention was given to this area. Our findings may be summarized as follows:

Variable	*95 Percent Confidence Limits of R.R. (If Not Overlapping 1)*			
	Retrospective Interview	*Retrospective Examination*	*Prospective Interview*	*Prospective Examination*
History of temporary weakness (arm or leg)	3.7 – 7.3		1.1 – 5.1	
History of temporary weakness (face)	3.8 – 10		NS	
History of sensory loss (arm or leg)	2.4 – 4.5		NS	
History of loss of eyesight (general)	1.2 – 2.1		1.3 – 3.4	
History of decreased binocular vision (non-refractive)		1.7 – 4.9		NS

Variable	*95 Percent Confidence Limits of R.R. (If Not Overlapping 1)*			
	Retrospective Interview	*Retrospective Examination*	*Prospective Interview*	*Prospective Examination*
History of decreased monocular vision (non-refractive)		NS		1.6 – 13
History of double vision	2.4 – 4.5	1.8 – 8.0	1.1 – 3.9	2.2 – 22
History of fainting or blackouts	1.9 – 3.5		NS	
History of vertigo		1.6 – 5.0		1.2 – 9.1
History of dizziness	1.5 – 2.5		1.5 – 3.5	
History of headaches	1.8 – 2.9		NS	
History of deafness	NS		1.1 – 3.0	
History of incoordination	2.0 – 3.7		NS	
History of speech disturbances	2.1 – 3.8		NS	
History of choking	1.3 – 2.9		NS	
History of confusion	NS		NS	
TIA			3.0 - 8.2	NS

Of those variables showing a significantly increased relative risk in the prospective interviewer study, loss of eyesight (for thrombosis only) and double vision are of importance in older white females, deafness is of importance in whites only, and dizziness relates to cerebral hemorrhage in males (especially nonwhite). Temporary weakness of the arm or leg does not relate to any particular subcategory. Speech disturbances, while not having a significantly increased relative risk overall, do have a significantly increased relative risk when young nonwhite males only are considered. Of the four variables with significantly increased relative risks in the prospective examination study, only a history of vertigo still has a significant relative risk when thrombotic strokes only are considered.

Considering first the two interviewer studies and looking at those variables which have a significant relative risk retrospectively but not prospectively, we find that although the relative risks have decreased (sensory loss 3.04 to 1.32, fainting 2.43 to 1.63, headaches 2.22 to 1.55, incoordination 2.59 to 1.40, speech disturbances 2.67 to 1.65, choking 1.91 to 1.34, facial weakness 5.37 to 0.95), they have not (with the exception of facial weakness) dropped below 1. This suggests that although these variables are of the type one would expect to find overestimated in a retrospective study (preferential recall, confusion of before-and-after effects, and so on), they may tangentially serve as indicators for a more general stroke-prone syndrome.

Few of the variables looked at in the interview study were, however, of much significance by themselves. The best at forecasting a stroke of these single variables in the prospective interviewer study was dizziness, with a relative risk of 2.22, a sensitivity of 41 percent and a specificity of 99.2 percent. The more accurately defined "vertigo" in the prospective examination (physician) study had a similar relative risk (2.92) but a lower sensitivity (22%). Of interest was a history of double vision, which gave a statistically significant relative risk in all four studies. A history of double vision was obtained twice as often by the lay interviewers as by the study physician (6% against 3%). The more careful questioning by the physicians was associated with a much higher relative risk (5.98 against 1.94) but the sensitivity of both approaches was poor (17% and 11%).

When the definition of TIA (in effect, a "Yes" answer to any three of the questions dealing with neurological function) for the interviewer study was decided on, it was as much for convenience in deriving the diagnosis on the computer as for anything else. It was thus a pleasurable surprise when this amorphous composite variable yielded the highest relative risk (4.97) of any variable looked at in the prospective interviewer study. In addition, the sensitivity of this variable in predicting stroke (24%) was higher than is usual with a composite variable. Unfortunately, from a practical viewpoint (at this stage of development), the usefulness of this variable as a screening tool is limited because of the large number of questions (20) that need to be asked to elicit it.

The number of new strokes (18) in the prospective examination study is still small, but within these limits, persons diagnosed as having had a TIA (whether doubtful, mild, moderate, or severe) by our staff physicians did not have an increased relative risk of developing a stroke. We have noted, however, that the 95 percent confidence limits of this relative risk extend up to beyond 3.6, so this finding may well be pure chance.

Miscellaneous Conditions

Relatively little good data have been published on other risk factors which may increase an individual's probability of developing a stroke. Our findings may be summarized as follows:

Variable	*95 Percent Confidence Limits of R.R. (If Not Overlapping 1)*			
	Retrospective Interview	*Retrospective Examination*	*Prospective Interview*	*Prospective Examination*
History of gout	1.2 – 2.8		NS	
History of cigarette smoking	NS		NS	
History of drinking alcohol	1.2 – 1.9		1.1 – 2.7	
Family history of stroke	1.1 – 1.7		NS	
History of hypothyroidism		NS		NS

A history of gout had a significant relative risk in the prospective study only for cerebral hemorrhage among older nonwhite females. A history of the use of alcohol was associated with a significantly increased relative risk, both for cerebral hemorrhage (in particular) and cerebral thrombosis among younger males. Among white males aged 50 to 59 years, this variable had the highest relative risk (10.6) for all strokes of any variable looked at (except for hardened arteries and memory loss, which involved very few persons), with a sensitivity of 83 percent. For nonwhite males aged 50 to 59 years, the relative risk was lower (1.88) but the sensitivity (62%) was much the best of any variable looked at. For all hemorrhagic strokes, the use of alcohol carried a relative risk of 3.14 with (along with "dizziness") the highest sensitivity (50%) of any variable studied.

The above findings with regard to alcohol are of particular interest because they relate to a younger age group and because they fit in with the old belief relating alcoholism and "apoplexy." What is remarkable is that these findings held even though our definition of an alcohol user (a person taking an alcoholic drink at least once a month) does not, in any sense, define an alcoholic.

It appears from what we have discussed that a simple screening test could be developed which would pick out an at-high-risk-for-stroke group among males with a relatively small margin of error and among females with less surety. For cerebral thrombosis, a history of ischemic heart disease, the finding of ST changes on the ECG, and the finding of K.W. fundi > grade 2 are reasonably specific, especially for males. For cerebral hemorrhage, a history of dizziness and of using alcohol are reasonably specific, especially for persons under 60 years of age. For all strokes, a history of treated hypertension and a history of several minor defects of neurological function (taken together) would round out the picture. It is notable that information collected without the use of physicians would give us an almost complete picture of the risk status of any individual or group.

To prevent strokes, the most logical and economically practical program would appear to be a community effort directed at the control of already diagnosed hypertension. The steps in this program might be (a) ascertainment (using volunteer help) on a yearly basis from every person aged 40 years or older in the community whether they had ever been told that they had high blood pressure, (b) notification to a central agency of this information, (c) checking (by the central agency) with the physician (if any) of those persons named whether the information was correct and whether the physician wished to assume continued responsibility for the supervision and treatment of his hypertensive patients, (d) providing assistance to physicians in the routine recall of their hypertensive patients and to the patient (through his physician) in the purchase of appropriate medication, and (e) for those persons without a private physician or whose private physician did not wish to provide routine supervision, the provision of decentralized clinic services where medical supervision could be provided, treatment given, and a follow-up recall system developed.

Findings from the Rehabilitation Study

Sixty-six patients with a diagnosis of completed stroke and who had indicated their willingness to enter the study were submitted from the University Hospital to the rehabilitation study for consideration (Table 8.12). Of these, nine were considered by

TABLE 8.12
DISTRIBUTION AND SELECTED CHARACTERISTICS OF STROKE PATIENTS CONSIDERED FOR ADMISSION TO THE REHABILITATION STUDY

	Selected for inclusion			*Excluded*
	Experimental group (all completed)	*Control group*		
		Completed trial	*Lost or dropped*	
Number in group	29	18	5	14
White males	7	2	0	1
White females	5	2	1	1
N/White males	8	6	3	8
N/White females	9	8	1	4
Oldest (in years)	66	64	63	66
Youngest (in years)	43	45	52	48
Number aged 60 or over	11	10	2	9
Number aged under 60	18	8	3	5
Average age (in years)	574	58.3	57.0	60.9
Died in hospital				
early in trial	0	0	1	4
late in trial	4	1	—	—
Moved away	0	0	3	—
Other major illness	0	0	0	9
Refusals	0	0	1	1
Average time under observation (months)	8.1	6.4	—	—

a staff neurologist and/or a staff physiatrist as being unsuitable for inclusion in the study because of other major illness (heart disease, severe chronic respiratory disease, profound mental deterioration, and a brain tumor). Four died before a final disposal could be made and one changed his mind and refused to be considered further. This was a somewhat older group than that which was accepted.

The remaining 52 patients were given a detailed total-rehabilitation evaluation (see earlier in this report) by a team of workers and a combined report was prepared which (a) recorded on a six-point scale the personal-care and vocational status of the patient at the time of this first evaluation and (b) recorded on this same six-point scale the projected level of improvement which (from previous experience with other similar patients) each patient might reasonably be expected to achieve with regard to personal-care and vocational status. Note that at this stage the patient concerned had not yet been allocated to the experimental or control group and thus the first evaluation was done "blind."

Following this evaluation, these 52 patients were randomized into two groups. The randomization was done using an excess of unmarked sealed envelopes (with equal numbers having the instruction "Experimental" or "Control" inside) prepared well ahead of time. By chance, 29 patients were allocated to the experimental group and 23 to the control group. It will be noted that the experimental group was not only larger than the control group but also included a larger proportion of white patients (41% compared to 22%), with rather fewer patients over the age of 60 years (38% compared to 52%) though the average age of the two groups was similar.

Within a few days of being allocated to the control group, four patients dropped out of this group (one refused further cooperation and three moved to distant cities) and one died. It was, of course, obvious to these patients at this stage that they had been allocated to the control group. This left 18 controls.

The subsequent progress of the patients in the experimental and control groups with regard to personal care is given in Table 8.13 and with regard to vocational status is given in Table 8.14.

TABLE 8.13

THE BIRMINGHAM REHABILITATION STUDY: THE PERSONAL CARE STATUS ON A CODED SCALE OF 29 EXPERIMENTAL SUBJECTS GIVEN INTENSIVE CARE AND 18 CONTROL SUBJECTS GIVEN ROUTINE CARE

(Showing Level at Time of First Exmination, Projected Level To Be Reached, Actual Level Reached, and Whether Further Improvement Might Still Be Possible)

Initial evaluation		*Number of persons in best level actually reached in study period: level*						*Further improvoment possible from this level*	
Level at time of first examination	*Projected level to be reached*	*1*	*2*	*3*	*4*	*5*	*6*	*Yes*	*No*
1	2	—	—	1	—	—	1	—	2
	3	—	(1)	4 (1)	—	1	1	1 (1)	5 (1)
	4	—	1	1 (1)	—	(3)	—	(3)	2 (1)
	5	—	—	(3)	1	—	2	1 (1)	2 (2)
	6	—	—	(1)	1	1	—	(1)	1 (2)
2	3	—	—	—	—	(1)	1 (1)	1	—
	4	—	—	—	1	1	1	—	3
	5	—	—	1	1	1	1	1	3
	6	—	—	—	—	—	3 (3)	—	3 (3)
3	5	—	—	—	—	—	(1)	—	(1)
	6	—	—	—	(1)	—	—	—	3
4	4	—	—	—	—	—	2	—	1
5	5	—	—	—	—	—	(1)	—	(1)
6	6	—	—	—	—	—	1	—	(1)

Note. For persons in the control group the numbers are given in parentheses.

TABLE 8.14

THE BIRMINGHAM REHABILITATION STUDY: THE VOCATIONAL STATUS ON A CODED SCALE OF 29 EXPERIMENTAL SUBJECTS GIVEN INTENSIVE CARE AND 18 CONTROL SUBJECTS GIVEN ROUTINE CARE

Showing Level at Time of First Examination, Projected Level To Be Reached, Actual Level Reached, and Whether Further Improvement Might Still Be Possible)

Initial evaluation		*Number of persons in best level actually reached in study period: level*						*Further improvement possible from this level*	
Level at time of first examination	*Projected level to be reached*	*1*	*2*	*3*	*4*	*5*	*6*	*Yes*	*No*
1	1	7 (3)	1	—	—	1	—	1	8 (3)
	2	3	1 (2)	(1)	1 (1)	2 (2)	—	1 (3)	7 (1)
	3	3 (1)	—	—	—	—	—	1 (1)	2
	4	(1)	—	—	1	1	—	(1)	2
	5	(4)	—	—	—	4 (2)	1	(2)	5 (4)
	6	—	—	—	—	—	(2)	—	(2)
2	2	—	1	—	—	—	—	—	1
3	3	—	—	(1)	—	—	—	(1)	—
5	6	—	—	—	1	—	—	—	1

Note. For persons in the control group the numbers are given in parentheses.

The results are given in terms of the point of maximum improvement that was noted while under observation, with an average time under direct observation of 8.1 months for the experimental group and 6.4 months for the control group. Of the experimental group, four regressed from their observed "best" while under observation and four more died in hospital. The corresponding figures for the smaller control group were two and one.

The evaluation made at this "best-to-be-reasonably-expected" point (the decision as to when this was reached was made by the senior staff physiatrist) was a replication of that done when the patient was being considered for admission to the study. This evaluation unfortunately could not be done "blind," and possible observer bias (especially with regard to potential future improvement when the evaluator knew what had been tried for the experimental group much more intimately than he knew what had been tried for the control group) could not be excluded.

The results show the following:

1. At the time of the original evaluation, proportionately fewer of those who became the experimental group were at level 1 (a completely dependent bed patient) with regard to personal care.

Actual level (start)	*Personal care*		*Vocational status*	
	Exp.	*Control*	*Exp.*	*Control*
1	14	12	27	17
2	11	3	1	0
3+	4	3	1	1

2. At the time of the original evaluation, the projected level expected to be reached by those who became the experimental group was lower than the expected level for those who became the control group, both with regard to personal care and with regard to vocational status.

Projected level (start)	*Personal care*		*Vocational status*	
	Exp.	*Control*	*Exp.*	*Control*
1	0	0	9	3
2	2	0	9	4
3	7	2	3	2
4	5	5	2	1
5	7	5	6	6
6	8	6	0	2

3. At the time of the original evaluation, the expected change in level (i.e. projected level minus starting level) was greater for those who became the control group both with regard to personal care and to vocational status.

Projected change in level (start)	*Personal care*		*Vocational status*	
	Exp.	*Control*	*Exp.*	*Control*
No change	1	2	10	4
+1	3	0	9	4
+2	9	3	3	1
+3	9	4	2	1
+4	6	6	5	6
+5	1	3	0	2

4. For personal care, a larger proportion of those in the experimental group reached or surpassed their projected goal. Regarded as a 2×3 table, the χ^2 value (= 1.85) is not statistically significant ($p < 0.05$).

Group	*Number and percentage of persons who*		
	Did not reach projected level	*Reached projected level*	*Surpassed projected level*
Experimental	6 (21)	13 (45)	10 (34)
Control	7 (39)	6 (33)	5 (28)

5. For vocational status, a larger proportion of those in the experimental group surpassed their projected goal. Regarded as a 2×3 table, the χ^2 value (= 1.83) is not statistically significant ($p < 0.05$).

Group	*Number and percentage of persons who*		
	Did not reach projected level	*Reached projected level*	*Surpassed projected level*
Experimental	7 (24)	14 (48)	8 (28)
Control	6 (33)	10 (56)	2 (11)

6. For both personal care and vocational status, the experimental group did better in terms of "best level reached" than did the control group.

Best level Reached	*Personal care* *Exp.*	*Control*	*Vocational status* *Exp.*	*Control*
1			13	9
2	1	1	3	2
3	7	6	0	2
4	3	1	3	1
5	5	4	8	2
6	13	6	2	2

7. For both personal care and vocational status in terms of change between their starting level and their best level reached, there was very little difference between the experimental group and the control group.

Change in level	*Personal care* *Exp.*	*Control*	*Vocational status* *Exp.*	*Control*
—1	0	0	1	0
No change	1	1	14	10
+1	2	2	2	2
+2	9	7	0	1
+3	6	0	2	1
+4	6	7	8	2
+5	5	1	2	2

8. For both personal care and vocational status, it was estimated that further improvement was potentially still possible (under ideal circumstances) for a larger proportion of the control group than of the experimental group. For both personal care ($t = 2.328$) and vocational status ($t = 2.676$) this difference is statistically significant ($p < 0.05$)

Group	*Personal care Further improvement possible*		*Vocational status Further improvement possible*	
	Yes	*No*	*Yes*	*No*
Experimental	4 (14%)	25 (26%)	3 (10%)	26 (90%)
Control	6 (33%)	12 (67%)	8 (44%)	10 (56%)

Earlier in this report, we have mentioned the 33 cases of stroke which occurred in our prospective study who did not die and who were not admitted to hospital but were treated at home. Thirty of these were brought in to have the diagnosis established more firmly by one of our staff neurologists. The opportunity was taken to have these same patients examined by a staff physiatrist and their rehabilitation potential investigated. It was reported that only 5 out of the 30 needed or would benefit from an organized rehabilitation program. For the remainder, home treatment appeared to be adequate.

While the objectives of the rehabilitation study were met in part, it cannot be said that the population used for the study was representative of all stroke patients within the city of Birmingham. The (understandable) failure of the private physicians to accept the randomization of their private patients into a control (standard care) or experimental (intensive rehabilitation) group limited the population to be randomized to "staff" patients. This group, in general, showed multiple pathology and a record of unstable occupational adjustment in the past, had a low socioeconomic and educational background, and lacked the motivation so necessary for full physical, social, psychological, and vocational restoration.

Even within the group made available for randomization, difficulty was experienced in achieving a good match between the experimental and control subgroups (*q.v.*). In view of our findings showing little or no advantage to that group receiving intensive rehabilitation, this difficulty is of limited importance (since one might have expected it to favor the experimental group), but if there had been a difference it would have been difficult to estimate the bias involved.

Our findings should not be taken to mean that rehabilitation of stroke patients is of no value. Both the experimental and control groups made substantial gains in their personal-care status (87% improved by two levels or more) and lesser gains in their vocational status (38% improved by two levels or more). It is important to appreciate that we were not comparing care with no care but rather routine care with intensive care.

However, on the basis of our present knowledge, it can be safely stated that the long-range relative effectiveness of lengthy and expensive physical medicine and rehabilitation as applied to this project and its patients has not proven to be of value. This is a negative significant finding, which is nonetheless of importance to social and rehabilitation services and state departments of vocational rehabilitation. We note the following:

1. Persons suffering from significant degrees of residual neurological impairment who are over 60 years of age, have other debilitating diseases or generalized vascular disease, and are of low education and low-skilled employment history are usually poorly motivated for vocational rehabilitation and lack the combined inner and outer resources which hold promise for personal rehabilitation. These persons require a different approach to socioeconomic restoration after their physical needs are brought as well under control as is possible.

2. This suggests that those stroke patients having the optimal chance for rehabilitation as presently conceived, and to be considered by the rehabilitation team, are those who have a reasonable life expectancy, are still employable in some phase of productive business or industry, who have a previous stable work history of progressive accomplishment, and who have psychological motivation to use their available personal resources to a maximum level.

3. These criteria can form a basis on which the rehabilitation counselor can realistically appraise their choices for candidates to receive services.

4. These criteria will also assist in the education of the medical community to make meaningful referral of stroke patients to appropriate agencies for rehabilitation services.

SUMMARY

The Birmingham Stroke Study (1965-70) was a five-year study designed to investigate (a) the magnitude of the stroke problem, (b) those (hopefully preventable) factors which predisposed to the development of a first stroke, and (c) the effectiveness of intensive rehabilitation procedures applied to the stroke patient.

A review of the literature showed the following: (a) Age-adjusted death rates from stroke (which are probably underestimates) within the U.S.A. are in the neighborhood of one per thousand, with higher rates in the Southeast and for Negroes. (b) Reported incidence rates for first strokes in the age group 50 to 69 years vary from 2 to 5 per 1000 per year (acceptable figures on whites only are available). (c) Negroes, persons who have had a transient ischemic attack (TIA), who have high blood pressure, diabetes, or ECG changes suggestive of ischemic heart disease are particularly liable to develop a stroke. (d) Little convincing evidence exists that stroke patients given intensive rehabilitative care did much better than patients given more routine care.

The planning provided for (a) a retrospective and prospective questionnaire study of a random sample of the population of Birmingham aged 50 to 69 years, administered by lay interviewers but with careful cross-checks to ensure that all strokes in the survey population were reported and with physician validation of any reported cases (10,000 patient-years of follow-up required), (b) a retrospective and prospective study of a random subsample of the questionnaire group, who would be given a complete medical examination with supportive laboratory and consultant services (2000 patient-years of follow-up required), (c) the interviewing of about 2200 new respondents and the examination of about 500 of these new respondents each year of the study, (d) the reinterview each year of the study of all those who had been interviewed or reinterviewed the previous year, and (e) stroke patients to be given a complete, scaled multidisciplinary evaluation and then randomized into two groups, one of which would receive standard hospital care and the other intensive rehabilitation care.

A pilot study in the small city of Fairfield (adjoining Birmingham) done in the first year of the study (a) provided a testing ground for the sampling procedures and a training opportunity for the lay interviewers and medical examiners, (b) provided a detailed check on the questionnaire to be used, with 29 of the final 84 questions being reworded and 11 new questions added, (c) yielded (on 278 possible respondents) an interviewer response rate of 96 percent and (on 80 who were called in for examination) an examination response rate of 80 percent, (d) led to changes in the physician-examination protocol, to closer contacts being established between team members and outside private physicians, and to further laboratory procedures, and (e) revealed some of the difficulties likely to be encountered in bringing private patients into the rehabilitation trial.

To obtain the population samples required, the sixty-one census tracts in Birmingham (in which, according to the 1960 census, there lived 61,500 people aged 50 to 69 years) were divided into seven strata on the basis of age, race, sex, and socioeconomic factors. Each year tracts were drawn from each stratum on a probability proportional to the population size of that tract, until the potential population drawn for that year exceeded 10,000. Twenty-five percent of the blocks in each selected tract were drawn on a random basis, and all persons aged 50 to 69 years in those blocks (their names being obtained by household listings) constituted the questionnaire sample. Thirty percent of the population actually interviewed were randomly selected for examination by a physician. In the first year, 10 percent of the physician-examined group were randomly selected for examination by a neurologist, and thereafter all "suspect strokes" were referred to a neurologist with a sufficient random sample from the "others" to bring the proportion up to 10 percent.

A "stroke" was defined as a localizing neurological deficit which persisted for longer than twenty-four hours, for which no other cause was detected, and which was confirmed by a physician. Information on new strokes was obtained through reinterviews, reexaminations, patient notifications, physician notification, hospital and nursing home records, and death records.

Definitions were established for the sixty-two independent variables investigated in the epidemiological study and for the six levels of personal-care status and vocational status used in the rehabilitation study.

It was found that the lay interviewer record by itself was substantially unclear in diagnosing the type of stroke. Thus 19 percent of strokes diagnosed from the interviewer record as being cerebral thrombosis and 71 percent of strokes diagnosed from the interviewer record as being cerebral hemorrhage were incorrectly assigned. For this reason, strokes diagnosed retrospectively were not further classified according to type.

In the four years of the main study, first interviews were successfully completed on 8802 (or 94%) of the persons drawn for the sample. Of these, 1991 (75% of those chosen for examination) were examined by a staff physician, with the poorest response being from nonwhites aged 50 to 59 years. Excluding persons who had already had a stroke, who had died from causes other than stroke, or who had moved out of Birmingham so that close control was no longer possible, 10,876 annual reinterviews on the interviewer group and 2674 annual reinterviews for the examination group were obtained.

Two hundred and eighty-three strokes were found in the retrospective study (75 in the physician-examined subsample), for a prevalence rate of 32 per 1000. By age-race-sex groups, prevalence rates were uniformly higher for persons aged 60 to 69 years, for nonwhites, and for males. In 343 patient-years of follow-up on this group of old strokes (excluded from the main prospective study), there were 11 recurrent strokes with 6 deaths and 21 deaths from other causes, for a nonstroke death rate of 61 per 1000 per year compared with 19 per 1000 per year (181 deaths) in the initially stroke-free main prospective study group.

Of the 75 "old strokes" (from the interviewer record) who were examined by staff physicians (who did not know what the interviewer had recorded), 49 were classified by the physicians as a "completed stroke" and 12 as a TIA. Another 21 "completed strokes" recorded by the physicians were not recorded as such by the interviewer.

Eighty-seven first strokes were found in the prospective study (18 in the physician-examined subsample), for an incidence of 8 per 1000 per year. Twelve died before admission to hospital, 42 were hospitalized (of these, another 12 died in hospital), and 33 were treated at home. The death rate in the nonhome-treated group (44%), the incidence in the age groups 50 to 59 years (3.8) and 60 to 69 years (6.2), in whites (2.7) and nonwhites (9.2), and in males (7.0) and females (3.6) all resemble those found in a large registry study covering the whole population of Jefferson

County being conducted at the same time as this survey. In contrast, the home-treated group were largely older white males with relatively mild thrombotic strokes.

Of the 87 strokes in the prospective study, 22 (10 deaths) were due to cerebral hemorrhage, 2 (1 death) were due to subarachnoid hemorrhage, 55 (13 deaths) were due to cerebral thrombosis, 1 was due to cerebral embolism, and 7 were unclassified.

Those variables most closely associated with the future development of a stroke can best be shown in the following simplified listing. In each case, the relative risk of developing a stroke was significantly ($p < 0.05$) greater than 1 and the sensitivity sufficiently high (more than 20% in the relevant subgroup) to give the variable practical importance.

Variable	*R.R. significant*		*Type of*	*Special subgroups*
	Retrospective	*Prospective*	*stroke*	*most effected*
History of high B.P.	Yes	Yes	Thrombotic Hemorrhagic	White males Females
Finding of high B.P.	No	Yes	All	—
Abnormal ST on ECG	Yes	Yes	Thrombotic	White males
History of cardiac infarct	No	Yes	Thrombotic	—
History of chest pain	Yes	Yes	Thrombotic	Old white males
History of diabetes	Yes	Yes	Thrombotic Hemorrhagic	Old white males Younger nonwhites
K.W. fundi > gr. 2	Yes	Yes	Thrombotic	—
Supraclavicular bruits	No	Yes	Thrombotic	—
TIA	—	Yes	All	—
Dizziness	Yes	Yes	Hemorrhagic	Males
Use of alcohol	Yes	Yes	Hemorrhagic	Younger males

Variables with a wide distribution in the population which were not found to be associated with an increased relative risk included a high blood glucose, a high serum cholesterol, overweight, a history of cigarette smoking, and a family history of stroke.

That group with a normal resting and exercise ECG had the lowest risk of developing a stroke of any group that was looked at.

Most of the information required to assess risk could be obtained without the need for medical examinations conducted by a physician.

Of 66 patients who had had a stroke and who were considered for the rehabilitation study, 14 had to be excluded. The remaining 52 were given a personal-care and vocational status evaluation and then randomized into 23 controls, who were to receive standard University Hospital care, and 29 in the experimental group, who were to receive intensive multidisciplinary rehabilitative care. Unfortunately, 5 of the controls were lost shortly after randomization and the control group as finally constituted had fewer whites and more persons aged 60 years or older, though the average age of the two groups was about the same. Both groups were generally from lower socioeconomic levels with a poor vocational record and little motivation.

For both personal-care and vocational status, a larger (but not significantly larger) proportion of those in the experimental group than in the control group reached or surpassed the projected goal which had been set (blind) at the time of their first evaluation. The final levels reached by the experimental group were also higher than for the control group, but the change in level (since the control group had started lower) was about the same for the two groups. At the final evaluation, a statistically significant ($p < 0.05$) larger proportion of the control group were considered not to have reached their optimum.

Despite these encouraging results, the final conclusion was that the long-range relative effectiveness of lengthy and expensive rehabilitation as applied to the type of population studied in this project had not been proven to be of value.

REFERENCES

1. Locksley, H.B. Hemorrhagic strokes. *Med. Clin. N. Amer., 52:*1193, 1968.
2. Lee, K.F., and Hodes, P.J. Intracranial ischemic lesions. *Radiol. Clin. N. Amer., 5:*363, 1967.
3. Meyer, J.S., and Ericsson, A.D. Definition and classification. In Borhani, N.O., and Meyer, J.S. (Eds.) *Medical Basis for Comprehensive Community Stroke Programs.* In collaboration with the Special Task Force of the Joint Council Subcommittee on Cerebrovascular Disease, 1968, p. 8.
4. Fisher, C.M., Dalal, P.M., and Adams, R.D. In Harrison, T.R. (Ed.) *Principles of Internal Medicine,* 5th ed. New York, McGraw-Hill 1962, p. 1147.

5. Kurtzke, J.F. *Epidemiology of Cerebrovascular Disease.* New York, Springer-Verlag, 1969.
6. Kannel, W.B., Dawber, T.R., and McNamara, P.M. Vascular disease of the brain: Epidemiologic aspects: The Framingham study. *Amer. J. Public Health, 55:*1355, 1965.
7. Resch, J.A. The epidemiology and geographic pathology of atherosclerotic cerebrovascular disease. *Current Concepts of Cerebrovascular Disease (Stroke), 5:*33, 1970.
8. Kuller, L. Cerebrovascular disease mortality among Baltimore residents aged 20-64. *Amer. J. Public Health, 57:*2091, 1967.
9. Editorial. Poll on medical practice: Stroke. *Modern Medicine,* May, p. 73, 1969.
10. Marquardsen, J. The natural history of acute cerebrovascular disease. *Acta Neurol. Scand., 45* (suppl. 38), 1969.
11. Loewenson, Ruth B. Stroke U.S. and Japan: Comparative morbidity and mortality. *Geriatrics, 24:*85, Oct. 1969.
12. Robinson, R.W., Demierl, M., and Le Beau, R.J. Natural history of cerebral thrombosis: Nine to nineteen year follow-up. *J. Chronic Dis., 21:*221, 1968.
13. Mahoney, Florence I., and Barthel, Dorothea, W. Rehabilitation of the hemiplegic patient: A clinical evaluation. *Arch. Phys. Med., 35:*359, 1954.
14. Boyle, R.W., and Scalzitti, P.D. A study of 480 consecutive cases of cerebral vascular accident. *Arch. Phys. Med., 44:*19, 1963.
15. Stallones, R.A. Epidemiology of cerebrovascular disease: A review. *J. Chronic Dis., 18:*859, 1965.
16. Heyman, A., Bartel, A., Cassell, J., Hames, C.G., Heyden, S., Karp, H.R., Stuart, W., and Tyroler, H.A. Cerebrovascular Disease in a Rural Southern Community. Distributed at American Heart Ass'n. Conference on Stroke Epidemiology, New Orleans, Mar. 4, 1970.
17. Eisenberg, H., Morrison, J.T., Sullivan, P., and Foote, F.M. Cerebrovascular accidents: Incidents and survival rates in a defined population, Middlesex County, Connecticut. *J.A.M.A., 189:*883, 1964.
18. Acheson, R.M., and Fairbairn, A.S. Burden of cerebrovascular disease in the Oxford area in 1963 and 1964. *Brit. Med. J., 2:*621, 1970.
19. Kurland, L.T., Choi, N.W., and Sayre, G.P. The epidemiology of cerebrovascular diseases. In Fields, W.S., and Spencer, W.A., (Eds.) *Stroke Rehabilitation: Basic Concepts and Research Trends,* 3, 1967.
20. Ostveld, A.M. Chicago Stroke Study: August 1965–January 1970. Distributed at American Heart Ass'n. Conference on Stroke Epidemiology, New Orleans, Mar. 4, 1970.
21. Yates, P.O. A change in the pattern of cerebrovascular disease. *Lancet, 1:*66, 1964.
22. Krueger, D.E., Williams, J., and Paffenbarger, R.S. Trends in death

rates from cerebrovascular disease in Memphis, Tenn. 1920-1960. *J. Chronic Dis., 20:*129, 1967.

23. Borhani, N.O. Changes and geographic distribution of mortality from cerebrovascular disease. *Amer. J. Public Health, 55:*678, 1965.
24. Takahashi, E. The geographic distribution of cerebral hemorrhage and hypertension in Japan. *Hum. Biol. 29:*140, 1957.
25. Johnson, B.C. Stroke Experience in a Total Community Study: Tecumseh, Michigan. Distributed at American Heart Ass'n. Conference on Stroke Epidemiology, New Orleans, Mar. 4, 1970.
26. Nefzger, M.D., Acheson, R.M., and Heyman, A. Stroke Mortality among U.S. Veterans in Georgia and Five Western States. Distributed at American Heart Ass'n. Conference on Stroke Epidemiology, New Orleans, Mar. 4, 1970.
27. Meyer, B.J., Peples, W.J., Meyer, A.C., and Theron, J.J. Atherosclerosis in Europeans and Bantu. *Circulation, 29:*415, 1964.
28. Yablonski, M., Behar, A., Ungar, H., Resch, J., and Alter, M. Cerebral atherosclerosis among Israeli Jews of European and Afro-Asian origin. *Neurology, 18:*550, 1968.
29. Resch, J.A., Okabe, N., Loewenson, Ruth B., Kimoto, K., Katsuki, S., and Baker, A.B. A comparative study of cerebral atherosclerosis in a Japanese and Minnesota population. *J. Atheroscler. Res., 7:*687, 1967.
30. Gordon, T. Mortality experience among the Japanese in the United States, Hawaii and Japan. *Public Health Rep., 72:*543, 1957.
31. Friedman, G.D., Wilson, W.S., Mosier, J.M., Colandrea, M.A., and Nichaman, M.Z. Transient ischemic attacks in the community. *J.A.M.A., 210:*1428, 1969.
32. Paffenbarger, R.S., and Wing, A.L. Characteristics in youth predisposing to fatal stroke in later years. *Lancet, 1:*753, 1967.
33. Baker, A.B., Resch, J.A., and Loewenson, Ruth B. Hypertension and cerebral atherosclerosis. *Circulation, 39:*708, 1969.
34. Friedman, G.D. Seal Beach Study. Distribution at American Heart Ass'n. Conference on Stroke Epidemiology, New Orleans, Mar. 4, 1970.
35. Johnson, K.G. Cerebral vascular disease in Hiroshima, Japan. *J. Chronic Dis., 20:*555, 1967.
36. Friedman, G.D. Relationship of stroke to other cardiovascular disease. *Circulation, 38:*536, 1968.
37. Aronson, S.M., and Aronson, Betty E. Ischemic cerebral disease: Frequency in autopsy population. *New York J. Med., 66:*956, 1966.
38. Chapman, J.M. Epidemiology of vascular lesions affecting the central nervous system: The occurrence of strokes in a sample population under observation for cardiovascular disease. *Amer. J. Public Health, 56:*197, 1966.
39. Pearce, J., and Aziz, H. Uric acid and plasma lipids in cerebrovascular

disease. Part 1; Prevalence of hyperuricaemia. *Brit. Med. J., 4:*78, 1969.

40. Ettinger, M.G., Kusonoki, R., and Fujishima, H. Coagulation studies in cerebrovascular disease: II. Cooperative study of stroke patients in Minnesota and Japan. *Neurology, 17,*797, 1967.
41. Stoica, E., Costa-Foru, D., and Cherciulescu, F. The reactivity of the clotting mechanism and fibrinolysis in cerebral thrombotic disease. *J. Neurol. Sci., 4:*491, 1967.
42. Cole, M. Strokes in young women using oral contraceptives. *Arch. Intern. Med., 120:*555, 1967.
43. Sartwell, P.E., Masi, A.T., Arthes, F.G., Green, G.R., and Smith, H.E. Thromboembolism and oral contraceptives: An epidemiologic case-control study. *Amer. J. Epidem. 90:*365, 1969.
44. Grant, Ellen C.G. Venous effects of oral contraceptive. *Brit. Med. J., 4:* 73, 1969.
45. Inman, W.H.W., Vessey, M.P., Westerholm, Barbro, and Engelund, A. Thromboembolic disease and the steroidal content of oral contraceptives: A report to the Committee on Safety of Drugs. *Brit. Med. J., 2:*203, 1970.
46. President's Commission on Heart Disease, Cancer and Stroke. *Report to the President. A National Program to Conquer Heart Disease, Cancer and Stroke.* Washington, D.C., Dec. 1964, Vol. I.
47. Peacock, P.N.B. Relative risk for multifactorial studies. *Biometrics,* in press.
48. Cornfield, J. A method of estimating comparative rates from clinical data: Applications to cancer of the lung, breast and cervix. *J. Nat. Cancer Inst., 11:*1269, 1951.
49. Haldane, J.B.S. The estimation and significance of the logarithm of a ratio of frequencies. *Ann. Hum. Genet., 20:*309, 1956.
50. Woolf, B. On estimating the relation between blood groups and disease. *Ann. Hum. Genet., 19:*251, 1955.
51. Sheehe, R.R. Combination of log relative risks in retrospective studies of disease. *Amer. J. Public Health, 56:*1745, 1966.
52. Dunnett, C.W. A multiple comparison procedure for comparing several treatments with a control. *J. Amer. Stat. Ass., 50:*1096, 1955.
53. Dawber, T.R., Moore, F.E., and Mann, G.V. Coronary heart disease in the Framingham Study. *Amer. J. Public Health, 47:*4, 1957.
54. Kahlstorf, A. Über eine orthodiagraphische Herzvolumenbestimmung. *Fortschr. Röntgenstr., 45:*123, 1932.
55. Evans, D.W., and Carpenter, P.B. Errors involved in radiological heart volume determination by the ellipsoid-approximation technique. *Brit. Heart J., 27:*429, 1965.

Chapter 9

COMMUNICABLE DISEASES

GORDON T. STEWART

EVEN THOSE who despair of human progress in other fields usually concede that the conquest of the major communicable diseases is one of the great and lasting achievements of the present century. For, until very recently, conquest was the word. The developed countries of the world had eliminated all the disaster epidemics, like cholera, yellow fever, smallpox, and malaria, and were grappling with techniques to control influenza, measles, and numerous lesser infections.[1-3] In the underdeveloped world, measures for local and international surveillance and control of smallpox,[4] malaria,[5] and cholera[6-8] were being generally observed and were effective insofar as very few major epidemics had spread beyond national boundaries between 1930 and 1960, though localized and sporadic outbreaks were common and, in some countries, smallpox, malaria, cholera, typhoid, and plague remained endemic.[9] However, recent epidemics in various parts of the world have demonstrated sharply the difference between conquest and the power to conquer. Infectious disease never respects national frontiers unless positive efforts are made to restrict immigration of cases, carriers, and vectors. Thus, smallpox has been excluded from the United States since 1900 by vaccination and quarantine, but plague still occurs in New Mexico and elsewhere where immigrants and rodents can act as carriers of infection. Influenza and other respiratory viral infections are always widespread in distribution because they can be transmitted so easily by travelers. Epidemiologically, infectious disease must be viewed geographically and regionally and, in this regard, the local culture and level of administrative competence are often as important as the germ itself in determining whether or not infectious disease will vanish, remain, or increase.

MALARIA

In many parts of the world and notably in Ceylon, Cyprus, Crete, and other insular places, malaria had been vigorously attacked during and after World War II and had been greatly reduced in mortality and morbidity by 1960.[10] Subsequently, recrudescences and sometimes increases were reported[11] and malaria is now regarded once again as a serious cause of morbidity and death even in locations where control had been achieved. An increase in the prevalence and severity of malaria in South Vietnam is also reported,[12] not only among local inhabitants but also among combatant and noncombatant U.S. military personnel, some of whom have carried infection back to the continental United States on repatriation, there to initiate small secondary outbreaks.[13] Since there is no evidence in either of these instances that biological changes in the malaria parasites or the vectors have contributed significantly to the recrudescence of disease, we have to conclude that conquest remains a technical possibility but that the will to conquer or the application of techniques, or both, are weaker than formerly despite intensive reexamination of the problem.[13a]

CHOLERA

In cholera, also, we are witnessing resurgence and spread of infection in epidemic form from Southeast Asia to the Middle East, Crimea, North and West Africa, in most of which zones it had been absent for fifty years or more. Cholera is always a revealing epidemic, the investigation of which by John Snow, in 1849-56, marked the opening of an epidemiological era. Also, there are few major epidemics which are better understood or more easily controllable. It is therefore instructive to recall the recent history of cholera insofar as it relates to its recurrence now in lands in which it once was under control.

The present pandemic, which began in 1961 in Southeast Asia, is the seventh[14] in the long and catastrophic history of cholera. It probably originated from endemic infection in the Celebes Islands of Indonesia, where an outbreak, now known to be due to the same *el Tor* biotype which is mainly responsible for the present pandemic, was reported in 1935. From Indonesia, the disease spread to the Philippines, Taiwan, Korea, and Southeast Asia in 1961. It attained pandemic proportions soon afterwards, reaching a peak with 94,000 recorded cases in 1964,[15] mainly in India, Pakistan, and then Afghanistan, Iran, Iraq, Saudi Arabia, Syria, and Egypt, following trade routes more or less in geographic sequence. Most of the governments concerned reported the isolation of classical and *el Tor* cholera vibrios[16] and the number of known cases, but in 1965, Iran and Iraq stopped reporting cholera shortly after a refusal by the Soviet Union to accept shipments of citrus fruits from Iran.[17] Between 1965 and 1967, the number of reported cases fell substantially[15] but rose in 1968-69 because of a resurgence in Southeast Asia and again, in 1970, when cholera was officially reported in the area of the Black Sea and Volga basin despite vigorous quarantine and control measures by the Russian health authorities. Reports from the World Health Organization confirmed that cholera was present in that year in fourteen countries, while unofficial reports of vaccination and quarantine programs suggested that it had erupted also* in Iran, Iraq, Jordan, Saudi Arabia, Tunisia, Turkey, and Egypt.[18] The disease had therefore reached North Africa via the Near East, but it then spread to Guinea, in West Africa, where it had not been reported since 1893.[19] Following confirmation of its presence in Guinea by W.H.O., the government of Guinea followed the precedent set by some other countries affected by the pandemic and stopped reporting cholera.[20] From there, it was obvious that the disease would spread to adjacent countries in West Africa (as indeed it did), and W.H.O. set up a regional training center in Ibadan, Nigeria.

Against this background and the admitted complexity of factors favoring geographic spread—or interfering with control, which is the same thing—should be set the story (pp. 353-357) by Dr. Roger Simon of the spread of the pandemic to a village in Ghana. In this instance, a localized but intense outbreak with a

*The spread of cholera into Spain in 1971 has now been confirmed. Sporadic cases have also been reported elsewhere in Europe. *Brit. Med. J. 2*:266, 1971.

high mortality rate was brought under control very quickly by simple measures, without specialized equipment or expert personnel. From the evidence presented, it seems likely that a more elaborate or formal approach through official channels might have been much less effective in the short term, at least. Whether or not this is so, the lesson is clear enough when the Ghana outbreak is considered along with the history of the spread of the infection into Africa: confirmation of diagnosis, reporting of cases, and quarantine measures are not in themselves sufficient; an emergency center for isolation and early treatment of cases also is essential. It is clear from this seventh pandemic that early and continuous rehydration by oral or parenteral infusion can control the disease by replacement of water, sodium, potassium, and bicarbonate, and reduce mortality to less than 1 percent,[21] especially if combined with oral tetracycline, streptomycin, or dihydrostreptomycin in the treatment of severe cases and all carriers.[9,22] Control depends also upon the provision of safe water, prohibition of eating uncooked vegetables, and the sanitary disposal of feces. The experience reported on pp. 353-357 shows that elaborate facilities and expert staff are not required for this purpose, provided one or two individuals in the locality have the necessary knowledge, drive, and backing to initiate simple preventive and therapeutic measures. Protection by vaccine, which is short-lived and only partially effective,[15,16] is probably unnecessary if hygienic eating, drinking, and sewage disposal are ensured. Identification and treatment of carriers with streptomycin given orally is an important measure;[22] the cholera vibrio, like other bacteria, can develop resistance to this antibiotic in 24-48 hours, so treatment need not be continued beyond this period, after which alternative drugs (paromomycin, neomycin, kanamycin, tetracycline) should be given orally to chronic carriers.

From the wider, international viewpoint, the development and spread of the sixth pandemic illustrates additional lessons and gaps in the epidemiology of cholera. The sixth pandemic (1899-1922) spread from the Ganges delta throughout India eastward to Southeast Asia, Pacific Islands, and China, and westward to the Near East, Balkans, and Eastern Europe.[16] The remainder of

Europe and the Americas were unaffected, as was Africa except for minor outbreaks in Egypt. In 1922, the pandemic subsided but infection remained endemic in India and Southeast Asia, with local epidemics there still accounting for over 40,000 reported cases per year.[15] During this time, it became apparent that vaccination, even by improved methods, could not give more than 30 to 50 percent protection[7-9,15,16] and that control depended upon early diagnosis, reporting, quarantine, and sanitary precautions with food, water, and feces. Carriers were not thought to be of any long-term importance, and the use of antimicrobial agents was debatable. Treatment consisted essentially of rehydration and electrolyte replacement.

From the seventh pandemic, new epidemiological facts of considerable practical importance have emerged. The long-held beliefs[3,9,19] that there are no long-term carriers of the vibrio and that even the contact or convalescent carrier states are comparatively unimportant are dispelled by work in the Philippines which showed that 41 percent of infants in households of cases of cholera were infected, often asymptomatically. The convalescent and subclinical carrier states are, in fact, now known to be very common indeed and often of long duration,[23] involving the biliary as well as the intestinal tract. In endemic zones such as Calcutta, the vibrio may be found in 1.5 percent of the healthy population,[24] while intermittent but long-term carriage, especially in children, is now known to be a hazard which continues after an epidemic subsides,[16] though it may be controlled, as in Calcutta,[25] by attention to water supply and disposal of feces. However, a high carrier rate is not necessarily accompanied by an outbreak or even a high case rate. In Hong Kong, for instance, the carrier rate between 1961 and 1963 was estimated to be relatively high,[26] one in three hundred of the crowded population having been infected at one time or another; yet the case incidence was low (1:30,000) and the occurrence of a case in a household seemed to protect rather than endanger the rest of the household. Similar studies in households in Calcutta[27] disclosed the presence of many carriers without overt disease.

It may be that only a minority of persons are susceptible to cholera in its classical clinical form[9] or it may be that preexisting or contemporaneous subclinical infection confers protection against disease. Since infection is, as far as is known, acquired only by the oral route, there may be a dose factor if small numbers of vibrios are destroyed at some level in the gut. The possible role of gastric secretion and of the competitive gastrointestinal flora in this regard is poorly understood. But a simpler and possibly more important clue to the seeming anomaly between high carrier rates and low case rates in some communities is offered by the finding, reported from Iran,[16] that purgative doses of magnesium sulfate increased the yield of positive fecal cultures from supposedly negative persons. If, as in typhoid infection, such individuals excrete vibrios only when biliary secretion is stimulated or when diarrhea is provoked, intermittent carriage and hence sporadic infectivity would be explained. In cholerous areas, nonspecific gastroenteritis with diarrhea is notoriously common and it would be reasonable to postulate that such attacks in carriers of the cholera vibrio would provoke spread of infection whenever personal hygiene, disposal of feces, or purification of water is defective. This danger is increased because of the proven viability of the vibrio in water, uncooked food, utensils, kitchen furniture, and on human hands.

It is also apparent, from press reports[17,20,28] much more than from medical or public health agencies, that commercial, administrative, and political factors operate powerfully in the spread of cholera. Commercial considerations such as tourism and exports of fresh foods may delay or even prevent the reporting of cholera and the intervention of international health agencies. Administrative and fiscal repercussions may impete the application of quarantine and international sanitary regulations; even when existing quarantine measures are applied, there is no provision in international sanitary regulations to place any restriction upon carriers,[4,9,29] who are clearly important in transmitting infection from one locality to another.[30] Political attitudes or changes, especially in developing countries relying upon international assistance in their health programs, may delay or wholly prevent the application of control measures which necessarily entail some intervention or change in local procedures and customs.

On the scientific front, the seventh pandemic reveals more clearly than ever the inadequacy of strategy based upon the widely held assumption that infectious diseases can be eliminated by vaccines and chemotherapeutic agents. Despite considerable advances in the production of purified, strain-specific vaccines and in the laboratory diagnosis of the biotypes of the vibrio, prevention of disease and control of spread by vaccination has been, at best, only partially successful. Intramuscular vaccination with the *el Tor* biotype protects only 30 to 50 percent of susceptible subjects and immunity lasts only three months.[15,29,30] It is necessary to include at least two serotypes (Ogawa and Inaba) of *el Tor* in the vaccine[9,30] and it is uncertain how much protection this gives against other variants or against classical strains of *V. cholerae*, which have been isolated along with *el Tor* in recent outbreaks. Recent work by teams from the University of Maryland and elsewhere have shown that attenuated living organisms can give some protection to volunteers who ingested cholerogenic vibrios, but the duration of immunity and the risk of induced disease have not been fully investigated nor has the vaccine been tested in the setting of a natural epidemic. The combination of vaccination with chemoprophylaxis offers promise but has not been adequately tested in the field and would, in any event, be extremely expensive to apply in cholerous areas. The main successes, scientifically, during the past decade have been the development of more rapid and efficient methods for microbiological diagnosis and biotyping[31] and possibly some minor improvements in chemotherapy, like the introduction of furalazine.[32]

With the seventh pandemic still smouldering at the time of writing, the inescapable conclusion epidemiologically is that control of cholera is still dependent upon the application of traditional methods and that failure to control the disease is almost invariably due to human failure to apply existing knowledge rather than to any serious gap in knowledge.[33] Even in the hyperendemic areas and in the midst of epidemics, persons who follow hygienic principles in eating, drinking, and in other personal habits are rarely, if ever, attacked by the disease; likewise, the developed countries of the world have been untouched by the pandemic, as have privileged communities or individuals within the epidemic zones. It is abundantly clear from the foregoing and from the literature cited here that epidemics can be prevented or stopped by attention to water supplies, food, feces, carriers, case reporting, quarantine, symptomatic treatment, and other simple, relatively inexpensive methods, including health education of vulnerable communities. It is less clear that this is a practicable possibility unless enlightenment is conveyed to the said communities at all levels and, for this purpose, personal and governmental ignorance or inaction must be regarded and named as major causal factors in the spread of the disease, as much a part of its etiology as contamination of water.

AN EXPERIENCE IN EMERGENCY MANAGEMENT OF A CHOLERA EPIDEMIC

ROGER SIMON

"Strange Disease, Doctors Rushed to Ada; Cholera Suspected as Dozens Die" (headline, *Daily Graphic,* Dec. 1970, Accra, Ghana). When the seventh cholera pandemic reached Ghana during November and December 1970, I happened to visit that country for five weeks of my senior year at Cornell University Medical College. A chance meeting with Dr. Charles Herron, of the U.S. Public Health Service, attached to the Ghana Smallpox-Measles Program in the Epidemiology Division of the Ministry of Health, led to my visiting Akplabanya, a cholera-infested coastal village not far from Accra. The prevalence and severity of the outbreak in the village demanded that someone with medical training take charge of treatment and control of infection. Since individuals with personal experience in treating the disease were nonexistent locally and since Ghanaian physicians were not immediately available for dispatch to outlying areas, I found myself responsible for one of the first rural treatment facilities in Ghana and, later, for organizing treatment of cholera at a rural mission hospital.

My expertise was that of a senior medical student at a good American school; this was supplemented by the rapid reading of applicable sections in two standard texts and a twenty-page abstract of important recent data on cholera treatment taken from the publications of the World Health Organization. Diagnostic equipment available to me consisted of my hands and a stethoscope. Bacteriologic confirmation was available in Accra within the limits imposed by meager communication and transportation facilities. Intravenous fluid, antibiotics, and salts for oral electrolyte replacement were dispensed through the pharmacy at Korle Bu Hospital, of the University of Ghana, Accra; but availability of these supplies was a function of the same logistic considerations. No other supportive facilities were available.

Cholera was known to be moving down the West African coast, and humerous positive cultures were being reported in the Ivory Coast. Ghanaian monitoring efforts were focused in the western part of the country, since the migratory habits of fisherman in that area made spread along the coast likely. There was some surprise, then, when suspicious cases were reported several hundred miles to the east in a group of primitive fishing villages around Ada. A local fisherman had become ill in Togo and had returned to his village to die. After the funeral, many of the villagers, who presumably had touched the body, developed the same disease.

A treatment facility was rapidly established at the fishing village of Akplabanya in the tin-roofed schoolhouse, one of the few permanent structures in the village. The building was shared with omnipresent guana-producing bats. Fourteen previously prepared cholera cots* and a group of hastily calibrated buckets completed the furnishings. Coconuts and oranges provided a small but safe source of food; in addition, the former were valuable as a potassium supplement in children. Patients were carried or came on foot from as far as six hours away since reliable vehicles and roads were few. Approximately fifty to seventy-five patients were "admitted" to our facility—usually obtunded, with markedly decreased turgor, cold skin, absent peripheral pulse, and other

*A simple canvas bed with an opening for the buttocks, through which excrement is voided and collected for measurement and sanitary disposal.

signs of severe hypovolemic shock. Dehydration was estimated almost exclusively on the basis of skin turgor and pulse. Rapid replacement of volume was accomplished with sodium lactate Ringer's solution or normal saline administered by large-bore needle in the femoral vein. Intake and output were strictly recorded for each patient: fluid loss was determined from measured volume of stool, urine, and vomitus collections. Due to the shortage of IV fluid, resulting from communication and transportation problems, patients were switched to oral fluid as soon as the initial rehydration was complete. Oral replacement contained NaCl, $NaHCO_3$, and glucose* in preweighed amounts, measured for dissolution in fifteen liters of water. Rainwater was purchasable from the villagers and could be boiled for a fee. Because of adequate HCO_3 replacement in the oral solution and the unavailability of sterile bicarbonate for injection, this oral regimen, via nasogastric tube or p.o., became a critical factor in treatment. Acidosis proved fatal in several patients well rehydrated but without base replacement. In only rare cases was vomiting so severe after initial rehydration as to make oral therapy ineffective. Tetracycline 2000 mg/d p.o. was begun as soon as vomiting ceased, and patients were ready for discharge by the second or third day.

With very limited facilities, a large number of patients were of necessity treated as outpatients; at least fifty new cases were screened and treated daily. These patients were asked to stay in the vicinity until they either felt well enough to return home or became ill enough to require IV treatment. Oral fluid supplement was made available to mildly dehydrated patients; and all patients with a suspicious history were placed on tetracycline, if available, while they remained in the area. Unfortunately, complete courses of antibiotics were often interrupted by a shortage of drugs or the patient's unwillingness to continue medication after a feeling of well-being had returned.

At Akplabanya, two of approximately seventy-five critically ill

---

*90 mEq/liter Na, 60 mEq/liter Cl, 30 mEq/liter HCO_3 120 m-mol/liter glucose (Johns Hopkins University Medical Research Training Center, School of Tropical Medicine, Calcutta).

patients died during my brief tenure. (The first three patients treated at Korle Bu Hospital died). This rapidly established and immediately effective treatment center could not have functioned had it not been for the fact that in nearly every village the local schoolteacher was in residence and spoke English, the official language, as well as native dialects. The schoolteachers were strikingly intelligent and literate individuals who commanded respect in their villages. They quickly accepted the facts of the pathogenesis of the disease and were active over long hours daily as translators, clerks, and nurses. Their assistance in transcending cultural, social, and language barriers was invaluable. On several occasions, I drove to villages in which it was rumored that many deaths were occurring and was able to dispense emergency care quickly by locating the teacher and the "gong-gong" man (town crier).

The villagers could observe that the offered treatment was effective, since many people had died before but only two after the therapy became available. People walked great distances to bring a few oranges or some coconuts, not because they wanted medicine but because they had learned of the facility's existence. It was striking, then, that the villagers retained their traditional customs for dealing with disease and other undesirable aspects of life over which they had no control. Not only did the customs and ceremonies continue, but the belief in their effectiveness remained unaltered. One ceremony in particular was of interest: the men of the village gathered palm branches and sticks and walked through the village dragging these implements behind them. After a suitable time, the men then attacked the "presence" of the disease with the sticks and, beating the ground, literally "drove" the disease out of the village and into the sea. In addition, various fetishes were routinely placed on the beach to guard against intrusion. A dead cock was a favorite symbol of protection.

Vaccination has become a major facet of the Ghanaian government's program against cholera. The effectiveness of vaccination in combatting smallpox and yellow fever is well known to the most rural of Ghanaians; in fact, smallpox has been virtually unheard of for the past two years. In much the same manner as

Americans visiting their local physician, Ghanaians do not feel they have received complete treatment for any complaint until an injection of something has been given. Vaccination against cholera, therefore, is much sought after.

As fear of the disease spread, the desire for vaccination became nearly a panic. Vaccination sites were mobbed; police used their clubs routinely in an effort to maintain order. The vaccine used was quoted as approximately 30 percent effective, i.e. some 70 percent of vaccinated persons would contract the full-blown disease if adequately exposed. The vaccinated population, however, reflecting on their past experiences, felt that an injection was tantamount to immunity. A most difficult situation existed, therefore, with regard to initiation of public health measures against the disease. The government's educational program was essentially limited to the newspapers, and the few attempts made to persuade the rural population to adopt basic protective measures met striking skepticism. Boiling of water obtained from the same source for generations seemed unreasonable to the villagers, particularly because firewood was expensive. Handwashing was customarily performed after eating, not before. Vaccination undoubtedly saved some lives, but strict adherence to simple measures of hygiene *alone* might have been more effective. Little effort in public health education was made by the government.

My final week in Ghana was spent establishing a treatment facility at the Mission Hospital in Apam. Dozens of cholera cases were reported from the nearby government hospital at Winneba, and Apam was without a physician. Modern buildings and a group of Dutch nurses with incredible endurance differentiated Apam from the fishing villages. Treatment facilities were identical: cholera cots, volume replacement, oral electrolytes, and antibiotics. A larger facility permitted admission of less critically ill patients. At Apam, one of the first one hundred patients died; the fatality rate at the Winneba Hospital was considerably greater.

My experience in Ghana leads me to suggest that even a small core of information, barely adequate supplies, and primitive conditions, together with enthusiasm, constitute an effective combination against cholera.

SMALLPOX

(Chapter 9, by G.T. Stewart, continued)

Apart from minor sporadic and localized outbreaks, usually attributed to admission of an infective immigrant or visitor, the developed countries of the world have remained free from smallpox since 1920 or earlier. The disease has, however, remained endemic in most parts of the underdeveloped world, especially, but not entirely, in tropical and subtropical zones. Smallpox was one of the first of the major communicable diseases to receive recognition as an international health problem, and legislative measures[4] for control have been accepted, if not fully enforced, by most countries for many years past. Despite this, high case-prevalence rates (i.e. 5-30 per 100,000) were regularly reported in the Indian subcontinent, equatorial Africa, South America, and some of the larger Pacific Islands.[34] The international health agencies focused attention on these areas from 1947 onward, laying emphasis upon indisputably sound measures like early diagnosis, isolation, quarantine, case reporting, and extensive vaccination. But the disease persisted in the regions mentioned and even increased in some countries (Table 9.1), causing an overall increase in the total number of cases (337,613) reported for the three years 1965-67 over the number (308,612) reported in 1962-64. There was no sign in these regions of the classical epidemiological cycle described by Burnet,[4] in which, as protection increases and prevalence diminishes, the pattern of disease changes from an epidemic disease of young children to a sporadic disease of young adults. It was therefore obvious that smallpox was at a static level of endemicity in large areas of South America, Africa, the Indian subcontinent, and the Pacific, and that cases were being transmitted from there to adjacent areas and occasionally to nonendemic zones in Asia, North America, Australia, and Europe. In 1967, 131,164 cases were reported from forty-three countries; the true incidence, including undiagnosed and subclinical cases, was obviously much higher. In that year, WHO began a program aiming at eradication of smallpox.

TABLE 9.1
CASES OF SMALLPOX REPORTED BETWEEN 1962 AND 1970

	1962	*1963*	*1964*	*1965*	*1966*	*1967*	*1968*	*1969*	*1970*
Africa									
North	1	5	—	—	—	—	—	—	—
West and Central	17,235	6687	3565	6257	7570	10,818	5408	482	64
East and South	7542	10,162	9017	10,683	6986	4460	5544	3095	3113
America									
North	—	—	—	—	—	—	—	—	—
Central	1	—	—	—	—	—	—	—	—
South	10.031	7385	3713	3632	3670	4537	4375	7394	1795
Asia (excluding China)	63,692	108,405	58,906	91,532	76,184	111,344	64,766	42,725	26,324
Europe	136	129	—	1	72	5	2	—	22
Australia	—	—	—	—	—	—	—	—	—
Totals	98,638	132,773	75,201	112,155	94,482	131,164	80,095	53,696	31,318
Number of countries reporting cases	61	55	46	44	43	43	38	29	23

In the years 1947-67, laboratory work had led to improvements in diagnostic methods and especially to great accuracy in the differentiation of the virus of variola major from the related viruses of alastrim, chickenpox, and vaccinia. The vaccine and technique of vaccination had also been improved,[35] and N-methylisatin-β-thiosemicarbazone was available for passive prophylaxis, as were hyperimmune sera and globulins. No other measures for control of smallpox had been made in the interim, so the eradication program was based upon closer surveillance, early diagnosis, case reporting, and mass vaccination. The result was, in the first instance, an apparent increase in case incidence, due to the detection through field surveillance of numerous cases which would otherwise have escaped attention. This increase was especially noticeable in Brazil, the Democratic Republic of the Congo, Indonesia, and West Pakistan—and is a very usual finding when statistics from a well-planned surveillance are compared with those obtained by routine case reporting. Thereafter, however, improvement began and was most striking in western and central Africa and in Asia, reaching by 1969 in both regions a lower number of recorded cases than ever before. It should be remembered that the method of surveillance had led to the detection of greater numbers of cases than formerly, so that the true reduction was much greater than that shown in Table 9.1. There was also a fall in eastern and southern Africa, which included the Congo, a country in which the disease had been hyperendemic for a long time but in which, despite size and social turbulence, a very vigorous vaccination program had been extended to cover about half of the country's population, including for the first time many preschool children. The fall in that country and the apparent elimination of the disease from most of the other countries of West, Central, and East Africa by the end of 1970[36] indicated a remarkable movement toward regional control of the disease by well-coordinated national and international action. To counterbalance this, however, serious outbreaks persisted in South Africa, at one pole of the continent, and in Ethiopia and the Sudan, at the other. There is no evidence to indicate that effective eradication programs have been implemented in these countries, and it has been estimated by W.H.O.[34] that the number of actual cases in Ethiopia may be ten to fifty times the recorded number.

In South America, smallpox seems to have been eradicated from all countries except Brazil, where, in 1969, there was a sharp increase to a level exceeding the 1962-67 peak. This may have been due to more intensive surveillance, because variola minor is common in Brazil and was probably unsuspected prior to 1967.

The position in Asia is uncertain, partly because intensive eradication measures and surveillance were not initiated until 1968-69, since when there has been a real or apparent decrease in India, East Pakistan, Afghanistan, and Nepal, no change in Indonesia, and probably a real increase in West Pakistan.[34]

These efforts and results suggest that perhaps, for the first time since the growth of civilization in Asia Minor in pre-Christian times,[37,38] the eradication of smallpox from the traditional endemic zones is a practical possibility. In the assessment of results, however, especially in the short term, it has to be remembered that smallpox in its natural pattern in endemic zones tends to become epidemic every five to six years,[1,9] which is the period required in various diseases of high infectivity for the accumulation of newborn children to produce a population of susceptibles high enough to sustain the spread of infection, according to the principles described on pp, 375-381. The countries affected by smallpox all have high birth rates and infant mortality rates. Each rate is influenced by many factors, largely imponderable but nevertheless so relevant to epidemiology and control as to demand attention for future strategy. Birth-control and family-planning programs have not, so far, led to appreciable reduction in the birth rates or natural increase in population even in countries where figures are available, as in India and Pakistan; in other countries the position is entirely speculative but it is not unreasonable to suppose that traditional population trends will continue so that, unless the infant mortality rate remains high, there will be a natural increase in population, which will be intensified as smallpox is eradicated. This will create, in a few years, a huge population of susceptibles unless the present rate of vaccination of preschool children is accelerated. With large supplies of dried vaccine from the U.S.A., U.S.S.R., and elsewhere now available, such an accomplishment is not impossible if problems of personnel and access in the affected countries are overcome. We shall then, by our epidemiological strategy and priority, have released population growth from yet another natural inhibitor.

One of the arguments in favor of the total eradication of smallpox from endemic zones is that the disease is liable to be spread to other countries by travelers. Such transmissal certainly happens periodically but it need not. Five outbreaks were initiated in the United Kingdom in 1962 by immigrants from Pakistan,[34] but there were no outbreaks in Europe in 1964, 1965, 1967-69, although individual cases were detected, nor were there any cases reported from South America in 1969-70 except for 3 in Uruguay, despite the hyperendemicity of the disease in Brazil. In 1970, one outbreak affecting 24 persons occurred in West Germany[39] following admission of an infected immigrant from West Pakistan. The patient was isolated and treated with standard precaution and had no direct contact with any of the other 74 patients in the hospital. But the patient had extensive cutaneous and oral lesions and a cough, and the disease was transmitted, almost certainly by airborne medium, to 13 (18%) of the 74 patients and also to 6 other persons. This epidemic, the first in which the virus of variola major has been shown convincingly to have spread by airborne routes instead of by direct face-to-face contact with a case or by indirect contact via infected fomites, reveals how a single case can initiate an outbreak even when conventional isolation measures are applied. If, as is likely, such transmission occurs more easily in less hygienic settings, there will be an obvious difficulty in eradicating smallpox from a community if even one person develops the disease amid an incompletely vaccinated population. The variola virus is thought to have a capacity to survive outside the body in dry atmospheres.[40] Hence, even if all the other factors are controlled, as is theoretically possible, it is hard to see how the difficulty of airborne transmission will be avoided except by extraordinary methods of isolation and repeated vaccination, not only of contacts but of more remote persons.

There are important differences between smallpox and other lethal epidemics. For various reasons, tuberculosis, influenza, plague, malaria, and yellow fever have all become modified in their biological history so that, without intervention, the pattern and virulence have tended to ameliorate as susceptible populations have adapted themselves. These diseases, however devastating they may be to a nonimmune population, have left in their wake surviving generations with some degree of natural immunity or resistance to the disease. Cholera leaves no appreciable immunity but it can be controlled by attention to food and water and by prompt treatment. With smallpox these benefits are not available. Historical incidents as well as numerous outbreaks have placed its infectivity and lethality on record in grim terms: historically, it has decimated nonimmune populations again and again,[1,2,38] and in recent epidemics mortality rate in nonimmune subjects has always been high—often 70 percent, sometimes almost 100 percent. This consistent virulence, together with the susceptibility of newborn infants even in hyperendemic zones, places smallpox in a special category: unlike all the other diseases mentioned, it can be controlled only by inducing and maintaining a high degree of artificial immunity by vaccinating large numbers of persons, whether or not smallpox is present, wherever it is likely to be present. In addition, measures for suspected cases and immigrants are essential as long as even one endemic zone remains on the trade or passenger traffic routes of the world. This fact is unpleasant to contemplate, for it involves restrictions on individual liberty and right of protest, but it is the inescapable epidemiological conclusion and the price of eradication of smallpox, if that is our aim. This means that the efficiency, risks, and complications[41,42] of vaccination have to be weighed against the alternative dangers of contracting and transmitting smallpox, which in developed countries is almost negligible. Hence, in the absence of an epidemic or scare of one, vaccination rates of infants fall, which means that the complication rate of vaccinations performed subsequently rises, since the vaccine is not tolerated so well after infancy. There is therefore a need for constant surveillance not only of the endemic zones but also of vaccination rates in disease-free countries, on traffic routes, in travelers, and in personnel in airports, immigration ports, hospitals, and points of first contact.

As an explanation of the persistent localization of smallpox in Asia Minor, India, and tropical Africa, it has been suggested that the virus possesses an antigen related to the antigen of blood group A.[43] In these parts of the world, blood group A is less common than elsewhere, but smallpox scars are more common in persons with blood of group A than in other persons.[44] Hence, it is claimed that group A individuals stand at a disadvantage because they lack anti-A antibody or cannot manufacture anti-A when infected by smallpox virus. In contrast, persons of groups B and O have a biological and survival advantage in that they already possess anti-A and can produce more in response to infection. Historically, this would mean that the disease gained ascendance by eliminating susceptibles of group A, but there are weaknesses in this reasoning, which has been refuted by Downie *et al.*[45] in a study of ABO groups in smallpox zones. There is, however, a geographic association between smallpox and the predominance of A and B genes in the Old World[46] and in the high frequency of the O gene in the Old and New Worlds,[47] from which it would appear that, biologically, smallpox may have influenced the survival or distribution of peoples in certain parts of the world. This aspect of epidemiology of communicable and other diseases joins with anthropology and genetics (see Chap. 3) in leading to important information about human survival, evolution, and population growth.[48,49]

VENEREAL DISEASE

Syphilis and gonorrhea, the two chief forms of venereal disease, enjoy the dubious distinction today of being epidemic in scale in developed as well as in undeveloped countries. Both diseases are increasing rapidly in prevalence, especially among young people in cities, in a "silent epidemic"[50] or pandemic whose dimension is still unmeasured and perhaps unmeasurable unless additional information and more efficient use of it is obtained (pp. 385-387).

This increase has occurred in the face of technical conquest of the responsible microorganisms and widespread knowledge and recognition of the other etiological factors concerned in the two diseases. The organism responsible for syphilis, *Treponema pallidum,* is killed rapidly by penicillin in dilutions of 10^{-8}, which makes it as sensitive to this nontoxic, cheap, universally available antibiotic as any other germ, and still much more sensitive than most; drug resistance on the part of *T. pallidum* is unknown[51] and probably biologically impossible; the only contraindication to the use of penicillin is allergy to the drug[52] in a minority of patients and, when this occurs, substitute antibiotics such as tetracycline, erythromycin, cephalosporins, and others are available and are almost as effective. *Neisseria gonorrhoeae,* the gonococcus, also is highly sensitive to penicillin, being inhibited usually by dilutions of 10^{-7} and invariably by 10^{-5}, a concentration at which even the so-called resistant strains are killed.[53] Other antibiotics such as ampicillin, erythromycin, tetracyclines, and cephalothin also are effective in high dilution (10^{-5} to 10^{-7}),[53] and drug resistance by the organism is comparatively rare. The antibiotics are effective prophylactically when given immediately before or within forty-eight hours after exposure to infection; used therapeutically after symptoms have appeared, they are strikingly effective in acute cases and reasonably effective even in late chronic cases[52] in that they at least render patients noninfectious. In males, a single dose of 2.4 megaunits of procaine penicillin G cures both diseases in their acute stages in over 90 percent of cases, while in females, 4.8 megaunits has comparable efficacy.[52-54] Except in allergic cases, penicillin treatment is harmless, and in allergic cases there are alternatives; one shot is usually enough. Both diseases are easy to recognize or, at least, to suspect. Routine serology in pregnant women leads to correct diagnosis and successful treatment of syphilis in 95 percent of cases.[54]

There are few, if any, communicable diseases for which medical science has produced such powerful antagonists. That the problem remains with us at all is disappointing; that it should grow almost uncontrollably in developed communities would be incredible were it not for the fact that it does. In the U.S.A., venereal disease is now second only to the common cold in annual incidence[55] and in some areas exceeds the average total annual incidence of all other communicable diseases. The increase in New Jersey in the first six months of 1970 was 55 percent over the 1969 incidence,[56] and the general rate throughout the nation was graphically described by an expert as "a teenager infected every 75 minutes."[55]

Because of the advent, widespread use, and proved efficacy of antibiotics in treatment, syphilis, and gonorrhea decreased in incidence in many countries between 1950 and 1957. A reverse trend then became apparent[57] and has continued, with few interruptions, through 1970. The chief numerical increase internationally is due to gonorrhea but a rising incidence of syphilis also is reported in many countries.[58] Large metropolitan areas and seaports always show higher rises of both diseases than do smaller urban or rural districts but the difference in this respect is smaller than might be imagined in U.S. cities. This and other demographic aspects of venereal disease are well documented in a series of reports issued by the World Health Organization,[59] the American

Social Health Association,[60] and numerous other international and national bodies concerned with the problem.[55,60]

In these reports the facts speak for themselves and point accusingly at the real determinants of disease and the obstacles to cure: the personal, social, educational, and administrative factors which can never be countered by episodic therapy and traditional practice. Of special importance in this respect is the conflict between therapy and prevention. Therapy requires efficient and immediate treatment and follow-up of each patient or each episode of infection. If the physician does this confidentially, as his conventional ethical role demands, he is doing nothing to prevent the spread of disease except insofar as his patient is rendered non-infectious for a shorter or longer period. If the physician notifies the public health authorities of his patient's infection, confidentiality is violated but contact tracing and preventive action (Fig. 9.1) can follow and are known to be effective in proportion to the zeal of implementation. In the U.S., at least 75 percent of cases are treated by private physicians,[55,58,61] but only about 11 to 18 percent of that total are reported.[58] In 1970, the number of reported cases of gonorrhea in the U.S. was over 500,000. If it is

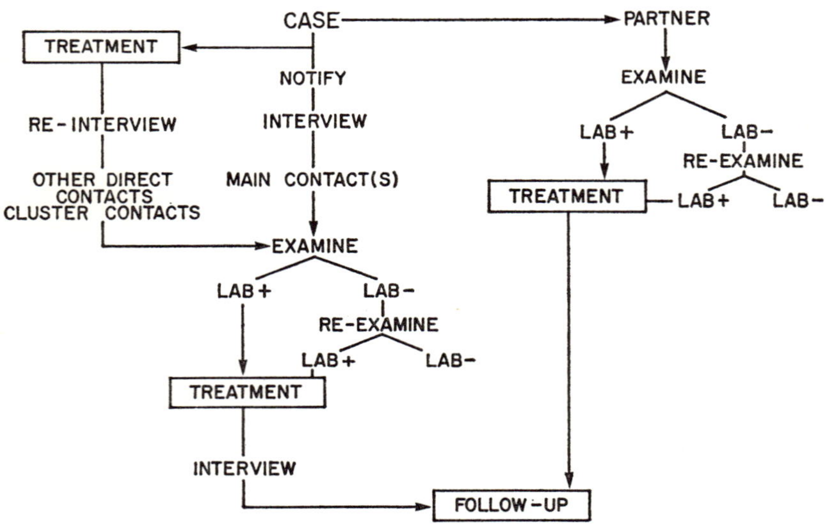

Figure 9.1. Source tracing in venereal disease.

assumed that, as in 1968, 70 percent of this total were reported and treated by private physicians, the real total of new cases receiving treatment from private or public sources can be estimated at nearly two million. Similarly, the projected incidence in infectious syphilis receiving treatment in 1970 can be estimated at about 70,000.

To these totals should be added the numbers not seeking or receiving specific treatment, as follows: (a) children with unrecognized congenital infection, (b) teenagers unaware of manifestations, (c) persons with asymptomatic infections, (d) persons inadequately treated, (e) persons reinfected shortly after therapy, and (f) travelers, seamen, and immigrants. There are no reliable figures, at present, giving the numbers of persons in these categories but there is plenty of collateral evidence to suggest that they might be considerable: the occurrence of disease in adolescents and school children, greater sexual freedom and promiscuity, abandonment of the condom in favor of the contraceptive pill, more premarital intercourse and pregnancy, widespread ignorance about the nature and symptoms of venereal disease and about the availability of treatment. It is well known, also, that infection may be unrecognized in women, who can easily infect many male contacts, and in homosexual males.

More so than in any other communicable disease, control of venereal disease requires prompt notification and source tracing. Notification is statutory in most countries but is seldom checked or enforced, partly because to do so necessitates breaching confidentiality and individual privacy. Even when cases are notified, there are wide discrepancies in different communities in the extent to which source tracing is practiced or is practicable. It is estimated, for instance, that in the U.S. in 1969 about 93 percent of reported cases of syphilis were interviewed, 83 percent reinterviewed, and 71 percent cluster-interviewed; this led to location and examination of about 45 percent of contacts, of whom 15 percent were treated.[58] But the range within each heading between states varied considerably, as did the provision for diagnosis, treatment, follow-up, and premarital and prenatal tests. A special problem is created by the need, in some states, to obtain parental consent for the treatment of minors, and by the reluctance of some of the teenage population to visit established centers for treatment. In addition to syphilis and gonorrhea, lymphogranuloma venereum, chancroid, granuloma inguinale, *Trichomonas* infection, and candidiasis are endemic in some communities and can be transmitted venereally.

If we accept the premise that the main forms of venereal disease are controllable by modern technology, we have to accept, as determinants of the contemporary epidemic, the various nontechnical factors listed above—failure of notification, of contact tracing, of education of teenagers, of implementation of safeguards and regulations. These factors are difficult to assess because of personal and professional reticence, and research is required to examine the extent to which conventional attitudes impede common objectives. But much of the impediment is obvious and need not be measured. Since venereal disease obviously cannot be controlled by conventional practice, the problem is to gain acceptance of the need for multifactor trials and, in so doing, to assess the relative weight of the various social, behavioral, administrative, and educational factors which are responsible for the maintenance and spread of these diseases.

Of the many factors conducive to the spread of venereal disease, four would appear to be of prime importance:

1. The failure or imperfection of notification and source tracing, as described above. This is a measurable factor, the extent of which can be estimated from published reports.[57,60,61]

2. The substitution of the birth-control pill for the condom in contraception. That this has occurred on an immense scale in most developed countries and in many developing countries is not in doubt, nor is there any doubt that the condom is a relatively efficient prophylactic against infection of female by male or vice versa. It seems highly probable that this change in habit together with the current increase in premarital and extramarital intercourse is a major factor—perhaps the principal factor—in the spread of venereal disease.

3. The third factor is ignorance: despite some health education in schools and frequent presentation of health problems in

news media and popular magazines, ignorance about venereal disease is still widespread in all age groups and especially among the young.[58,60] The uninhibited teenagers who "do their own things" are often surprisingly unaware of the symptoms and contagiousness of venereal disease. Even when aware, they are sometimes reluctant to attend official clinics for treatment and follow-up.

4. This brings us to the fourth factor, which is the revolt of youth. During the past two decades, youthful groups and sometimes youth generally, in Western countries at least, have shown growing discontent, expressed by rejection of traditional dress, proprieties, and mores. Superficially, this change is accompanied by a loosening of moral standards, but in actuality there is a real moral nucleus in the revolt insofar as it signifies distrust of double-talk, double standards, and dubiousness generally in the deteriorating world fashioned and upheld by their elders and betters, possibly fostered in no small measure by the permissiveness which their elders have accorded them. Paradoxically, it is the younger generations that are hankering after personal freedom and a retreat from organized societies in which technical triumphs are underscored by recurring failures in human understanding. This is the positive philosophy of revolt. The negative ideations—fatalism, indifference, *anomie,* indiscriminate tolerance—are much more familiar and constitute the nihilistic credo of a sizable slice of today's youth. In either case, the effect of the belief is a severance of traditional restrictions and a do-as-you-please attitude. Sexual taboos and hurdles were amongst the first to go, accelerated by the birth-control pill and then by abortion-on-demand. Sexual symbols and performance dominate trade as well as entertainment; the emotional power and meaning in sexual relations have been overshadowed, if not devoured, by the dollar power of sensation and pornography developed, not by youth, but by an accommodating elder society which may disapprove while in church but not in everyday life.

These mixed motives create a societal drive and incentive to greater and more diverse sexual activity not only in youth but at other ages, homosexually as well as heterosexually. The consequences are promiscuity, perversion, fetishism, and at the same time, an inability or unwillingness on the part of many young people to seek treatment from the establishment against which they are rebelling, and a disinclination on the part of the establishment itself to probe the complex moral, economic, and administrative facets of the problem. Hence we have an epidemic of unprecedented size, clinical diversity, and etiologic complexity.

Viewed thus, venereal disease is a behavioral disorder in which the behavior of society, including physicians who fail to report the disease or teachers and parents who ignore its presence, is at fault equally with the behavior of persons who contract it, carry it, and spread it. In this respect, venereal disease is a leading symptom of a deeper and graver psychosocial malady, reflected also in drug abuse (Chap. 12) and alienation (p. 567), which are collectively responsible for the biggest of the contemporary epidemics because it is destructive of human values and progeny as well as of health. Medical science can prevent or cure the infection without touching the behavior which causes it. Social science has expanded, like the problem, without offering effective answers. As in all multifactor diseases, analysis of the problem is basically epidemiological—but standard works and journals and, therefore, contemporary investigators in epidemiology seldom reflect much interest and show little sign of meeting the greatest challenge in their field today.

MAN-MADE FACTORS AFFECTING SUSCEPTIBILITY TO INFECTIOUS DISEASES

Everyone knows that some people are relatively immune to infectious agents whereas others are highly susceptible, both to infection and to the ensuing diseases. But there is a big difference between knowing this and knowing exactly what is meant by susceptibility except in experiments with well-standardized animal-model infections, which are seldom applicable to human situations.

The increasing therapeutic uses of immunosuppressive and cytotoxic drugs during the past decade for grafts, transplants, and neoplasms have shown convincingly (and sometimes disastrously) that practically any type of commensal microorganism can produce severe infection if defensive cellular and humoral responses are inhibited. Definitive pathogens, like pyogenic cocci, *Pseudomonas,* and *Enterobacter-Klebsiella,* become more troublesome under these circumstances but even diphtheroids, *Serratia, Herrelea,* and yeasts can readily and increasingly cause autogenous or secondary infection, especially in hospitals (pp. 382-386). Apart from specific interference with immune mechanisms, there are many other less specific ways in which nutritional[62,63] or metabolic deficiencies depress resistance, leading in some communities to lethality in diseases, like measles in West Africa.[64] The competitive microflora in the skin, nasopharynx, alimentary canal, and vagina also is a factor which limits invasion by extraneous microorganisms and is, in turn, influenced by antimicrobial therapy.[65,66] The percise mechanisms by which these various defenses operate are incompletely understood but the facts are plain, and it is easy to depict the chain of events leading to or interfering with disease as opposed to infection (Fig. 9.2). In assessing other factors, it is

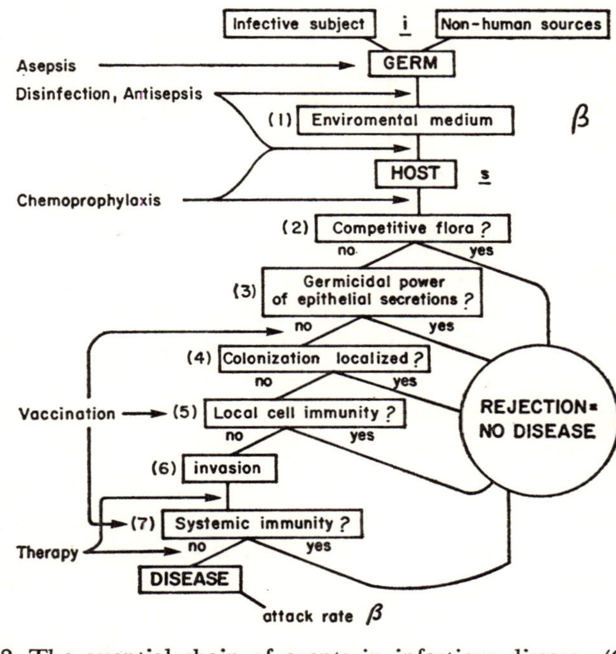

Figure 9.2. The essential chain of events in infectious disease. (Courtesy of the *Lancet.*)

necessary to draw a sharp distinction between major, minor, and facultative pathogens.

The major pathogens are, in general, those in which the germ is dominant, displaying high infectivity and causing severe disease in healthy populations: the obvious examples are *V. cholerae* (pp. 347-357), smallpox virus (pp. 359-364), influenza A viruses, plague bacilli, *N. gonorrhoeae,* and *T. pallidum* (pp. 364-370). These germs are so dangerous that intervention is effective only if it kills the organism at source, interrupts contact, or makes the host immune. The pathogens which are minor in the epidemiological sense include many familiar organisms, like staphylococci, *M. tuberculosis,* and respiratory viruses, which possess high virulence in certain cases but relatively low infectivity. Infections caused by these germs are strongly influenced not only by well-described sociocultural[2,48,67] and ethnic factors[65] but also by less well known behavioral factors, as described below. The facultative pathogens include practically all members of the indigenous human commensal microflora and the normally harmless microbes in air, water, and soil. Until now, these organisms have been unimportant, but the increasing use of grafts, transplants, endoprostheses, parenteral infusions, dialyses, immunosuppressive agents, and antimicrobial and cytotoxic drugs is giving rise to new types of infection and iatrogenic disease.[68,69] In this unexplored and portentous field, latent or persisting germs are stirred into activity[70] and may acquire unprecedented virulence.[71] Apart from their effect on the individual's microflora, antimicrobial agents have altered infectious disease epidemiologically in three ways: (a) by eliminating or diminishing major diseases,[51,65] like scarlet fever, which were once common, (b) by creating thereby a zymotic vacuum, in which latent pathogens like *Mycoplasma*[72] have gained pathogenic prominence, and (c) by creating new populations and subspecies of drug-resistant variants[65,70-76] of pathogens and nonpathogens with unfamiliar and sometimes unmanageable disease pattern (Table 9.2). At the time of writing, primary and secondary infections caused by *Enterobacter-Klebsiella, Pseudomonas, Serratia, Herrelea,* and fungi are responsible for some of the most serious outbreaks in U.S. hospitals.[68] In Europe, infections caused by staphylococci which have become resistant to the newer penicillins are increasing in prevalence.[76] Drug resistance and resistance-transfer constantly limit the usefulness of antimicrobial agents;[68-76] and so the story continues as an unending race between the ingenuity of man and the genetic adaptability of microbes.

TABLE 9.2
MICROORGANISMS RESPONSIBLE FOR IATROGENIC AND NOSOCOMIAL INFECTION

Viruses	Herpes simplex	*Fungi*	Aspergillus
	Varicella-zoster		Candida spp.
Bacteria	Aerobacter spp.*		Coccidioides
	Diphtheroids		Cryptococcus
	Enterobacter spp.*		Histoplasma
	Klebsiella spp.		Mucor
	Listeria		Nocardia spp.*
	Mimea-herrelea	*Protozoa*	Pneumocystis
	Pseudomonas spp.*		Toxoplasma
	Serratia		
	Staphylococci		
	Streptococcus moniliformis		

*In recent years, unfamiliar varieties and sources of these organisms have become increasingly common in hospital-acquired infections. The outbreaks of sepsis due to *Enterobacter erwinia* in many hospitals in 1971 have been traced to the presence of the organism in supposedly sterile intravenous infusions.

The spread of these infections, inside and outside of hospitals, is determined partly by artificial or man-made susceptibilities in special-risk groups. This leads to the consideration of other aspects of human behavior as determinants of infectious disease.

BEHAVIOR AS A FACTOR IN HOST SUSCEPTIBILITY

The psychological connection between behavior and disease is examined expertly in Chapter 4. The points discussed here are less complex but no less potent as determinants. It is obvious that certain infections (venereal disease, hepatitis in heroin addicts) can be entirely avoided by avoidance of personal exposure or abandonment of a habit. Exposure to many other infections is also optional, though less personal: zoonoses, enteritides, certain skin and respiratory infections, among others, can be circumvented by deliberate avoidance of exposure or contact. Alternatively, calculated exposure to infection is deliberately adopted as a Spartan policy in some cultures and by individuals, irrespectively of their cultural environment, on philosophic grounds, albeit with varying and unpredictable success. But such attitudes should not be ignored, for they provide examples of empirical prophylaxis and immunity which was once and might be again, one day, man's only defense against the competing forces of the microbial world.

Epidemiologically we can recognize if we cannot entirely harness such forces of survival. We concern ourselves more with things which can be measured or exploited and, in this connection, new facts are emerging which disclose some of the behavioral factors associated with susceptibility or resistance to infection. To establish these facts, we have to look at the minor pathogens (because they give the host an option) acting amid healthy human populations that can exercise the option. Thus Plag and Phelan[77] found that less than a tenth (8.7%) of healthy naval enlistees accounted for over a third (34.2%) of all illnesses, including many infections, during training. Similarly, Voors *et al.*[78-80] in a series of studies on naval and marine recruits found that personal attitudes and response to training appeared to influence susceptibility to respiratory infection as well as to other disabilities, the difference between persons and platoons in this respect being seen less in the acquisition of infection than in complaints and illness attributable to infection.[79] Unexpectedly, this was not linked to hypochondria or other personality attributes as measured by the MMPI scale,[80] but social disparities, status incongruity, and the maladaptation which resulted from a change in life situation were influential factors,[78] as noted also by Hinkle *et al.*[81] and Jackson.[82] Specifically, such factors may operate by affecting the hormonal pattern of the Selyean stress reaction[83] or the physiological response of the nasopharynx in a manner described by Holmes and his colleagues,[84] who have made a special study of the interaction of physiological, psychological, and infectious mechanisms in various respiratory infections.

In more general terms, it is a matter of common experience that disruption in lifestyle and personal insecurity increase anxiety and predispose to illness. We might therefore postulate, if not define, a personal threshold to microbial disease, below which the infectivity of the organism makes the stake but above which defensive personal and behavioral attributes determine the odds for and against disease, thus

$$\text{Severity of disease} = \frac{\text{Number of germs} \times \text{virulence}}{\text{Defensive response of host}}$$

Personal behavior in this respect is obviously partly individualistic but partly a reflection of group behavior; this, in turn, is a product of sociocultural[85] as well as interpersonal factors,[86,87] the study of which is one of the important growing edges of epidemiology,[88-91] especially insofar as it defines changes in the pattern of existing disease and emerging new diseases.[92] The sum total of all these complex genetic, personal, behavioral, and social interactions in all the individuals in a community constitutes the susceptibility or resistance of that community to infectious disease. It is impossible to compute such a total, but comparisons between populations and subpopulations are natural experiments which reveal differences which can be used as pointers for preventive intervention and convincing precedents for changes in policy. If an infectious or any other disease is a product of multifactorial etiology (pp. 379-381), it can only be prevented or controlled by attention to each of the accessible factors, in proportionality (Table 9.3), and by acceptance of the need for multifactor programs (see Chap. 7).

THE APPLICATION OF EPIDEMIC THEORY TO SURVEILLANCE AND CONTROL

In theory, data required for efficient surveillance and prediction can be classified into simple input categories, as follows:

Infective persons or sources	i
Susceptible persons at risk	s
Effective contact rate between s and i	β
Time period of effective contact	t
Persons removed by isolation, immunity, or death	z
Removal rate	γ

TABLE 9.3

EXAMPLES OF CONTROL MEASURES APPLIED TO COMMUNICABLE DISEASES IN TERMS OF EPIDEMIC MODELS

Disease	*Infectives (i)*	*Susceptibles (s)*	*Contact (β)*	*Time (t)*	*Removals (z)*
Smallpox	Recognition of case	Vaccination	Quarantine	Quarantine	Disinfection of clothes, etc.
Cholera	Diagnosis of cases; identification of carriers	Personal attention to food and water	Disposal of feces	Quarantine	Identification of carriers
Influenza	Voluntary withdrawal	Immunization	Propaganda	Seasonal awareness	—
Venereal disease	Condoms; chemotherapy	Education; chemoprophylaxis	Education	Notification data bank	Contact tracing
Malaria	chemotherapy	Chemoprophylaxis; mosquito nets and repellents	Vector	Control	Treatment of relapses
Hospital infection	Ward surveillance	Recognition of high-risk sectors	Ward design; review of medical, surgical, and nursing procedures	Regulation of admissions and transfers	Awareness of transfer potential, drug resistance, bandit organisms

By definition, the total population is

$$s + i - z = n \quad \text{(1)},$$

the number of new infections in the period t is given by

$$\frac{ds}{dt} = -\beta si \quad \text{(2)},$$

the changes in the number of infective persons is

$$\frac{di}{dt} = \beta si - \gamma i \quad \text{(3)},$$

and the change caused by removal is

$$\frac{dz}{dt} = \gamma i = \gamma (n\text{-}s\text{-}z) \quad \text{(4)},$$

while $\rho = \frac{\gamma}{\beta}$ is the relative removal rate of infectives.

An epidemic obviously cannot start unless

$\rho < s_0$ (the original number of susceptibles)

and $[\frac{di}{dt}]_{t=0} > 0$, which define the base-line conditions mathematically. In the absence of any sudden change in population by influx or withdrawal, a community reaches the threshold level of susceptibles when $\rho = s_0$.[93] An approximate solution of equations (2), (3), and (4) is obtained by eliminating i and integrating, to give

$$s = s_0 e^{-z/\rho} \quad \text{(5)}$$

From (4) and (5) can be obtained a new differential equation for this difference caused by removals,

$$\frac{dz}{dt} = (n - z - s_0 e^{-z/\rho}) \quad \text{(6)}$$

Bailey[94] offers a solution to this equation on the assumption that s_0/ρ or $(z/\rho) - 1$ are small, as $\rho = s_0$. It must also be assumed that the exposure and contact process, whereby susceptibles become infective, is independent of the susceptible process or state s_0; $t \geqq 0$.

The first solution offered by Bailey to equation (6) is a standard mathematical procedure involving expansion of the exponential factor to give an approximation of z, with introduction of the hyperbolic secant to give the epidemic curve (Fig. 9.3)

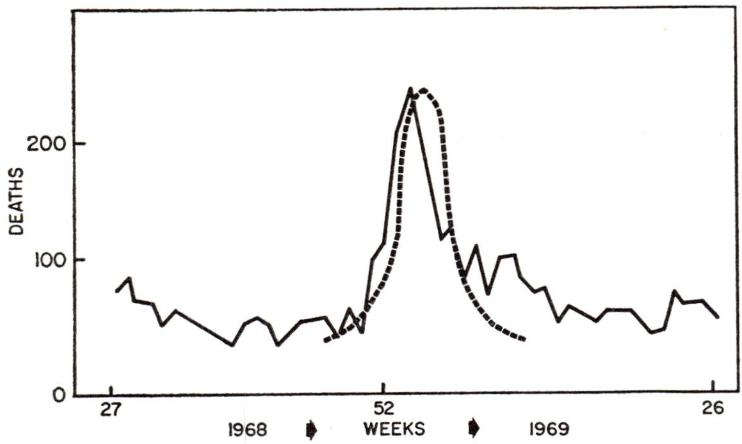

Figure 9.3. Deaths from pneumonia and influenza in New York City, 1968-69. The rise in December 1968 indicates the epidemic of Hong Kong (A_2) influenza and the actual epidemic (continuous line) is compared with a mathematical model of an epidemic of similar intensity (interrupted line).

$$\frac{dz}{dt} = \frac{\gamma d^2 \rho^2}{z s_2} sech^2 \left(\tfrac{1}{2}\alpha\gamma t - \Phi\right) \ldots\ldots\ldots\ldots\ldots\ldots\ldots\ldots \quad (7)$$

where α and Φ are transformations of parameters within the expanded equation (6). This curve is symmetrically bell-shaped and approximates to outbreaks of infection spread explosively by face-to-face contact, like smallpox and influenza in populations with no immunity or low immunity. As can be seen from the equation, the shape of the curve, i.e. the rate of development and subsidence of the epidemic, are strongly governed by α, which expresses the proportion of susceptibles who become infective, and by ρ, the relative removal rate of infectives. These rates are influenced primarily by β, which is the effective contact rate between infectives and susceptibles. If the removal rate changes (v), so that $s_0 = \rho + v$, there will be a severe outbreak only if the population at risk is appreciably greater than the threshold population—a condition which is obviously met in the current cholera pandemic, in the influenza epidemics of 1957 and 1969, and in cyclical epidemics of measles in young children (Fig. 9.4).

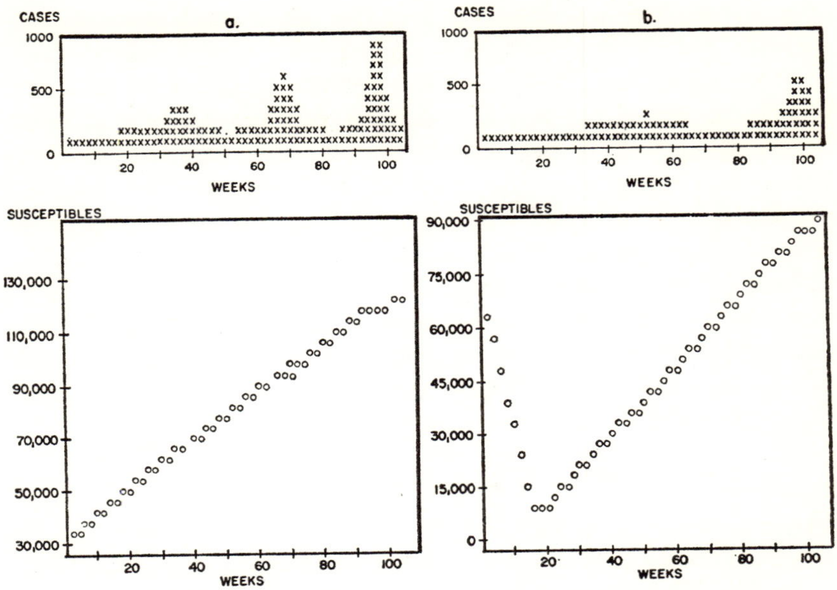

a. with high birth rate and linear increase in susceptibles. Three outbreaks in two years.

b. with low birth rate or immunized population. One epidemic in two years.

Figure 9.4. Mathematical model of an epidemic of measles. The data were printed by a Datel 30 computer from a program devised by Professor Walter Lynn, of the Center for Environmental Quality Management, Cornell University.

The ultimate size of such outbreaks, proceeding unchecked, is given by the equation

$$z\infty = \frac{\rho^2}{s_0}\left(\frac{s_0}{\rho} - 1 + \alpha\right) \dots\dots\dots\dots\dots\dots\dots\dots \quad (8)$$

which can be simplified to

$$z\infty \sim 2\rho\left(1 - \frac{\rho}{s_0}\right), \text{ if } \alpha = \frac{s_0}{\rho} - 1.$$

If the new value $s_0 = \rho + \nu$ is then substituted, $z\infty \sim 2\nu \left(\frac{\rho}{\rho+\nu}\right)$ and the total size of the epidemic is approximately 2ν. The number of susceptibles $\rho + \nu$ is thus reduced to $\rho - \nu$, which is the condition governing the termination of the outbreak, when the final number of susceptibles is as far below the threshold as the original number was above it and the curve tends toward symmetry.

The model described above has definite applications to a community in which the effective contact rate is relatively uniform over a given period. But it is in concept deterministic and may underestimate the infection rate, which tends to increase after the threshold is passed, and therefore the total size of the epidemic. The approximations introduced into equation (8) also lead to inaccurate predictions, though these can be overcome by more complicated mathematical methods described by Kendall[95] and Bailey.[94] Essentially, Bailey suggests that some of the inaccuracy can be overcome by shifting the mathematical origin to the center ("central epoch") of the outbreak to give a value

$$\frac{dz}{dt} = \gamma[i - z + \rho\,(1 - e^{-z/\rho})\,] \quad \ldots\ldots\ldots\ldots\ldots\ldots\ldots\ldots \quad (9)$$

where $-\infty < t < \infty$ is the interval containing an epidemic with an origin at the peak of a curve which is not necessarily symmetrical, as in (7). The intensity is now more realistically expressed as the proportion [α in equation (7)] of susceptibles who become infected and infectious in the given period.

Bailey's deterministic model, as described, provides a basis for calculating how an epidemic will develop from a small number of infectives if the total population exposed exceeds the relative rate of removal of infectives. It discounts intermediate variations in contact rate and removal rate. The number of susceptibles falls first to the threshold value when the number of new cases reaches a peak and then continues to fall more gradually. The model shows, also, how in the absence of any major change in total population the spread of an epidemic can be arrested simply if an adequate number of infectives are isolated during a period before the "central epoch" is reached. The governing condition of the model, the uniform contact rate, is applicable to certain diseases of high infectivity (e.g. smallpox, influenza, cholera) attacking closed communities; it is especially relevant to institutional infection and to a teenage population exposed to venereal disease.

If the community is large enough, intermediate variations in infection rate do not necessarily change the intensity of the epidemic,[37] but allowance must be made in smaller communities for such variation by using a stochastic model to provide differing possibilities of susceptible persons becoming infected.[95] To meet this condition, it is helpful to assume in the first instance that the total number of infectives and susceptibles does not change appreciably and to limit consideration to nonlethal infections in which infectives remain in contact with susceptibles, like persons with common colds circulating in households. The probability p of susceptibles becoming infected may follow a Poisson, geometric, or a binomial chain function, according to how the action variable (β) responsible for contact operates. In the basic model, given the probability that at any given time (t) a residue (r) of susceptibles remains uninfected, the chance of a new infection occurring over a period of time (dt) in a sample population (n) is $\beta r\ (n - r + 1)$ dt, i.e. the general probability is again a function of the number of susceptibles and infectives while the chance of a new infection is $\beta rsdt$ and of a removal, βsdt. The relative removal rate can be expressed in the same way as in the deterministic model, γ/β. If contact follows a binomial distribution, the probability of infection occurring is given by the general formula which is the binomial expansion of the $(q+p)^n$, viz.:

$$\binom{n}{r} p^r q^{n-r} = \frac{n\,(n-1)\ (n-2)\ \ldots.\ (n-r+1)}{r\,(r-1)\ (r-2)\ \ldots\ (2)\ (1)}\ p^2 q^{n-r} \qquad (10)$$

where $p + q = 1$ represent, respectively, the likelihood of a person remaining uninfected or becoming infected. At small values of n, the binomial distribution is skew but as n increases and p approaches 0.5, the distribution tends to become normal. If n is large and p is small—as in diseases of high infectivity—the Poisson distribution is appropriate,[96] thus

$$p\,(r) = \frac{np^r}{r!}\,e^{-np} \ \ldots\ldots\ldots\ldots\ldots\ldots \qquad (11)$$

where $r = 1, 2\ldots$ The distribution, even with a small n, is markedly skew.

Thus far, the reasoning and the mathematics are straightforward, but calculation of the generation of the epidemic involves more complicated mathematical treatment, for which the reader is referred to Bailey,[94] Karlin,[97] Daniels,[98] and others.[10,99,100] By constructing curves for varying populations and variable infection rates under stochastic conditions, it can be shown that when $n \leqq p$, the distributions are J-shaped and the epidemics subside quickly; whereas when $n > p$, the curves are U-shaped or bimodal. The average chance of one new infection in time t is $\beta rsdt$, which lies between the extreme possibilities $\beta nsdt$ and $\beta n (1-i) sdt$. Various other manipulations, employing chain-binomial and Poisson distributions, are necessary to allow for continuous infection. Classical models for this purpose have been devised by Reed and Frost,[101] Greenwood,[37,102] Lidwell and Somerville,[103] Whittle,[104] Markov,[105] Siskind,[106] and Becker.[107]

The studies of Bartlett[99] on measles and of Robson *et al.*[108] on bovine diarrhea deal with the mathematical problems caused by recurrence and periodicity. Of particular interest in relation to cholera, in which natural or artificial immunity is short-lived, is a model analagous to a reversible catalytic curve, first described by Muench.[109] If ϵ is the reversion rate of infective and post-infective immune persons to the susceptible state, then

$$\frac{di}{dt} = \beta (1-i) - \epsilon i \quad \ldots\ldots\ldots \quad (12)$$

Where i is, as before, the proportion of the population in an infectious state, solved as

$$i = \frac{\beta}{\beta+\epsilon} + ce^{-(\beta+\epsilon)t} \quad \ldots\ldots\ldots \quad (13)$$

in which c is a constant with different values at different points of time, different populations, and so forth. Plotting (13), we get a simple catalytic curve with movable asymptote indicating the interplay of the force of infection, producing immunity, and reversion to the susceptible state (Fig. 9.5).

MONITORING OF INFECTION: HOSPITAL INFECTION

Infections acquired in hospital are a major hazard to the safety and comfort of patients and to accomplishment of medical and surgical objectives.[110,111] Advances in medical science, in surgical techniques, in hospital design, in chemotherapy, and in general awareness of the problem have contributed toward great improvement during the past decade[112,113] but have been to a large extent

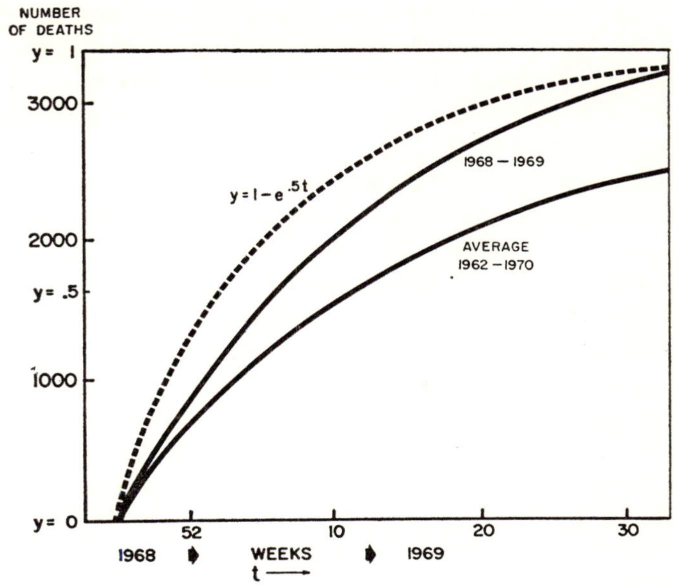

Figure 9.5. Cumulative mortality from penumonia and influenza, New York City, 1968-69 (Hong Kong influenza A_2) and 1962-70 (average). The corresponding catalytic curve is shown as an interrupted line.

neutralized by other factors[65,68-76,114]—mutant, drug-resistant and upstart bacteria, immunosuppressive therapy, shortage of trained staff—which often operate rapidly and cumulatively, creating serious clinical and economic problems before the danger is realized. Increasing use of dialysis, circulatory shunts, catheters, transplants, implants, inserts, grafts, and surgical prosthetic devices has created special catchment points in which resident or upstart organisms emerge as pathogens. Because the sources and pattern of infection are so variable, surveillance has to be flexible as well as prospective[115] to accommodate changes in local conditions.

Efficient monitoring requires a continuous flow of information[111-118] about all bacteria isolated from patients, appliances, and locations;[116] about all high-risk patients, whether or not infection has been reported in their vicinity; about use of immunosuppressive and chemotherapeutic drugs;[119] and about surgical and other therapeutic procedures.[68,110] Such information must be obtained regularly in the *absence* of known hospital infection but should be greatly increased should an infectious incident occur.

In practice, data are collected continuously in the following input categories:[68,111-113]

i—Computation of data from wards and clinical microbiology laboratory of pathogens isolated from patients, hospital personnel, equipment, dust, surfaces, and so on by location.

s—Enumeration of the patients at risk, proximity to an infectious case, surgery, immunosuppression, location, and so forth.

t—Duration of known or estimated contact between *i* and *s*.

r, z, n—From hospital census.

These frames of reference provide numerators (infected persons) and denominators (persons at risk) as follows:

1. *Sources of infection*—human and environmental (numerator *i*).

   Patients admitted with or acquiring infection.

   Carriers of latent infections: patients, visitors, hospital personnel.

   Utensils and materials: bedpans, handbasins, crockery, antiseptics[120] (e.g. *Pseudomonas*), dressings, soap, foods.

   Apparatus: inhalation tubes and catheters.

   Antibiotic-resistant, mutant, and upstart germs: *Staphylococci, Aerobacter-Klebsiella, Herrelea,* coliforms, yeasts, and so on, in any of the above categories (Table 9.2).

Microbiological information relating to *patients* and *carriers* forms the main numerator *i* in mathematical models. Information about other sources of infection is usually collateral or retrospective. It is especially important to "flag" and trace drug-resistant organisms, especially if high-risk patients are in the vicinity, as in surgical and medical intensive-care units. Microorganisms isolated from equipment and parenteral infusions should also be "flagged" in case similar material is being used elsewhere.

2. *Persons at risk* (denominators *n, r, s,* and *z*).

   Total number of patients in hospital.

   Number of patients in high-risk categories (see below).

Number of patients in infected locations (see below).
Number of removals and transfers.

3. *Risk factors in patients* (subsets of *s* and *r*).
   Therapy: immunosuppressive drugs, antibiotics, grafts, transplants, prostheses, major surgery, radiotherapy, infusions, catheters, shunts, dialyses.
   Concurrent disease: malignancy, debilitating conditions, immobility, paralysis, deformities.
   Prolonged stay in hospital.
4. *Environmental factors affecting contact* (β).
   Intensive care areas, burn wards.
   Areas with high patient intake or density.
   Contaminated materials: dressings, body fluids and discharges, garbage.
   Hospital design: ventilation, air conditioning, condition of walls and surfaces, passage of infected persons or materials through uninfected areas.

Computation is simplified and surveillance made more effective by in-progress evaluation of any changes in policy or hospital design,[112,113,121,123] and of the data generally. Thus, if a dangerous infection occurs in a high-risk area, patients in the high-risk category are excluded from that area; continuous monitoring of such interventions provides, in time, built-in standards. Even in the absence of overt cross-infection, the antibiotic sensitivity profiles of microbial isolates provides an indication of potential danger, as does a watch in the laboratory for transfer of R-factors between bacteria.[74,122]

A necessary feature of the plan outlined above is that surveillance must be continuous and *positive,* that is, the hospital must maintain a system and support trained personnel to look for infection even where none is apparent.[68] Reliability and regularity of input and effective retrieval of stored data are essential and are more important for the development of an effective system than elaborate programs for mechanized computation. Given these prerequisites, any one of several computerized or card-sorting programs can easily be applied to provide continuous information for detection, prevention, and control of infection.[68,111-113,117,123-128]

The value of an infection control program in a hospital, especially in a teaching hospital, is more than utilitarian. Any hospital is a microcosm full of factors and problems analogous to those which maintain infection or create epidemics in the larger world outside its walls.[129] Yet, within a hospital, all the main factors—intake and disposal of infectives, identification of susceptibles, contact factors, administration, policy generally—are under continuous professional scrutiny and largely under medical control. If, in this setting, we cannot assess and control infection, we can be sure that the defect is in ourselves or our system. A control program in hospital therefore furnishes a challenge which, if effectively met, is a test of local efficiency and a continuous educational experience for professionals at all levels and students, and an invaluable data-based ecological exercise.

MONITORING OF INFECTION: THE GENERAL CASE

In concept, the models described above and curves constructed from them (Figs. 9.3-9.5) are useful for teaching epidemiology and disease control. In practice, they are useful only insofar as input of data and monitoring of events are organized for purposes of defining thresholds, predicting outbreaks, and providing strategic information for health programs and economic deployment of resources. Like the basic model (p. 377), the basic input of information is classified under four main headings, as follows:

1. *Infective source or subject (i).*
   - Clinical case or subclinically infectious person (s).
   - Human carrier (s).
   - Infectious animals, excreta, materials, water, and so forth.
2. *Susceptible person or persons(s).*
   - Subpopulations at risk: household, institution, defined subgroup, finite community.
   - Population at risk: city, nation, region.
3. *Factors contributing to contact (β).*
   - Face-to-face: crowding, coughing, touching, . . .

Intermediate: contaminated materials.
Environment: air flow, humidity, dust, . . .
Personal behavior and hygiene.
Community behavior and hygiene.
Vector (s) : presence and removal.[37]
Pattern of transmission: deterministic, random, random chain, others.[94,95,101,105]
Isolation.
Immunization.
Therapy.
Cure.

4. *Duration of contact (t).*
   Discrete.
   Continuous.
   Intermittent.
   Seasonal factors.

Information collected under these main headings will vary according to the infection under scrutiny and local circumstances. Such information can be used for projections, predictions, estimates of costs, and assessments of efficacy of intervention. Major epidemics like malaria, cholera (p. 347), venereal disease (p. 364), and influenza can be monitored to accumulate a "data bank" in computers programed to integrate past experience with current input for planning purposes (Figs. 9.4 and 9.5). Continued programmed surveillance on a systematic basis is especially appropriate in checking institutional infection and in laying a basis of information for chemoprophylactic and vaccine trials. But a system is good only insofar as it simplifies and facilitates procedure. Complex forms, survey protocols, code sheets which have to be decoded, and other standard paraphernelia cause irritation and inefficiency. Essential information can often be given in a few minutes by telephone, teletype, or check-list in the course of other routine duties.

In this regard, there is a gap between the moving front of biomedical information systems and the static rear guard of traditional practice.* The newer systems can accommodate and process multiple inputs of data in minutes or, at most, a few hours; in customary medical and public health practice, diseases are notified retrospectively on forms by mail, often incompletely, permissively, and long after the event, while contributory information on immunity, contacts, transmission, and other highly relevant matters is not recorded at all unless a special surveillance or regulation has been applied in which case elaborate protocols are usually required. In the light of what is available and is being done in banking, accountancy, newspapers, weather forecasting, aerospace flights, and political elections, medicine and public health seem to be struggling to keep themselves in the rear: it is by no means uncommon to find that a hospital which computes every charge on patients' bills by the hour cannot compute nosocomial infection, iatrogenic disease, or adverse drug reactions by the month, if at all, though adequate, appropriate procedures have been described and can be applied.[110-128] The same weaknesses are seen in the search for, notification of, and action concerning the presence of infectious disease or other hazards to health in communities at large: an aircrew and ground staff alike can be notified instantly of changes or forecasts affecting weather, airports, personnel, and numerous other features of their destinations; public health personnel are rarely so informed about relevant parameters unless they get the information for themselves or adopt, as emergencies, measures which should be routine.

The fact that exceptions exist in the international networks maintained for surveillance of influenza and a few disaster dis-

*It is now known that over 600 cases of septicemia due to *Enterobacter cloacae* and *erwinia* with at least 200 fatalities occurred in a number of hospitals in America between January and April of 1971. The organisms were present as contaminants in the sealed caps of supposedly-sterile dextrose-containing replacement solutions and were transmitted to patients by intravenous infusion. All the contaminated solutions came from one manufacturer, the contaminants having been introduced during the manufacturing process. The facts were apparent, epidemiologically, early in February and were confirmed microbiologically by March 2nd. More than a month passed before information was conveyed effectively to all users. During that time, the contaminated infusions were widely used and many new cases occurred. This incident, which is not exceptional, shows how the absence of defined channels for information and regulation can lead to disaster, even when the source and means of spread of an infection are recognized.

eases like cholera does not even begin to meet the need for rapid action at the local level, where infections develop and spread, and where information is often spread by its newsworthiness rather than its data content. In retaining some of the epidemics of the past, we seem therefore to have retained, also, obsolete practices and an unreadiness to apply either the simpler measures which past experiences have shown to be effective or to adopt the modern techniques of communication, which are virtues of our technology no less relevant to epidemic control than are vaccination and chemoprophylaxis.

REFERENCES

1. Burnet, M. *The Natural History of Infectious Disease,* 3rd ed. London and New York, Cambridge University, 1962.
2. Dubos, R. *Man Adapting.* New Haven and London, Yale, 1965.
3. Gordon, J.E. *Control of Communicable Diseases in Man,* 10th ed. New York, American Public Health Ass'n., 1965.
4. *International Sanitary Regulations,* 2nd annotated ed. Geneva, World Health Organization, 1961.
5. Expert Committee on Malaria. *Technical Report Series No. 272.* Geneva, World Health Organization, 1964.
6. Christ, W. (Ed.) *Aspects of Water Pollution Control.* Geneva, World Health Organization, 1962.
7. Parrish, H.J. *Antisera, Toxoids, Vaccines and Tuberculins in Prophylaxis and Treatment,* 6th ed. Baltimore, Williams & Wilkins, 1963.
8. Zhdanov, V.M. *The Role of Immunization in Communicable Disease Control.* Geneva, World Health Organization, 1961.
9. Felsenfeld, O. *The Epidemiology of Tropical Diseases.* Springfield, Thomas, 1966.
10. Macdonald, G. *The Epidemiology and Control of Malaria.* London, Oxford University Press, 1957.
11. Gabaldon, A. *Amer. J. Trop. Med., 18:*641, 1969.
12. Symposium on Malaria. *Bull. N.Y. Acad. Med., 45:*997, 1969.
13. Panel on Malaria (49th Annual Session of American College of Physicians). *Ann. Intern. Med., 70:*127, 1969.

13a. See also Black, R.H. *Manual of Epidemiology and Epidemiological Services in Malaria Programmes.* Geneva, World Health Organization, 1968; *Technical Report Series Nos. 38, 63, 205, 242, 272, 291, 357, 374, 396.* Geneva, World Health Organizations; Frederiksen, H. *Popul. Stud., 24:*111, 1970.

14. *Lancet, 1:*827, 1967.
15. *Lancet, 2:*195, 1969.

16. *W.H.O. Chronicle, 20:*262, 1966.
17. *New York Times,* Aug. 16, 1970.
18. *Morbidity and Mortality Weekly Report, 19:*349, 1970.
19. Pollitzer, R. *Cholera.* Geneva, World Health Organization, 1959.
20. *New York Times,* Sept. 8, 1970.
21. Hirschhorn, N., Chowdury, A.K.M., and Lindenbaum, J. *Lancet, 1:* 1230, 1969.
22. Forbes, G.I., Lockhart, J.D.F., Robertson, M.J., and Allan, W.G.L. *Bull. W.H.O., 39:*381, 1968.
23. Azurin, J.C., Kobari, K., Barna, D., Alvarez, M., Gomez, C.Z., Dixon, J.J., Nakano, E., Suphdo, R., and LaDesma, L. *Bull. W.H.O., 37:* 745, 1967.
24. Sinha, R. *Lancet, 1:*1162, 1967.
25. Sen, R., Sen, D.K., Chakrabarty, A.N., and Ghosh, A. *Lancet, 2:*1012, 1968.
26. Van de Linde, P.A.M., and Forbes, G.I. *Bull. W.H.O., 32:*515, 1965.
27. Joint ICMR-GWB Cholera Study Group, Calcutta. *Bull. W.H.O., 43:* 379, 1970.
28. *Newsweek,* Sept. 7, 1970.
29. Felsenfeld, O. *Bull. W.H.O., 34:*161, 1966.
30. Joint ICMR-GWB Cholera Study Group, Calcutta. *Bull. W.H.O., 43:* 389, 1970.
31. Cholera: Summary of recent abstracts. *Trop. Dis. Bull., 67:*1, 1970.
32. Kobari, K., Takakura, I., and Nakatomi, M. *Bull W.H.O., 43:*365, 1970.
33. Stewart, G.T. *Lancet, 1:*1077, 1968.
34. *W.H.O. Chronicle, 24:*301, 1970.
35. Expert Committee on Smallpox. *Technical Report Series No. 382.* Geneva, World Health Organization, 1964.
36. *Weekly Epid. Rec., 46,* No. 3, 1971. Geneva, World Health Organization.
37. Greenwood, M. *Epidemics and the Crowd Diseases.* London, Williams & Norgate, 1935.
38. Hare, R. *Pomp and Pestilence.* London, Victor Gollancz, 1954.
39. *W.H.O. Chronicle, 24:*311, 1970.
40. Harper, G.J. *J. Hyg. (Camb.), 59:*479, 1961.
41. Kempe, C.H. *Pediatrics, 26:*176, 1960.
42. Report from public health lab. serv. *Brit. Med. J., 1,* Jan. 9, 1971.
43. Muschel, L.H. *Bact. Rev., 30:*427, 1966.
44. Pettenkoffer, H.J., Stross, B., Humbold, W., and Vogel, F. *Nature, 193:* 445, 1962.
45. Downie, A.W., Meiklejohn, G., St. Vincent, L., Rao, R., Sundara Babu, B.V., and Kempe, C.H. *Bull. W.H.O., 33:*623, 1965.
46. Livingstone, F.B. *Hum. Biol., 32:*17, 1960.

47. Mourant, A.E. *Distribution of the Human Blood Groups*. Springfield, Thomas, 1954.
48. May, J.M. *Ecology of Human Disease*. New York, MD Publications, 1958.
49. Salzano, F.M. *The Ongoing Evolution of Latin American Populations*. Springfield, Thomas, 1971.
50. *Health News*. Albany, N.Y. State Dept. of Health, Jan. 1971.
51. Stewart, G.T. *The Penicillin Group of Drugs*. London and New York, Elsevier, 1965.
52. King, A. *Recent Advances in Venereology*. London, Churchill, 1964.
53. In Beeson, P., and McDermott, W. (Eds.) *Textbook on Medicine*. Philadelphia and London, Saunders, 1967 pp. 186 and 327.
54. *Syphilis: Modern Diagnosis and Management*. Washington, D.C., U.S. Public Health Service, 1960.
55. *A.M.A. News,* Feb. 1, 1971.
56. *New York Times,* July 13, 1970.
57. Nichol, C.S. *Brit. J. Vener. Dis., 40*:96, 1964.
58. *Amer. J. Public Health, 53*:1835, 1963.
59. *Today's V.D. Control Problem*. American Social Health Foundation, 1970.
60. V.D., the challenge to man: A report on research priorities. *Social Health Papers*. American Social Health Ass'n., 1969, Vol. 4.
61. Mackenzie-Pollock, J.S. *Brit. J. Vener. Dis., 46*:414, 1970.
62. Scrimshaw, N.S., Taylor, C.E., and Gordon, J.E. *Amer. J. Med. Sci., 237*: 367, 1959.
63. Scrimshaw, N.S., Behar, M., Gusman, M.A., and Gordon, J.E. *Arch. Environ. Health (Chicago), 18*:51, 1969.
64. Kilbourne, E.D. In Beeson, P., and McDermott, W. (Eds.) *Textbook of Medicine*. Philadelphia and London, Saunders, 1967, p. 37.
65. Kilbourne, E.D., and Smillie, W.G. *Human Ecology and Public Health,* 4th ed. London, Macmillan, 1969, Chaps. 3 and 10.
66. Berntsen, C.A., and McDermott, W. *New Eng. J. Med., 262*:637, 1960.
67. Kass, E.H. *J. Infect. Dis., 123*:110, 1971.
68. U.S. Public Health Service. *International Conference on Hospital Infection*. Atlanta, Nat'l. Comm. Dis. Center, Aug. 1970.
69. Finland, M. *J. Infect. Dis., 122*:419, 1970.
70. McDermott, W. *Amer. Rev. Resp. Dis., 102*:857, 1970.
71. Wilfert, J.N., Barrett, F.F., Ewing, W.H., Finland, M., and Kass, E.H. *Appl. Microbiol., 19*:345, 1970.
72. Denny, F.W., Clyde, W.A., and Glezen, W.P. *J. Infect. Dis., 123*:74, 1970.
73. Stewart, G.T. In Kagan, B.M., (Ed.) *Antimicrobial Therapy*. Philadelphia, Toronto, and London, Saunders, 1970.
74. Symposium on Epidemiology of Drug-resistant Infections, 1966. In

Stewart, G.T. (Ed.) *Antimicrobial Agents and Chemotherapy.* Washington, D.C., American Society for Microbiology, 1967, pp. 245-296.

75. Hayes, W. *The Genetics of Bacteria and their Viruses.* London, Blackwell, 1964.
76. Benner, E.J., and Kayser, F.H. *Lancet, 2:*741, 1968.
77. Plag, J.A., and Phelan, J.D. *Amer. J. Epidem., 92:*1, 1970.
78. Voors, A.W., and Stewart, G.T. *Amer. Rev. Resp. Dis., 97:*515, 1968.
78a. Voors, A.W., Stewart, G.T., Gutekunst, R.R., Moldow, C.F., and Jenkins, C.D. *Amer. Rev. Resp. Dis., 98:*801, 1968.
79. Stewart, G.T., Voors, A.W., Jenkins, C.D., Gutekunst, R.R., and Moldow, C.F. *Amer. J. Epidem., 89:*254, 1969.
80. Voors, A.W., Rytel, M.W., Jenkins, C.D., Pierce, W.E., and Stewart, G.T. *Amer. Rev. Resp. Dis., 99:*420, 1969.
81. Hinkle, L.E., Christenson, W.N., Kane, F.D., Ostfeld, A., Thetford, W.N., and Wollf, H.G. *Psychosom. Med., 20:*278, 1958.
82. Jackson, E.F. *Amer. Sociol. Rev., 27:*469, 1962.
82a. Holmes, T. In Roessler, R., and Greenfield, N. (Eds.) *Physiological Correlates of Psychological Disorders.* Madison, University of Wisconsin Press, 1962.
83. Wolff, H. *Stress and Disease.* Springfield, Thomas, 1953.
84. Holmes, T.H., Goodell, H., Wolf, S., and Wolff, H.G. *The Nose.* Springfield, Thomas, 1950.
85. Susser, M.W., and Watson, W. *Sociology in Medicine.* London, Oxford, 1962.
86. Rahe, R.H., Meyer, M., Smith, M., Kjaer, G., and Holmes, T.H. *J. Psychosom. Res., 8:*35, 1964.
87. Stewart, G.T., and Voors, A.W. *Amer. J. Epidem., 91:*273, 1970.
88. Cassel, J.C. In Paul, B.D. (Ed.) *Health, Culture and Community.* New York, Russel Sage Foundation, 1955.
89. Jenkins, C.D. *Amer. J. Sociol., 71:*417, 1966.
90. Densen, P. *Environ. Res., 1:*265, 1967.
91. Mechanic, D. *Medical Sociology.* New York, Free Press, 1968.
92. Cassel, E.J. In Kilbourne, E.D., and Smillie, W.G. (Eds.) *Human Ecology and Public Health.* London, Macmillan, 1969, Chap. 12.
93. Kermack, W.O., and McKendrick, A.G. *Proc. Roy. Soc. Med., 115:*700, 1927.
94. Bailey, N.T.J. *The Mathematical Theory of Epidemics.* London, Griffin, 1957.
95. Kendall, D.G. In *Proceedings of the Third Berkeley Symposium on Mathematical Statistics and Probability.* Berkeley, University of California, 1956, vol. 4, p. 149.
96. Snedecor, G.W., and Cochran, W.G. *Statistical Methods,* 6th ed. Ames, Iowa State University Press, 1967.

97. Karlin, S. *A First Course in Stochastic Processes.* New York, Academic, 1966.
98. Daniels, S.E. In *Proceedings of the Fifth Berkeley Symposium on Mathematical Statistics and Probability,* Berkeley, University of California, 1968. vol. 4, p. 281.
99. Bartlett, M.S. *J. Roy Statist. Soc., 120:*48, 1957.
100. Dietz, K. *J. Roy. Statist. Soc., 130:*502, 1968.
101. Abbey, H. *Hum. Biol., 24:*201, 1952.
102. Greenwood, M., *J. Roy. Statist. Soc., 109:*85, 1946.
103. Lidwell, O.M., and Somerville, T. *J. Hyg. (Camb.), 49:*365, 1951.
104. Whittle, P. *Biometrika, 42:*116, 1955.
105. Markov, A. In Smith, C.E.D. *Biomathematics.* New York, Harper, 1969.
106. Siskind, V. *Biometrika, 52:*613, 1965.
107. Becker, N.G. *Biometrika, 55:*1007, 1968.
108. Robson, D.S., Kahrs, R.F., and Baker, J.A. *J. Theor. Biol., 17:*47, 1967.
109. Muench, H. *Catalytic Models in Epidemiology.* Cambridge, Mass., Harvard University Press, 1959.
110. Altmeier, W.A. *Ann. Surg., 147:*770, 1958.
111. Greene, C.F. *Canad. Hosp., 47:*34, 1970.
112. Williams, R.E.O., and Shooter, R.A. *Infection in Hospitals: Epidemiology and Control.* Oxford, Blackwell Scientific Publications, 1963.
113. leRiche, W.H., Balcom, C.E., and van Belle, G. *The Control of Infections in Hospitals,* Springfield, Thomas, 1966.
114. Sherris, J.C., and Lancaster, J.L. *J. Chronic Dis., 15:*743, 1962.
115. Brachman, P. In *Institutionally Acquired Infections.* Atlanta, Nat'l. Comm. Dis. Center, 1963.
116. Bidwell, O.M., and Williams, R.E.O. *J. Hyg. (Camb.), 58:*449, 1960.
117. Hughes, W.H. *J. Hyg. (Camb.), 68:*379, 1970.
118. Sanders, C.V., Luby, J.P., Johanson, W.G., Barnett, J.A., and Sanford, J.P. *Ann Intern. Med., 73:*15, 1970.
119. Voors, A.W., and Stewart, G.T. *J. Hyg. (Camb.), 64:*507, 1968.
120. Lowbury, E.J.L. *Brit. J. Industr. Med., 8:*22, 1951.
121. Smylie, H.G., Davidson, A.I.G., MacDonald, A., and Smith, G. *Brit. Med. J., 1:*67, 1971.
122. Roe, E., Jones, R.J., and Lowbury, E.J.L. *Lancet, 1:*149, 1971.
123. Coe, R.M. (Ed.) *Planned Change in the Hospital.* New York, Praeger Special Studies in U.S. Economic and Social Development, 1970.
124. *British Hosp. J. and Social Service Review, 80:*1886, 1890, 1939, 1944, 1994, and 1999, 1970.
125. Kanz, E. *Gesundheitswesen u. Desinfektion, 62:*129, 1970.
126. Haefliger, E., and Elasser, V. (Eds.) *Krankenhausprobleme der Gegenwart.* Bern and Stuttgart, Huber, 1969, vol. 3.
127. Lewis, C.E., and Hussanein, K.M. *Med. Care, 7:*379, 1969.
128. Laurence, C.A., and Block, S.S. *Disinfection, Sterilization and Preservation.* Philadelphia, Lea and Febiger, 1968.
129. Top, F.H. *Arch. Environ. Health, 21:*678, 1970.

Chapter 10

THE EPIDEMIOLOGY OF THE PATTERNS OF CANCER

David Schottenfeld

In 1900, only 3.7 percent of the deaths recorded in the United States were attributed to cancer, whereas in 1967, the proportion had increased to 16.8 percent.* In 1969, 323,000 persons died from cancer in the United States, or approximately 31,000 more deaths than our total battle deaths in World War II and 5.4 times our fatal civilian casualties in 1969 due to auto accidents. Since 1937, cancer has been the second leading cause of death in white and black men and women in the United States. A projection of age-specific mortality rates to the estimated population expansion over the next thirty years has predicted 510,000 cancer deaths by the year 2000 (Fig. 10.1).[1,2]

In 1966, approximately 40 percent of all cancer deaths in men and 43 percent in women occurred between 35 and 64 years of age (Table 10.1). Within these three decades of life, the proportion of all deaths attributed to cancer was approximately one-third in women and one-fifth in men (Fig. 10.2). Total cancer mortality rates in women exceeded that in men only during the age interval 30 to 50 years (Fig. 10.3). In 1930, the age-adjusted cancer death rate per 100,000 population was 111.9; by 1969 it had increased to 127.9. For men, age-adjusted cancer mortality increased from 101.3 in 1930 to 150.2 in 1965; for women, cancer mortality decreased from 122.4 in 1930 to 109.9 in 1965.

Cancer mortality statistics have been derived from standard death certificates codified as to the one underlying disease leading directly to death. Prior to 1949, the cause of death was selected

*In 1900, 26 percent of the United States population was encompassed by the states with death certification; the proportional population increased to 51 percent in 1910, 81 percent in 1920, and 95 percent in 1930. Mortality statistics became available for the entire nation in 1933.

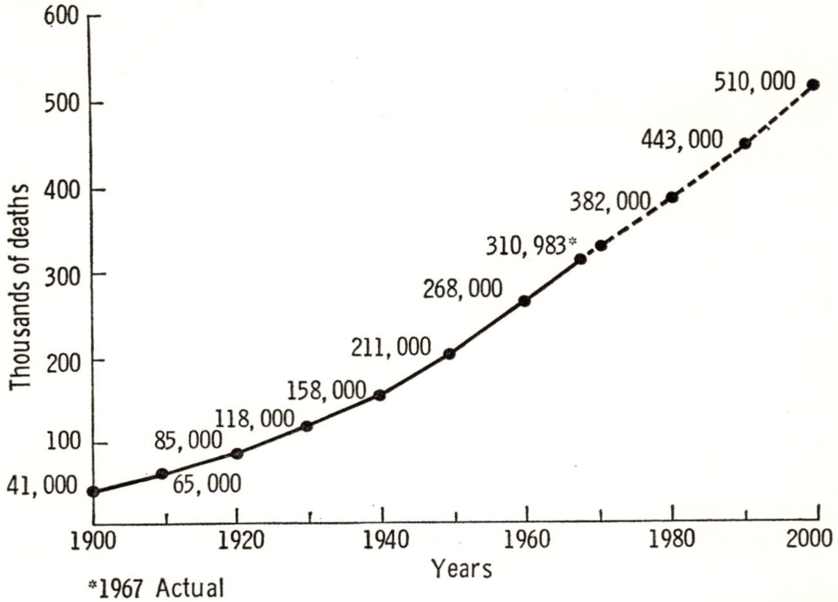

Figure 10.1 Forecast of cancer deaths, if present trends continue. Source: The American Cancer Society, Inc., Epidemiology and Statistics Department.

among an ordered listing of diseases embodied in the *Manual of Joint Causes of Death.* This ranking system was abandoned in 1949 and the underlying cause certified by the physician was subsequently codified. In a review of death certificates in 1955, the diagnosis of cancer was selected as the underlying rather than contributory cause in 93 percent of deaths and consequently, very little diagnostic information was excluded from the reports of the National Vital Statistics Division. In other diseases, however, the proportion of diagnoses assigned as the underlying cause varied considerably—coronary artery disease 75 percent, tuberculosis 69 percent, hepatic cirrhosis 66 percent, diabetes mellitus 41 percent, emphysema 31 percent, and so on.[3]

How reliable are the death certificates for interpreting cancer mortality trends for specific sites? The study in Saskatchewan of over 8000 death certificates by Barclay and Phillips[4] noted for all cancer sites an average overdiagnosis ratio of 11 percent and, after

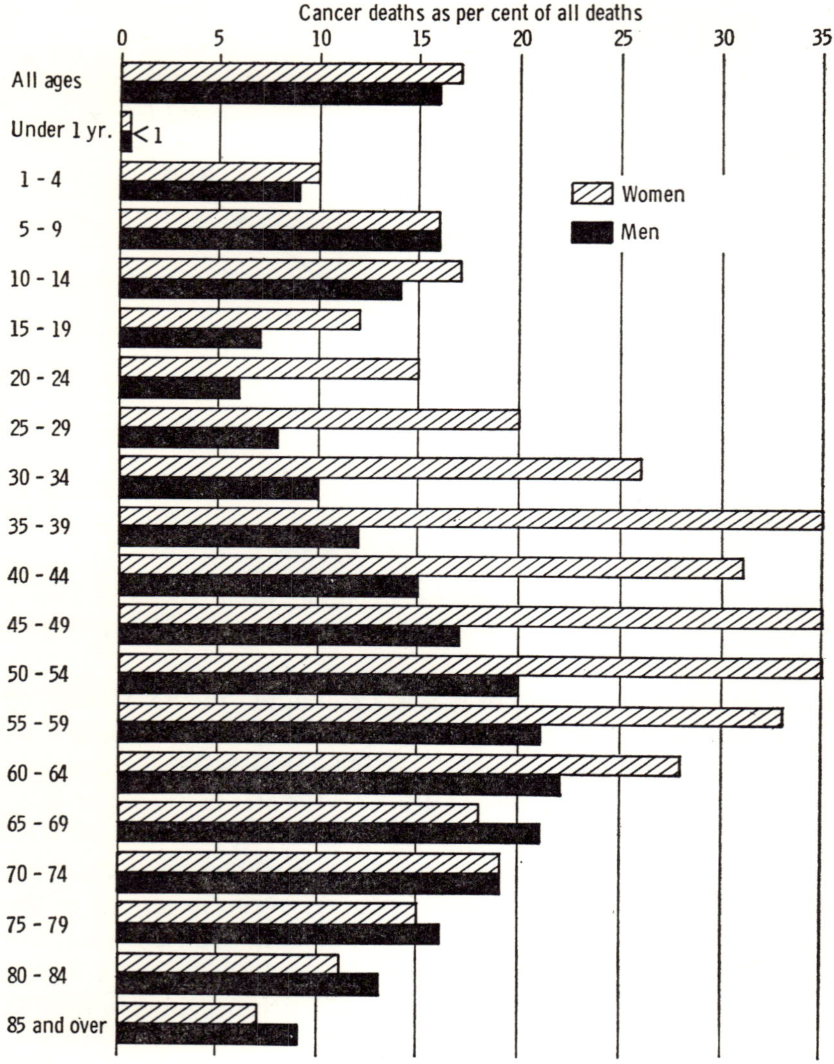

Figure 10.2. Cancer deaths in men and women as percent of all deaths by age, United States, 1966.

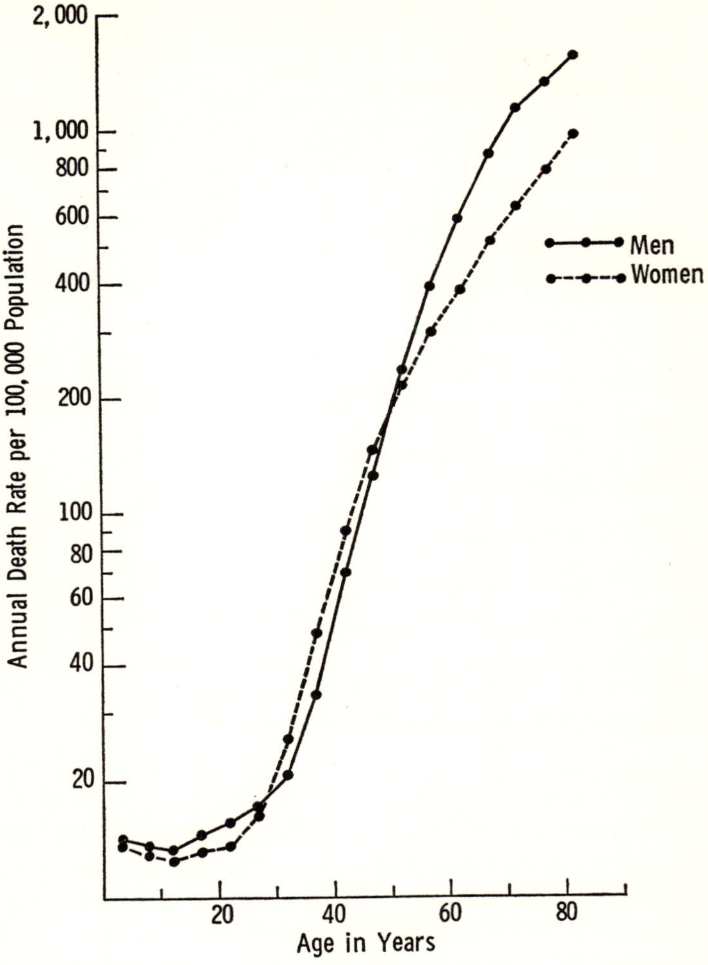

Figure 10.3. Annual cancer death rates per 100,000 population by age and sex, United States, 1966.

TABLE 10.1
NUMBER OF CANCER DEATHS AND CANCER DEATH RATES PER 100,000 POPULATION BY SEX AND AGE, UNITED STATES, 1966

	Both Sexes		Male		Female	
Age	Number	Rate	Number	Rate	Number	Rate
All Ages*	303,736	154.9	164,975	171.6	138,761	138.8
Under 5	1,547	7.8	827	8.2	720	7.4
5-9	1,432	6.9	826	7.8	606	5.9
10-14	1,155	5.9	673	6.8	482	5.0
15-19	1,366	7.7	820	9.2	546	6.2
20-24	1,262	9.3	754	11.3	508	7.3
25-29	1,529	13.3	796	14.1	733	12.5
30-34	2,563	23.6	1,145	21.5	1,418	25.6
35-39	4,994	42.3	2,104	36.2	2,890	48.2
40-44	9,728	78.2	4,163	68.6	5,565	87.3
45-49	15,841	136.1	7,109	125.6	8,732	146.0
50-54	24,313	227.4	12,363	237.9	11,950	217.4
55-59	31,953	342.4	17,594	391.5	14,359	296.7
60-64	38,249	482.2	22,469	597.6	15,780	378.0
65-69	43,196	676.7	25,275	869.8	17,921	515.6
70-74	44,444	855.5	25,698	1135.1	18,746	639.6
75-79	37,871	1025.8	21,221	1355.1	16,650	783.5
80-84	25,459	1226.3	13,318	1572.4	12,141	987.9
85 & Over	16,789	1500.4	7,793	1820.8	8,996	1301.1

Source of data: *Vital Statistics of the United States, 1966,* and the American Cancer Society, Inc., Epidemiology and Statistics Department.
*"All Ages" includes 45 deaths of unknown age, 27 male and 18 female.

excluding skin and lip cancers, an underdiagnosis ratio of 6 percent. The sites with a relatively high frequency of overdiagnosis, or where the certified cause of death could not be substantiated after a special review of all clinical records, included pancreas (23%), stomach (15%), large intestine (15%), lung (14%), urinary organs (12%), and prostate (12%). For each remaining site the ratio of overdiagnosis was less than 10 percent. A partial assessment of the frequency of underdiagnosis was possible by reviewing the death certificates for those persons treated in two large cancer clinics, where more than 90 percent of all cancer patients were treated. The analysis by site indicated that the ratio of underdiagnosis was 14 percent for prostate and 12 percent for breast. Excluding skin and lip, where the error factor was over 60 percent, the ratio of underdiagnosis was less than 10 percent for each remaining site.

In cooperation with the Pennsylvania State Department of Health, Moriyama *et al.*[5] validated the cause-of-death statements on a representative sample of more than 2000 death certificates. In 68 percent of 443 deaths attributed to cancer, the diagnostic information included microscopic examination of tissues. Among the deaths attributed to some malignant neoplasm, 15 percent were later characterized as "in doubt" or "probably wrong." The quality of supporting diagnostic information was least satisfactory for stomach and pancreas, and particularly good for urinary organs and lymphatic and hematopoietic tissues.

The most precise measure of risk of a disease within a population is incidence—the number of new cases diagnosed during a specified period of time. For those neoplastic diseases of brief duration between diagnosis and death and where rates of survival have not changed materially over the years—e.g. acute leukemia in adults, carcinomas of the lung, esophagus, stomach, pancreas, biliary passages and liver, and ovary, and so forth—rates of mortality are approximate indices of incidence.

Although cancer incidence statistics are not available for the United States, they are provided by central cancer registries comprised of cooperating hospital registries that are maintained in such states as Connecticut, California, upstate New York, and Iowa. By serving a defined geographic area, the central registry can describe disease frequency in the resident population at risk. Through the analysis of secular or temporal trends in the incidence of cancers of different anatomic sites and cell types, and the variations in frequency with respect to age, sex, race, social class, residence, and occupation, central cancer registries and national cancer morbidity surveys* provide important epidemiologic data

---

*The Third National Cancer Survey is now being conducted by the National Cancer Institute. During the survey period 1968-71, the records of over 200,000 new cancer cases will be analyzed. The geographic areas include the seven standard United States metropolitan statistical areas that were covered previously in 1937-38 and 1947-48. In addition, the population of Iowa, Colorado, and Puerto Rico are being surveyed.

for formulating causal hypotheses and facilitating the planning and evaluation of programs for cancer control.

CANCER AMONG INFANTS AND CHILDREN

In the United States in 1966, cancer in children between 1 and 4 years of age accounted for one-fourth as many deaths as accidents and approximated the mortality rates attributed to congenital malformations, influenza, and pneumonia; in children between 5 and 15 years of age, cancer was the second major cause of death, accounting for one-third as many deaths as accidents.[6] Between 1 and 15 years of age, the annual cancer mortality rate was 7.1 per 100,000. Under 5 years of age, the males exhibited an 11 percent relative excess in cancer mortality, 32 percent excess between 5 and 9 years, and 36 percent excess between 10 and 14 years. Between 15 and 19 years of age, the annual cancer mortality rate was 7.7 per 100,000 and the excess male-female cancer mortality ratio was 1.48 (Table 10.1). While carcinomas of the breast, lung, colon and rectum, stomach, pancreas, uterine cervix, ovary, and prostate bear most of the responsibility for mortality among adults, this is not true of infants and children. The majority of cancer deaths in this country in children were attributed to leukemia, tumors of the brain and central nervous system, lymphoma, neuroblastoma, Wilms's tumor of the kidney, and bone and soft tissue sarcomas (Fig. 10.4).

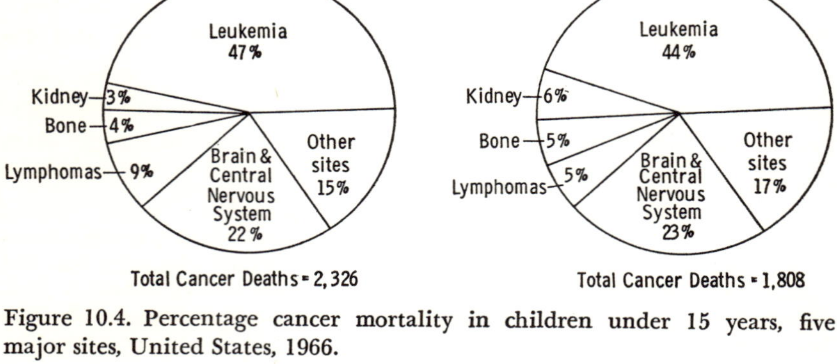

Figure 10.4. Percentage cancer mortality in children under 15 years, five major sites, United States, 1966.

Leukemia is the most common cancer in childhood. In white children in the United States during 1940-55, the prior rate of increase for total leukemia mortality began to diminish, and during 1955-60 the rates were stable. From 1961-65, there was a general decline in total leukemia mortality that was most pronounced among children 1 to 4 years of age. In black children, leukemia mortality since 1930, although increasing, was less than in white children, and since 1940 the relative rate of increase has diminished.[7-9]

In England and Wales, a comparably sustained decline occurred in younger children, 1 to 4 years of age, while in older children since 1955, leukemia mortality has been stable.[10] Since 1920 in England and Wales, and 1940 in the United States, acute lymphoblastic leukemia mortality rates peaked prominently at 3 to 4 years of age and then descended precipitously until about age 10 (Figs. 10.5 and 10.6). Slocumb and MacMahon[11] indicated

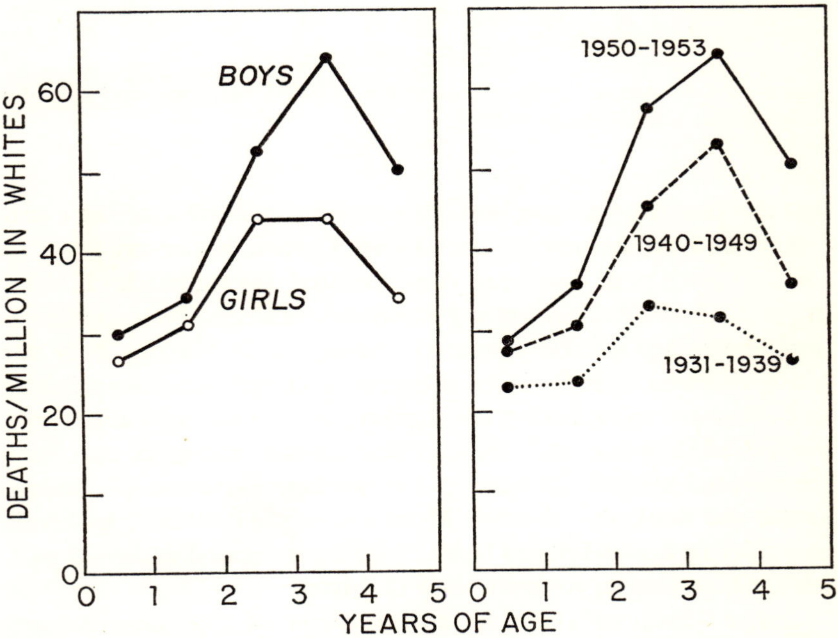

Figure 10.5. Mortality from leukemia in children under 5 years of age in England and Wales, 1931-53.

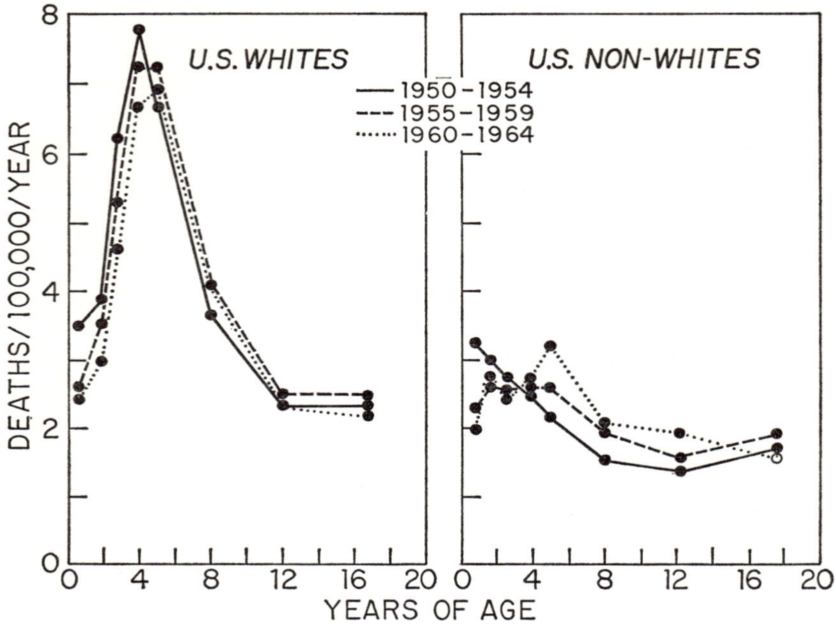

Figure 10.6. Childhood leukemia mortality rates by age, race, and calendar period in the United States, 1950-64.

that the peaking was due both to a decline in death rates at 1 and 2 years and an increase at ages 3 and 4 years. However, prior to 1960, no such peak had been demonstrated among black children in the United States or among Japanese children. This configuration of the age-specific mortality curve that is evident only for white children could reflect differences in genetic susceptibility and exposure to leukemogenic agents, or it could also arise from the availability and utilization of therapeutic measures that have contributed toward increasing the average duration of preleukemic and leukemic disease. More recently (1960-64), leukemia mortality in United States black children increased at ages 3 to 4, while decreasing in younger black children.

Since 1958, with the seventh revision of the International Classification of Diseases, the leukemia deaths have been codified by cell type. In the United States, the age distribution for the acute leukemias was bimodal, with a smaller peak during adolescence which was specific for acute myeloblastic leukemia, whereas the rates for chronic myeloid, lymphatic, and monocytic leukemias increased progressively after age 35 (Fig. 10.7). In the United States, Canada, Denmark, and England and Wales, chronic lymphatic leukemia was more prevalent than chronic myeloid leukemia; in Japan, Norway, and Sweden, the reverse was true.[12]

Whereas the sex mortality ratio for chronic myeloid leukemia was approximately 1.00, chronic lymphatic leukemia was associated in the various countries with the highest male-female leukemia mortality ratio (1.30-2.00). In contrast to chronic lymphatic leukemia, acute leukemia and chronic myeloid leukemia have been induced experimentally and associated epidemiologically with exposure generally in excess of 100 rads to therapeutic,[13,14] diagnostic,[15,16] and whole-body irradiation.[17,18] The decreasing likelihood of excessive exposure by the fetus or infant to irradiation has been offered as one explanation for the apparent decline or diminished rate of increase in leukemia mortality. The decreasing leukemia mortality evidenced by radiologists in the United States[19] and the United Kingdom[20] would be consistent with this hypothesis.

Epidemiologists have attempted to identify case clustering in leukemia. The rare demonstration, however, of low intensity but nonrandom clustering of leukemia cases has posed interpretive problems. A cluster or "microepidemic" is characterized by excessive aggregation of cases within a defined unit of space and/or time. In the epidemiology of acute communicable diseases, clustering may arise within a peculiarly susceptible population or within a normally susceptible population among whom there is an unusual degree of exposure or mode of communicability. The inability to detect human leukemia clusters with epidemiologic models that are, by contrast, sensitive to clustering in viral hepatitis and polio does not exclude the likelihood of a widely disseminated infectious etiologic agent in a highly resistant population. Our focus should then be on those events or predisposing conditions that alter the human host's immune system and the regulatory or repressive DNA-related functions. On the other hand, the demon-

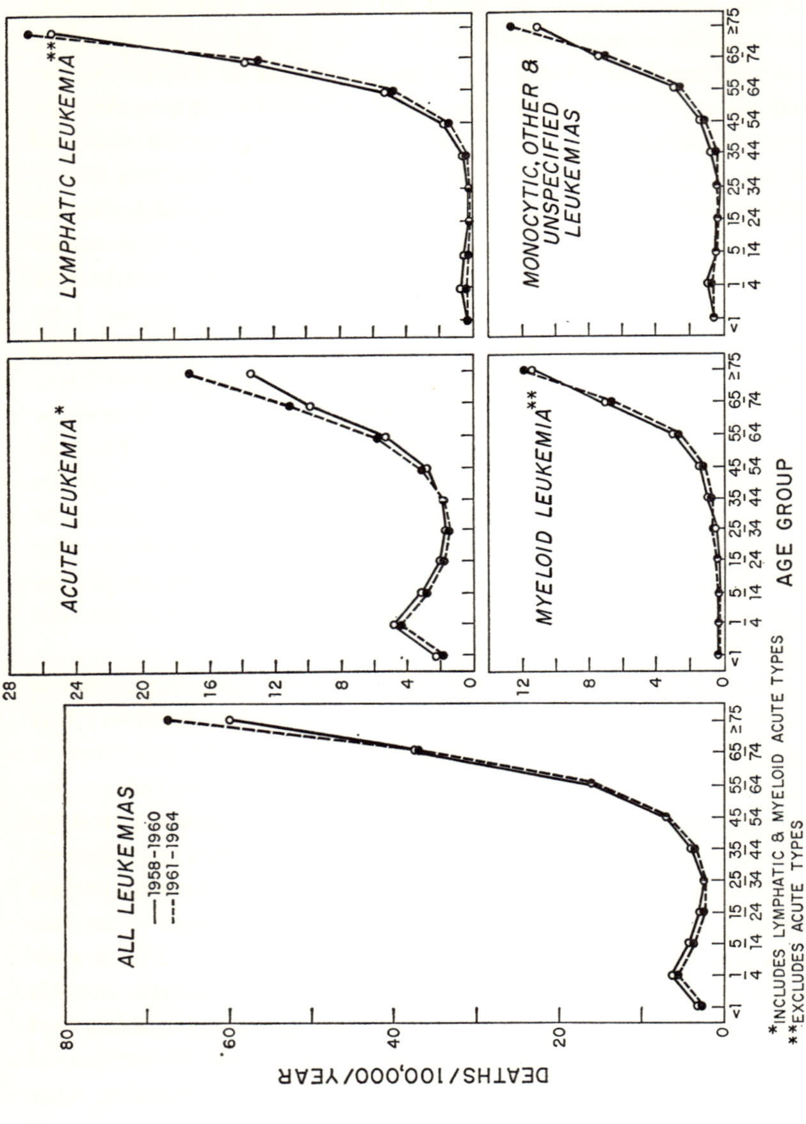

Figure 10.7. Leukemia mortality rates for United States white male population by cytologic type and age, 1958-60 and 1961-64.

stration of clustering, although consonant with a viral etiology, might occur also after a common exposure to radiation or other environmental leukemogens.[21-24]

There has been general agreement on the significant spatial-temporal clustering of children with Burkitt's lymphoma. The latter was recognized as a clinical entity by Denis Burkitt in 1958, and later classified as a malignant lymphoma characterized by a predominance of undifferentiated lymphoreticular cells. In well-defined areas of Central Africa, this malignant neoplasm accounted for 50 percent of all cancers in children. Burkitt[25,26] has recently summarized the salient epidemiologic relationships:

> (1) the distribution has not been restricted to specific racial or tribal groups; (2) the tumor is very rare in patients younger than one year; from the second year of life, the incidence rises progressively to a peak at age 6 and then declines precipitously to age 15; cases in persons older than 20 are uncommon; the distribution of cases tends to be at older ages in areas of lower incidence. There appears to be a higher incidence of adult cases among populations migrating from low incidence areas to endemic areas; (3) the disease occurs in a broad belt across equatorial Africa and in New Guinea and specifically in areas with a mean temperature over 60° F and with annual rainfall over 20 inches; (4) Dalldorf and his associates in Kenya have emphasized that the endemicity of Burkitt's lymphoma and malaria were highly correlated. This observation has given rise to the hypothesis that Burkitt's lymphoma is the result of a viral infection (i.e. Epstein-Barr virus and/or Reo virus, type 3) superimposed on a reticuloendothelial system which has been conditioned by chronic malaria.

Epidemiologic research has identified genetic syndromes, usually associated with chromosomal aneuploidy and fragility (i.e. Down's syndrome or mongolism, Bloom's syndrome, Fanconi's syndrome, and ataxia telangiectasia) that predispose to leukemia.[27] The risk of leukemia of various cell types in mongolism is increased at all ages and is at least twenty times greater than the rate for the general population. As is true for acute leukemia, the risk for mongolism increases with increasing maternal age. In approximately 90 to 95 percent of instances, Down's syndrome is characterized by trisomy 21. Observations from chromosomal studies in other species have demonstrated that such trisomies develop as a result of nondisjunction occurring during the first or second meiotic division. The genetic defect in mongolism has caused other hematopoietic disturbances such as defective lobing of polymorphonuclear leukocytes, and in several instances at birth, a "leukemia-like" disorder. The latter leukemoid disorder is believed to result from transiently ineffective maturation of granulocytes. Another abnormality of chromosome 21, with shortening of the long arm (the Philadelphia or Ph^I chromosome), is found in most patients with chronic myelogenous leukemia.[28]

Of interest is the work of Miller and Todaro[29] with the transformation of human fibroblasts in tissue culture with the oncogenic virus, SV 40. The transformed cells have the cytopathogenic properties which are associated with tumor production in animal systems, and thus may provide an index of *in vivo* susceptibility to cancer. Through the use of this technique, the skin fibroblasts from individuals with mongolism and Fanconi's anemia displayed a greater tendency to *in vitro* transformation than did normal cell cultures. Thus both diseases, predisposing to leukemia and associated with chromosomal abnormalities, exhibited increased sensitivity to transformation by an oncogenic virus. Other congenital cytogenetic disorders considered predisposing to leukemia are being surveyed in this manner. Such information would be valuable in family studies of leukemia.

The role of genetic factors in the etiology of human leukemia has been considered in the studies of twins and familial aggregation. In the national survey of cancer deaths in children in the United States, Miller[30] reported on seven presumably identical twins who died of acute leukemia. All but one of the twin pairs died within eight months of each other. The concordance for leukemia in monozygous twins under 6 years of age, was estimated to be 1:6 (16.7%). In their study of 3472 children who died of leukemia, MacMahon and Levy[31] observed three instances in which twins died of leukemia. When combining their series with three other cooperative studies, they concluded that the concordance for leukemia in like-sex twins was 1:9 (11.1%). One limitation of twin studies, however, is that although the relative degree of genetic predisposition may be determined, there is little insight afforded into the pattern of transmission or into the gene (s) concerned and the mechanism of gene action or interaction in a disease process.

In the study by Miller,[30] acute leukemia mortality in nontwin sibs did not occur with significantly greater frequency, and the leukemia deaths, unlike those observed in identical twins, did not concentrate in the first six years of life or within months of each other. Other surveys have shown that the occurrence of chronic forms of leukemia in first-degree adult relatives was significantly greater than expected.[32] The reports of multiple cases of leukemia within a given family without a history of consanguinity have, however, neither excluded nor clarified the nature of any interaction between immunogenetic factors predisposing to leukemia and common exposure to one or more leukemogenic agents.

Of interest in the national survey of cancer deaths in children was the observed ninefold excess of brain tumors among nontwin sib pairs; similarly, there was a ninefold excess in the concurrence of neuroepithelial brain tumors (i.e. glioblastoma, astrocytoma, or medulloblastoma) with an osteogenic sarcoma or soft tissue sarcoma in the nontwin brother or sister.[30]

Brain, spinal cord, and peripheral neurogenic tumors aggregate in families with genetic syndromes such as von Recklinghausen's neurofibromatosis, tuberous sclerosis, von Hippel-Lindau's disease, and multiple nevoid basal cell carcinoma syndrome. Conceivably some instances of the familial aggregation of brain and musculoskeletal neoplasms represent the varying phenotypic expression of a hereditary syndrome.

Neuroblastoma, retinoblastoma, embryonal rhabdomyosarcoma, hepatoblastoma, nephroblastoma or Wilms' tumor of the kidney shared with leukemia the characteristic of a peak mortality prior to 5 years of age. A syndrome of congenital bilateral aniridia, hemihypertrophy, mental retardation, microcephaly, craniofacial malformations and anomalies of the genitourinary tract was described in children with Wilms' tumor. In those children with Wilms' tumor and aniridia, the mean age at diagnosis (1.8 years) was earlier than in those children with Wilms' tumor without apparent congenital anomalies (3.6 years). The genitourinary anomalies included renal hypoplasia, bifid renal pelvis or double renal artery, hypospadias, and bilateral cryptorchidism.[33,34] Hemihypertrophy and sibship aggregation have been described in children with hepatoblastoma or embryonal hepatoma, adrenocortical carcinoma, and neuroblastoma; the neoplasms have occurred in organs manifesting congenital visceromegaly.[35-38] The association of specific congenital anomalies with cancers of infancy and early childhood would indicate their genesis prior to birth.

Death rates in children with sarcomas of bone increase progressively with age and are maximal at 16 to 17 years in females and at 18 years in males. There is a close correlation of age-specific bone cancer incidence, in particular osteogenic sarcomas, with growth changes during adolescence. Maximal growth velocity occurs somewhat earlier in girls (12 years) than in boys (14 years), and precedes, by approximately four years, the peak in bone cancer mortality.[31] Osteogenic sarcoma develops most frequently in long bones at the sites of maximal growth. Children with osteogenic sarcoma were found to be significantly taller at the time of diagnosis than a hospital control group of children with nonosseous cancers.[40] By analogy, canine osteosarcomas affected selectively large-sized breeds of dogs; the risk of primary bone sarcoma in dogs weighing over eighty pounds was between 60 and 185 times the risk in dogs less than twenty pounds.[41]

Hodgkin's disease in the United States has a bimodal age-specific incidence and mortality curve, with the first peak occurring at 15 to 34 years and the second after age 50 years. The disease is relatively uncommon before 5 years of age. The second mode is more prominent and its configuration similar to that of the other malignant lymphomas. In the southern United States, the relative risk of dying from Hodgkin's disease for young adults is about half that in the rest of the country; for the older adults, there is no apparent difference.

Bimodality is also evident in Great Britain, Norway, France, Italy, and Switzerland; these countries have higher rates than the United States under 40 years of age and lower rates after that age, but resemble the United States in having a more prominent second mode. In Denmark and the Netherlands, the two modes are equally prominent; in Japan, age-specific mortality until age 40 is rare, but the resultant unimodal mortality curve in the older age group is comparable to the second mode observed in Denmark and the Netherlands.[42-44]

The sex ratio comparing incidence rates for Hodgkin's disease under 11 years of age indicates that 75 percent of cases occur in boys. After age 11, the increasing incidence rates in boys and girls tend to converge so that 54 percent of the cases between 15 and 34 years of age occur in men; subsequently the incidence rates comprising the second mode diverge so that 63 percent of the cases occur in men.[42] There appears to be a high relative frequency of Hodgkin's disease in children during the first decade of life in various countries of South America, Africa, and the Middle East; boys are disproportionately affected in areas having an increased frequency of childhood disease. It has been suggested that the disease in children under 15 years tends to be clinically more severe and histopathologically less favorable in the lower socioeconomic countries.[45] On the other hand, the risk of Hodgkin's disease in adult men and women of the highest socioeconomic class is significantly increased; in this respect Hodgkin's disease is similar to other lymphoid neoplasms, i.e. lymphosarcoma, reticulum cell sarcoma, chronic lymphatic leukemia, and multiple myeloma.

In correlating age and sex distribution with histopathologic classification, Smithers[46] noted that the prognostically more favorable nodular-sclerosing type of lesion occurred with relatively greater frequency in women and primarily within young adults. The bimodal distribution and the age-specific differences in incidence in men and women by socioeconomic class, regionally, country of birth, and histopathologic type have suggested that Hodgkin's disease is heterogeneous with respect to etiology and clinicopathologic behavior.

In Hodgkin's disease, the Reed-Sternberg cell is assumed to be the principal malignant element, although there is a proliferation of other mononuclear or reticuloendothelial cells and the lymphocytes are defective in mediating cell-dependent immune responses. Little is known about the histogenesis of the Reed-Sternberg cell or the precursor morphologic stages of Hodgkin's disease. The immune system undoubtedly functions to prevent or restrict the proliferation of neoplastic cells. In fact, congenital syndromes associated with immunologic deficiency have been identified, which are predisposing to malignant neoplasia of the lymphoid system.* The risk of primary lymphoma, especially reticulum cell sarcoma and to a lesser degree primary carcinoma in various organs, is enhanced in patients receiving immunosuppressive therapy following kidney transplantation; secondary cancers have been inadvertently transplanted to recipients on immunosuppressive therapy from donors with unsuspected tumors of the breast, bronchus, lung, kidney, thyroid, and larynx. In the viral induction of neoplasms of lymphoid tissue in animals, prior impairment of immunological competence by whole-body irradiation, thymectomy, antimetabolites such as azathioprine, and prednisone has significantly enhanced tumorigenesis. Depression of the immunosurveillance system, therefore, may be viewed as having primary and secondary pathogenic significance in neoplasia of the lymphoid system.[47-49]

CANCER AMONG ADULTS

Cancer of the Digestive System

In 1970, cancers of the digestive system will account for approximately 98,000 deaths, or 30 percent of cancer deaths in the United States. In 1968 in New York State, exclusive of New York City, newly reported cases of cancers of the digestive system accounted for 24 percent of all cancers (excluding skin cancers other than melanoma) in women and 29 percent in men. In 1965 in Connecticut, a similar ratio for incident cancers of the digestive system to all cancers (25% in women and 30% in men) was reported. When combining the statistics for men and women in the United States, cancers of the digestive system account for the larg-

*1. Wiskott-Aldrich syndrome characterized by sex-linked recessive inheritance, recurrent infections, chronic eczema, and thrombocytopenia.

2. Congenital sex-linked agammaglobulinemia of Bruton.

3. Ataxia telangiectasia of Louis-Bar, which is a chronic and progressive multisystem disease with autosomal recessive inheritance, recurrent infections, oculocutaneous telangiectasia, mental retardation, progressive ataxia, choreo-athetosis, and nystagmus.

est proportion of cancer deaths and incident cases (Figs. 10.8 and 10.9).

Currently about 5 percent of all cancer deaths at ages 35 and older are reported to be from cancer of the stomach (Figs. 10.8 and 10.9). Since 1950, the age-adjusted mortality for stomach

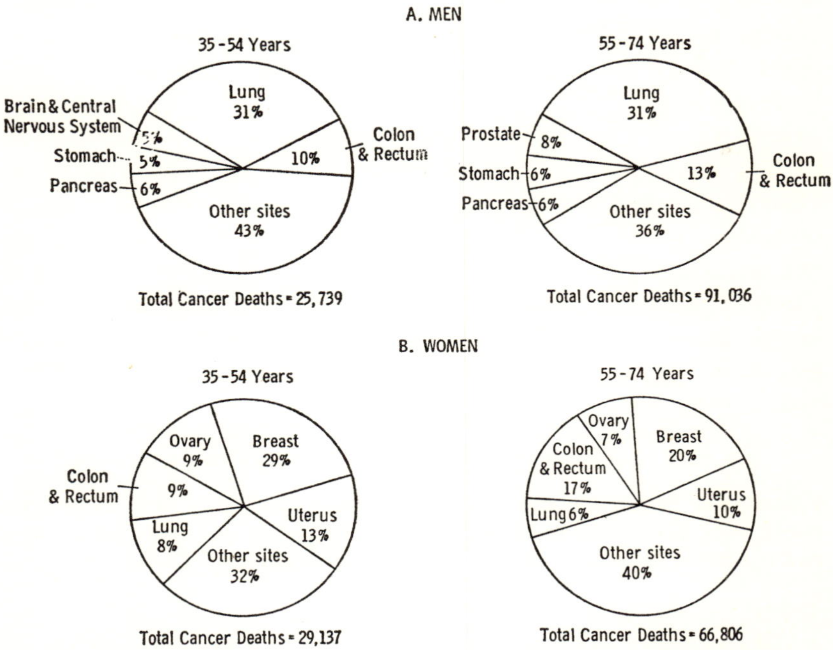

Figure 10.8. Percentage cancer mortality in adults, 35-54 and 55-74 years, five major sites, United States, 1966.

cancer in the United States diminished relatively over a fifteen-year period by 49 percent in women and 46 percent in men (Figs. 10.10 and 10.11); similarly, age-adjusted incidence diminished relatively by 42 to 44 precent in women and by 40 to 48 percent in men (Fig. 10.12). Among men, both white and black, the largest percentage decrease in incidence and mortality since 1950 occurred in the age group 55 to 64 years; in white women, the maximum reduction was exhibited at ages 55 to 74, while in black women at ages 45 to 54 years.

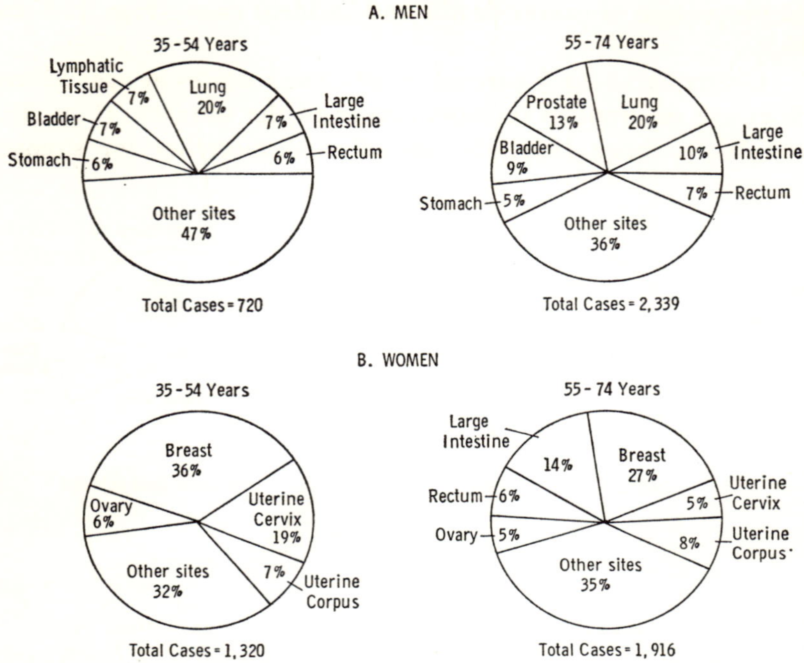

Figure 10.9. Percentage cancer incidence in adults, 35-54 and 55-74 years, major sites (including those with relative frequency of 5 percent or more and excluding cancers of the skin other than melanoma) Connecticut, 1965.

Mortality in this country has declined at a greater rate among those groups with lower initial rates, namely in women and native-born whites, and for men and women in successively younger generations. In industrialized countries, the incidence of cancer of the stomach, like that of the oral cavity, pharynx, and esophagus is generally highest in men and women of lowest social status.[50-53]

The study of patterns of cancer mortality by selected anatomic sites in migrant populations and their offspring, when compared with those existing in the countries of origin and destination, provides a unique opportunity to consider the etiologic role of changing environmental factors. In first-generation Japanese men and women (Issei) who have migrated to the United States,

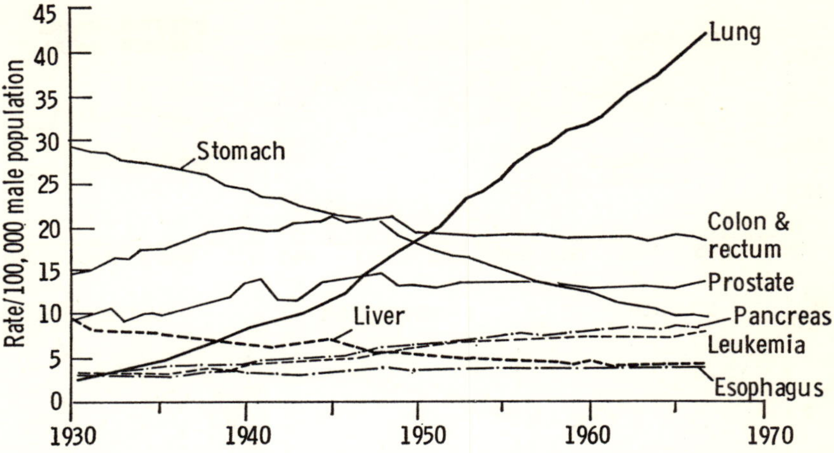

Figure 10.10. Male cancer death rates (standardized for age on the 1940 U.S. population) by site, United States, 1930-67.

stomach cancer mortality rates under age 75 years were considerably higher than in the United States white population but somewhat lower than those in Japan, which reported one of the highest rates for gastric cancer mortality in the world.[54] Among the male second-generation Japanese offspring (Nisei), age-specific stomach cancer mortality rates were lower than in the Issei. Therefore, for the older first-generation Japanese migrants, stomach cancer mortality related more to the country of origin than to the country of

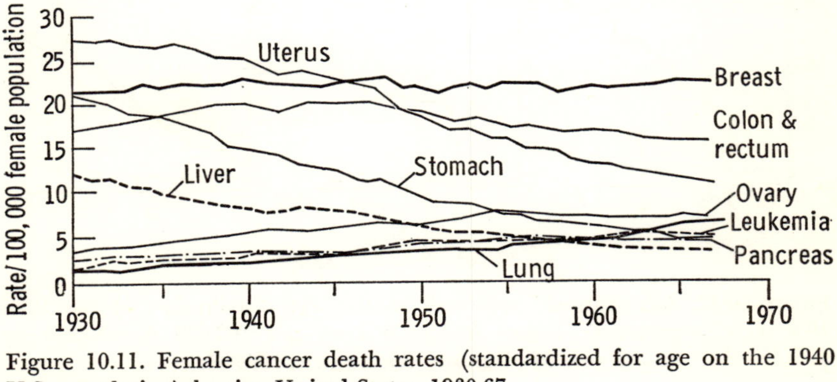

Figure 10.11. Female cancer death rates (standardized for age on the 1940 U.S. population) by site, United States, 1930-67.

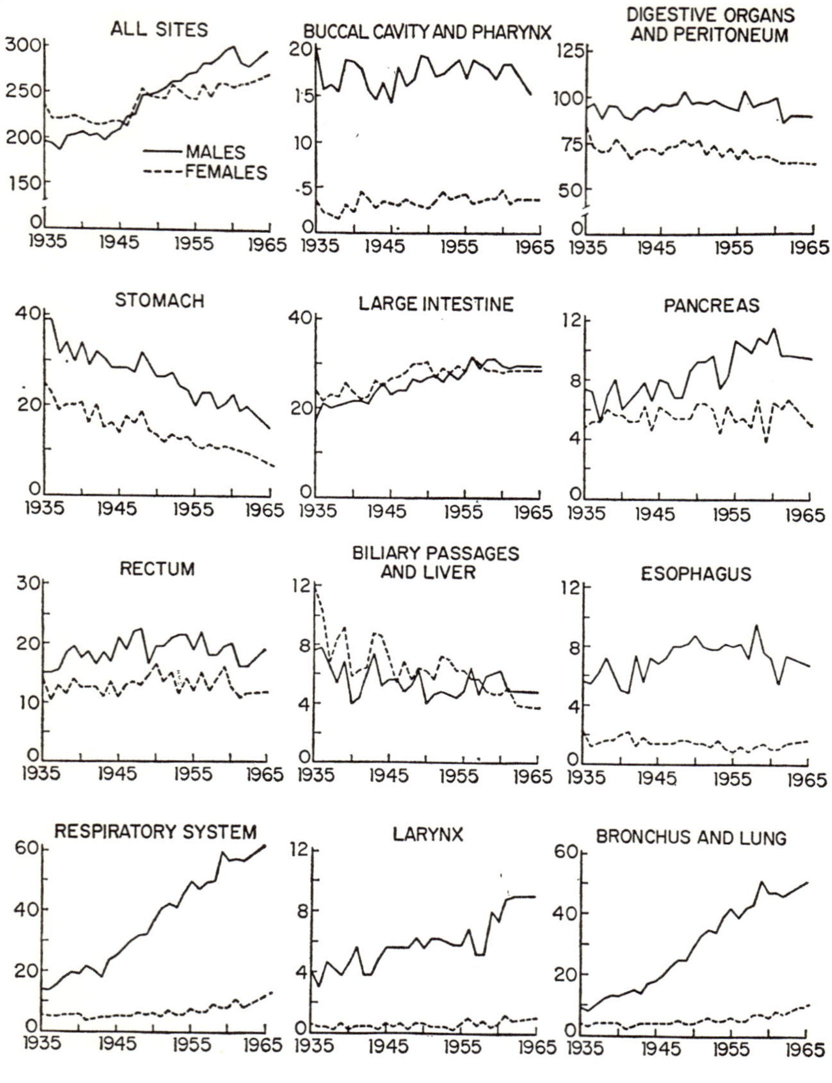

Figure 10.12. Age-adjusted (adjusted on the age distribution of the total 1950 U.S. population) cancer incidence rates per 100,000 population by primary site, sex and year of diagnosis, Connecticut 1935-65.

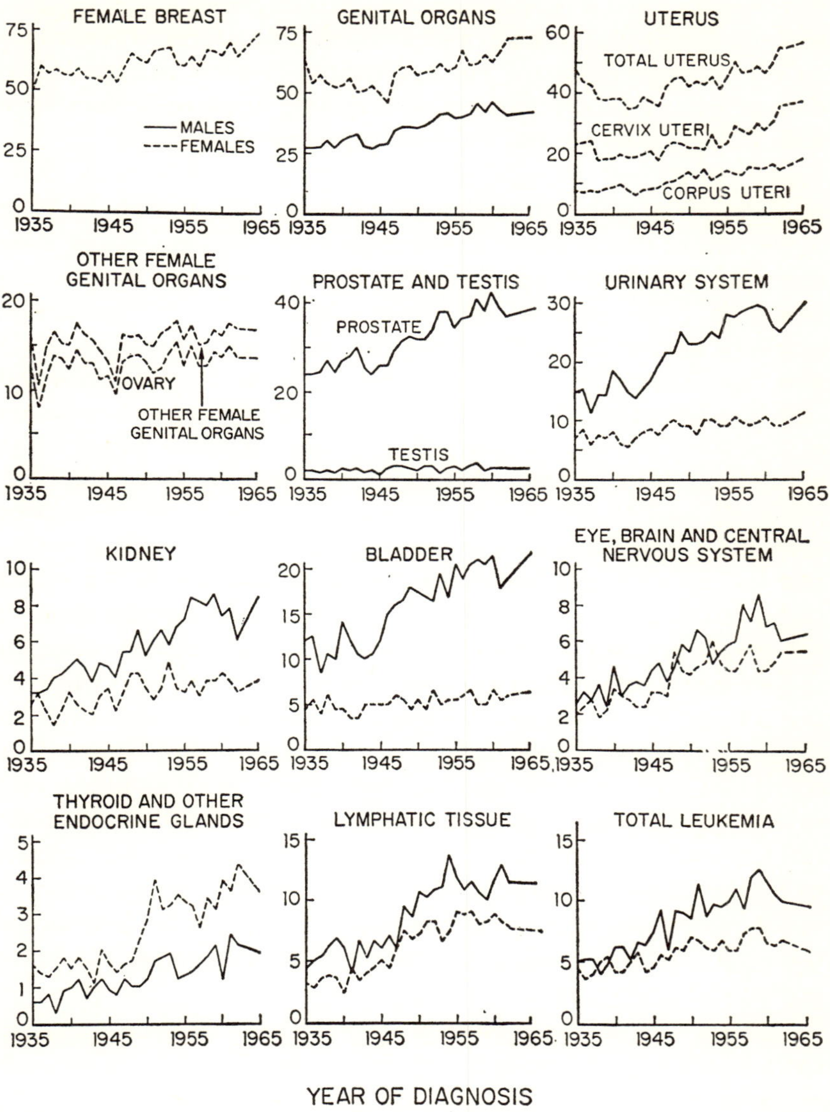

Figure 10.13. Age-adjusted (adjusted on the age distribution of the total 1950 U.S. population) cancer incidence rates per 100,000 population by primary site, sex, and year of diagnosis, Connecticut, 1935-65.

destination; this was also observed in migrants from Poland, Ireland, England, Norway, and Sweden. Long-term observations on the younger Nisei and their offspring (Sansei) are needed to determine any future pattern of declining age-specific incidence with changing social and cultural practices.

In the United States, England and Wales, and western European countries, stomach cancer mortality in women is about 50 to 67 percent of that in men. The average sex mortality ratio in these countries varied with age, however, beginning with 1.0 in young adults 25 to 29 years of age, rising regularly to the maximum excess in men of 2.2 at 55 to 59 years, and then decreasing to 1.5 after age 70 years.[55] The relationship between the sex ratios and ages was reflected similarly in countries where the secular trend of mortality has been diminishing sharply (United States white population, New Zealand, Australia), or declining more gradually (England and Wales, Scotland, western Europe), or remaining constant (Japan and eastern Europe). Flamant *et al.*[56] reported that the sex ratio was higher for cancers originating in the cardia or fundus of the stomach (3.0 to 5.0) when compared with those of the pyloric region (1.4 to 2.0); the sex ratios were intermediate for those cancers originating along the lesser or greater curvatures of the corpus of the stomach. In general, the highest sex ratios for cancers in the alimentary tract were observed for those sites highly correlated with tobacco and alcohol. These sites included oral cavity, supraglottic region or extrinsic larynx and esophagus* (middle one-third). The epidemiology of carcinoma of the cardia or fundus of the stomach should be distinguished from carcinoma of the more distal segment of the stomach and may be determined by some carcinogens that are common for cancers of the more proximal digestive tract.

Wynder *et al.*[57] suggested that nutritional factors operating early in life play a dominant role in the development of stomach

---

*The high correlation with tobacco and/or alcohol with cancers of these sites has been noted in the United States, England, France, Sweden, India, and Japan. However, in several geographic areas which reported very high incidence rates for cancer of the esophagus, such as Transkei in South Africa, the rates in Bantu men and women were nearly equal. Other etiologic factors that are suspect in this endemic area are carcinogens in the food (i.e. nitrosamines and aflatoxin).

cancer. The importance of early nutritional deficiency or exposure to dietary carcinogens leading to an irreversible sequence of histopathologic events is consistent with the relative persistence of gastric cancer risk within first-generation migrating cohorts. A common dietary profile in high-risk areas was one relatively high in carbohydrates and low in proteins, fats, fruits, and vegetables. In Iceland, where the incidence of stomach cancer is high, meat and fish were commonly preserved by smoking. Because of heavier and more prolonged exposure, home-smoked foods contained higher amounts of polycyclic hydrocarbons, including 3:4 benzpyrene, than commercially smoked foods.[58,59] Although the consumption of smoked foods might be of etiologic importance, other dietary practices and methods of preparation and cultivation of foods need to be totally evaluated and compared in populations with markedly divergent gastric cancer incidence. Dietary histories obtained retrospectively within a given region have not been sufficiently reliable or quantitatively meaningful.

Endogenous host factors—pernicious anemia, achlorhydria, atrophic gastritis, adenomatous polyps, gastric ulcer, intestinal metaplasia, familial aggregation, and blood group A—either are indicators of mucosal disease that may arise from common etiologic factors or inherently predispose to gastric carcinogenesis.[60-64] While pernicious anemia is significantly associated with benign adenomatous polyps and carcinoma of the stomach, it cannot account for the high rate of stomach cancer in Japan, since the condition is quite rare among the Japanese.[65-69] In Finland, Chile, and Japan, high mortality is reported for both gastric ulcer and carcinoma, but in western Europe and North America, there is no apparent correlation.[70,71] Japanese migrants have demonstrated diminishing mortality from gastric ulcer, even more substantially than for gastric cancer.[54] Migrant groups with high cancer risk also exhibit a high prevalence of intestinal metaplasia of the stomach, while those with low cancer risk have a low prevalence of metaplasia.[72,73] (In this context, intestinal metaplasia is the morphological and histochemical transformation of the epithelial elements of the stomach into elements resembling the epithelium of the small intestine. As is true for achlorhydria, the degree and frequency of intestinal metaplasia increase with age.)

It is estimated for the United States that in 1971 there will be 46,000 deaths from cancer of the colon and rectum, of which 35,700 (77.6%) deaths will be colonic and 10,300 (22.4%) rectal in origin.[74] As determined from the incidence rates of cancer recorded by the upper New York State registry (1957-59) in relation to age-specific mortality from all causes, the lifetime probability from birth of developing cancer of the colon and rectum is about 3.5 percent (1:30) in males and 4.0 percent (1:25) in females. In men 40 to 74 years of age, mortality from cancer of the colon and rectum is second only to lung cancer, and in older men it ranks only below that of prostate and lung. In women 55 to 74 years of age, mortality from cancer of the colon (excluding the rectum) is second only to breast cancer and is the leading cause of cancer mortality in women over 75 years.

Mortality from colon cancer (1965-67) in white men was slightly higher than in white women for the ages under 30 and over 60 years; the mortality for the age interval 30 to 59 years, however, was somewhat higher in the women. A similar relationship was noted for black men and women. As was true for carcinomas of the lung and stomach, the death rates for colon cancer increased exponentially with increasing age; the mortality in black men and women exceeded that in white men and women at all ages up to 70 years, after which they were lower than the constantly increasing mortality in the elderly white population.

The age-adjusted death rates for cancer of the colon (exclusive of the rectum) during the period 1930-45 increased 48 percent for white men and 22 percent for white women; since 1950, colon cancer mortality in white men has been stable, while for each age group in white women there has been a regular, slow decline in mortality. All age-specific colonic mortality rates in black men increased regularly from 1930-67; the age-adjusted mortality in black women exhibited a slow, regularly increasing trend since 1930, with the more apparent, sustained increases limited to the age groups 55 to 84 years.

The incidence rates for colon cancer are higher than for cancer of the rectum in all age groups in both men and women, and in most age groups the male colon cancer incidence rates are higher than the female rates. In both men and women, the highest proportion of cases of colon cancer are diagnosed in the age interval 60 to 74 years. In Connecticut, the age-adjusted incidence in men increased regularly from 1935-56 (17.5-31.5 per 100,000) but varied little in the subsequent ten-year period; the age-adjusted incidence in women was 30.3 in 1950 and 28.6 in 1965, but has been stable since 1958. In upper New York State, the age-adjusted incidence in men increased regularly from 18.0 per 100,000 in 1949-51 to 24.1 in 1967, while in women the age-adjusted incidence was 20.7 in 1949-51 and remained at this level through 1967 (21.2).

With the increasing use after 1950 of extirpative surgery for colon cancer, the relative survival rates increased; whereas the overall survival at five years for the period 1940-49 was reported by the End Results Evaluation Program* as 31 percent, this ratio increased to 42 percent in 1950-54 and 46 percent in 1955-59. The overall relative survival at ten years increased from 28 percent in 1940-49 to 39 percent in 1950-54. The survival in women was superior to that in men. For example, during the period 1955-59, the overall relative survival at five years in women was 49 percent as compared with 43 percent in men; for those women receiving surgery for localized tumors the five-year relative survival was 81 percent as compared with 76 percent for men. Since 1960, there has been some indication of further improvement in the three-year relative survival rate. The mortality trends over time will reflect both the patterns of incidence and the impact of treatment methods. For the white women, the stable incidence and improving survival resulted in the regularly declining age-adjusted mortality after 1950; in the white men, the stable mortality trend after 1950 resulted from the canceling of gains in survival by increases in incidence, particularly in men over 64 years of age. (Figs. 10.10, 10.11, and 10.12).

*The End Results Evaluation Program was an outgrowth of the Third National Cancer Conference in 1956 and was sponsored by the Cancer Chemotherapy National Service Center; the program is presently supported by the National Cancer Institute. The analyses of survival reflect the collaborative experiences of more than one hundred hospitals from various sections of this country and therefore, describe one fifth of all of our cancer patients. The cooperating hospitals and central registries were selected on the basis of their ability and willingness to participate. The extent to which they are representative of all hospitals treating cancer patients in the United States is not known.

The mortality rates for carcinoma of the rectum, like those for the colon, increase exponentially as the population at risk becomes older. The mortality rates (1965-67) in white men were higher in all age groups than those in women. In black men over age 49 years, the mortality from carcinoma of the rectum was consistently higher than that in black and white women; the mortality under age 70 years was higher in each sex for the black population, whereas the mortality in the elderly white population exceeded that in each sex for the elderly black population.[74]

For each age group in white men and women and in black men, mortality in the United States from cancer of the rectum, after increasing from 1940-49, decreased regularly from 1950-67. In black women, for the age interval 35 to 44 years, there was a consistent decline in mortality since 1940; for the age interval 45 to 64 years, the black women simulated the pattern in white men and women, but in black women 65 years and older, the mortality since 1950 has been stable.

In Connecticut, the age-adjusted incidence for cancer of the rectum in men was 19.6 per 100,000 in 1950 and 18.6 in 1965; the age-adjusted incidence rates between these points in time displayed only minor fluctuations. Prior to 1950, the age groups 35 to 54 and 75 to 84 years demonstrated regular increases in incidence; subsequently only the age group 75 to 84 years continued to manifest increasing incidence, whereas the other age-specific rates were either stable (55-74 years) or diminished (35-54 years). Similarly in women, where the age-adjusted incidence was 16.5 in 1950 and 11.8 per 100,000 in 1965, there were no consistent interval changes. Since 1950, the age-specific incidence rates in women have been stable for the age groups 45 and older; for the age group 35 to 44 years, the incidence declined from a peak in the late 1940's to its lowest point around 1957, after which the rates have been stable. In upper New York State, the age-adjusted incidence in men for cancer of the rectum was 14.2 in 1949-51 and 13.0 per 100,000 in 1967; in women the age-adjusted incidence diminished slowly from 9.7 in 1949-51 to 8.0 in 1967.

The survival trends for cancer of the rectum were similar to those for cancer of the colon; namely, that the major improvement occurred between 1940-49 and 1950-54. The declining mortality since 1950, therefore, occurred because of improving survival in the absence of major shifts in incidence (Figs. 10.10, 10.11, and 10.12).

While there were no important gradients in risk for colon and rectum cancer by social class or occupation, the incidence data from this country as well as from Denmark and Norway indicated a greater risk among urban residents, and particularly those residing in the more northern or industrialized regions.[75,76] Cancer of the large intestine is relatively rare in those countries with high frequency of gastric cancer. In the first-generation Japanese migrants to the United States, the mortality rates from colon cancer (excluding rectum) were more nearly those of the host country rather than the country of birth. The Japanese experience was consistent with that in other migrant populations, although quantitatively the first-generation migrants did not make the transition as completely as migrants from Norway and Poland.[54] The migrants from Poland and Norway exhibited a substantial rise for colon *and* rectum cancer.[77] The experience in the second-generation Japanese migrants suggested a further shift to the higher United States risk levels. In contrast to cancer of the colon, age-specific mortality rates from cancer of the rectum in native-born Japanese and the United States white population are comparable. The differences noted in Japanese migrants were limited to the remaining segments of the large intestine. The epidemiologic pattern of transition for colon cancer in migrants contrasts with that for gastric cancer, where the first-generation migrant population, particularly the older age groups, retain the risk level closer to the country of origin.

The mortality rates for colon cancer were approximately 30 percent higher in Jewish men and women than in non-Jewish white residents of New York City.[78] In a migrant study of Israeli Jews, the age-adjusted incidence of cancer of the colon and rectum in Jewish men born in Europe was 3 to 3.5 times that observed in male Jews born in Asia or Africa; the age-specific rates were more divergent with increasing age. A similar pattern was exhibited by the Jewish women born in Europe and the differences were demonstrated for colon as well as rectum cancer. The epidemiological pattern was interpreted as consistent with the higher incidence in more highly developed countries and the excess in urban versus rural frequency.[79]

The extremes of colon cancer incidence throughout the world differ by a ratio of approximately 8:1. The incidence is low throughout most of Africa, and the South African Bantu illustrates important differences with respect to the pattern of normal function and pathologic predisposition of the large intestine. The South African Bantu is characterized by minimal risk of carcinoma and adenomatous polyps of the large intestine. As is true for other low-risk populations, colon cancer in the Bantu tribe originates with significantly greater frequency in the cecum and ascending colon than in the sigmoid and rectosigmoid.* Associated non-neoplastic disorders of the large intestine such as ulcerative colitis, diverticulosis, appendicitis, and constipation are uncommon.[80,81]

The diet of the Bantu is distinguished by its high bulk, consisting mostly of starch in the form of a maize porridge, beans, and sour milk, and being relatively low in animal proteins and animal fat. Because of a positive correlation in the various industrialized countries of mortality due to atherosclerotic heart disease with colon cancer, a current etiologic consideration is the role of dietary fat in intestinal carcinogenesis.[82] The low residue, low natural fiber, and higher fat content of the Western diet would tend to inhibit spontaneous intestinal motility and prolong transit time. Intestinal physiology may serve to modify through physicochemical or biochemical means the action of ingested or enterically excreted carcinogens.

The intestinal microflora have been shown experimentally to influence metabolically the potency of various types of chemical carcinogens.[83,84] For example, the glucoside of cycasin when given orally to germ-free rats was excreted in the feces and urine almost entirely within forty-eight hours in its conjugated form and in a manner as if it were administered intravenously. When fed to conventional rats with indigenous intestinal microflora, only 18 to

*In countries at high risk, at least 60 to 65 percent of all cancers of the large intestine are within the view of the proctosigmoidoscope.

35 percent of the conjugated compound was recovered and in a number of instances, within a two-year period, adenocarcinomas appeared in the large intestine, kidney, liver (in association with diffuse centrilobular necrosis), and biliary passages. It was later shown that the cycasin glucoside had been hydrolyzed or deconjugated and converted to its aglycone, methylazoxymethanol. This product of cycasin hydrolysis was then demonstrated to be a potent carcinogen in germ-free animals.[85]

It has been postulated that intestinal bacteria produce carcinogens from bile steroids, dietary fats, or other ingested substrates, and that the geographic variations in colon cancer incidence reflect the interacting differences in diet and indigenous intestinal microflora.[86]

Cancer of the Lung and Bronchus

Lung cancer is the leading cause of cancer mortality in United States men between the ages 35 and 74; in women between the ages 35 and 54 it is the fourth leading cause of cancer mortality (breast > uterus > colon and rectum), while between the ages 55 and 74 years it is the fifth leading cause (breast > colon and rectum > uterus > ovary) (Fig. 10:8). Excluding basal and squamous carcinomas of the skin, which represent the most frequently reported cancers in men, carcinoma of the lung and bronchus is the leading incident site in men (Fig. 10.9).

In the United States, the age-adjusted death rate for cancer of the lung almost doubled between 1950 (11.1 per 100,000) and 1964 (20.7 per 100,000). In this fifteen-year period, deaths from lung cancer totaled approximately one-half million (467,442). The ratio of age-adjusted death rates in men compared to women increased regularly from 4.7 in 1950 to 6.8 in 1960; subsequently this ratio declined to 6.4 in 1964, reflecting the greater relative rise in mortality from lung cancer in women. The ratio of age-adjusted death rates in the white population compared to the nonwhite population indicated a 20 to 30 percent excess from 1950-54; the ratio then leveled off at 10 percent from 1955-58, and then remained at 1.0 after 1959, demonstrating the greater relative increase in lung cancer mortality in the nonwhite population during 1950-64.[87]

For each year of the period 1950-64, the lung cancer death rates in white and nonwhite men increased with increasing age from 25 to 74 years. However, lung cancer mortality (and incidence) increased almost exponentially throughout life as demonstrated in the various five-year cohorts (Fig. 10.14). The increasing steepness of succeeding curves indicated that lung cancer mortality rose more rapidly in each subsequently born cohort of men. A similar but less pronounced cohort displacement was evident for women. These patterns were also evident in England and Wales, Scotland, Denmark, Belgium, and the Netherlands.

Lung cancer incidence increases approximately in proportion to the fifth or sixth power of age, i.e. when age is doubled the incidence is increased about 32 to 64 times. The linear relationship that is derived when plotting lung cancer incidence on a probability scale against the logarithm of age has been interpreted as illustrating the effects of repeated exposure to one or more carcinogenic stimuli over a period of years, assuming that host susceptibility does not vary significantly with age.[88]

The incidence data reported from Connecticut and upper New York State reflected the secular trends observed for the mortality data. In Connecticut, the age-adjusted incidence in men increased from 28.5 per 100,000 in 1950 to 50.4 in 1965, and in women from 4.3 to 9.4 per 100,000. In upper New York State, age-adjusted incidence increased in men from 22.9 per 100,000 in 1949-51 to 41.9 in 1963-65; the corresponding data in women demonstrated an increase from 3.1 to 6.4 per 100,000.

In 1957, a study group[89] appointed by the National Cancer Institute examined the scientific evidence on the effects of cigarette smoking on health and concluded that cigarette smoking was a causative factor in the rapidly increasing incidence of human epidermoid and anaplastic small cell or oat cell carcinomas (Kreyberg Group I* tumors) of the lung. Later, in its 1964 report, the Advisory Committee to the Surgeon General[90] reported:

*The contribution of cigarette smoking to the development of Kreyberg Group I in man is significantly greater than to the development of adenocarcinoma and terminal bronchiolar carcinoma (Kreyberg Group II).

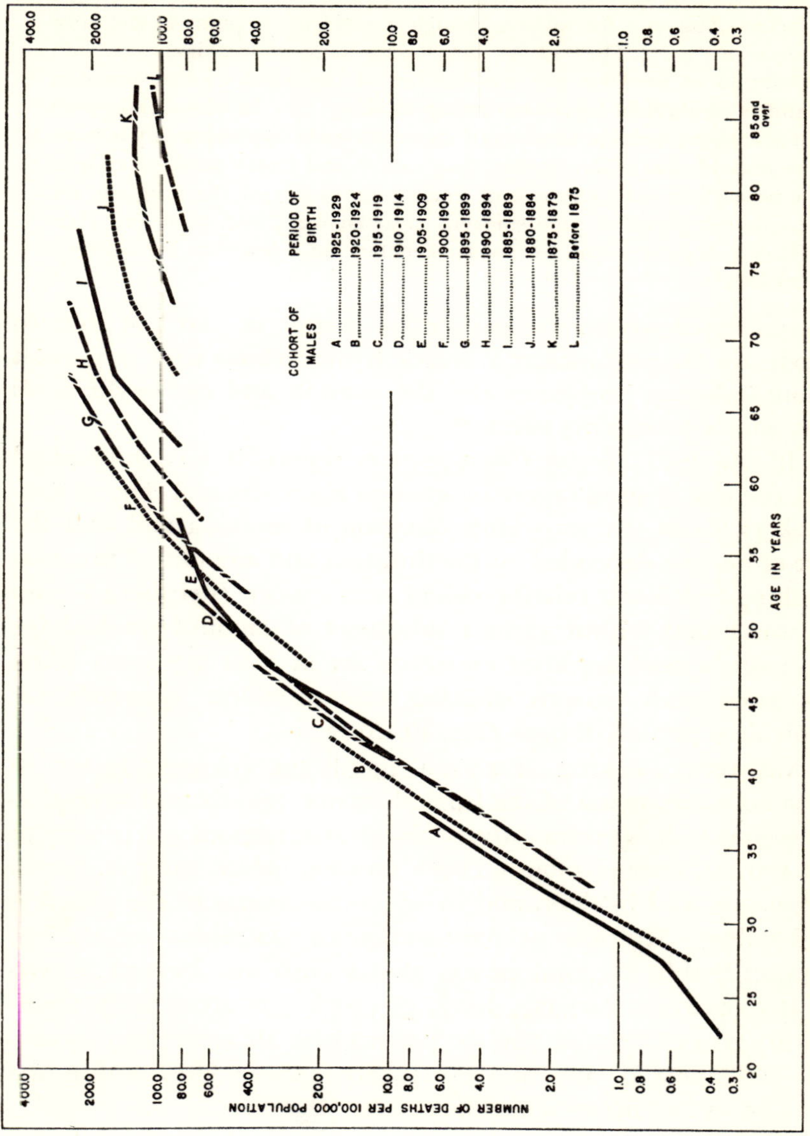

Figure 10.14. Cancer of the lung among men, by birth cohort and age at death: 1949, 1954, 1959, and 1964.[87]

> Cigarette smoking is causally related to lung cancer in men; the magnitude of the effect of cigarette smoking far outweighs all other factors. The data for women, though less extensive, point in the same direction. . . . The risk of developing lung cancer increases with duration of smoking and the number of cigarettes smoked per day, and is diminished by discontinuing smoking. . . . In comparison with nonsmokers, average smokers of cigarettes have approximately a nine- to tenfold risk of developing lung cancer and heavy smokers at least a twentyfold risk. The risk of developing cancer of the lung for the combined group of pipe smokers, cigar smokers, and pipe and cigar smokers is greater than for nonsmokers but much less than for cigarette smokers.

Concentrated within the particulate matter or "tar" of tobacco smoke are the polynuclear aromatic hydrocarbons with important tumor-inducing properties and the phenols and carboxylic acids with tumor-promoting effects.[91]

In the 1967 *Health Consequences* report, it was emphasized that the risk of lung cancer in smokers approximated that in nonsmokers about ten years after cessation of smoking and that the rate of decline depended on the duration and amount of previous smoking.[92] A lower relative risk of lung cancer (Kreyberg Group I) was found within various subclasses of amount smoked for individuals smoking filter cigarettes for at least ten years when compared with persons smoking only nonfilter cigarettes for equivalent periods of time (Fig. 10.15).[93]

Cigarette smoking is also a significant etiologic factor in squamous carcinoma of the lip and larynx (glottic and supraglottic regions); it is presumptively causal in squamous carcinomas of the tongue, floor of mouth, cheek mucosa, palate, gingiva, tonsil, esophagus, and bladder, and in adenocarcinomas of the pancreas and kidney. Multiple primary squamous carcinomas of the lip, subsites within the oral cavity, glottis (intrinsic larynx), supraglottis (extrinsic larynx), lung, or esophagus occur with significantly greater frequency in the patient with an antecedent squamous carcinoma of any of these tobacco-related sites within the respiratory and upper alimentary tracts.*[94]

*Cancers of the nasal cavity, paranasal sinuses, and nasopharynx do not share with these regional epithelial tissues in their enhanced risk for developing multiple primaries.

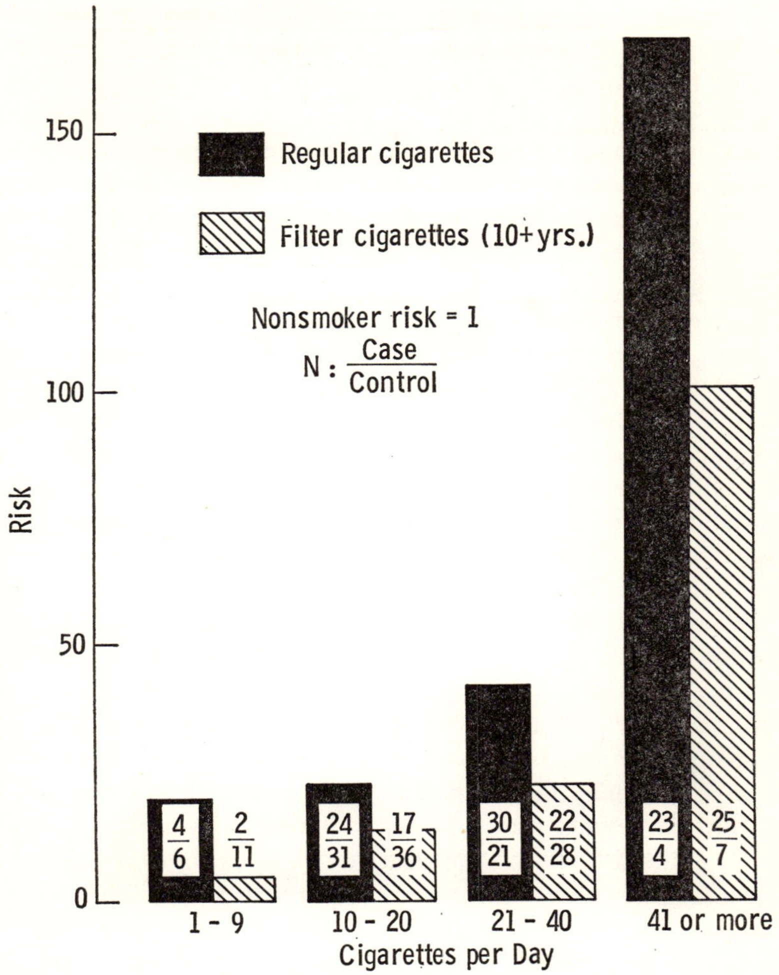

Figure 10.15. Lung cancer (Kreyberg I) risk in men by number and type of cigarettes smoked daily.[93]

The magnitude of the relative risk of incurring lung cancer among heavy cigarette smokers overshadows other risk factors such as urban residence,[95] air pollution,[96-99] decreasing socioeconomic class,[100] ionizing radiation,[101] occupational exposures,[102] and family history.[103]

The risk of developing lung cancer is apparently enhanced in men who are employed in uranium mines,[104,105] in the manufacture of hexavalent chromium compounds from chromite ore,[102] or are exposed to asbestos.[106-108] The induction in man of lung cancer by cumulative exposure to airborne ionizing radiation was suggested in studies of uranium miners. In the studies among uranium miners in the Colorado Plateau, Wagoner *et al.*[104] described excess mortality attributable to lung cancer. The principal radiation hazard was considered to be alpha radiation from the radon-daughter-decay products, isotopes of polonium, lead, and bismuth, which deposited on the bronchial epithelium. Working conditions in the mines probably contributed to excessive exposures. The inference of causality, after adjusting for cigarette consumption, was based upon a quantitative and site-specific relationship between increasing levels of exposure and the increasing incidence of lung cancer; in addition, with increasing radiation exposure, there was a higher relative frequency of small cell, anaplastic carcinomas.[104,105]

Asbestos miners and insulation- and textile-manufacturing asbestos workers are at increased risk of developing carcinoma of the lung and the relatively rare mesothelioma of the pleura and peritoneum.[106-108] Cancers of other sites—ovary, stomach, and colon—may be associated with exposure to asbestos, but the evidence is inconclusive. Selikoff *et al.*[107] noted that there was an extraordinary synergism between asbestos exposure and regular cigarette smoking in that the relative risk of dying from carcinoma of the lung was ninety-two times that in men who neither worked with asbestos nor smoked. In the absence of any smoking history, the risk of lung cancer in the asbestos worker was not excessive, suggesting a cocarcinogenic effect for the various asbestos fiber types. It has been suggested that the carcinogenicity of the asbestos silicate fibers may be related to associated hydrocarbon oils, iron complexes, or trace metal complexes rather than to the physicochemical properties inherent in the fibers. The occurrence of neoplasia does not correlate with the extent of pulmonary asbestosis. The interval from initial exposure to diagnosis generally exceeded twenty years.[108]

Tokuhata and Lilienfeld,[103] in evaluating the interaction of endogenous host factors and lifetime smoking history, noted that the factors of smoking and a positive family history of lung cancer were mutually reinforcing in increasing the familial aggregation of lung cancer as well as mortality from nonmalignant respiratory diseases. The familial aggregation of nonmalignant respiratory diseases suggested the possibility of an underlying host susceptibility to diseases of the bronchopulmonary system.

Breast Cancer in Women

Among the United States women 25 to 74 years of age, breast cancer is the leading cause of cancer mortality, and in women 40 to 44 years of age it is the leading cause of death. In 1966, of the 27,304 deaths in women due to breast cancer in the United States, 1.6 percent occurred in women under 35 and 41.5 percent occurred in women over age 64. For all United States women, the lifetime probability for developing breast cancer approaches 6 percent. Breast cancer mortality and incidence rates increase with age, but the rates of increase are greater during the reproductive years (Fig. 10.16). The data of Levin *et al.*[109] indicated that the increasing risk of incurring breast cancer during the menstrual years was 5 percent greater than during the postmenopausal years. Among all nonwhite women in the United States, 92 percent of whom are black, the mortality tends to be somewhat higher than in white women during the reproductive years and somewhat lower during later life. The age-specific mortality rates in nonwhite males exceed those of the white males in almost every age group (Fig. 10.16).

Apart from the 14 percent relative increase in mortality in women 45 to 54 years of age, the age-specific annual mortality rates from breast cancer in white women have been stable over the past thirty-five years in the United States. Stable rates of mortality over a period of time, however, may reflect the temporal balance between age-specific incidence and survival. Between the years 1935-39 and 1960-64, and presumably independent of major shifts in reporting practices and concepts, the incidence rates in Connecticut for breast cancer increased by about 45 percent

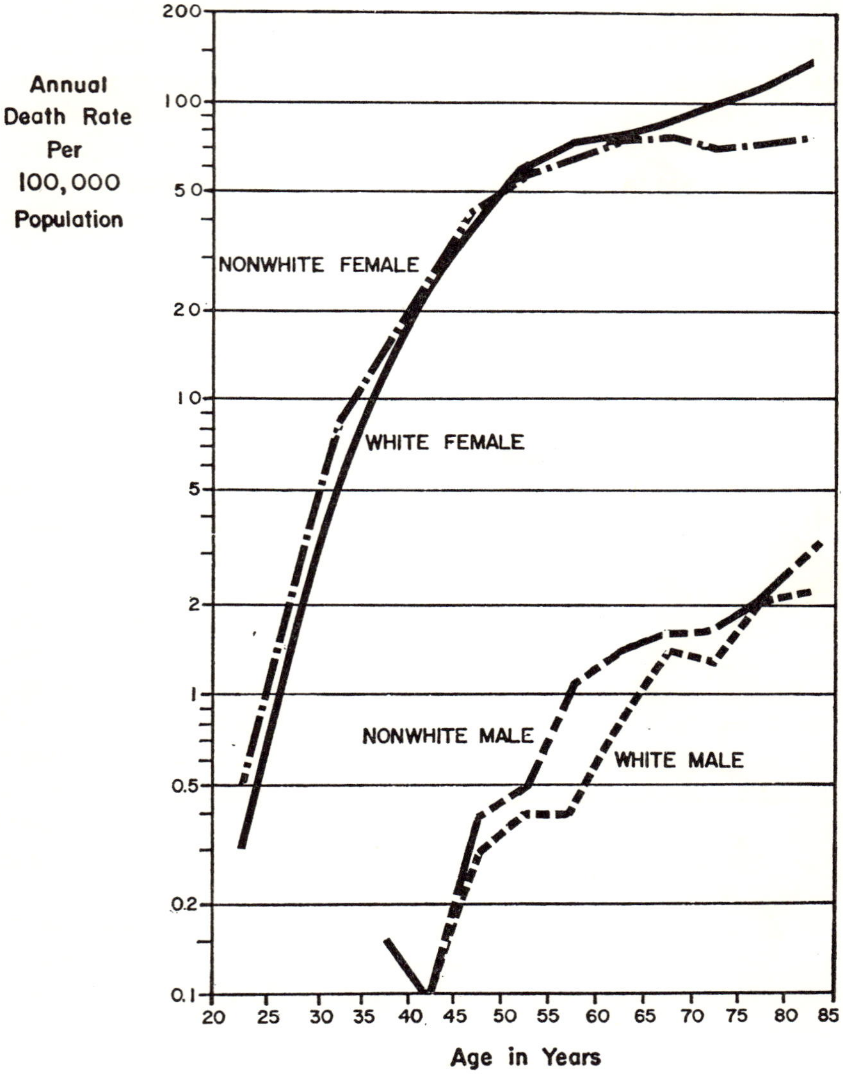

Figure 10.16. Breast cancer death rates by age, race, and sex, United States, 1964-66.

among women less than 55 years of age and did not change in older women.[110] The recent report of the End Results Evaluation Program indicated that there has been substantial improvement in the proportion of successfully treated breast cancer patients. When comparing those patients who were treated in 1940-49 with those in 1950-54, the overall ten-year survival rate, after adjusting for normal mortality expectation, increased subsequently from 39 percent to 47 percent; in patients with localized disease, survival increased from 66 percent to 72 percent and in patients with regional disease, from 28 percent to 33 percent.[111] If these data can be generalized, then the stable United States death rates over time have resulted from the canceling of gains in breast cancer survival by increases in incidence.

The age-specific incidence and mortality rates for breast cancer beyond 40 years of age are consistently higher in women who never marry.[112] In general, breast cancer patients marry and experience their first pregnancy at a later age and have fewer children. The risk of breast cancer in single women is about 40 percent higher than in women who marry but approximates the risk in married women who are never pregnant. The relative risk in married women who are first pregnant at age 30 or older is at least double that for women who are first pregnant under age 20. Women with four or more children are at about one-half the risk of nulliparous women.[113,114] Cohort life-table studies among Catholic nuns demonstrated excessive breast cancer mortality.[115]

Breast cancer patients tend to experience natural menopause at a later age and artificial menopause with lesser frequency.[116-118] As compared with the frequency in all white women, artificial menopause occurs 40 percent less frequently in single white women.[119] Women who undergo hysterectomy and bilateral oophorectomy before age 40 have one-quarter the risk of developing breast cancer. This beneficial effect is observed independently of parity. Surgical castration after age 40 and other surgical procedures that do not involve castration but permanently interrupt menstruation do not diminish significantly the risk of developing breast cancer.[120]

There has been considerable interest about whether prolonged nursing of each child or the total lactation experience influences the risk of breast cancer. In 1926, Lane-Claypon[121] reported that 15 percent of the children of breast cancer patients as compared with 7 percent of the children of controls had never been nursed. In their study with hospital patients and carefully matched controls, MacMahon and Feinleib[117] found no appreciable differences in lactation history. Levin *et al.*[109] indicated that the influence on relative risk of cumulative lactation was complex and that any protective effect became apparent only after thirty-six months. Shapiro *et al.,*[122] in their study of a population of women participating in the breast cancer screening program of the Health Insurance Plan of Greater New York, did not demonstrate any relationship with the aggregate number of months of breast feeding. In their international study, after adjusting for age, parity, and socioeconomic status (duration of schooling), MacMahon *et al.*[114] and Yuasa and MacMahon[123] were unable to demonstrate any protective effect of lactation.

Comparative population studies demonstrate that the age-adjusted mortality rates for adenocarcinomas of the breast and ovary are significantly and positively correlated.[124] When compared with women from the United States and Europe, Japanese women have substantially lower age-adjusted mortality rates for cancers of the breast, ovary, and endometrium and manifest age-specific differences that are increasingly divergent after the fifth decade.[125]

The age-standardized incidence data compiled by the Israel Cancer Registry (1960-64) indicated that the highest rates for breast and ovary were in Jews from middle and eastern Europe, when compared with immigrating Jews from Asia or Africa, native-born Jews, and non-Jews. With respect to epidermoid carcinomas of the uterine cervix, oral cavity, pharynx, and esophagus, that reflect epidemiological characteristics quite different from those observed in patients with adenocarcinoma of the breast, these neoplasms occurred with relative infrequency in the European Jews.[126]

In first-generation Japanese (Issei) who have migrated to the United States, Haenszel and Kurihara[54] did not observe significant increases in age-specific breast cancer mortality; among their second-generation offspring (Nisei), age-specific breast cancer mortality has persisted at significantly lower rates than those exhibited by United States white women. Assuming that the social and cultural practices of the second-generation Japanese offspring are reflecting to a greater degree those of their new host country, then the sustained resistance to breast cancer manifested by Japanese women in the United States would underscore the etiologic significance of genetic or endogenous factors. In this regard, Japanese men manifest a similar resistance to breast cancer mortality.[127,128]

The prevalence of breast cancer has been determined among the relatives of breast cancer patients and compared with general population statistics or the frequency among family members of index persons without breast cancer. Lilienfeld[112] reviewed the results of eight studies of the relative prevalence or mortality of breast cancer among mothers and sisters of breast cancer patients. In six studies there was at least a twofold excess of breast cancer among the mothers and/or sisters of breast cancer patients. Tokuhata[129] described the excessive prevalence of malignant and benign neoplasms of the breast in the daughters of white and nonwhite mothers with breast cancer. Macklin[130] noted that the excessive risk of breast cancer exhibited by close relatives of breast cancer patients was highest (at least threefold) in those who were never pregnant. The demonstration of the familial occurrence of breast cancer delineates an important subsegment of the population who should benefit from periodic screening.

Clinical studies[131] have described the apparently significant coexistence or prior occurrence of benign breast disease in patients with breast cancer. When compared with the age-specific incidence of breast cancer in the general population, women with benign cystic dysplasia have demonstrated 1.7 to 4.5 times the normal risk of developing breast cancer. Although Foote and Stewart[132] did not describe any specific type of benign breast lesion that was peculiarly "precancerous," more recent reviews[133] have given emphasis to the association of carcinoma with foci of cellular atypia with large duct or lobular hyperplasia or duct papillomatosis. The tendency of these benign proliferative lesions of the breast to be multicentric has been repeatedly emphasized. Although specific benign dysplastic lesions may be viewed as precancerous, the pathogenetic relationship may be an indirect one in that the same causal factors may be stimulating a spectrum of benign and malignant neoplasia.

In searching experimentally for endocrine factors in breast cancer, investigators have studied those hormones that regulate mammary growth and lactation and their relationship to the induction of tumors. The gonadal and adrenal steroid hormones, pituitary prolactin and somatotrophin, and thyroid hormone have been studied in various experimental models. Substantial exposure to ionizing radiation increases the risk of human breast cancer[134-138] and, at least experimentally, these radiation effects are potentiated by exogenous estrogens.[139]

Bulbrook *et al.*[140] indicated that in patients under 65 with metastatic breast cancer who excreted subnormal concentrations of etiocholanolone relative to 17-hydroxycorticosteroids, that their response to adrenalectomy or hypophysectomy was less than one-half that of patients with higher androgen ratios. However, the empirical application of these prognostic biochemical discriminants was sensitive to success in only 35 to 40 percent of patients and falsely negative in 16 percent. In those patients with negative discriminants or low androgen excretion who demonstrated recurrent disease in less than two years after mastectomy or were within six years postnatural menopause, the response rate to endocrine ablation was least favorable—only 5 percent.

In their prospective study of 4850 women 35 to 55 years of age, Bulbrook and Hayward[140] are attempting to identify the patterns of steroid excretion in women who later develop breast cancer. During the initial five and a half years of the study, 76 percent of the women who developed breast cancer excreted, either preceding or at the time of diagnosis, abnormal concentrations of 17-hydroxycorticosteroids and etiocholanolone. The aberrant excretion patterns were multidirectional, although generally the levels of etiocholanolone were subnormal. Urinary steroids were also measured in twelve ostensibly normal sisters of the women who developed breast cancer, and nine of these women had abnormal steroid patterns; two of these nine women later developed breast cancer.

Antecedent obesity and associated glucose intolerance enhance the relative risk of endometrial carcinoma. DeWaard[141,142] hypothesized that in Occidental countries of high breast cancer incidence, the adrenergic triad of obesity, diabetes, and hypertension was peculiar to breast cancer women who were postmenopausal. Obesity was viewed as a primary event leading to increased adrenal secretion of cortisol and estrogens. Dao *et al.*[143] postulated, based upon induction of mammary tumors in rats, that adipose tissue functioned as a storage depot for fat-soluble polynuclear hydrocarbons. Increasing the dietary fat in experimental animals potentiated the incidence of spontaneous and steroid-induced breast carcinomas.[144]

Assuming that ovarian hormones play an essential initiating and/or maintaining role in the natural history of human breast cancer, how may the apparently protective effects of early age at first pregnancy, number of pregnancies, or castration before age 40 be reconciled with the induction of a disease process extending over one or more decades? Cole and MacMahon[145] hypothesized that the relative concentration among at least three estrogen fractions—estrone, estradiol 17B, and estriol—was of paramount importance. Prior to any hormonal or ablative therapy and remote from any stressful procedure, the majority of breast cancer patients excrete subnormal concentrations of estriol relative to estrone and estradiol. During pregnancy and the luteal phase of the normal ovulatory cycle, estriol production is increased to a much greater degree than the other two estrogen fractions.[145,146] The stimulation by estradiol of cellular proliferation in the breast, uterus, and related target organs is related to ribonucleic acid synthesis and interaction with specific intracellular receptor molecules. Current experimental data would suggest that the estriols, with impaired tumor- or growth-promoting effects, compete with estradiol for these essential intracellular receptor sites.[147] Smith and Smith[148] broadened these considerations of estrogen fractions so as to assess their essential inhibitory or stimulatory effect on pituitary gonadotrophins and somatotrophin.

By identifying groups or individuals at increased risk of incurring breast cancer, the epidemiologist facilitates the selective application of optimal screening methods. With respect to cost-benefit considerations, the principle would be to concentrate the greatest proportion of potentially new cases in the smallest proportion of the total population at risk. By way of illustration, Dunn[149] has selected the variables age, marital status, and fertility. Among single women, we would expect to find 11 to 15 percent of the cases within 7 percent of the United States population of women 35 years of age and older. Among married infertile women, we would expect to find 10 to 20 percent of the cases among 16 percent of the United States population of women 35 years of age and older. By combining the subcategories of women who are single with those who are married with two or fewer children, we would expect to find 73 to 78 percent of the cases among 60 percent of the population. The same principle would apply to the screening of the sisters and daughters of a breast cancer patient, or patients with previous benign breast disease characterized by cellular atypia with ductal or lobular hyperplasia or papillomatosis. In our present ambiguous posture with respect to oral contraceptives, these same risk relationships should guide discriminatory use of estrogens and progestogens.

Epidermoid Carcinoma of the Uterine Cervix

It has been estimated for 1970 in the United States that there will be 9,400 deaths from cancer of the uterine cervix, which ranks only below breast cancer as a cause of cancer deaths in white women 35 to 54 years of age. Between 1950 and 1957, the age-adjusted incidence of invasive cancer of the uterine cervix declined relatively by 27 percent and the overall age-adjusted mortality by 50 percent. The diminishing trends for invasive cancer and total mortality began to level off after 1963. Concurrently, the age-adjusted incidence of *in situ* carcinoma increased almost tenfold and for all cancers of the uterine cervix by 50 percent. Because of the decreasing incidence of invasive cancer of the uterine cervix during the period 1950-57, the upper New York State registry estimated that 2600 deaths were averted (Table 10.2). The ad-

TABLE 10.2
AGE-ADJUSTED INCIDENCE AND MORTALITY RATES PER 100,000 WOMEN FOR CANCER OF THE UTERUS, NEW YORK STATE EXCLUSIVE OF NEW YORK CITY, 1950-67

	Incidence				Mortality	
	Cervix†					
Year	Total	Invasive	In Situ	Uterus except Cervix‡	Cervix†	Uterus except Cervix‡
1950	23.3	21.4	1.8	15.5	11.4	6.0
1955	22.4	17.3	5.1	15.8	9.2	4.6
1960	24.2	14.9	9.3	13.5	7.1	4.7
1963	29.9	14.6	15.3	13.3	6.3	4.2
1964	32.5	14.2	18.2	13.2	5.8	3.9
1965	32.9	15.7	17.3	14.5	6.5	4.1
1966	33.0	14.8	18.2	14.9	6.4	4.1
1967	35.2	15.7	19.5	15.7	5.7	4.0

Source: Cancer Control and Registry Report, New York State Department of Health.
*Age-adjusted to the total 1940 U.S. Population Census figures.
†ICD 7th, 1955 (171)
‡ICD 7th, 1955 (172-174)

vances in earlier diagnosis and diminishing mortality are due in part to the examination of cervicovaginal cytology in populations at risk; the leveling in the rate of decline in mortality in recent years is disturbing and suggests that subsegments at high risk in the population are not being reached.

In Connecticut, the relative increase in age-adjusted incidence for all cancers of the uterine cervix between 1950 and 1965 was about 40 percent. During these years the most significant increases with respect to age-specific incidence occurred under 35 years. The proportion of all registered patients with *in situ* disease increased from 16 percent (1950-54) to 50 percent (1960-62); currently in both Connecticut and Alameda County in California approximately two thirds of all registered carcinomas of the uterine cervix are diagnosed in the *in situ* stage.

With declining mortality and increasing incidence there was significant improvement in the management of patients reported by the End Results Evaluation Program. For all patients registered with carcinoma of the uterine cervix, the five-year relative survival rate increased from 45 percent (1940-49) to 60 percent in 1955-59. More than two-thirds of the patients were treated primarily with radiation and their relative survival at five years improved from 45 percent to 55 percent; in those irradiated patients with invasive carcinoma which was limited to the uterine cervix, the five-year relative survival improved from 60 percent (1940-49) to 73 percent (1955-59).

At all ages, the mortality rates in the United States were significantly higher in black women; for those age groups under 65 the magnitude of excess was approximately 2.6-fold, while in the older black women their mortality was at least double that in white women. The downward trend in age-adjusted mortality over the past twenty years has been 26 percent in black women, and uterine cancer has remained the leading cause of cancer mortality.[150]

The natural history of carcinoma of the uterine cervix evolves insidiously over a period of years. The earliest event that has been identified affects most commonly the squamous epithelium of the portio vaginalis (as distinguished from the columnar epithelium of the endocervical canal) and consists mainly of nuclear enlargement and hyperchromasia. This initial cytologic abnormality was described by Papanicolaou as "dyskaryosis" and corresponds histopathologically to the "dysplasias" of varying severity or the "borderline" lesions.[151] Depending on the severity, length of follow-up, and age- and race-related host factors, perhaps 18 to 50 percent of the incident cases of dysplasia will progress to carcinoma *in situ*.[152]

By means of periodic cytologic screening it has been possible to estimate the prevalence, incidence, and average duration of intraepithelial and preclinical squamous carcinoma of the uterine cervix. As determined by the initial screening examination, the age-specific prevalence of carcinoma *in situ* is bimodal, with a major peak between 30 and 44 years of age and a minor peak at age 60; the prevalence of preclinical invasive carcinoma becomes appreciable after age 30, increasing gradually until age 50 and then rising precipitously during the next decade until it reaches a peak at age 60. Kashgarian and Dunn[153] estimated that the average duration of carcinoma *in situ* was 10.7 years in white women and 8.5 years in black women. The average duration was longest in women 25 to 35 years of age (16 years) ; in women with a lesion developing at a younger age, the average duration was approximately ten years; while in women 40 to 49, it was approximately five years. The average duration of preclinical invasive carcinoma in white women was estimated to be five years, with little variation at different ages of onset. At each age level, the average duration of *in situ* and invasive carcinoma was shorter in black women.

The risk factors associated with carcinoma of the uterine cervix contrast with those described for breast cancer. Various indices of increased sexual and reproductive activity have been correlated with cancer of the uterine cervix (invasive and *in situ* carcinoma). The more significantly discriminating variables were early age at first coitus and at first pregnancy, and the total number of pregnancies. The inverse relationship with socioeconomic status was highly correlated with earlier sexual activity.[154-157] With adjustment for socioeconomic factors, Christopherson and Parker[158] demonstrated that the frequency of uterine cervical cancer was comparable in black and white women.

The low incidence of cervical cancer among Jews and Moslems stimulated the hypothesis that exposure to uncircumcised males was an important mechanism for transmitting the disease. Conceivably human smegma could be carcinogenic and its concentration on the glans or beneath the foreskin would be regulated by personal cleanliness; circumcision is an effective preventive measure against carcinoma of the penis. Experimental studies have demonstrated some carcinogenicity of human smegma when applied to the skin, vagina, or prepuce of mice.[159-161] However, epidemiologic studies of uterine cervix cancer in Israeli Jews, non-Jewish women in New York City,[162] an Amish population in Ohio,[163] women in East Africa,[164] and comparing Lebanese Christians and Moslems[165] have not confirmed a significant association with uncircumcised male partners. In other retrospective studies, there have been discrepancies in the statements by wives about the presence or extent of circumcision of their partners, and these errors have been of sufficient magnitude to obscure any association.

A significant association between antibodies to herpes virus hominis type 2 and invasive carcinoma of the cervix has been reported. Preliminary studies demonstrated antibodies to the virus in approximately 80 percent of patients as compared with a frequency of zero to 20 percent in other groups tested. The presence of viral infection with genital herpes (as distinguished from the nongenital herpes type 1) was positively correlated with low socioeconomic status and sexual promiscuity.[166-169] However, the proportion of patients with dysplasia or *in situ* carcinoma who had elevated titers was reported to vary between 32 and 100 percent. In a study in New Zealand there was no significant difference from normal controls in the occurrence of antibodies to type 2 herpes in patients with invasive or *in situ* carcinoma.[170]

The etiologic role of any infectious agent in uterine cervical cancer needs to be identified in population subgroups of varying risk and in relation to ethnicity, age, and socioeconomic status. Several models have been proposed to describe the sequence of events leading to invasive cancer. The initiating event would appear to be temporally related to age at first coitus. Exposure to a chemical and/or viral agent may generate a clone of mutant cells within the susceptible epithelium of the adolescent lower genital tract. As suggested by Barron and Richart,[157] invasive carcinoma of the uterine cervix is a multistage process requiring a succession of promoting events that are related to the pregnancy history of women in whom the process has been initiated. Hygienic practices and endocrine, nutritional, and metabolic factors may influence the mucosal susceptibility of the genital tract and in this manner promote carcinogenesis. The prevalence of these tumor-enhancing factors may vary with age, ethnicity, and socioeconomic status.

REFERENCES

1. Progress Against Cancer 1970. A Report by the National Advisory Cancer Council.
2. American Cancer Society, Inc. Cancer Statistics 1970.

3. Dorn, H.F. *Nat. Cancer Inst. Monogr., 19:*421, 1966.
4. Barclay, T.H.C., and Phillips, A.J. *Cancer, 15:*5, 1962.
5. Moriyama, I.M., Baum, W.S., Haenszel, W.M., and Mattison, B.F. *Amer. J. Public Health, 48:*1376, 1958.
6. United States National Center For Health Statistics. The Health of Children—1970.
7. Fraumeni, J.F., Jr., and Wagoner, J.K. *Public Health Rep., 79:*1093, 1964.
8. Fraumeni, J.F., Jr., and Miller, R.W. *Science, 155:*1126, 1967.
9. Fraumeni, J.F., Jr., and Miller, R.W. *J. Nat. Cancer Inst., 38:*593, 1967.
10. Court-Brown, W.M., and Doll, R. *Brit. Med. J., 1:*981, 1961.
11. Slocumb, J.C., and MacMahon, B. *New Eng. J. Med., 268:*922, 1963.
12. Fraumeni, J.F., Jr., Manning, M.D., and Mitus, W.J. *J. Nat. Cancer Inst., 46:*461, 1971.
13. Court-Brown, W.M., and Doll, R. *Brit. Med. J., 2:*1327, 1965.
14. Lilienfeld, A.M. *Yale J. Biol. Med., 39:*143, 1966.
15. MacMahon, B. *J. Nat. Cancer Inst., 28:*1173, 1962.
16. Graham, S., Levin, M.L., Lilienfeld, A.M., Schuman, L.M., *et al. Nat. Cancer Inst. Monogr., 19:*347, 1966.
17. Bizzozero, O.J., Jr., Johnson, K.G., and Ciocco, A. *New Eng. J. Med., 274:*1095, 1966.
18. Bizzozero, O.J., Jr., Johnson, K.G., Ciocco, A., Kawasaki, S., and Toyoda, *S. Ann. Intern. Med., 66:*522, 1967.
19. Seltser, R., and Sartwell, P.E. *Amer. J. Epidem., 81:*2, 1965.
20. Court-Brown, W.M., and Doll, R. *Brit. Med. J., 2:*181, 1958.
21. Heath, C.W., Jr., and Hasterlik, R.J. *Amer. J. Med., 34:*796, 1963.
22. Ederer, F., Myers, M.H., and Mantel, N. *Biometrics, 20:*626, 1964.
23. Mantel, N. *Cancer Res., 27:*209, 1967.
24. Glass, A.G., Hill, J.A., and Miller, R.A. *J. Pediat., 73:*101, 1968.
25. MacMahon, B. *Cancer, 21:*558, 1968.
26. Burkitt, D.P. *J. Nat. Cancer Inst., 42:*19, 1969.
27. Fraumeni, J.F., Jr. *Nat. Cancer Inst. Monogr., 32:*221, 1969.
28. Lilienfeld, A.M. *Epidemiology of Mongolism.* Baltimore, Johns Hopkins Press, 1969.
29. Miller, R.W., and Todaro, G.J. *Lancet, 1:*81, 1969.
30. Miller, R.W.: *J. Nat. Cancer Inst., 46:*203, 1971.
31. MacMahon, B., and Levy, M.A. *New Eng. J. Med., 270:*1082, 1964.
32. Gunz, F.W., and Veale, A.M.O. *J. Nat. Cancer Inst., 42:*517, 1969.
33. Miller, R.W., Fraumeni, J.F., Jr., and Manning, M.D. *New Eng. J. Med., 270:*922, 1964.
34. Fraumeni, J.F., Jr., and Glass, A.G. *J.A.M.A., 206:*825, 1968.
35. Fraumeni, J.F., Jr., and Miller, R.W., and Hill, J.A. *J. Nat. Cancer Inst., 40:*1087, 1968.

36. Fraumeni, J.F., Jr., and Miller, R.W.: *J. Pediat., 70:*129, 1967.
37. Sy, W.M., and Edmonson, J.H. *Cancer, 22:*234, 1968.
38. Fileppi, G., and McKusick, V.A. *Medicine, 49:*279, 1970.
39. Hems, G. *Brit. J. Cancer, 24:*208, 1970.
40. Fraumeni, J.F., Jr. *Cancer, 20:*967, 1967.
41. Tjalma, R.A. *J. Nat. Cancer Inst., 36:*1137, 1966.
42. MacMahon, B. *Cancer Res., 26:*1189, 1966.
43. Cole, P., MacMahon, B., and Aisenberg, A. *Lancet, 2:*1371, 1968.
44. Newell, G.R. *Amer. J. Epidem., 91:*119, 1970.
45. Burn, C., Davies, J.N.P., Dodge, O.G., and Nias, B.C. *J. Nat. Cancer Inst., 46:*37, 1971.
46. Smithers, D.W. *Lancet, 2:*1285, 1970.
47. Editorial. *Lancet, 1:*505, 1969.
48. Penn, I. *Malignant Tumors in Organ Transplant Recipients.* New York, Springer-Verlag, 1970.
49. Walker, D., Gill, T.J., and Corson, J.M. *J.A.M.A., 215:*2084, 1971.
50. Logan, W.P.D. *Public Health Rep., 69:*1217, 1954.
51. Case, R.A.M. *Brit. J. Prev. Soc. Med., 10:*172, 1956.
52. Haenszel, W. *J. Nat. Cancer Inst., 21:*213, 1958.
53. Terris, M., and Hall, C.E. *J. Nat. Cancer Inst., 31:*155, 1963.
54. Haenszel, W., and Kurihara, M. *J. Nat. Cancer Inst., 40:*43, 1968.
55. Griffith, G.W. *Brit. J. Cancer, 22:*163, 1968.
56. Flamant, R., *et al. J. Nat. Cancer Inst., 32:*1309, 1964.
57. Wynder, E.L., Kmet, J., Dungal, N., and Segi, M. *Cancer, 16:*1461, 1963.
58. Thorsteinsson, T., and Thordarson, G. *Cancer, 21:*390, 1968.
59. Thorsteinsson, T. *Cancer, 23:*455, 1969.
60. McConnell, R.B. In Shivas, A.A., (Ed.) *Racial and Geographical Factors in Tumor Incidence.* Edinburgh University Press, 1967, pp. 108-113.
61. Edwards, F.C., and Coghill, N.F. *Brit. Med. J., 2:*1409, 1966.
62. Berg, J.W. *Cancer, 11:*1149, 1958.
63. Ming, S., and Goldman, H. *Cancer, 18:*721, 1965.
64. Glass, G.B.J. *Amer. J. Dig. Dis., 10:*376, 1965.
65. Kaplan, H.S., and Rigler, L.G. *Amer. J. Med. Sci., 209:*339, 1945.
66. Mosbech, J. *Acta Med. Scand., 148:*309, 1954.
67. Jorgenson, J. *Acta Med. Scand., 139:*472, 1951.
68. Zamcheck, N., Grable, E., Ley, A.B., and Norman, Z.R. *New Eng. J. Med., 252:*1103, 1955.
69. Hoffman, N.R. *Geriatrics, 25:*90, 1970.
70. Hirohata, T. *J. Nat. Cancer Inst., 41:*895, 1968.
71. Hirohata, T., and Kuratsune, M. *Brit. J. Cancer, 23:*465, 1969.
72. Stemmermann, G.N., and Hayashi, T. *J. Nat. Cancer Inst., 41:*627, 1968.

73. Correa, P., Cuello, C., and Duque, E. *J. Nat. Cancer Inst., 44:*297, 1970.
74. Silverberg, E. *Cancer of the Colon and Rectum: Statistical Data,* New York, The American Cancer Society, Inc., 1970.
75. Haenszel, W., and Dawson, E.A. *Cancer, 18:*265, 1965.
76. Wynder, E.L., Graham, S., and Eisenberg, H. *Cancer, 19:*1561, 1966.
77. Staszewski, J., and Haenszel, W. J. *Nat. Cancer Inst., 35:*291, 1965.
78. Newill, V.A. *J. Nat. Cancer Inst., 26:*405, 1961.
79. Mass, N., and Modan, B. *J. Nat. Cancer Inst., 42:*529, 1969.
80. Higginson, J. *J. Nat. Cancer Inst., 37:*527, 1966.
81. Bremner, C.G., and Ackerman, L.V. *Cancer, 26:*991, 1970.
82. Wynder, E.L., Kajitani, T., Ishikawa, S., Dodo, H., and Takano, A. *Cancer, 23:*1210, 1969.
83. Spjut, H.J., and Spratt, J.S., Jr. *Ann. Surg., 161:*309, 1965.
84. Stewart, H.L. *Nat. Cancer Inst. Monogr., 25:*199, 1967.
85. Laqueur, G.L. In Burdette W.J. (Ed.) *Carcinoma of the Colon and Antecedent Epithelium.* Springfield, Thomas, 1970, pp. 305-313.
86. Hill, M.J., Drasar, B.S., Aries, V., Crowther, J.S., Hawksworth, G., and Williams, R.E.O. *Lancet, 1:*95, 1971.
87. National Center For Health Statistics. Mortality from Diseases Associated with Smoking: United States, 1950-64. Series *20,* (No. 4) 1966.
88. Doll, R. *Cancer Res., 23:*1613, 1963.
89. Joint report of the study group on smoking and health. *Science, 125:* 1129, 1957.
90. *Smoking and Health.* Report of the Advisory Committee to the Surgeon General of the Public Health Service. U.S. Public Health Service Publication No. 1103, 1964.
91. Wynder, E.L., and Hoffman, D. *Science, 162:*862, 1968.
92. *The Health Consequences of Smoking.* U.S. Public Health Service Publication No. 1696, pp. 34-37 and 127-145, 1968.
93. Wynder, E.L., Mabuchi, K., and Beattie, E.J., Jr. *J.A.M.A., 213:*2221, 1970.
94. Berg, J.W., Schottenfeld, D., and Ritter, F. *J. Nat. Cancer Inst., 44:* 263, 1970.
95. Hammond, E.C., and Horn, D. *J.A.M.A., 166:*1159 and 1294, 1958
96. Kotin, P. *Cancer Res., 16:*375, 1956.
97. Wynder, E.L., and Hammond, E.C. *Cancer, 15:*79, 1962.
98. Buell, P., and Dunn, J.E. *Arch. Environ. Health, 15:*291, 1967.
99. Lave, L.B., and Seskin, E.P. *Science, 169:*723, 1970.
100. Cohart, E.M. *Cancer, 8:*1126, 1955.
101. Seltser, R. *Arch. Environ. Health, 10:*923, 1965.
102. Doll, R. *Brit. J. Industr. Med., 16:*181, 1959.
103. Tokuhata, G.K., and Lilienfeld, A.M. *J. Nat. Cancer Inst., 30:*289, 1963.

104. Wagoner, J.K., Archer, V.E., Lundin, F.E., Jr., Holaday, D.A., and Lloyd, J.W. *New Eng. J. Med., 273:*181, 1965.
105. Saccomanno, G., Archer, V.E., Auerbach, O., Kuschner, M., Saunders, R.P., and Klein, M.G. *Cancer, 27:*515, 1971.
106. Selikoff, I.J., Bader, R.A., Bader, M.E., Churg, J., and Hammond, E.C. *Amer. J. Med., 42:*487, 1967.
107. Selikoff, I.J., Hammond, E.C., and Churg, J. *J.A.M.A., 204:*106, 1968.
108. Wright, G.W. *Amer. Rev. Resp. Dis., 100:*467, 1969.
109. Levin, M.L., Sheehe, P.R., Graham S., and Glidewell, O. *Amer. J. Public Health, 54:*580, 1964.
110. Feinleib, M., and Garrison, R.J. *Cancer, 24:*1109, 1969.
111. Cutler, S.J., and Heise, H.W. *Cancer, 24:*1117, 1969.
112. Lilienfeld, A.M. *Cancer Res., 23:*1503, 1963.
113. Salber, E.J., Trichopoulos, D., and MacMahon, B. *J. Nat. Cancer Inst., 43:*1013, 1969.
114. MacMahon, B., Lin, T.M., Lowe, C.R., Mirra, A.P., Ravnihar, B., Salber, E.J., Trichopoulos, D., Valaoras, V.G., and Yuasa, S. *Bull. WHO, 42:*185, 1970.
115. Fraumeni, J.F., Jr., Lloyd, J.W., Smith, E.M., and Wagoner, J.K. *J. Nat. Cancer Inst., 42:*455, 1969.
116. Lilienfeld, A.M. *Cancer, 9:*927, 1956.
117. MacMahon, B., and Feinleib, M. *J. Nat. Cancer Inst., 24:*733, 1960.
118. Hirayama, T., and Wynder, E.L. *Cancer, 15:*28, 1962.
119. National Center For Health Statistics Age at Menopause, United States: 1960-1962. Series *11,* (No. 19) 1966.
120. Feinleib, M. *J. Nat. Cancer Inst., 41:*315, 1968.
121. Lane-Claypon, J.E. *Public Health and Medical Subjects, No. 32.* London, British Ministry of Health, 1926.
122. Shapiro, S., Strax, P., Venet, L., and Fink, R. *Amer. J. Public Health, 58:*820, 1968.
123. Yuasa, S., and MacMahon, B. *Bull. W.H.O., 42:*195, 1970.
124. Wynder, E.L., Hyams, L., and Shigematsu, T. *Cancer, 20:*113, 1967.
125. Wynder, E.L. In Forrest, A.P.M., and Kunkler, P.B. (Eds.) *Prognostic Factors in Breast Cancer.* Baltimore, Williams & Wilkins Co., 1968, pp. 32-49.
126. Steinitz, R. *5-Year's Morbidity from Neoplasms in Israel's Population Groups (1960-1964).* Jerusalem, Israel, Ministry of Health, Division of Chronic Diseases and Rehabilitation, 1967.
127. Schottenfeld, D., and Lilienfeld, A.M. *J. Chronic Dis., 16:*71, 1963.
128. Schottenfeld, D., Lilienfeld, A.M., and Diamond, H.D. *Amer. J. Public Health, 53:*890, 1963.
129. Tokuhata, G.K. *Amer. J. Epidem., 89:*139, 1969.
130. Macklin, M.T. *J. Nat. Cancer Inst., 23:*1179, 1959.
131. Davis, H.H., Simons, M., and Davis, J.B. *Cancer, 17:*957, 1964.

132. Foote, F.W., and Stewart, F.W. *Ann. Surg., 121*:6 and 197, 1945.
133. Kern, W.H., and Brooks, R.N. *Cancer, 24*:668, 1969.
134. Mackenzie, I. *Brit. J. Cancer, 19*:1, 1965.
135. Myrden, J.A., and Hiltz, J.E. *Canad. Med. Ass. J., 100*:1032, 1969.
136. Tamplin, A.R., and Gofman, J.W. *Lancet, 1*:297, 1970.
137. Mettler, F.A., Jr., Hempelmann, L.H., Dutton, A.M., Pifer, J.W., Toyooka, E.T., and Ames, W.R. *J. Nat. Cancer Inst., 43*:803, 1969.
138. Wanebo, C.K., Johnson, K.G., Sato, K., and Thorslund, T.W. *New Eng. J. Med., 279*:667, 1968.
139. Segaloff, A., and Maxfield, W.S. *Cancer Res., 31*:166, 1971.
140. Hayward, J. *Recent Results in Cancer Research*. New York, Springer-Verlag, 1970, pp. 52-68, 121-135.
141. DeWaard, F. *Int. J. Cancer, 4*:577, 1969.
142. Mirra, A.P., Cole, P., and MacMahon, B. *Cancer Res., 31*:77, 1971.
143. Dao, T.L. *Progr. Exp. Tumor Res., 11*:235, 1969.
144. Carroll, K.K., Gammal, E.B., and Plunkett, E.R. *Canad. Med. Ass. J., 98*:599, 1968.
145. Cole, P., and MacMahon, B. *Lancet, 1*:604, 1969.
146. Lemon, H.M. *Cancer, 23*:781, 1969.
147. Wotiz, H.H., Shane, J.A., Vigersky, R., and Brecher, P.I. In Forrest, A.P.M., and Kunkler, P.B. (Eds.) *Prognostic Factors in Breast Cancer*. Baltimore, Williams & Wilkins Co., 1968, pp. 368-382.
148. Smith, O.W., and Smith, G.V. *Lancet, 1*:1152, 1970.
149. Dunn, J.E., Jr. *Cancer, 23*:775, 1969.
150. Stamler, J., Fields, C., and Andelman, S.L. *Amer. J. Public Health, 57*: 791, 1967.
151. Koss, L.G. *Obstet. Gynec. Survey, 24*:850, 1969.
152. Hulka, B.S., and Redmond, C.K. *Amer. J. Epidem., 93*:23, 1971.
153. Kashgarian, M., and Dunn, J.E., Jr. *Amer. J. Epidem., 92*:211, 1970.
154. Christopherson, W.M., and Parker, J.E. *New Eng. J. Med., 273*:235, 1965.
155. Stern, E., Lachenbruch, P.A., and Dixon, W.J. *Cancer, 20*:190, 1967.
156. Wynder, E.L. *Obstet. Gynec. Survey, 24*:697, 1969.
157. Barron, B.A., and Richart, R.M. *Cancer, 27*:978, 1971.
158. Christopherson, W.M., and Parker, J.E. *Cancer, 13*:711, 1960.
159. Plaut, A., and Kohn-Speyer, A.C. *Science, 105*:391, 1947.
160. Pratt-Thomas, H.R., Heins, H.C., Latham, E., Dennis, E.J., and McIver, F.A. *Cancer, 9*:671, 1956.
161. Reddy, D.G., and Baruah, I.K. *Arch. Path. (Chicago), 75*:414, 1963.
162. Stewart, H.L., Dunham, L.J., Casper, J., Dorn, H.F., Thomas, L.B., Edgecomb, J.H., and Symeonidis, A. *J. Nat. Cancer Inst., 37*:1, 1966.
163. Cross, H.E., Kennel, E.E., and Lilienfeld, A.M. *Cancer, 21*:102, 1968.
164. Dodge, O.G., Linsell, C.A., and Davies, J.N.P. *E. Afr. Med. J., 40*:440, 1963.

165. Abou-Daoud, K.T. *Cancer, 20:*1706, 1967.
166. Josey, W.E., Nahmias, A.J., and Naib, Z.M. *Amer. Obstet. Gynec., 101:* 718, 1968.
167. Rawls, W.E., Tompkins, W.A.F., Figueroa, M.E., and Melnick, J.L. *Science, 161:*1255, 1968.
168. Rawls, W.E., Laurel, D., Melnick, J.L., Glicksman, J.M., and Kaufman, R.H. *Amer. J. Epidem., 87:*647, 1968.
169. Rawls, W.E., Tompkins, W.A.F., and Melnick, J.L. *Amer. J. Epidem., 89:*547, 1969.
170. Rawls, W.E., Iwamoto, K., Adam, E., Melnick, J.L., and Green, G.H. *Lancet, 11:*1142, 1970.

Chapter 11

RADIOACTIVE ISOTOPES IN EPIDEMIOLOGICAL STUDIES

OSCAR FELSENFELD

THE MISSION of the public health laboratory is to support the epidemiologist by rendering reports that may help him to ascertain if a disease is present in a given area, if the population and its components are susceptible to an infection for lack of antibodies against the causative agent, and if the illness afflicted the population in the past. Serological methods admirably serve as indicators of numerous present and past diseases as well as in the determination of the absence of protective antibodies. Serological investigations are frequently carried out in conjunction with a search for the causative agent in man, animals, birds, insects, and other hosts. There is no doubt that many of the presently employed tests are reliable within variations that can be determined with the aid of statistical methods. A great number of them can be carried out on a large scale, principally when the respective procedure is adaptable to semiautomatic or automatic means. When *in vitro* tests are used, micromethods are preferred provided that the results are not significantly different ($P < 0.05$) from those achieved with macromethods.

The majority of bacterial, rickettsial, viral, protozoan, and metazoan disease can be investigated with the aid of immunological *in vitro* or skin tests. However, there is a trend to substitute laboratory methods for skin testing, so that the person has to be seen by the epidemiological team only once and not two or more times to "set up" the skin test, and then to "read" it at intervals. The investigation of susceptibility to diptheria and attempts to develop a reliable *in vitro* procedure instead of the tuberculin test, as well as the estimation of susceptibility to smallpox, belong in this category.

Modern *(sit venia verbo)* epidemiology does not concern itself only with transmissible diseases. True, in developing countries this group of ills still represents a formidable array of the pressing problems faced by the practicing epidemiologist because of the frequent outbreaks of such diseases. Practically all other pathological conditions, including aberrations transmissible by heredity, lack of enzymatic factors, other metabolic disturbances and hunger itself, endocrine irregularities, accidents, aging, tumors, environmental influences, and other factors that may predispose or cause disease, fall within the range of activities of the up-to-date epidemiologist. This elevated the public health laboratory from a limited microbiological and food-and-water chemistry workshop to a multipronged agency dealing with microbiological, biochemical, histopathological, entomological, and agricultural problems as well as delving into developmental physiology, hematology, toxicology, radiation, and other physicochemical factors affecting health, as well as other branches of subjects of pathology relegated only to hospital laboratories in the past. Naturally, only properly equipped, manned, and conducted laboratories are in a position to carry out all these tasks.

First, the methods used must be reliable and reproducible. Quality control, carried out with the aid of outside agencies or by an internal arrangement, must yield satisfactory results. Admittedly the interpretation of the reports may not be easy. Few "normals" have been established, and an aberration from the means > 2 S.D. is not significant for the epidemiologist when observed only in a few individual instances but only proves that the examined population yields data that can be plotted on the probability distribution curve. The same aberrant data will, however, invite the attention of the clinician for whom they may be pathognomic. But what is "normal"? How to explain vibriocidal titres, say, up to 1:200 in persons who never were in cholera-infested areas nor were vaccinated against that disease? What about the numerous "cross-reactions," for instance, in arboviral infections? Does a titre of 0.01 or 0.02 antitoxin units per ml serum really assure us that the person is not susceptible to tetanus? Needless to say that in search for "normal" values the first thought which comes to the mind is that a standardized technique has to be used and carried out punctually to the letter. One has to recall the statement of Dr. Reuben Kahn, who used to say that if a serum has to be inactivated at 56° C, that does not mean that the waterbath thermometer may show 55.5° C or 56.5° C but the method calls for exactly 56° C.

When radioactive isotopes are employed, the problem of standardization acquires added dimensions: How much of the isotope was taken up? What was the rate of deterioration? How much was lost during the processing? What amount was bound to substances other than the immunologically active participants in the reaction mixture? What kind of apparatus was used to measure the radioactive emission? What was the background count? What was the efficacy of the measuring device? How good was the standard? How did light, heat, and moisture influence the counter? and so forth. There are no generally accepted standards, as yet, to indicate when the reaction is "positive" in immunological tests employing radioactive isotopes. As a rule of the thumb, in our laboratory we consider counts at least twice as high as the background count plus that of the negative control as "borderline," but much further investigation is necessary before this method of evaluation can be considered valid, principally when working with such complicated antigenic materials as those prepared from tissues.

Another prerequisite for a laboratory test is that it should be simple, especially if destined for use in mass-examination, so that it can be carried out by persons with minimal erudition and experience as is often necessary in underdeveloped countries, as well as in other areas when sudden accumulation of requests for laboratory examinations (e.g. a typhoid outbreak) necessitates the emergency transfer of technicians to a different type of work assignment. The employment of radioactive isotopes requires special precautions. We have been concentrating on the use of ^{14}C, that has a long half-life but its soft beta emission is stopped by ordinary glass tubing and even by surgical gloves when they are employed in small amounts, as e.g. in the internal labeling of bacteria. The disposal of wastes from such operations does not pose specific problems. Detergents available from a number of radioactive isotope supply houses and subsequent autoclaving or incineration of amounts containing less than 1 mCi is considered a safe procedure according to most state atomic energy commissions. ^{14}C-labeled materials give relatively low counts. However, if used in autoradiography, its zigzag pattern of their trace may be more confusing than ^{3}H-produced granules. We recommend both isotopes for serological work. Liquid scintillation counters are feasible for the determination of the emission of both radioactive isotopes, but this machinery is not recommended in some tropical laboratories that have few facilities and inexperienced personnel. The low-beta, low-background gas counters give lower counts but require less service and are easy to work with. For instant labeling of proteins particularly antibodies, radioactive iodine, the short-lived ^{131}I or ^{125}I with a longer half-life, is generally employed. We have found ^{51}Cr quite useful for external labeling. All three isotopes require the use of gamma emission analyzers, and their handling rigid adherence to proper precautionary measures. The short half-life of these labels prevents the dispatch of labeled materials to other laboratories from a central labeling station, which is a distinct disadvantage in field-work. The uptake of the radioactive label by antigens may vary from one batch to another, which militates against the consideration of this method as a simple procedure.

The results of all laboratory tests have to be delivered to the epidemiologist within the shortest time possible after the samples are submitted. The pressure of a threatening or already present epidemic, the evaluation of a vaccination campaign, the assessment of the state of immunity of a population, and other questions demand the use of rapid methods. Many simple agglutination, precipitation, bacteriolysin, and related tests can be carried out within a few hours. Mass-examination with radioactively labeled reactants is also rapid. A low-beta gas flow counter or a liquid scintillation counter equipped with an automatic elevator or turning device can "count" one hundred samples in about two hours. If the precipitation is carried out on a feasible filter pad, if the incubation requires less than two hours, and if the filters are set up connected in series, it is possible to render a numerical result within five hours after the sample reaches the laboratory. In mass-surveys, it is possible either to collect exactly 0.1 ml serum on a filter pad and send the pads to the laboratory in a sealed plastic envelope, or the blood may be delivered to the laboratory, where 0.1 ml serum will be separated and applied to the filter. In recent hitherto unpublished experiments, we have been using laked full blood instead of serum, but this method is feasible only for the low-beta gas counter, in which we have not yet observed interference due to the color of the blood.

It should be pointed out that the public health laboratory must adhere to the rules of economy. The services are usually rendered free of charge. The budget may be heavily burdened by the necessity of purchasing expensive diagnostic bacteriological media during an epidemic outbreak. The methods employed should conform to the principles of cost consciousness. Radioactive isotopes, with the exception of ^{131}I, are by no means cheap. Nevertheless one has to hope that the increasing demand for such materials will result in lower prices of the other radioactive isotopes also. However, ^{125}I and ^{51}Cr used in autoradiographic demonstrations of immunological reactions also are available at a reasonable cost today.

The training of the personnel handling radioactive isotopes is a serious but not unsurmountable difficulty. One can always find a little slot in the teaching schedule of technologists for radiation safety measures. Printed teaching materials are cheap (from the various atomic energy committees) and often available without charge. A small fee may have to be paid for the permission to reproduce pertinent paragraphs that may be kept by the student for later reference if pamphlets without cost cannot be acquired. It must be added that "tolerated doses" listed in various tests are often estimated and not derived from observation. Therefore it is advisable to exert more than the minimal required care with gamma and/or alpha emitters.

It is evident that the use of radioactive isotopes in epidemiological surveys is in its early childhood. Simpler and less costly methods have to be developed. Recent interest and research in this field raises hopes that such a goal is not unattainable.

It is not feasible to label each serum separately in epidemiological investigations. Radioactive labeling of the antigens is, therefore, the preferred method. This can be accomplished by internal labeling, i.e. culturing the organisms in the presence of a radioactively labeled metabolite, or by external labeling, adding radioactive I or Cr to the antigenic extract. Undoubtedly more efficient labels will be developed in the future.

LABELING BACTERIA

A simple procedure, particularly feasible for gram-negative bacteria, has been described by our group.[1,2] The organisms are grown in a medium containing ingredients necessary for a luxuriant growth. For instance, *Enterobacteriaceae* may be cultured in the presence of 1 percent Trypticase® *or* Tryptose®, 0.5 percent NaCl, and 0.2 percent yeast or meat extract. After adjusting the pH to 7.2 and sterilization, enough ^{14}C-labeled yeast protein hydrolysate *or* ^{14}C amino acid mixture is added to give 2 mCi per liter medium. After inoculation, the broth is incubated for 18 to 24 hours at 37° C, the growth harvested by centrifuging at 15,000 $\times$ *g* and +2° C, the sediment mixed with an equal amount (v/v) of the supernate, and the bacterial bodies disintegrated in a colled ball mill or French press. The antigen is prepared by centrifuging off all particulate material at 25,000 $\times$ *g* and +2° C. The supernate may be concentrated in viscose bags on which commercial confectionery sugar powder or polyvinyl pyrrolidine is heavily dusted to absorb surplus water. The radioactive emission of the antigen is checked in the counter. Then the antigen is stored in the cold. The pH of the antigen should be adjusted if it exceeds the range of 6.8 to 7.8.

We have been using equal amounts (v/v) of antigen and antibody (serum) in the precipitin reaction. Complete antigen-antibody complex formation would require about four days at +2° C. Sufficient binding can be achieved by adding the antigen to the serum on a millipore or equivalent filter paper with pore size of 0.45 n. The papers are incubated at 50° C for one to two hours in a moist chamber, then placed into the millipore filter apparatus or its equivalent. The unreacted antigen and antibody are carefully washed out under mild suction with phosphate-saline buffer pH 7.2. The papers are rapidly dried with a fan, immersed first into 10 percent, then into 5 percent trichloracetic acid, finally into ether, and, when dry, affixed to planchets with starch paste. It is essential that the filter papers are completely flattened out. The planchets are put into the low-beta, low-background counter, together with the necessary controls, and the radioactive emission determined.

We compared the results of this test with routine tube agglutination, hemagglutination, bentonite precipitation, the capillary tube precipitation test, and rapid antigen-antibody electrophoresis[2] in typhoid patients, symptomless carriers, vaccinated individuals, and controls. We correlated also the efficacy of agglutination, vibriocidal activity, and circulating antitoxin levels in cholera in man and artificially infested laboratory animals, as well as in monkeys with *Pasteurella* infections.[1] A greater proportion of the sera of symptomless but infected individuals gave significantly higher counts than did positive tests with other methods. It became apparent that the radioactive-isotope-labeled antigen reacted with high-molecular-weight immune globulins, principally of the class IgM, more readily than with IgG (7S) because of the greater number of binding sites on the former and larger complexes produced that emit more beta radiation than the small IgG-antigen complexes. This appeared to be advantageous in the early stages of those infectious diseases in which first IgM is discharged into the blood circulation, as e.g. in typhoid. Since IgG is considered the more stable immune globulin and frequently the representative of a longer-lasting immunity, longer incubation time (2 hrs.) and filters with smaller pores and/or with greater absorptive capacity (as Whatman's 3MM paper) were employed in later experiments.

Figure 11.1 demonstrates the results of the examination of two hundred sera from cholera patients, convalescents, postconvalescents, contact, and controls. The last group was never immunized against cholera, lived in Louisiana where that disease did not appear for more than sixty years, and never left the area. The curve shows that the number of counts per minute is higher during the

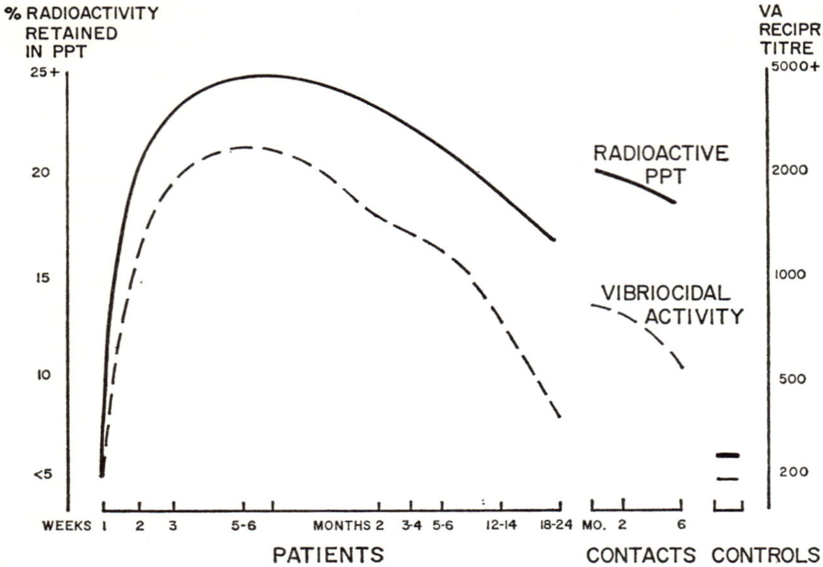

Figure 11.1. Comparison of vibriocidal activity titre in patients and contacts infected with *Vibrio cholerae,* and controls, with the radioactive isotope precipitation test.

early days of the disease and remains longer at an elevated level than the frequently used vibriocidal titre determined according to the very reliable opacity method. It appears that the use of radioactive isotopes potentiates this titre, as does absorption of the precipitinogens on some serologically inactive materials, e.g. bentonite.

Either internal or external labeling produced useful antigens from tubercle bacillus fractions. The microorganisms were grown in the presence of ^{14}C yeast extract containing TB Broth Base without Polysorbate (Baltimore Biological Laboratory). The non-dialyzable protein fraction of the culture fluid was treated according to Chaparas *et al.,*[3] by precipitation with 1 percent acetic acid at pH 4.0 and +4° C, clarified by centrifugation at 5000 × *g* and +2° C, passed through a Sephadex G-50 column, the protein-rich fractions collected, concentrated *(vide Enterobacteriaceae),* and used in the co-precipitation test after one hour's incubation at 37° C, overnight at +4° C. Rabbit antihuman serum was employed as the co-precipitating agent, and incubated for eight hours.

External labeling of the precipitinogen was carried out with ^{51}Cr by the method of Braude *et al.*[4] or with ^{125}I according to Gruber and Wright.[5] In both instances the radioactive emission of the supernatant was determined in the single-channel gamma analyzer. The counts were deducted from that given by labeled antigen and rabbit antihuman serum alone. We[6] found that the results were positive in 17 of 20 patients with fibroulcerous and in 16 of 20 with nodular parenchymatous tuberculosis but in only 7 to 20 early parenchymatous lesions. The test was positive also in 23 of 25 patients with lepromatous leprosy of more than one year's duration but negative in 16 instances of tuberculoid leprosy. On the other hand, it was positive in 5 patients simultaneously afflicted with fibroulcerous tuberculosis and tuberculoid leprosy. The radioactive emission count of the antibody-antigen precipitate was reduced by 72 to 78 percent in lepromatous leprosy after the absorption of the sera with *Nocardia brasiliensis* carried out according to Salazar Mallén *et al.*[7] This method gave good results also when the sera were labeled either with ^{125}I or with ^{51}Cr, and may be helpful in the differentiation of lepromatous and tuberculoid leprosy as well as assist in the determination of the presence of both tuberculosis and leprosy. The importance of further work on this subject does not have to be stressed because of the common observation that patients with Hansen's disease often die of tuberculosis that may not be recognized *intra vitam.*

So-called bacterial toxins can be labeled with ease using the procedure of Braude *et al.*[4] We have utilized it for labeling diphtheria and tetanus toxoid and found a significant correlation between this test and the precipitation of the same antigens adsorbed on tanned-sheep red cells. The results are shown in Figure 11.2. While sheep red cells with adsorbed anatoxin cannot be kept for a long time, radioactive-isotope-labeled antigens remain usable for the half-life of the internal or external label or until the antigen deteriorates, whichever comes first.

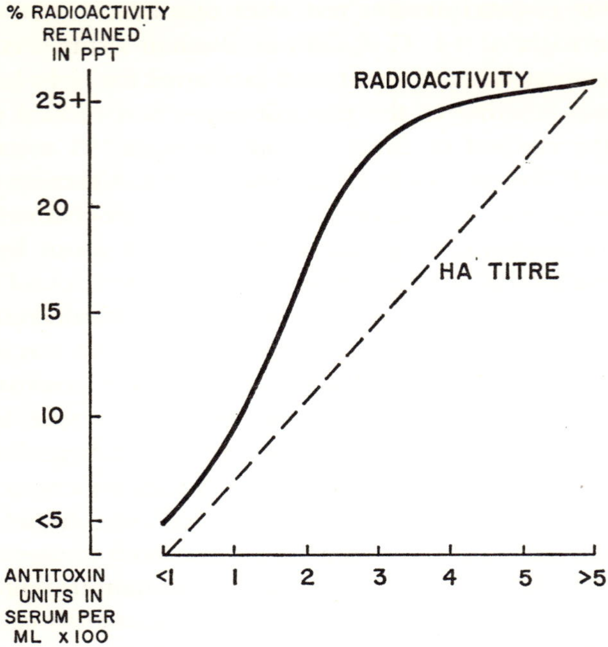

Figure 11.2. Comparison of antitoxin units × 100 per ml serum and the results of radioactive isotope precipitation test with tetanus toxoid.

VIRUSES

Two approaches are possible. One is their internal labeling by adding to the tissue on which the virus is to be cultured or injecting newborn mice with a feasible radioactive isotope at the time of the infection. The other method is external labeling of the RNA or DNA extracted from the respective virus. A modification of the latter procedure is to permit the reaction between the respective ribonucleic acid and the serum to take place, then determine the unbound nucleic acid by co-precipitation with radioisotope-labeled methylated albumin—RNA or DNA rabbit antiserum, respectively. The procedure may be inverted by labeling the examined sera.

Gerloff *et al.*[8] were the first to experiment with labeled poliovirus. They used ^{32}P, 0.1 mCi per ml tissue culture. We substituted ^{14}C or ^{3}H-labeled nucleosides and either DEAE-Sephadex 50 column chromatography or sucrose gradient centrifugation for the purification of the viral material. The incubation time of the serum-antigen mixture was 30 minutes at 37° C, followed by addition of rabbit antihuman globulin serum for co-precipitation, reincubation for one hour at 37° C, and centrifugation at 1000 × *g* for 10 minutes at +2° C. The radioactivity of the supernate was determined and the amount bound in the antibody-antigen reaction calculated.

^{3}H thymidine for DNA viruses and ^{3}H uridine for RNA viruses gave higher readings than the respective preparations internally labeled with ^{14}C. Of the RNA viruses, rheovirus 3 and California encephalitis virus were tested; of the DNA viruses, human herpes and vaccine virus.[9] The latter gave results of special interest to the epidemiologist. When sera of persons vaccinated against smallpox were tested by this method, the results remained positive for more than two years, whereas the hemagglutination-inhibition and the complement-fixation tests showed increased titres only for about 12 to 14 months after vaccination. However, experience indicates that the protective value of smallpox vaccine lasts longer than one year.

OTHER APPLICATIONS

The precipitation of radioactively labeled antigens or antibodies can be demonstrated also with the aid of autoradiography applied to antigen-antibody reactions in agar gel. For instance, Heiner *et al.*[10] applied sera to be tested to commercial immunodiffusion plates used for the determination of the groups of immune globulin in the sera. After these reactions were completed, the plates were carefully washed free of serum and ^{125}I-labeled δ-gliadin, *Aspergillus fumigatus* extract, or diphtheria toxoid were deposited in the respective reservoir holes. After incubation, the agar gel plates were dried, stained with Thiazine Red R to record the immune globulin precipitation rings, then covered with x-ray film for two hours to seven days. The blackening of the film after development permitted the determination of the antigen-binding capacity of the sera.

This method can be shortened in our experience by using Polaroid film. It gives good results and is feasible for the simultaneous examination of great numbers of serum samples. The method of Heiner *et al.*[10] is recommended for testing allergens, (lipo-) polysaccharides, venoms which are difficult to precipitate, and in autoallergic conditions.

Autoallergic conditions with or without clinical manifestations are worthy of studying in various population groups. The development of demonstrable autoallergic (autoimmune) antibodies with progressing age is an interesting and hitherto little-explored field. Autoallergic phenomena have been observed after vaccination and for not well understood reasons in so-called autoimmune diseases. Few surveys have been carried out in selected population groups to determine the frequency of autoallergy and its relationship to internal and external factors. Especially more epidemiological surveys are desirable in autoimmune diseases affecting the gastrointestinal tract, the central and peripheral nervous system, the liver, and the sensory organs. Most of the past studies have been summarized by Gell and Combs.[11] Radioactively labeled antigens are feasible for such mass-examinations in several ways, including the method of Heiner *et al.*,[10] which is applied with ease when using agar gel diffusion plates containing antihuman serum active also against immune globulins of the classes A and E for the screening procedure.

Endocrinological surveys may require the application of radioactive isotopes because the analytical methods used in the assay of hormones are often based on such procedures. The proceedings of a symposium held under the aegis of the U.S. Atomic Energy Commission[12] summarized the principles as well as gave several technical details for such determinations. Those hormones which are antigenic can be estimated by immunoprecipitation with antisera, employing radioactive isotope labels as indicators in radioautography or other procedures. Competetive binding of proteins also may be used. Nonantigenic hormones, as e.g. thyroxine and steroids, can be coupled to proteins and a radioactive label attached. Most methods employ ^{131}I or ^{125}I today. Detailed description of the techniques are beyond the scope of this chapter.

We merely wish to ascertain at this point that the development of endocrinological techniques is also aimed in the direction of simplicity that may lead to the development of methods usable in public health laboratories. Furthermore, these procedures are highly specific. For instance, thyroxine determination with the aid of ^{125}I-labeled thyroxine gives results comparable to those of protein-bound iodine but it seems that there is no interference in the radioactive isotope test from the effect of iodine preparations, salicylates, heparin, and other drugs administered to the patient.

Projecting possible future developments, it is possible that chromosomal labeling will find its way into epidemiological studies, widening the potentialities of family and group surveys for chromosomal aberrations. In view of the numerous gaps in our knowledge of heredity and "inborn" diseases, as well as our attempts to accumulate more data in this field, such a development would not be surprising.

REFERENCES

1. Felsenfeld, O., and Parrot, M.W. Antigens labelled with radioactive isotopes in epidemiological surveillance. Proceedings of the symposium on *In Vitro Procedures with Radioisotopes in Medicine*. Vienna, International Atomic Energy Agency, 1969, p. 213.
2. Felsenfeld, O., and Parrot, M.W. Comparison of radioactive tracer and other methods in epidemiologic surveillance. *Health Lab. Sci., 7*:24, 1970.
3. Chaparas, S.D., Baer, H., and Godfrey, H. In vitro and in vivo studies on tuberculin active polysaccharide and protein fractions. *Z. Immun. Allergieforsch., 137*:234, 1969.
4. Braude, A.I., Carey, F.J., Southerland, D., and Zalesky, M. Studies with radioactive endotoxin. *J. Clin. Invest., 34*:850, 1955.
5. Gruber, J., and Wright, G.G. *I labeling of purified microbial antigens by microdiffusion. *Proc. Soc. Exp. Biol. Med., 126*:282, 1967.
6. Felsenfeld, O., and Dutta, R.N. *J. Nucl. Biol. Med.,* in press.
7. Salazar Mallén, M., Amezcua Chavarría, E., and Escobar Gutiérrez, A. Estudios de immuno-precipitación en la lepra. *Rev. Inst Salud Públ., 27*:3, 1967.
8. Gerloff, R.K., Hoyer, B.H., and McLaren, L.C. Precipitation of radiolabeled poliovirus with specific antibody and antiglobulin. *J. Immun. 89*:669, 1962.
9. Felsenfeld, O., Felsenfeld, A.D., and Brannon, R.H. Comparison of

phage inhibition and radioactive isotope methods in sero-diagnosis. *Amer. J. Clin. Path.,* 1970.

10. Heiner, D.C., Hague, G.M., and Rose, B. A method for the measurement of the antigen-binding activity of immunoglobulins precipitated in commercially available radial immunodiffusion plates. *Clin. Exp. Immun. 6:*773, 1970.
11. Gell, P.H.G., and Coombs, R.R.A. *Clinical Aspects of Immunology,* 2nd ed. Oxford and Edinburgh, Blackwell Sci. Publ., 1968.
12. Hayes, R.L., Goswitz, F.A., and Murphy, B.E.P. (Eds.) *Radioisotopes in Medicine: In Vitro Studies.* Proceedings of the symposium of the Oak Ridge Assoc. Univ., 1967. Springfield, Va., U.S. Atomic Energy Commission, U.S. Dep't. of Commerce, 1968.

Chapter 12

EPIDEMIOLOGIC DRUG TRENDS IN SAN FRANCISCO

GEORGE R. GAY

SINCE THE DAYS of the Gold Rush, San Francisco has proven a sympathetic haven to the disillusioned, the disenfranchised, the psychopathic, the runaway, and many poor souls who felt psychologically out of tune with society for whatever reason.

In the 1950's a neo-Bohemian group of artists, poets, dropouts, and hangers-on (the "beats," or "beatniks") moved into the coffeehouse, bar, and brothel "Northbeach" area of San Francisco to paint, to write their poetry, to act out their particular problems, and generally to reject the unexciting but affluence-success-oriented Eisenhower post-Korean years. San Francisco took note, and shrugged, and smiled, and so this rather negative element of society, the "beat generation," entrenched itself into the legend that was San Francisco.

As we moved into the early 1960's, however, a new social phenomenon was noted to be emerging. A new and exhilarating social optimism was felt as the Kennedy years began: indeed many young people were becoming actively politically involved within the existing political structure; this included the civil rights movement, the Peace Corps, and many nonviolent campus activities through which they hoped to bring about social betterment through peaceful means around a nucleus of new, young, appealing political and social leaders (the Kennedys, Martin Luther King, Jr., the maturing Malcolm X).[1]

A parallel social evolvement was also noted, however, as a new subculture appeared—the "hippies" or "flower children," reminiscent of the "beats" but much more positive and aggressive. Followed and generally lauded by an exuberant press, this new social phenomenon suddenly moved en masse into the previously staid, integrated Haight-Ashbury area at the beautiful green borders of Golden Gate Park.

In a breakdown of this new community or subculture, basically four subgroups could be identified.[2] They were, first, the "hard-core" committed hippies who had a particular, consistent philosophical system, one of "turning on chemically." The two drugs used almost exclusively at this time were marijuana (the hippies' social drug) and LSD-25 and other psychedelic agents (their religious drugs).[3]

The San Francisco *Chronicle*[4] reported:

> What do Viet Nam, the Flying Nun, detergent, and marijuana have in common? . . . Magic, for one thing, and each in its own way illustrates an American return to a primitive faith in the black arts . . . The alchemists of the present day are the members of the drug cult. With LSD or something else exotic from the chemical retort, they believe this leaden old world can be turned into instant gold. They talk about it in terms of "expanding consciousness" or "turning on" as though their minds were light bulbs, but what they are really talking about is acquiring a love of life that will give them the strength to go on.

Peripheral to the "core" hippies were the hangers-on, the "weekenders," the "plastic hippies," or the "Clark Kent hippies."

The second major element of the new Haight-Ashbury was that of the sociopathic element, which contained the "Hell's Angels," "Gypsy Jokers" (the leather, bully boys), radicals (both black and white), amphetamine or "speed" dealers, and criminals of varying types.

The third major element was that of the prepsychotic individuals who "could not make it" in a more regulated society and indeed often had a long record of institutionalization. These individuals were not particularly violent, but on occasion an "ambulatory schizophrenic" could have a disastrous response to the "mind-altering" drugs now indigenous to the area.

The fourth and last major group of the new Haight was that of the "teeny-boppers," particularly impressionable youngsters no longer drinking beer on Fort Lauderdale's beaches but often taking excessive quantities of drugs because it was the "in" thing to do.

THE CONCEPT OF THE FREE CLINIC

Conceived as a social statement that "Love needs Care,"[5,6] the Haight-Ashbury Free Medical Clinic was founded and opened during the "Summer of Love" of 1967. Many of the new community of the Haight—indeed, neither the new nor the old had access to or desire to utilize existing psychosocial and medical facilities, so it was determined that the Free Clinic would offer unrestricted (and unscreened) free medical and psychosocial treatment for all of the community. Founded by Dr. David Smith and others and managed almost entirely by a volunteer staff, this ethic of free care has been maintained and has served as the prototype for over 150 free clinics throughout the world.

THE CHANGING POPULATION PATTERNS AND THE EVOLUTION OF THE HAIGHT-ASHBURY JUNKIE

The initial psychedelic phase of the hippie community has been mentioned. At that time, the use of amphetamines and heroin was negligible. With the summer of 1967, however, came the influx of thousands upon thousands of young people, transients of widely divergent background, motivation, and drug experience, drawn to the "Mecca of the Psychedelic World," as the mass media called it. Each week, as hundreds came seeking this psychedelic experience, and as other hundreds moved on, the "core" hippie influence was seen to be diluted and waning. The population of the Haight-Ashbury might normally be three to four thousand people, yet on each day of that disastrous summer might be found twenty to twenty-five thousand young adventurers. Haight Street on a weekend was literally wall-to-wall kids. The "core" psychedelic hippie moved away or he moved "underground." The neighborhood was now noisy and crowded; the quiet, pastoral, nonthreatening environment appropriate to a "good" trip was no longer available, nor were there an adequate number of experienced LSD "guides" or "gurus" for those seeking "mind expansion" or "cosmic awareness." Abortive or "bad" trips or "bummers" (acute anxiety reactions) resulted. The use of amphetamines tended to help relieve the anxiety so produced, and barbiturates and heroin were turned to more and more often as "downers" for a bad trip.

By the time of Shick's first survey (1968)[7] of the Haight-Ashbury population, a trend toward "speed" was to be noted. One hundred and forty (34.1%) of his total sample of 413 respondents had tried using amphetamines by intravenous administration at least once. Thirty of those (7.3% of the total population sample) were at that time "abusing" the drug. Thus the summer explorers and the thrill seekers had moved on, and the purist, ritual psychedelic users were being replaced by a population rapidly turning to amphetamines.

Certainly the "multiple drug abuse" theory (the person who abuses one drug is likely to abuse others, either concurrently or at a later time) must be considered as being integral to the Haight-Ashbury population. The LSD abuser (quiet, mystical, introspective, nonviolent) in many cases later developed an abusive amphetamine habit, whereupon he became gregarious, talkative, hyperactive, and as his intravenous habit developed and continued, often became paranoid and violent (that is, he might develop a true toxic psychosis, a major break with reality, which might have many of the characteristics of a paranoid or schizophrenic reaction). If the same individual later became habituated or addicted to barbiturates, he would develop the signs of the "doper"; he would become lethargic, withdrawn, and dull, develop sloppy mannerisms of dress and posture; he might drool, "nod out," or burn holes in his clothing with his cigarette. The "doper," with the possible exception of the "glue sniffer," is the least highly regarded of all drug abusers.

Following the psychedelic scene, then, came the "speed" scene, and right on its heels the "barb" scene—indeed we regard this as the "upper-downer" phase. This is pharmacologically quite predictable (sociologically as well, if we take a look at the ads on TV or take a peek into our own medicine cabinet, where a microcosm of the "street" drug scene can be found in Mom's reducing pills and sleeping pills). Indeed, the compulsive use of barbiturates (with the life-threatening convulsions and hyperpyrexia of its abstinence or "kicking" syndrome) was increasingly seen, as was the ominous appearance of an increasing use of heroin. (Barbiturates and heroin are recognized by the street-wise drug user as natural "downers" for coming off a bum acid trip or a "speed run.")

The composition of the population of the Haight-Ashbury has proven to be a selective end-process in itself; as one type of drug user appeared, another was pushed out or pushed "underground." As Smith[8] has noted, "Speed *always* drives out acid, as in the broader society the violence dominates the higher aspirations of nonviolence, peace, and love." The psychedelic scene proved vulnerable in its inability to withstand crowds, curiosity seekers, and the violent characteristics innate in an urban area (also the LSD advocate discovered that repeated use led to tolerance and decreased psychedelic experience) ; so also the "speed" scene was self-limited by its own intensity. Also to be considered is the very real hippie-engendered slogan that "speed kills," with the ravages of malnutrition and hepatitis. The very exhaustion of a "speed run," with the ultimate profound depression after "crashing" and the knowledge of possible amphetamine psychoses,[9] led many users into a "speed-barb" sequence and others to experiment increasingly with heroin.

The dynamics of drug abuse in the Haight-Ashbury has shown an undeniable and escalating swing to heroin since August of 1969. Before that time, an average of from two to four heroin addicts were seen at the clinic each week with symptoms of withdrawal and were subsequently treated. This number has gradually increased, when sometimes sixty such patients are seen each afternoon. In an effort to respond to this tremendous increase in patients seeking heroin detoxification, we have now established a heroin clinic with around the clock services and have brought together a specialized volunteer team of physicians, nurses, psychologists, job rehabilitation experts, social workers and ex-addicts, to provide as complete a psycho social and medical facility as possible.

THE CONCEPT OF OUTPATIENT ADDICT CARE

Several factors led us to the conclusion that ambulatory outpatient treatment was not only feasible but perhaps ideal for our population. These were (a) the emergence, almost *de novo,* of heroin use of epidemic proportion, creating a need for treatment facilities far in excess of existing and traditional institutional facilities (b) the nature of the patient population, generally an individual with a small, short-term habit (if Dole and Nyswander's group[11-14] of screened hard-core, mainline New York addicts were ideal for long-term or life-term methadone maintenance treatment, surely our group was ideally suited for a trial of short-term outpatient detoxification), (c) the acceptance of the Haight-Ashbury Free Clinic as an integral part of the "hip" community.

With the passage of the Harrison Tax Act in December 1914, the opiate addict was effectively cut off from his heretofore unrestricted purchase of drugs. This revenue act, originally intended as a means to abolish opium smuggling and indiscriminate over-the-counter sale of narcotics, was soon to assume a much more significant and ominous role in creating the "criminal addict" (and it is a postulate that the length of the criminal record of each addict is directly proportional to the length of time he has been into the drug scene and is isolating him from medical and psychosocial supervision and care.[15-17]) The addicts affected at that time were (a) individuals with chronic painful disease (rheumatism and so forth), (b) users of patent nostrums or "cure-alls" containing opiates (this included a lot of middle-American housewives), and (c) some Chinese opium smokers. Public concern for these people led to the setting up of public clinics (some forty-four were in operation between 1919 and 1923) to offer outpatient narcotic therapy.[18] The clinics of Florida, Louisiana, and California could be considered reasonably successful; however, the New York clinics were a disaster of poor organization and supervision, creating such adverse publicity (aided by the open criticism of the Federal Bureau of Narcotics and crusading newspaper editors eager to draw on this "scandal") that all such clinics were forced to close by 1923. The "hard line" of the Federal Bureau of Narcotics, picturing the addict as a thankful "dope fiend" unwilling to respond to humane medical treatment and a threat to society (therefore deserving of the harshest penal sanctions), helped to complete the transformation of victim to criminal. Cut off from outpatient medical care, the addict was faced with the choices of locked institutionalization, "cold turkey" withdrawal, or turning to the underworld for his drug supply.

Although imperfect in many ways, it would appear that the clinics certainly did not receive fair or adequate trial. Edwards[19] has stated: "The American system of 'ambulatory' treatment failed because of lack of resolute determination to implement it." The A.M.A. stated, in a resolution of 1924 (which it reaffirmed in 1957), that both federal and state governments should exert their full powers and authority to put an end to all manner of so-called ambulatory methods of therapy. (In 1957, however, the A.M.A. pondered the fact that the reasons for closing the clinics originally were "obscure.")

Today, some forty-eight years later, the time is long overdue to reexamine our past failures and to reconsider the efficacy of multiple methods of outpatient treatment of addiction. It is abundantly clear that (a) institutional programs have failed to establish a broad base of effective treatment; the recidivism rate is appalling—out in the morning and 'back on the spoon' before "noon"—and (b) law enforcement has failed either to stop the flow of drugs or to incarcerate all users. We are left with a medical and social problem of staggering dimensions.

In the past seven years, an increasing number of outpatient programs utilizing methadone as a heroin substitute have proven their practicability.[14,15,20] Patients in such programs are encouraged to pursue their jobs, their education, and in general to stretch their capabilities to the limit.

Merry[16] has stated that "the outpatient centre is not just a place where drugs are prescribed—it should also provide the very important preparatory stage of a formidable treatment programme." We at the Haight-Ashbury Free Clinic have adopted this as a working philosophy for our approach to outpatient heroin detoxification.

THE YEAR OF THE MIDDLE-CLASS JUNKIE

1970 has been called the year of the emergence of the "Middle-Class Junkie."[10] As we have been evolving for several years into a full-blown heroin scene, we can see how this phenomenon has been silently evolving for several years in white middle America. No longer is heroin abuse safely hidden in urban ghettos, the drug of economically underprivileged ethnic minorities. We find that this new-style addict consists largely of alienated youth of white and blue-collar background.

This new population is reflected in the Haight-Ashbury subculture by the now disenchanted "flower children" of the sixties and by their younger brothers and sisters who have followed them. The Haight-Ashbury, along with New York's East Village, has proven to be an epicenter of youthful drug abuse.[3,7,10,21] In such centers, patterns are established and then predictably "ripple" out to involve other parts of the country. The drug user in the Haight has traditionally been six to eighteen months ahead of his counterparts elsewhere in the country. We have seen this pattern repeat itself with heroin abuse (the heroin epidemic).

We have now moved full-blown into the heroin scene. Heroin is regarded by rebellious youth as the ultimate in drug abuse; it is the drug of the black ghetto and of the underworld. Heroin is Nirvana, offering surcease of all pain, discomfort, and frustration. The "stoned" feeling induced by heroin is likened to the peaceful, withdrawn feeling after a satisfying meal or the total-body warmth and relaxation induced by a hot bath. It is a protopathic sensation similar to the most satisfying sexual orgasm but many times longer-lasting and achieved virtually instantly with little physical effort and no intense personal involvement (viz. the giving or receiving of love). As a tranquilizer it is nonpareil[22] smoothing out the hassles and anxieties of everyday living. Certainly there is a new widespread availability of heroin in our particular drug-prone society. Also, because of the excellent tranquilizing and analgesic properties described, heroin is repeatedly turned to as a "social anesthetic" by many of our patients.[1] In an environment which, for whatever reason, has become intolerable to them, it affords a most convenient and effective escape mechanism.[23] As one of our young patients noted, "It's like a finance plan which allows you to consolidate all of your problems into one—Junk!—and then the injection in your arm makes them all go away."

Since 1967 the Haight-Ashbury Free Clinic has provided the primary (and often the only) available source of health care to the young people of the dope scene in the Haight. It is not surprising, therefore, that we were the first to detect and institute outpatient treatment for the rising tide of heroin addiction.[10] Over 90 percent of all patients now seen in our drug unit are heroin addicts; we employ no "screening" or other social service devices designed to discourage utilization of the program by the patient.[21]

NONNARCOTIC OUTPATIENT HEROIN DETOXIFICATION[10]

The junkie's whole day is given over to the "hassle" for heroin. He steals, deals (sells), or prostitutes to get it.[24] Psychologically, the rapidity of the downward spiral into the criminal-sick self-image is truly remarkable. He usually "shoots up" two to three "bags" or "balloons" per day. A $15-$25 bag in the Haight-Ashbury weighs about 350 to 400 mg and is between one to ten percent pure heroin—the remainder of the "junk" (aptly named) being quinine, powdered sugar, powdered coffee, or you-name-it; if he is "marked" for a "hot shot" it might be strychnine or arsenic. Thus a $75-a-day heroin habit might be (generously speaking) about 20 to 50 mg of pure heroin. Considering the recommended medical dose for surgical pain relief to be about 3 or 4 mg, we see a person who has literally anesthetized himself; so it is little wonder that he fails to recognize the warning pains of abscessed teeth, pelvic inflammatory disease, or even ruptured appendix.

All patients are accepted for a trial of ambulatory treatment. Since methadone is illegal in California except in certain designated research centers, withdrawal is treated symptomatically with various nonnarcotic medications. Each patient is seen daily, re-evaluated, and his medications readjusted accordingly. He is questioned about the intensity of each symptom (experienced now and in previous withdrawals), and this history forms the rough basis for his therapeutic regime. There exists a subtle sophistication among "street" drug users, and often they have firmly fixed ideas about what sleeping pill or tranquilizer "works" for them; they are subsequently encouraged (within logical limits) to name their own drugs.

Our medical regime of detoxification is thus aimed at providing symptomatic treatment via multiple "mild" medications. We recommend "sick leave" if the patient has a job that requires coordination and manual dexterity. This has not been a major problem since 75 percent of our patients are unemployed at the time of treatment.

Basically, we treat four symptom complexes. (One articulate patient described his symptoms as those of "super-flu.") In general we must treat (a) pain (muscle, joint, and bone "aches"), (b) sleeplessness, (c) nervousness or jitteriness, and (d) gastrointestinal complaints.

For the young patient without other major medical complications, abrupt withdrawal from heroin may be discomforting in the extreme, but nonetheless presents no life-threatening crises (such as the convulsions and hyperpyrexia occasionally seen with alcohol-tranquilizer-barbiturate withdrawal). During acute heroin withdrawal, the patient may experience sialorrhea with runny eyes and nose; fever, chills, and diaphoresis; nausea, vomiting, abdominal cramps, and diarrhea; photophobia due to dilatation of the pupils; musculoskeletal pains and cramps; jitteriness and insomnia to a marked degree. These symptoms make their appearance from 6 to 8 hours after the last "fix," are maximal at from 24 to 36 hours, and in the main, have largely subsided after five days. Insomnia, general irritability, and muscular aches and pains gradually lessen over the ensuing days and weeks.

As the physical symptoms subside, every effort is made to involve each patient in the available psychiatric and social aftercare services.

The agents employed for pain relief have been Darvon® (propoxyphene) 130 mg, or Talwin® (pentazocine) 100 mg every 4 hours. The patient is warned not to take Talwin until at least 12 hours after his last "fix," lest the narcotic antagonist properties of this drug throw him into "instant cold turkey." It has also been our experience that when we have prescribed Talwin in conjunction with Thorazine® (chlorpromazine), a high incidence of hallucinations and "spaciness" has been noted. In some milder cases of withdrawal (and symptomatology *is* very often time and dosage related), various aspirin compounds have been successfully utilized. For muscle spasms we have on occasion employed Soma® (carisoprodol) in recommended dosage.

To combat sleeplessness, two hypnotic agents have been employed with good results: chloral hydrate in doses up to 2.5 gm, and Noludar® (methyprylen) in doses up to 900 mg. Doriden® (glutethimide) was tried initially but was discovered to be a desired drug of abuse.

For nervousness, phenobarbital 30 mg, Valium® (diazepam) 5 to 10 mg, or Librium® (chlordiazepoxide) 10 to 25 mg are given to be taken three or four times daily. Meprobamate is avoided because of its addicting and abuse potential.

For gastrointestinal symptoms our patients are treated with Bel-Phen #3 (8 mg belladonna and 15 mg phenobarbital) or Bentyl® (10 mg dicyclomine and 15 mg phenobarbital) or Antrenyl® (5 mg oxyphenonium and 15 mg phenobarbital), two tablets to be taken every 4 hours. For patients with a real "stomach habit" (pronounced nausea and vomiting) Compazine® (prochloroperazine) 5 mg is given every 4 hours.

The drugs that we recognize as those of special abuse potential (Doriden, Valium, Talwin) are usually dispensed by day-to-day small-quantity prescription. If dispensed more indiscriminately, these drugs soon find themselves on the open street market.

In accordance with the "Madison Avenue" approach to the marketing and dispensing of street medications and perhaps as an extension of the great American ethic of "pills for all ills," many of our patients are found to be self-medicating their symptoms of withdrawal with marijuana, beer, wine, barbiturates ("reds," "yellows," or "rainbows"), codeine, or any number of varieties of narcotic preparations.

From the inception of our therapy, psychosocial intervention is mandatory if we are to hope to restructure a useful lifestyle. Thus we utilize *whatever* facilities are available, whether they be halfway houses, group or individual psychotherapy, or job-placement services.

INTERVIEW AND PSYCHOSOCIAL SURVEY

On his initial visit, each patient is asked a series of questions by a clinic staff member (usually a graduate student in psychology) regarding his social situation and drug usage. Heavy use of other drugs is particularly questioned, as are simultaneous and sequential drug patterns. The figures presented in this report are based on evaluation of 1254 of these medical records, gathered between November 1969 and January 1971.[21]

RESULTS

In reviewing the statistics (Fig. 12.1), one thing that became immediately apparent was the large number of patients with a history of relatively recent addiction: 76.2 percent of our addict population first began using heroin after January 1964 and 56.2 percent first began using after January 1967.

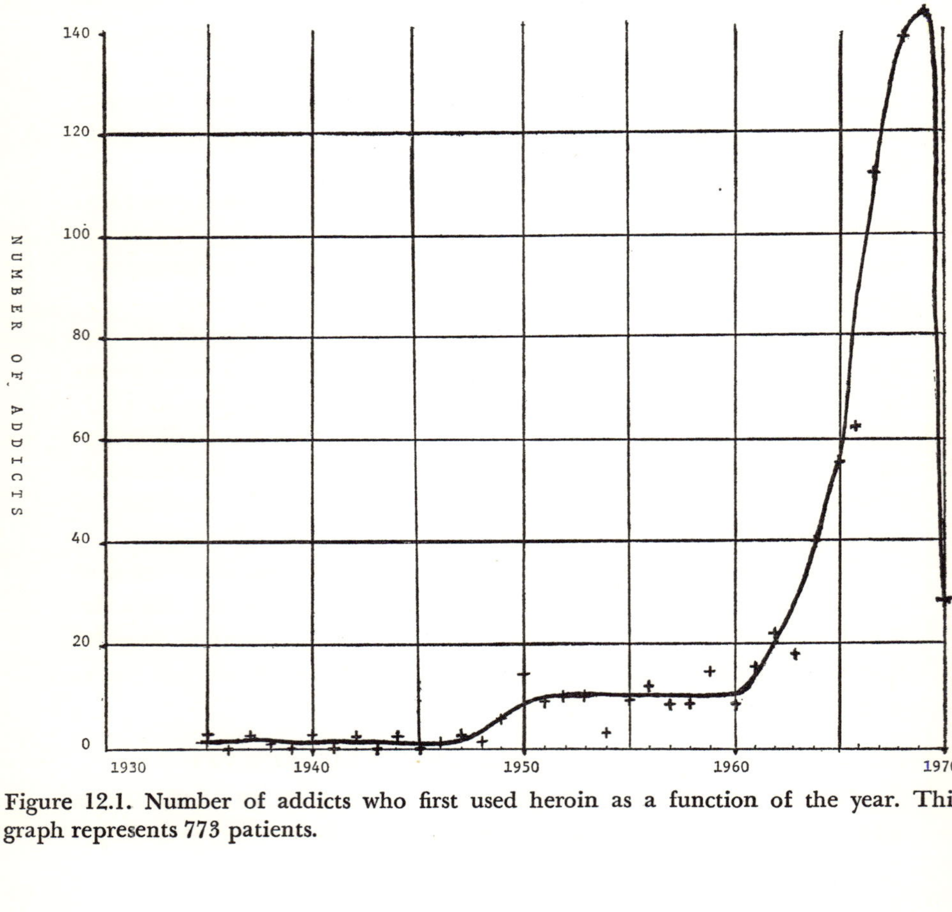

Figure 12.1. Number of addicts who first used heroin as a function of the year. This graph represents 773 patients.

The subsegments noted were as follows (Table 12.1) :

1. The "New Junkie" (NJ), who began using heroin after January 1967.

TABLE 12.1
TOTAL ADDICT SUBSEGMENT

New Junkie (NJ)	704	(56.2%)
Transitional Junkie (TJ)	251	(20.0%)
Old-Style Junkie (OSJ)	299	(23.4%)

2. The "Transition Junkie" (TJ), who first began using between January 1964 and January 1967.

3. The "Old-Style Junkie" (OSJ), who began using prior to January 1964.

The largest segment (704) is made up of those addicts who first used heroin after January 1967 ("New Junkie," or NJ). These addicts have a mean age of 23.5 years, 74.4 percent were first "hooked" on the West Coast (mainly San Francisco or Los Angeles), and 91.5 percent have habits of less than $100 a day (Table 12.2). The NJ's were generally rather heavily involved with other drugs prior to using heroin, with 67 percent reporting heavy prior use of marijuana, 51.1 percent having used "speed" (amphetamines) heavily, and 30 percent having used "barbs" heavily (mainly Seconal® and Nembutal®) (Table 12.3). They average only 1.2 withdrawals each prior to their first clinic visit; of these, 50 percent were done "cold," 18.1 percent were self-treated, and only 9.8 percent were attempted with the help of a physician (Table 12.4).

TABLE 12.2
NUMBER OF ADDICTS (PERCENTAGE OF SUBSEGMENT) WITH EACH RANGE OF HABIT SIZE

		Size of Habit (Dollars per Day)									
		Less than $60		*$50-$99*		*$100-$200*		*More than $200*		*Total*	
Addict	NJ	474	(67.5%)	169	(24.0%)	57	(8.0%)	4	(0.5%)	704	(100%)
Subseg-	TJ	133	(53.0%)	73	(29.1%)	41	(16.3%)	4	(1.6%)	251	(100%)
ment	OSJ	142	(47.5%)	100	(33.4%)	51	(17.0%)	6	(2.0%)	299	(100%)

TABLE 12.3
DRUGS USED HEAVILY PRIOR TO HEROIN

		Marijuana		*LSD*		*Amphetamines*		*Barbiturates*		*Alcohol*		*Cocaine*		*Opium*	
Addict	NJ	471	(67.0%)	311	(44.2%)	359	(51.1%)	211	(30.0%)	186	(26.4%)	41	(5.9%)	6	(0.9%)
Subseg-	TJ	165	(66.0%)	112	(44.6%)	128	(51.0%)	69	(27.6%)	73	(29.2%)	18	(7.2%)	6	(2.4%)
ment	OSJ	145	(48.5%)	42	(14.1%)	84	(28.2%)	62	(20.8%)	70	(23.2%)	15	(5.0%)	7	(2.2%)

TABLE 12.4
METHOD USED TO WITHDRAW

		Cold		*Methadone*		*Self Rx'd*		*M.D. Rx'd*		*Total*		*Withdrawals per addict*
Addict	NJ	425	(50.0%)	186	(22.1%)	152	(18.1%)	83	(9.8%)	846	(100%)	1.20
Subsegment	TJ	250	(48.0%)	102	(19.7%)	133	(25.0%)	38	(7.3%)	523	(100%)	2.32
	OSJ	435	(52.9%)	168	(20.4%)	123	(14.9%)	98	(11.8%)	824	(100%)	2.77

Note. Methadone includes both "street" and physician administered. Percentages refer to percentage of total withdrawals for each addict group.

The smallest (251), and in many ways the most ambiguous segment of our population, we have chosen to call the "Transition Junkie" (TJ). He began regular use of heroin between January 1964 and January 1967. He really has very little in common with the "Old-Style Junkie" (OSJ), his background being much closer to that of the NJ, but at the time he entered the "drug scene" the social attitude of his subculture was optimistic and very much into drug "experimentation and "mind expansion."[1]

In comparison with the OSJ, the TJ and the NJ have a significantly greater past history of heavy use of all the common "street" drugs (Table 12.3) (viz.: marijuana, "acid," "speed," barbiturates). In many cases the TJ first tried heroin as an experiment "to see what it felt like." Later, as both his personal and his subculture's fortunes took a downward course, and as heroin became readily available on the street, he turned to it as an escape.

The TJ also impresses us as a "self-treater." He treats or self-medicates his mental state in much the same way as the dominant culture treats colds and flu. Unfortunately, he is self-medicating himself with much more potent medications. One of the recurrent stories related by these patients is that they first began regular use of heroin to treat depressions following a long "speed run," or as a "downer" for a "bum acid trip."

Upon examination of the methods used to withdraw (Tables 12.4 and 12.5) the TJ figure becomes distinctive in that he has a lower percentage of "cold" withdrawals (48.0% of his withdrawals are "cold" vs. 50% for the NJ and 52.9% for the OSJ), and he has more "selfmedicated" withdrawals (25% vs. the NJ's 18.1% and the OSJ's 14.9%). He self-treats almost 25 percent of these withdrawals (which is one-half as many as the percentage treated by the OSJ and one and one-half times the percentage treated by the NJ).

TABLE 12.5
NUMBER OF WITHDRAWALS PRIOR TO SEEKING HELP AT THE HAIGHT-ASHBURY FREE CLINIC

		0		*1*		*2*		*3*		*4*	
Addict	NJ	251	(35.5%)	180	(25.6)	116	(16.5%)	45	(6.4%)	112	(16.0%)
Sub-	TJ	30	(12.0%)	47	(18.7%)	47	(18.7%)	37	(14.6%)	90	(36.0%)
segment	OSJ	29	(9.7%)	30	(10.0%)	39	(13.0%)	28	(9.3%)	173	(58.0%)

TABLE 12.6
NUMBER OF ADDICTS (PERCENTAGE OF SUBSEGMENT) IN EACH FAMILY SITUATION

		Family Status											
		Single		*Married*		*Cohabitation*		*Divorced*		*Widowed*		*Separated*	
	NJ	351	(50.0%)	178	(25.0%)	113	(16.1%)	26	(3.7%)	4	(0.6%)	32	(4.6%)
Addict	TJ	127	(50.6%)	60	(24.0%)	31	(12.4%)	22	(8.8%)	1	(0.4%)	10	(3.8%)
Subsegment	OSJ	97	(32.4%)	96	(32.2%)	21	(7.0%)	48	(16.0%)	10	(3.4%)	27	(9.0%)

The TJ is less apt to be divorced or separated than the OSJ but is more apt to be single (Table 12.6). That is, the TJ is less apt to have established family ties or permanent relationships.

The third segment (299 addicts) is that of the "Old-Style Junkie" (OSJ), who has a long-term "heavy" habit and who first used heroin regularly prior to January 1964. Of the OSJ's, 63.6 percent were hooked on the West Coast and 19.0 percent have a habit of more than $100 a day. They are more apt to be divorced or separated but less likely to have remained single, with the breakup occurring during an attempted withdrawal, when the couple discovers that their only common bond is a heroin life style.[24]

The OSJ has more children to support (Table 12.7) than do the other groups (25.7% have two or more children vs. 12.0% for the NJ and 13.8% for the TJ). This group is predominantly ghetto-bred (Table 12.8), with a higher proportion of nonwhites (38.8% are nonwhite vs. 33.6% of the TJ's and 19.4% of the NJ's).

The OSJ was significantly less involved (Table 12.3) in heavy prior use of marijuana, "acid" (also mescaline and other psychedelics), and "speed" than were their more contemporary counterparts. Interestingly, the OSJ has less prior involvement with heavy alcohol usage. Several have expressed the feeling that "alcohol is a downer" which increases their feelings of depression, and it may be this feeling that accounts for this lesser degree of involvement.

The OSJ's habit (Table 12.2) is more likely to be over $100 a day than the NJ (19.0% vs 8.5%) or the TJ (17.9%) and less apt to be less than $50 a day (47.5% vs. 67.5% for the NJ and 53.0% for the TJ). There does appear to be a limiting factor as to habit size, because in all three groups only 1 percent to 2 percent of the habits were greater than $200 a day. This is a reflection

TABLE 12.7

NUMBER OF ADDICTS (PERCENTAGE OF SUBSEGMENT) WHO ARE SUPPORTING VARIOUS NUMBERS OF CHILDREN

		0		*1*		*2*		*3*		*4 or more*	
	NJ	504	(71.4%)	115	(16.4%)	45	(6.4%)	22	(3.1%)	18	(2.5%)
Addict	TJ	172	(67.8%)	46	(18.4%)	14	(5.8%)	10	(4.1%)	9	(3.9%)
Subsegment	OSJ	162	(54.2%)	60	(20.1%)	29	(9.7%)	24	(8.0%)	24	(8.0%)

TABLE 12.8
RACIAL DISTRIBUTION OF HEROIN POPULATION IN HAIGHT-ASHBURY

		White		*Black*		*Mexican-American*		*Oriental*		*Indian*		*Mixed*	
Addict	NJ	561	(80.6%)	103	(14.7%)	33	(4.7%)	5	(0.7%)	2	(0.2%)	0	
Subsegment	TJ	167	(66.4%)	60	(24.0%)	20	(8.0%)	3	(1.2%)	0		1	(0.4%)
	OSJ	183	(61.2%)	78	(26.2%)	33	(11.0%)	4	(1.3%)	0		1	(0.4%)

of the social and economic reality that in order to sustain a habit of this size, the addict must become a substantial "dealer," resort to extensive burglary, or engage in daily prostitution (all of which greatly increase risks of arrest).

This limiting effect on cost leads to a relatively fixed habit ceiling for most addicts. Under these conditions (coupled with the predictable development of tolerance), the addict is soon "fixing" not for a "high" or euphoria but rather only to prevent the development of an abstinence syndrome (or withdrawal state). "I just fix enough to stay well now, doc."

There are several areas in which changes are seen to progress in an orderly manner from the OSJ through the TJ to the NJ. One of these areas is the increasing percentage of female addicts (Table 12.9). A similar progression is seen in the decreasing number of dependent children from the OSJ to the NJ (Table 12.7).

TABLE 12.9
SEX DISTRIBUTION OF ADDICTS

		Male		*Female*	
Addict Subsegment	NJ	467	(66.3%)	237	(33.7%)
	TJ	197	(78.5%)	54	(21.5%)
	OSJ	253	(84.5%)	46	(15.5%)

The NJ averages 1.2 withdrawals each, the TJ averages 2.32, and the OSJ averages 2.27 (Ttable 12.4). That is, with increasing duration of habit or earlier use there comes an increasing number of withdrawals.

The older addicts (TJ and OSJ) show a higher percentage of patients who were first "hooked" elsewhere than the West Coast (36.4% for the OSJ and 35% for the TJ vs. 25.6% for the NJ) (Table 12.10). This probably reflects the mobility of the American population rather than a fundamental difference in the addict group. Since, however, the drug scene differs in various parts of the country at different times, this mobility makes it more difficult to evaluate the effects of culture on the background of our patients.

In terms of therapeutic results (Table 12.11), the older addict (OSJ) has a lower "cure" rate but shows a higher percentage who

TABLE 12.10
LOCATION WHERE FIRST "HOOKED"

		West Coast	*East Coast*	*Southwest*	*Midwest*	*Foreign*	*Army*	*Unknown*
Addict	NJ	524 (74.4%)	56 (7.9%)	4 (0.6%)	15 (2.1%)	5 (0.7%)	2 (0.3%)	98 (14.0%)
Subsegment	TJ	163 (65.0%)	37 (14.8%)	2 (0.8%)	6 (2.4%)	2 (0.8%)	3 (1.2%)	38 (15.2%)
	OSJ	190 (63.6%)	44 (14.8%)	4 (1.3%)	8 (2.6%)	4 (1.3%)	7 (2.3%)	42 (14.1%)

Note. The West Coast is mainly San Francisco and Los Angeles, and the East Coast is mainly New York City.

TABLE 12.11
THERAPEUTIC STATUS OF THE VARIOUS SEGMENTS OF THE HAIGHT-ASHBURY HEROIN ADDICT POPULATION

		Clean		*Markedly Improved*		*Lost to Follow-Up*		*In Treatment*	
Addict	NJ	37	(5.3%)	120	(17.0%)	452	(64.2%)	95	(13.5%)
Subsegment	TJ	21	(8.4%)	31	(12.3%)	178	(70.9%)	21	(8.4%)
	OSJ	18	(6.0%)	67	(22.4%)	169	(56.5%)	45	(15.0%)

Note. "Clean" indicates those patients that have not used for at least one month. "Markedly improved" indicates using no more than once a week (i.e. use as a tranquilizer for relief of intolerable tension) and no evidence of abstinence syndrome.

remain in treatment and a lower "lost to follow-up" percentage. This tendency of the OSJ to stick with therapy longer is reflected in the number of clinic visits (Fig. 12.2). The OSJ group has a higher percentage of patients with more than ten visits when compared with either of the other two groups. Of the OSJ group, 48.4 percent make less than three clinic visits (vs. 48.5% for the TJ and 53.4% of the NJ's). In more concise terms, the OSJ is a more "faithful" patient and gives therapy a longer trial before rejecting it.

Figure 12.2 demonstrates a definite (but statistically nonsignificant) trend toward increasing age of first use of heroin. This is rather startling in view of the rather widely reported drug usage (including heroin) in the high-school and younger populations[25,26] and would seem to indicate that these younger patients are not seeking help at our clinic. There are several possible explanations for this phenomenon: First, the younger drug users may not be seeking help; indeed, we believe that there is a "lag phase" of about one year between the first use of heroin and that time when socioeconomic desperation and psychological pain drives the young addict to seek professional help. Secondly, as a characteristic of adolescence, this group will have a distrust of all adults, even in such an accepted community project as the Haight-Ashbury Clinic. Thirdly, their main motivation to seek medical help may be parental and this is more likely to lead to private medical or psychiatric help than to a clinic. Finally, it is unlawful in

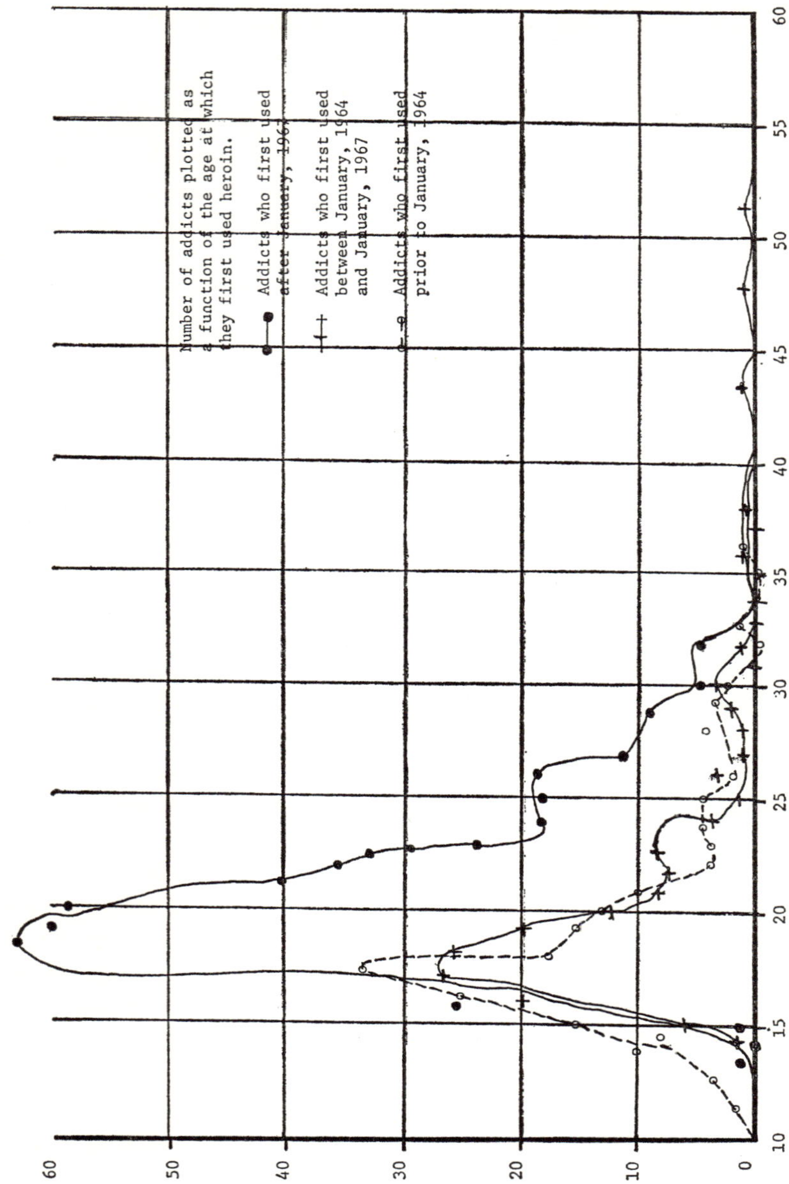

Figure 12.2. Age of first heroin use. This graph represents 773 patients.

California to treat patients under 18 without parental consent; thus very many underage patients report their age as 18 or older.[27]

DISCUSSION

In the population of heroin addicts seen by the Haight-Ashbury Drug Detoxification Section from its opening in November of 1969 until January of 1971, there have emerged three overlapping but distinct addict-group types (1254 medical and social histories are reviewed here). We call these subsegments "New Junkie" (NJ), "Transition Junkie" (TJ), and "Old-Style Junkie" (OSJ).

Because of similar background, age, and prior life style, we group the NJ and the TJ together as the "Middle-Class Junkie." Distinct differences in these two groups, however, are noted.

The "New Junkie" is one predominantly of white middle-class background who entered the drug scene at a time of sociological and political disillusionment (the "flower children" had gone and the Haight-Ashbury neighborhood had deteriorated) and who pharmacologically "dropped out" with the perfect drug of escape, heroin. "It's a womb trip." Contingent upon the law of supply and demand, heroin now has widespread availability; consequently, the more recent addict tended to get into heroin with less prior involvement in the heavy use of other drugs than did his TJ counterpart. The NJ has engaged in less drug "experimentation before settling" on heroin. He is more aware of some of the dangers of the "street" drugs (having seen the effects on the TJ) and he is less of a self-medicator than the TJ.

The "Transition Junkie," with a similar family and social background to the NJ, differs mainly in the effects of the social atmosphere of the drug subculture of the Haight-Ashbury that existed when he first came upon the scene. He passed through a period of multiple drug experimentation (e.g. the psychedelics, the "mind expanders," and the amphetamines). He has "tried all drugs" and he tends to be a self-medicator.

The TJ has an attitude of distrust of the medical profession in general (this couples with the medical profession's lack of interest in treating him: he is unreliable and he cannot pay). This leaves the addict with little recourse except withdrawing either by "cold turkey" (which is the method of the OSJ), by institutionalization in a state hospital, or by self-medication. The TJ has been raised in a culture in which the mass media advertise, and the public swallow, a theory of multiple medication; therefore he finds available a wide range of potent "street" medications. This attitude may be summarized by relating a typical case. The patient is a 20-year-old female who began using heroin in 1966. She related a history of two previous withdrawals which she had self-medicated with "speed," which tended not to alleviate her symptoms but indeed made them much worse. "But I *had* to use something and 'speed' was all I had." Once again we see the belief that a pill, any pill, will make one better.

The older addict (OSJ) is distinguished from both the NJ and the TJ by many factors, including background, prior use, duration of habit, number of withdrawals, family status, percentage of females, and race. They also differ in therapeutic response, with the older addict being a more "faithful" patient but one who is less likely (not statistically significant) to get "clean" than his newer counterparts.

SUMMARY

Since November of 1969, we at the Haight-Ashbury Medical Clinic have noted a marked increase in patients seeking relief from symptoms of heroin withdrawal. The results of a review of 1254 of these charts reveal three groups with rather distinctive characteristics. We have titled these groups or subsegments the "New Junkie" (NJ), who began using heroin after January 1967, the "Transition Junkie" (TJ), who began using between January 1964 and January 1967, and the "Old-Style Junkie" (OSJ), who began using heroin prior to January 1964.

Hopefully, these classifications will provide useful insight into the background and attitudes of the heroin addicts being seen today. They should prove useful to the local physician as the "ripple" effect from such drug abuse centers as the Haight-Ashbury reaches his area. In the future, these classifications may be significant in terms of program and therapy designs. They may

TABLE 12.12

NUMBER OF PATIENTS (PERCENTAGE OF SUBSEGMENT) MAKING A GIVEN NUMBER OF CLINIC VISITS

		Number of Clinic Visits											
		1		*2*		*3*		*4*		*5-10*		*10 or more*	
Addict	NJ	234	(33.4%)	143	(20.0%)	88	(12.6%)	58	(8.2%)	125	(17.8%)	56	(8.0%)
Subsegment	TJ	84	(33.4%)	39	(15.5%)	35	(13.5%)	11	(4.3%)	55	(21.9%)	27	(10.8%)
	OSJ	99	(33.1%)	46	(15.3%)	37	(12.3%)	20	(6.7%)	56	(19.0%)	41	(13.6%)

also serve as a useful predictive function in patient selection for various follow-up therapies, allowing for better medical care for this long neglected and ignored patient population. The current trend in treatment of the narcotics abuser is a "multimodality" approach, but we feel that this concept can reach its full potential only if careful attention is given to selection of the proper modality for a particular style of junkie.

APPENDIX

HEROIN STATISTICS FOR 1254 PATIENTS
NOVEMBER 1969 TO JANUARY 1971

Sex		
Male	917	(73%)
Female	337	(27%)

Age		
Less than 20	95	(7.5%)
20 to 25	652	(51.7%)
26 to 30	254	(20.2%)
31 to 40	180	(14.7%)
Over 40	73	(5.8%)
Oldest patient was age 78		

Residence		
Haight-Ashbury	214	(17.0%)
San Francisco (other than the Haight)	745	(58.5%)
Out of town	284	(23.6%)
Unknown	11	(0.9%)

Size of Habit		
Less than $50 per day	749	(60.%)
$50 to $100	342	(27.4%)
$100 to $200	149	(11.8%)
Over $200	14	(1.1%)
Largest habit reported was over $400 per day		

Duration of Habit		
3 months or less	33	(2.6%)
3 to 6 months	77	(6.2%)
6 months to one year	281	(22.4%)
One year to three years	420	(33.4%)
Three years and over	433	(35.4%)

Race		
White	911	(73%)
Black	241	(19.3%)
Mexican-American	86	(6.9%)
Oriental	12	(0.95%)
American Indian	3	(0.24%)

Family Status		
Single	575	(46%)
Married	334	(26.6%)
Cohabitation	165	(13.2%)
Separated	69	(5.5%)
Divorced	96	(7.6%)
Widowed	15	(1.2%)

Dependent Children		
None	838	(67%)
One	221	(17.6%)
Two	88	(7.0%)
Three	56	(4.5%)
Four or more	51	(4.1%)

Age First Used Heroin		
Under age 15	38	(3.03%)
15 to 19	630	(51%)
20 to 25	442	(35.8%)
26 to 30	99	(8.0%)
Over 30	41	(1.9%)
Over 50	4	(0.3%)

Previous Withdrawal History		
None	310	(24.5%)
One	257	(20.3%)
Two	202	(16.2%)
Three	110	(8.6%)
Four	93	(7.5%)
Five or more	287	(23.0%)
2193 withdrawals reported		

How Withdrew

"Cold"	1110	(51%)
Methadone (both M.D.-administered and self-medicated	456	(21%)
Self-medication ("street drugs" other than methadone)	408	(18%)
M.D. medication (other than methadone)	219	(10%)

Job History

Regular job	318	(25.2%)
Not working	932	(74.8%)
Lost a job due to habit	332	(26.4%)

Withdrawal Symptoms Most Commonly Reported

NO SYMPTOMS	50	(4.0%)
Sleeplessness	866	(69.0%)
Jittery (nervousness)	773	(61.5%)
Nausea and/or vomiting	773	(61.5%)
Muscle cramps	768	(61.0%)
Abdominal cramps	665	(51.8%)
Runny eyes and nose	704	(56.1%)
Joint pains	575	(45.8%)
"Sweats"	506	(40.3%)
Diarrhea	436	(34.7%)
Muscle "twitches"	393	(31.3%)
"Hot and cold flashes"	393	(31.3%)
Headaches	314	(25.0%)
"Skin crawls"	249	(19.8%)
"Chills"	88	(7.0%)
"Bone aches"	72	(5.7%)
"Back aches"	61	(4.9%)
Anxiety	24	(1.9%)
Depression	21	(1.7%)

Symptoms Also Reported

"No energy, blahs"	11	(0.88%)
Generalized "shakes"	9	(0.71%)
Yawning	9	(0.71%)
"Spacey feelings"	9	(0.71%)
"Fever"	9	(0.71%)
Sneezing	7	(0.56%)
Weakness	7	(0.56%)
Convulsions	7	(0.56%)
No appetite	7	(0.56%)
"Foul body odor"	6	(0.48%)
"Body jerks"	6	(0.48%)
"Dry heaves"	6	(0.48%)
"Choking and/or gagging feeling"	5	(0.40%)
"Nerve thing"	5	(0.40%)
Leg cramps	5	(0.40%)
Cough	4	(0.32%)
Nightmares and general restless sleep	4	(0.32%)

"Bile in mouth"	3 (0.24%)
Blurred vision	3 (0.24%)
Stiffness	3 (0.24%)
Constipation	3 (0.24%)
"Suicidal feelings"	3 (0.24%)
"Body itch"	3 (0.24%)
"Gooseflesh"	2 (0.16%)
Toothaches	2 (0.16%)
"Bad attitude in general"	2 (0.16%)
"Irritable"	2 (0.16%)
Hallucinations	2 (0.16%)
"Pain in kidneys"	2 (0.16%)
Dizziness	2 (0.16%)

Other Symptoms Also Reported

"Head thing"	1 (0.8%)
"Fuzzy mind thing"	1 (0.8%)
"Pain in liver"	1 (0.8%)
"Mind short-circuits"	1 (0.8%)
Loss of balance	1 (0.8%)
Profuse menstrual bleeding	1 (0.8%)
"Nerves jump"	1 (0.8%)
"Super bad flu"	1 (0.8%)
"Burning inside"	1 (0.8%)
"Hot rushes"	1 (0.8%)
"Can't breathe"	1 (0.8%)
Bones and muscles "tingle"	1 (0.8%)
"Little wires pulling throughout body"	1 (0.8%)
"Motor running inside"	1 (0.8%)
Hands ache	1 (0.8%)
Toe spasms	1 (0.8%)
"Restless . . Want to get out of my body"	1 (0.8%)
"Paranoia"	1 (0.8%)
Slurred speech	1 (0.8%)
"Bad taste in mouth"	1 (0.8%)
Itchy nose	1 (0.8%)
Neck ache	1 (0.8%)
"Freaked"	1 (0.8%)

"Heavy" Use of Other Drugs Prior to Heroin

NO OTHERS	93 (7.4%)
"Grass"	781 (62.5%)
"Speed"	571 (46.0%)
"Acid"	465 (37.5%)
"Barbs"	342 (27.4%)
Alcohol	324 (26.0%)
Cocaine	74 (5.9%)
Mescaline or peyote	43 (3.4%)

Codeine	37	(2.9%)
Morphine	30	(2.4%)
Hashish	22	(1.7%)
Opium	19	(1.5%)
STP	13	(1.0%)
Doriden	10	(0.8%)
Methadone	9	(0.7%)
Psilocybin	8	(0.64%)
Numorphan®	4	(0.32%)
THC	4	(0.32%)
MDA	1	(0.08%)
PCP, "Peace-Pill"	1	(0.08%)
Nembutal	1	(0.08%)
Valium	1	(0.08%)
Stelazine®	1	(0.08%)
Belladonna	1	(0.08%)
Thorazine	1	(0.08%)
Mellaril®	1	(0.08%)

Other "Street" Drugs Taken When on Heroin, for Self-Attempted Withdrawal or Otherwise

NONE	55	(4.4%)
"Grass"	672	(53.6%)
"Barbs"	427	(33.7%)
Alcohol	401	(32.0%)
Cocaine	197	(15.7%)
"Speed"	113	(9.0%)
"Acid"	76	(6.1%)
Methadone	61	(4.9%)
Morphine	39	(3.1%)
Codeine	35	(2.8%)
Hashish	30	(2.4%)
Mescaline	28	(2.2%)
Opium	26	(2.1%)
Dilaudid®	17	(1.3%)
Valium	14	(1.1%)
Meprobamate	12	(0.96%)
Thorazine	12	(0.96%)
Percodan	10	(0.8%)
Mellaril	10	(0.8%)
Demerol	9	(0.71%)
Dilantin®	5	(0.40%)
Numorphan	4	(0.32%)
Doriden	3	(0.24%)
Darvon	4	(0.32%)
Paregoric	3	(0.23%)
STP	5	(0.40%)
MDA	5	(0.40%)

Robitussin®	2 (0.16%)
Stelazine	2 (0.16%)
THC	2 (0.16%)

Number of Clinic Visits

One	417 (33%)
Two	228 (18.2%)
Three	160 (12.8%)
Four	89 (7.1%)
Five to nine	236 (19.0%)
More than ten	124 (10%)

Aftercare

Drug Treatment Section of Haight-Ashbury Free Clinic (group sessions or "night raps")	161 (12.8%)
Psych. Annex of Haight-Ashbury Free Clinic (psychiatric or psychosocial counseling)	73 (5.8%)
San Francisco General Hospital (methadone detoxification)	43 (3.4%)
Mendocino State Hospital (methadone detoxification)	40 (3.2%)
Jail (intermediate to long-term sentences)	37 (3.0%)
Private physician (other than psychiatrist)	18 (1.4%)
"Fort Help" (Nonmethadone heroin detoxification, groups, and psychological counseling)	18 (1.4%)
Private psychiatrist	14 (1.1%)
Private Hospital	14 (1.1%)
Walden House (group residence house)	10 (0.80%)
Center for Special Problems (nonmethadone detoxification, group, and psychological counseling)	10 (0.80%)
Napa State Hospital (methadone detoxification)	9 (0.71%)
Reality House West (group residence house)	6 (0.48%)
San Francisco General Hospital (group sessions)	2 (0.16%)
Clayton House (group residence house)	2 (0.16%)
Langley Porter Neuropsychiatric Hospital	2 (0.16%)
Mendocino State Hospital "Family"	2 (0.16%)
Highland Hospital	1 (0.08%)
Moved out of state	4 (0.32%)

Results

Currently in treatment (seen in last two weeks)	161 (12.8%)
Whereabouts unknown (lost to follow-up for two weeks or more)	799 (63.5%)
Dead of heroin overdose	5 (0.4%)
Suicide	1 (0.08%)
Markedly improved (decreased habit to "chipping"; no more than once per week; no physical dependency; no withdrawal symptoms; follow-up for at least one month)	218 (17.4%)
"Clean" for one month or more	76 (6.6%)

REFERENCES

1. Gay, A.C., and Gay, G.R., *J. Psych. Drugs, 4,* 1971.
2. Yablonsky, L. *The Hippie Trip.* New York, Pegasus, 1970.
3. Shick, J.F.E., Smith, D.E., and Meyers, F.H. *J. Psych. Drugs, 2:*49, 1968.
4. Smith, D.E. *Clin. Tox., 2:*69, 1969.
5. Smith, D.E., and Luce, J. *Love Needs Care: A History of San Francisco's Haight-Ashbury Free Clinic,* Little Brown and Co., 1971.
6. Schubart, P., Smith, D.E., and Conrich, R. *J. Psych. Drugs, 1:*113, 1968.
7. Shick, J.F.E., Smith, D.E., and Meyers, F.H. *Clin. Tox., 3:*19, 1970.
8. Smith, D.E. *Clin. Pediat. (Phila.), 8:*185, 1969.
9. Smith, D.E., and Fischer, C.M. *J. Psych. Drugs, 2:*49, 1969.
10. Gay, G.R., Bathurst, W., Matzger, A.D., and Smith, D.E. *Int. J. Addict. 6:*241, 1971.
11. Dole, V.P., and Nyswander, M.E. *J.A.M.A., 193:*646, 1965.
12. Dole, V.P., Nyswander, M.E., and Kreek, M.J. *Arch. Intern. Med. (Chicago), 118:*304, 1966.
13. Dole, V.P., and Nyswander, M.E. *Arch Environ. Health, 14:*477, 1967.
14. Dole, V.P., Nyswander, M.E., and Warner, A. *J.A.M.A., 206:*2708, 1968.
15. Oppenheimer, G.B. *Lancet, 1:*1154, 1969.
16. Merry, J. *Brit. J. Addict., 63:*247, 1968.
17. Smith, R. *J. Psych. Drugs, 2:*93, 1968.
18. Terry, C.E., and Pellens, M. *The Opium Problem.* New York, Bureau of Social Hygiene, Inc., 1928.
19. Edwards, G. *Lancet, 1:*768, 1969.
20. Jaffee, J.H., Zaks, M.S., and Washington, E.N. *Int. J. Addict., 4:*481, 1969.
21. Sheppard, C.W., Gay, G.R., and Smith, D.E. *J. Psych. Drugs, 3:*22, 1971.
22. Meyers, F.H., Jawetz, E., and Goldfien, A. *A Review of Medical Pharmacology.* Los Altos, Calif., Lange, 1969, p. 269.
23. Von Hoffman, N. *We Are the People Our Parents Warned Us Against.* Greenwich, Conn., Fawcett World, 1968, p. 254.
24. Wellisch, D.K., Gay, G.R., and McEntee, R. *J. Family Process, 9:*425, 1970.
25. *Life, 63:*25, 1970.
26. *Time,* March 16, 1970.
27. Smith, D.E., Gay, G.R., and Ramer, B.S. Proceedings of the 3rd National Conference on Methadone Treatment, New York. 1970.

Chapter 13

A STUDY OF SOCIAL AND HEALTH NEEDS OF SELECTED FAMILIES LIVING IN THE BEDFORD-STUYVESANT HEALTH DISTRICT OF NEW YORK CITY

DEPARTMENT OF PUBLIC HEALTH
CORNELL UNIVERSITY MEDICAL COLLEGE

Students: William A. Donnelly, Monte E. Ikemire, Richard N. Lopatin, Michael A. Mustille, John E. Nees, William R. Raskin, Neil D. Ravin, and Ryan S. Searle
Preceptors: Kenneth G. Johnson, Jeanne F. Magagna, and Katsuhiko Yano

OBJECTIVES

AS THE POPULATION of this country becomes more and more concentrated into urban centers, the need to find solutions for the long-standing problems of the inner city community becomes a more and more pressing one. Every community, be it urban or otherwise, has certain rather specific needs. Ideally, these needs are converted to demands by a knowledgeable populace, and through individual motivation, coupled with efficient delivery of services by public and private agencies, these demands of the community are successfully met. But in the inner city ghetto this system has not worked; somewhere a link is missing in this chain of events. As a result, even the most pressing needs, in a community truly tortured with needs, are not met.

The Cornell Family Study (CFS) was designed to find out how some of the problems of such an urban ghetto might be successfully solved by a more productive use of the system which is presently responsible for delivery of services to the community. Our intent was to work directly with the people of the community on a personal basis, and our goals were threefold: first, we wished to assess the needs of the people in the ghetto; secondly, we wished to formulate a plan of action which could produce solutions to these specific needs; thirdly, we wished to implement this plan of action.

THE STUDY COMMUNITY

Bedford-Stuyvesant was, in part, the urban ghetto investigated in this study. It comprises an area of about 3.3 square miles in the center of Brooklyn, and contains about 285,000 people (Appendix 13A). In 1960, 59 percent of these people were black and 37 percent were white; in 1967, 83 percent were black and 12 percent were white; and in the northern one-third of Bedford-Stuyvesant, which was the area selected for the Cornell Family Study, 91 percent of the population in 1965 was black, 3 percent were Puerto Rican, and only 6 percent were white. The figures show a rather rapid demographic change in Bedford-Stuyvesant, from a predominantly white, well-to-do population to a predominantly black, poverty-level population during the past few decades.

As a result of this rapid change, the area is quite heterogeneous in its appearance, ranging from stately, well-preserved brownstones on relatively litter-free streets to dilapidated, wooden-frame apartments which give Bedford-Stuyvesant the appearance of a hard-core slum.* The smallest unit of homogeneity is the block. That is, most often the houses on the same block are in the same condition or stage of deterioration. This reflects, in part, the block approach of both government and community organization in combating the problems of the slum.

With one major exception, the dispersion of such "slum blocks" occurs in a generally increasing percentage from the Kings County and Brooklyn Hospitals at the southern tip northward. This gradient is also present in the race distribution of the populace—the Southern Health Area (#48) was 78.1 percent white and 19.4 percent black in 1965; and the Northern Health Area (#28) was only 8.3 percent white and 89.8 percent black.

The major exception to the gradient is the business district flanking Fulton Street. This street cuts transversely across the

*The Model Cities Foundation, in its *Report on Brooklyn* published July 1970, labeled Bedford-Stuyvesant one of the worst slums in the United States.

district, separating the upper one-third from the southern two-thirds and is the largest singly concentrated slum in Bedford-Stuyvesant. Most of the businesses are privately owned and consist primarily of small, crowded independent food stores, used furniture shops, new and secondhand clothing stores, and bars. While most of the smaller concerns appeared to be manned by blacks, the working force of the larger companies (i.e. gas company, building contractors) is overwhelmingly white. Similarly, the fire department, police department, and school teachers seemed to be predominantly white.

As more government agencies realize the need for local branch offices, and as the community itself increases its efforts to solve this problem, the number of social-service-related agencies is increasing in the area. In addition, the community has a large number of small independent churches interspersed with the usual businesses. Their abundance points out the importance of religion to the people of Bedford-Stuyvesant and indirectly demonstrates the failure of the larger, organized religious groups to satisfy this spiritual need.

The streets of Bedford-Stuyvesant are often in need of repair, almost universally cluttered with trash, and littered with the bodies of stripped and abandoned cars. Garbage is piled high in front of many buildings and often overflows onto sidewalks and streets before the Sanitation Department collects it. This garbage provides breeding grounds and food for innumerable insect and rodent pests.

Bedford-Stuyvesant has a modest number of public parks, which are poorly cared for. The grass is dying for lack of water, there is a tremendous amount of litter and broken glass, and much of the equipment is broken. The parks are used primarily by the unemployed or retired black males, drunks and drug addicts, and young adults. The only children present are those that are part of an organized group such as Headstart or Day Camp. Noticeably absent are individual mothers and their children, who are so commonly seen in Manhattan local parks.

The apartment houses themselves in this community often present a reasonably attractive facade to the casual observer; most of the buildings are brownstones, and from the outside appear to be well maintained. Once inside the universally unlocked door, however, the foyer and stairwell are often dimly lit, cluttered with trash and the remains of plaster long ago fallen from buckling ceilings. The stairways are generally in disrepair; the handrails offer little support. The apartment mail boxes and doors are rarely numbered, making it difficult to find someone once inside the building. The apartments themselves are generally dirty and poorly kept, the walls riddled with holes, and the kitchens swarming with roaches. In these buildings designed for two or three families, there are often six or seven now. Overcrowding has forced the tenants to use most of the rooms as bedrooms, and mattresses and dirty bedding are usually scattered around the floors. The bathrooms usually have a toilet with an overhead tank and chain; and in some cases, the apartments are frankly "cold water flats."

Before ending the description of the community, it must be stated that the greatest disfigurement of the community has been caused, ironically, by the Model Cities Program, which has razed blocks of housing, leaving acres of rubble-strewn lots.

THE STUDY POPULATION

For the purpose of our study, we selected two distinct subpopulations from the northern one-third of the community. One subpopulation consisted of one hundred "senior citizens" households made up of one or two persons 60 years of age or older. In order to maintain homogenity, senior citizens living with their children were excluded because it was assumed that they would receive aid from their children in solving their needs; and thus, the children constituted a resource not universally available to all senior citizens. No effort was made, however, to screen those with relatives living close by. The second subpopulation consisted of sixty "newcomer" families who have lived in New York City less than three years. Senior citizens and newcomers were selected for this study because it was felt that these groups of people would have the most needs and would be least able to meet these needs by themselves because of inability to utilize available community resources or lack of knowledge of their existence. Both subpopulations were selected from a group of families who had been surveyed by the New York City Health Department Health Guides Project between October 1969 and May 1970. Thus all these families had shown at least some willingness to cooperate with health workers, since all had furnished information to the health guides during the survey visit. The health guides themselves played an integral and essential part in the Cornell Family Study. These health guides are a group of women who live in the Bedford-Stuyvesant community. They do not hold professional certification, but they have been well trained in the collection of demographic information and the dissemination of health information on a personal basis to the community. During the past ten months they have visited many families in Bedford-Stuyvesant and referred hundreds of people to various health and social agencies in the area.

LITERATURE REVIEW

Review of Community Health Projects and Programs

As our Cornell Family Study program deals with the solution to needs in the Bedford-Stuyvesant community through a variation on family advocacy, it would be wise to survey briefly the literature in this area.

Family advocacy, broadly speaking, is an effort to bridge the gaps between the individual's problem and its solution, rendered within the realm of functioning agencies. As such, it automatically delineates the rights and needs to be sought by the advocate—those self-established by the community's social and health services. Further, the principle of the client's role in this problem-solving effort is paramount.

Robert Sunley,[1] in writing on this subject, discusses the important aspects of family advocacy: interviewing, casework, intervention and objectives, and agency structuring. Problems are encountered in obtaining accurate information from clients, relevant regulations and requirements from agencies, assessing value judgments and meeting frustrations, leading to mere "adjustment" solutions to environmental problems. Many forms of advocacy intervention are possible. Among them are studies and surveys as groundwork for further action by the advocacy program and education of others; case conferences with other agencies or even client groups to effect change and action on one's own behalf; educational methods, such as direct information, pamphlets, meetings, exhibits, press releases, and so forth; demonstration projects aimed at long-term methods of advocacy to develop communication awareness and leadership; client-group formation by advocates for social change; petitions for calling attention to an issue and mobilizing members around an action; persistent demands, a type of escalation of demands against figures who are inaccessible to personal contacts; demonstrations and protests. The concern for various goals for the family, in exposing different levels of agency contact, would dictate what means of intervention are appropriate.

The evaluation of home-oriented health and social aid, as utilized in the Cornell Family Study program, is one for which adequate precedence is not established in the literature. Much has been written, however, on the opportunity for service by "home health aides" and other paramedical personnel, usually working out of a conveniently located community health center. Such workers are trained and assigned tasks ranging from strictly education in community health facilities to becoming home health aides competent in the functions traditionally assigned to public health nurses and social workers.

As outlined by Young and Hamlin,[2] a health education aide can be trained by a city health department as an indigenous nonprofessional, extending the knowledge of the professional services of the community health agencies. Their emphasis, significantly, is on the total family. Henrich Blum[3] has described the "multipurpose worker," operating out of a "Neighborhood Multi-Purpose Center." The worker, in essence, is a counselor who, at present, is integrating the services of welfare, health, and probation. The unit helps the community members focus on their own problems, seek a solution, and participate in the solution. There is a goal of promoting community-city interaction, oriented toward a more active democratic process.

The development of a comprehensive family health workers program has been a project of the Montefiore Hospital Neighborhood Medical Care Demonstration since 1966.[4] The center, opened in July 1968, has trained family health workers as part of a goal for "intensive participation of the people in the operation of the health center." The family health workers are placed under the supervision of a public health nurse, who is given a mandate for the preventive care of neighborhood families. The family health worker is involved in a six-month training program in all areas of health care and social service, then becoming part of the physician-public health nurse-family health worker team. Her roles in health education, patient care, and social advocacy activities are carried out with forty to sixty assigned families from the clinic. The goal for these families has been a simplification of the complexities of health and social services now available to poor patients.

Work by Kent and Smith[5] has outlined many of the important considerations when a program to involve the urban poor in city health and social services is contemplated. Prospective patients can be reached if their particular cultural and economic aspects are taken into account; neighborhood representatives are uniquely suited to involve the disadvantaged. In utilizing neighborhood workers, their tasks need a component of social action which transcends health care values, for health care is a "latent consequence" of a more general problem-solving process. In short, people cannot be helped who cannot be reached. The worker can represent the community life and values to the professional, and health programs to the low-income client. In attaining more skills in social advocacy, the worker helps solve more immediate problems, thus lowering the barriers to health care. The worker, then, must be action oriented. By involving the disadvantaged in the accommodation process, neighborhood workers open an area through which the urban poor can move toward participation in the ongoing society. More effective patterns of behavior enable future problems to be met more competently.

There was no information on attempts by Kent and Smith to

document the effectiveness of neighborhood representatives' social efforts in a quantitative fashion, although health effects were estimated. Their Denver Clinic evaluations after implementation of health workers showed a 42 percent higher attendance, in the same time period, than clinics without health workers. Sixty percent of patients at a new Mother and Infant Care Clinic after four months were referred by neighborhood representatives. Twenty percent more unwed mothers than in comparable neighborhoods were served, and a positive trend appeared for mothers to be seen earlier in pregnancy. The success of neighborhood representatives in social areas of immediate need was described as "particularly effective," with a subsequent categorization of examples, i.e. welfare grants, food orders, and so on.

Quantitative evaluations of overall results attained by community teams in comprehensive social and health aid projects are difficult to find. A major documented effort involved the New York State Community Aid Association. Their preliminary work lead to a thirty-one-month social research study in Chemung County, New York, dealing with "multiproblem" families. These families were defined as suffering a "variety of health and welfare problems, with chronic dependence on community services, while nevertheless displaying apathy toward agency efforts, or actually resisting or rejecting the services." Their objective was to assess the effects of intensive social casework on a group of fifty multiproblem families, in contrast with the effects of normal public assistance services given a control group of fifty similar families. An emphasis was placed on using available community services. The entire family was considered the client.[6]

Casework, as defined in this study, entails a process by which the social worker attempted to promote a "successful and gratifying adaptation" between individuals and their social environment. All those involved in the study held degrees in social work.

The emphasis in evaluating the families revolved around dimensions of family function as developed by Dr. Ludwig Geisnar.[7] These parameters included family relationship and family unity, individual behavior and adjustment, care and training of children, social activities, economic practices, household practices, health conditions and practices, relationship to project worker, and use of community resources. The evaluation of success in the casework rested on the "movement" upward in family functioning as measured on a scale for each of the nine dimensions. But

> after two years of service to multi-problem families by trained caseworkers, operating with reduced caseloads, and with special cooperation of the community resources, but within the framework of public assistance policies and procedures, the demonstration group showed a small but statistically non-significant margin of improvement over the control group which received only routine service from regular public assistance workers.

Further, it was concluded that there was little difference in effectiveness between caseworkers with graduate degrees and "other workers," and there was a corresponding lack of progress by both groups demonstrated in the project. They qualified this conclusion by stating that "whatever was done by these workers for their clients cannot be demonstrated to have had a beneficial effect by the particular procedures we chose to apply."

Several other studies involving casework analyses are cited in the literature. A report by the Bureau of Public Assistance, Department of Health, Education, and Welfare, in 1953-54 concluded that skilled social workers had improved the family status in 141 out of 240 families selected through the Aid to Families with Dependent Children program.[6] The improved parameters involved were financial support from absent fathers (34 cases improved), marital relations (32 cases), health (51 cases), full-time employment (18 cases), and better housing (23 cases). A program sponsored by the San Francisco City and County Public Welfare Department concerning diagnostic and rehabilitation treatment for 5500 families showed that "improvement" was reported for only 17.5 percent of the problems identified.

Ludwig L. Geisnar,[7] in a research demonstration in New Haven involving a group of thirty multiproblem families versus fifty-one control families from comparable housing projects, concluded that "multi-service intervention can effect changes in social functioning which are measurable by subjective techniques."

The literature here supports several conclusions. Our family advocacy work will bring us in contact with various levels of agency functioning, depending upon the specific need, and thus the several possibilities for intervention should be foreseen. The lack of skilled, postgraduate-trained caseworkers should not handicap our possibilities to effect change in the conditions of multi-problem families in the Bedford-Stuyvesant area. On the contrary, the use of neighborhood representatives (health guides) would increase our potential for effectiveness. Finally, our "success" in the study will be largely dependent on how we define our criteria for having improved the conditions of our families, i.e. needs met versus unmet.

The Aged and Their Problems

The problems of the aged have been extensively documented.[8-12] Only slightly less voluminous are the writings devoted to ideas for meeting these manifold and interrelated problems. Far less space and verbiage have been devoted to evaluation of the programs and ideas which have been aimed toward solving the problems of the aged.

Many authors have correctly pointed out that one of the most frequent and debilitating infirmities of the aged is the limitation of mobility owing to arthritis, various forms of foot trouble, and to cardiovascular problems.[10] The most commonly seen solution to this problem is the nursing home, in which the aged person is placed in close proximity to resources which have been centralized and designed to meet all his needs, and the visiting home-care personnel, who visit the aged at home, bringing the resources to the aged. The latter ordinarily is the less expensive proposition. It is easier to provide people to visit other people than to provide a set of buildings and personnel to staff the buildings and to care for the residents. Unfortunately, caring for the aging in their own homes, which are not designed specifically to meet their needs, is often more difficult than caring for them in nursing homes which have been engineered clear of potential dangers (stairs, exposed fuel and heat sources, and so forth).[12] Considerations of expense have usually preempted considerations of efficiency: the nursing home may be more efficient, but the cost of providing nursing homes for everyone over 65 would be staggering. And many people would not want to live in homes, for cultural and psychological reasons. The future of the aged then seems to lie in home care.

That the population of the aged is a growing one may seem to be a surprising notion: the ranks of the old are usually thought to be growing smaller, being depleted faster by death than other groups. But the significant fact is that more people are living to be old, and once they arrive, they stay longer. Whereas the total population of the United States of America increased almost 100 percent in the fifty years since 1900, by 1950 the number of people in the 65-and-older group increased almost 500 percent. The numbers of people living to be old have meant that the nation has had to devote more of its resources toward providing for them. The group over 65 is not totally unproductive and dependent, but it is less productive and more dependent than, say, the group between 35 and 45. It is often difficult for Americans who are geared to devoting their input into the areas which promise the greatest proportionate return to devote a great input of energy to this segment of the population, which will not return as much for the dollar: pour money and time into the training and care of the young of the nation and they will produce more efficiently when they come of age. Pouring money into the aged seems to some Americans like a low-return proposition. The arguments against this kind of thinking range from outright moral diatribe to more calculating efforts, which have pointed out that beyond the question of what we owe to the aged, the aged are, if not the most valuable, at least a valuable asset to our society.[8,11] It is beyond the scope of this paper to argue the question of whether or not great sums of money and time should be directed toward solving the problems of the aged. This paper is concerned only with pointing out that the mere question of the worth of the aged is a problem of the aged, both in regard to their own conception of self-worth and with respect to the difficulty it causes when funding of programs for the aged is considered.

Nor is the question of self-worth the only problem for the

aged. In our society, especially among the poor, the aged have to rely more and more on government pensions and other pensions and less on their families. In other cultures and times, where the care of the aged was considered a matter of family honor, this was not so.[13] In America today, the aged are fast becoming the disinherited.

Vedder and Lefkowitz.[13] note, "The aged must look else than to their progeny for companionship and sociability to satisfy financial, health and social needs. The aged today turn to government and other organizations." American society today is highly mobile, and this mobility has led to the dispersal of relatives and friends. Whereas in earlier times a person could look forward to growing old in his home town with his friends to take care of each other, today his friends and family may be far flung by the time he is 60. Says Vedder, "They are deprived of the society of their family, and having lost associates on the job and friends by death or departure to other communities, find themselves with too much time on their hands."

Community Medicine: The Indigenous Approach

That the nursing home is not, for economic reasons, a viable solution for the care of the aged on a large scale has been suggested earlier. Psychological, cultural, and individual reasons are often even more compelling. The elderly person, already cut off from the friends and family he knows, may become disoriented if he is taken out of a familiar house or environment.[12] Individuals who were quite well adjusted in their own house may become depressed if transplanted into a new and uncomfortably unfamiliar environment.

The hospital is often not the optimal health center, tending to be to removed and aloof from ethnic considerations of local neighborhoods. Gibson[9] further feels that local or "primary" health centers should meet neighborhood health needs, including those of the aged, the young, and the newcomer of each locality. Says Gibson,[9(p1189)] "There is actually a sociologic difference in organization between the two institutions rendering it much more feasible for the health center to relate in a meaningful way to the community in which it is located."

The hospital tends to be oriented toward the identification and treatment of disease, i.e. it is what Gibson calls "lesion-oriented" rather than "person-oriented." This is perhaps necessary for the very ill, but for the chronically ill or marginally ill and for those who need preventive medicine this is not conducive to the rendering of the best medical care.[13]

The elderly then are a minority group with special problems.[13] One way of meeting these problems has been sought through the use of multipurpose community personnel who visit the homes of the aged.

METHODOLOGY

For the purposes of our study, each of eight medical students was assigned to one of the health guides to form a total of eight health teams, and each health team was assigned a group of twenty families, each senior citizens or newcomers, to work with during the six weeks spent in the community.

In order to realize the goals stated above, to assess the families' needs and then to formulate and implement a plan to meet these needs, a triphasic approach to the families was used. This approach consisted of at least three visits to each family by the health team.

During the initial visit, demographic information was collected on a form we had devised for this purpose (CFS Form 1, Appendix 13B). Data concerning the family makeup, home environment, education, employment, welfare status, and health status of the family members were recorded on this form. In order to assess the needs of each family in a consistent way, a problem-oriented resource list was compiled by the medical students and health guides (Appendix 13C). This list took almost a full week of work to compile; it contained the names, addresses, telephone numbers, and brief descriptions of sixty-seven public and private agencies in the Brooklyn area, most of which were visited by a health team to make sure of the accuracy of our information and the accessibility of the agency. These agencies were grouped under six main categories: housing, education, employment, health, welfare, and community organizations. This resource booklet was used much as a check-list by the health team during the initial visit in order to elucidate the needs of each family. In this way, some consistency was maintained in assessing the needs of the different families. In addition, a health check-list was designed to be used with senior citizen families since it was anticipated that this group would have a higher incidence of medical problems; the check-list consisted of thirty-eight questions, to be answered *yes* or *no,* concerning the presence of specific symptoms or medical facts important for people in this age group (CFS Form 3, Appendix 13B) . A similar list for the newcomers was not formulated because it was felt that the newcomers would have fewer health problems, and those that did present would be acute ones and easily recognizable by the family or team.

After the family's needs had been assessed, the remainder of this first visit was spent by the health team in educating the family about what kinds of services were available to them in the community. A preliminary plan of action was formulated at this first visit, and the family was told how they could implement this plan. Naturally, individuals varied in the amount of motivation with which they attempted to solve their needs, so this phase also included persuasion by the interviewers with emphasis on the importance of implementing the preliminary plan as soon as possible. Variability in the different teams' abilities to educate and persuade was also inevitably present, but each team made a conscious effort to be consistent in its approach to each family.

The second of the three phases was called the "minimal assistance" phase and consisted of a second visit to the family approximately one and one half weeks after the first visit. The health team discussed the plan of action they had offered on their first visit and found out if the family had followed up on their suggestions. If no progress had been made toward meeting the need, the health team aided the family directly in carrying out the plan, but still played a clearly minor role. For example, the health team might make an appointment with an agency for the family with limited mobility and no phone, or pick up an application form and bring it to the family.

The final stage of "maximal assistance" consisted of a visit one and one half weeks later. Once again the health team found out whether any progress had been made in meeting the family's needs. If not, then the health team aided the family directly and clearly played the dominant role in trying to meet the needs. For example, the health team would accompany the person to the clinic, making sure that the proper services were rendered. Or the health team might represent the family at an agency if they were confused or intimidated by the agency's procedures.

In order to record the information we had gathered concerning the needs of each family, we devised the Cornell Family Study Need Sheet (CFS Form 2, Appendix 13B), and one such sheet was kept for each need that we encountered. This form is subdivided into three sections corresponding to three visits. The visits ideally represent the three phases previously discussed—education, minimal assistance, and maximal assistance. It should be noted, however, that the phase overlap the visits, in that the result of the educational phase is recorded at the second visit, the results of the minimal assistance phase at the third visit, and the results of the maximal assistance phase either at the third visit or at a fourth one.

On this form, the nature of each need assessed during the initial visit, the individual's effort to meet the need, and the approach suggested by the health team were recorded. In recording the nature of the family's need on the need sheet, nine categories were used: none, housing, job, welfare, education, food, medicare care, other health, and social (specific descriptions of these categories are given later in this section).

With the individual's previous efforts, a brief statement as to their effectiveness was noted when possible. If the family did nothing, this was recorded, and a reason for their apathy was included when possible. The suggested approach included primarily referrals, but, of course, depended upon the need. For example, a senior citizen might know of an agency but he might be afraid to go there alone. The suggested approach here might have been to get another person (ideally from another of the team's families who had a similar need at the agency) to go with him.

Under "nature of contact/time spent," the amount of time with the family or representing it and how the time was spent was listed (i.e. 45 minutes—interview, 10 minutes—telephone call, and so on). This was absolute time and did not include time spent traveling or contemplating action in behalf of the family. It is obvious that an error in the time spent with a family would have been introduced if the total interview time were recorded with each problem. If the family had more than one need, the time spent on each need was recorded as a fraction of the interview, (i.e. 15/45 means that 15 minutes of the 45-minute interview was devoted to the particular need in question). Also, in this same area, a circled number indicated the number of visits needed to contact the family (actual contact visit included).

The second visit was one and one half weeks after the first, but was earlier if the situation allowed or required it—that is, if the individual was highly motivated and reliable or if the need was serious enough to require immediate follow-up. At the time, the results of the first phase were recorded and reasons for failure and changes in the plan of action were also noted. The suggested approach at this time might have included such things as making appointments for a family or arranging for a baby-sitter or transportation so the individual could go to a clinic or agency.

The final subdivision on the need sheet corresponded to the third visit (one and one half weeks, if necessary, after the second). It included two result sections, the first to record the outcome of the approach decided upon at the second visit, and the last to record the results of the maximum assistance phase (if needed). The documentation of the final results often involved a fourth visit when it was not feasible to go directly to the agency needed the same day as the third visit.

This sheet had several shortcomings; foremost was that not all needs fit into its mold. However, it was flexible enough to include most. For example, "agency" could be replaced by landlord, clinic, neighbor, and so forth, depending upon the suggested approach. Also, question 1 of the final results was interpreted loosely to include whether the family kept its appointment with the study team if the approach decided upon involved the team accompanying the family to an agency. In addition, some needs could not be stretched into three phases (e.g. half-fare cards) while others required more than three visits. In the case of the latter, the last subdivision was repeated as many times as needed.

In order to quantify the information gathered concerning the needs of the families under study, index cards which summarized the data from the demographic and need sheets were used (Appendix 13B, CFS Data Cards 1, 2, and 3). The demographic data card (Card 1) is self-explanatory, except possibly the listing of children's ages. If a son or daughter was under 21 but had children of her own, she was listed under "Other Adult" and the ages of her children recorded and identified as grandchildren to the head of the house. Also, under "Home Environment," the E, G, F, and P by "Phys. Plant" and "Housekeeping" stand for excellent, good, fair, and poor, respectively. As indicated, the family needs data card (Card 2) lists nine need categories.

The "None" category was checked if the family had no discernible needs.

The "Housing" category included all problems associated with maintenance of the family's living quarters, including apartment, halls and stairways, building, cellar, and back yard. Also included were needs arising because of inaccessibility, disinterest, or hostility on the landlord's part, and infestation of quarters with insect pests. Although very few families had satisfactory housing, only those who specifically requested help in moving were recorded as having a need for better housing. The exception to this was when the apartment was grossly overcrowded or the housing directly and immediately imperiled the family, such as the lack of hot water or the presence of crumbling ceilings. In those cases, new housing was listed as a need regardless of whether or not the family complained. This attitude was taken by the study team because of the reality of the housing shortage in New York City. This same type of subjective realism influenced the team's decisions in all of the nine basic need categories. No rigid criteria were established defining what constituted a need and what did not, and except for a weekly group meeting to compare cases, each team acted as they saw fit.

Those families subject to relocation because of urban renewal were also listed as having a housing need. With this particular need, it could be argued that if it went unmet, the failure was due to the individual's inability to find new housing. However, because the need was created by urban renewal, and because that agency should be better equipped to find new apartments, the failure was recorded under agency rather than individual.

The "Job" category was checked if any family member was seeking employment, if the family had needs arising from employment such as baby-sitters and/or day care centers, or if the family needed assistance from the Social Security Administration.

Under "Welfare," only those needs arising from Public Assistance payments from the Department of Social Services were included. Medicaid, Medicare, or Social Security problems were specifically excluded from this category.

All levels of educational need, from Headstart through high school to college level and vocational training courses, were listed under the "Education" category.

The "Food" category was designed to include specifically the Donated Foods Program of the Department of Social Services and the newly organized Food Stamp Program.

"Medical Care" was considered to include family health needs that require immediate medical or dental treatment.

The "Other Health" category included all needs for preventive or prophylactic medical care, including lead poisoning blood tests, immunizations, and dental and physical examinations. Also included in this category was rodent pest control.

Under "Social" needs were listed those stemming from lack of social contacts and loneliness among the senior citizens and difficulties in adjusting to a new community among the newcomers. Also included was the procurement of half-fare public transportation cards for the senior citizens.

In the next section of Data Card 2, information concerning efforts made to solve the needs was summarized. If the family itself had made any effort, even a minimal, unsuccessful one, to find solutions to its problems, "Yes" was checked under "Family Previous Efforts." The team considered a "contact" with a family as a personal or telephone conversation during which the family's need was discussed. Letters written to the family were also considered as "contacts." The number of "visits" included the number of personal, telephone, and letter contacts and also unsuccessful attempts to contact the family. The same criteria were used in listing contacts and visits to agencies. "Time" in hours spent in discussing each problem with the family was recorded; this time excluded the time taken to travel to and from the family's residence. "Time in Hours (Agency)" records the entire period spent at the agency (including waiting in lines) and the time taken to travel to and from the family's residence and the agency.

In the final section of Data Card 2, the status of each need at the end of the study was evaluated. If the need had been completely met during the team's contact with the family, "Need Met" was checked, and the amount of medical student-health guide team intervention required to meet the need was recorded on the last line of Data Card 2 ("If Met. . ."). In filling out the later information on the "If Met" line, one of the three categories "Education," "Minimal Assistance," or "Maximal Assistance" was checked according to the stage of intervention required, as has been discussed previously.

If, at the end of the study, the need had remained completely unmet, the "Unmet" category was checked, and the reason for the failure was recorded on the line beginning "If Unmet. . ." On the latter line, the reason for failure was attributed to one of four causes, the first being a lack of motivation on the family's part. "Agency Inaccessible" was checked if the attempted solution was foiled by excessive bureaucratic delay or by a series of "buck-passing" contacts with the agency during which no progress could be made. If an agency was too centralized so that the utilization of its services required an excessive expenditure of time and money it also became "Inaccessible." For example, the Division of Continuing Education provided adult classes in the English language, but they were offered either in schools too far from the families or were offered at night, both situations unappealing to many families. "Agency Ineffective" was checked if the agency did not fulfill its promises of action or if its action was not sufficient to meet the family's need. The category entitled "No Solution" was checked if the health guide-medical student team and the family had exhausted its resources without successfully meeting a need and if this failure was not attributable to lack of cooperation or action by an agency.

The third category describing the status of the need at the end of the study, "Partially Met," was checked if the need had been successfully met only in part. For example, if the family were unable to get the full amount of money desired from the Department of Social Services, or if a half-day Headstart program was accepted because a place in a full-day program was not available, this category was checked.

The last category, "In Progress," was checked if, at the end of the study, some concrete gain had been made toward a solution, but the solution had not yet been completed. This category included, for example, an instance in which a pest control inspector had visited a building at our request but an exterminator had not yet been sent, or an immunization program was started but not completed at the termination of the study.

In the case of the latter two categories concerned with evaluation of the status of a need at the end of the study, namely, "Partially Met" and "In Progress," the "If Met" line on the data card was also completed as described previously.

In order to summarize the data on all the needs of each family, Data Card 3 was devised, and one card was filled out for each family in the study. The categories on Data Card 3 are self-explanatory, being taken directly from the Data Card 2 for each family, with the exception of the column labeled "Total." In this column, "Number of Needs," "Time in Hours (Family)," "Time in Hours (Agency)," "Number Unmet Needs," "Number Met Needs," and "Number Needs in Progress" were summed.

At the conclusion of the study, the resource sheet was amended and corrected and copies of it were left with the health guides to be used in their future work. A shorter resources list was also prepared, which contained the names, addresses, telephone numbers, and short descriptions of seven agencies; this list was intended to be distributed to all the families visited by the health guides as a home reference list which could be used to meet needs arising in the future.

RESULTS

Demographic Characteristics of the Study Population

One hundred and thirty-two families were contacted during the course of the study. An additional 20 newcomer and 20 senior citizen families originally included were not reached. Of these, 14 newcomers and 8 senior citizens had moved, 5 senior citizens were deceased, and the remainder either refused contact or were continually not at home on repeated visits.

The sociodemographic characteristics of the 132 families are summarized in Table 13.1. The "typical" newcomer family is black, from the South, contains 4 to 5 individuals (with a range of 2 to 11), with a female as the head of the house who has completed ten years of schooling. These families are most likely on welfare and pay slightly more than one-fourth of their income for rent. The "typical" senior citizen family is also black and from the South, but has been residing in New York City for almost forty years. These families usually contain 1 to 2 people, have a female head of the house who has completed six years of school, are probably receiving welfare, and pay slightly less than 40 percent of their income for rent.

The 45 newcomer families contained 219 people whereas the 87 senior citizen families contained 178 people. The large size of the newcomers is obviously due to the large number of children (144/219 = 66%) in that group. This gave a total of 397 people actually contacted.

Nature of Needs

It should be remembered that we are dealing only with outstanding needs, and this should not be misconstrued to mean all the problems of the area. A certain number of existing needs were already being adequately handled by the families we encountered and we did not concern ourselves with them. How-

TABLE 13.1
SOCIODEMOGRAPHIC CHARACTERISTICS OF 132 STUDY FAMILIES

Characteristics	Newcomers	Senior Citizens
Total Number of Families	45	87
White	1	0
Black	38	86
Puerto Rican	6	1
Total Number of Persons	219	178
Male Adult	25	42
Female Adult	50	95
Children*	144	41
Place of Residence of Families prior to N.Y.C.		
Southern States, U.S.	29	59
Other States	0	10
West Indies	8	11
Puerto Rico	6	1
Other Countries	2	5
Unknown	0	1
Average Length of Residence in N.Y.C.	1.7 yrs. (45 Families)	38.4 yrs. (85 Families)
Average Length of Education†		
Male	7.9 yrs. (23 Persons)	6.4 yrs. (20 Persons)
Female	10.1 yrs. (43 Persons)	6.0 yrs. (53 Persons)
Average Income of Family per Week	$100.8 (43 Families)	$53.8 (62 Families)
Average Rent per Month	$118.5 (44 Families)	$88.1 (63 Families)
Number of Families on Welfare	29	30
Number of Families on Medicaid	31	51

*Includes individuals under 21 years of age (unless head of household).
†Includes all adults for whom information was available.

ever, they are problems nevertheless, and their exclusion from the study in no way implies that they are any less severe or less numerous. It is simply that we concentrated upon what was unresolved or uninitiated rather than documenting what was being cared for.

Newcomer needs, as shown in Figure 13.1, include 53 health needs, 44 housing, 22 medical, 22 educational, 11 welfare, 6 employment, 5 food, and 3 social.

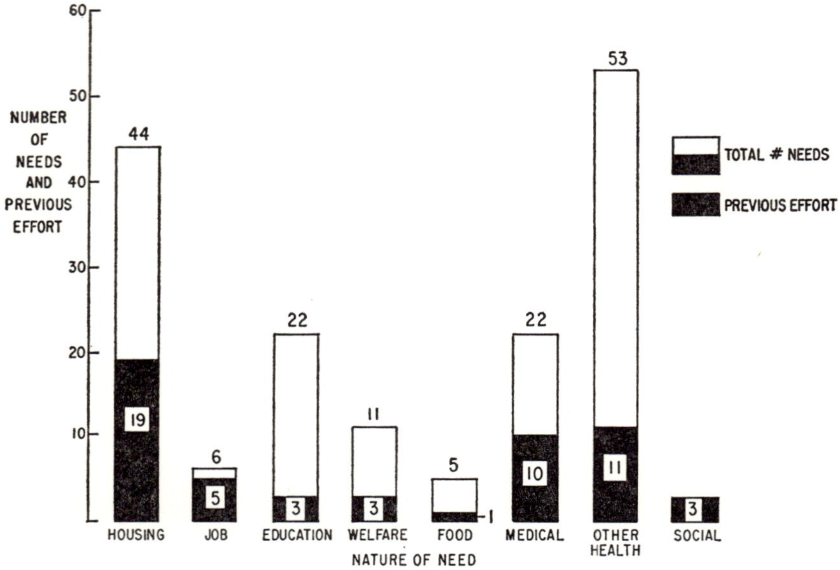

Figure 13.1. Number of needs by nature of need and family's previous effort to meet need for forty-five newcomer families.

A word of caution must be interjected here against assuming that "other health" needs are more pressing than housing. The graph represents only the *number* of needs and in no way expresses the *severity* of those needs. The health needs reflect, for the most part, prophylactic care available to the children of this group, and includes such things as immunizations and lead screening tests. In contrast, the housing needs are much more serious, representing such conditions as overcrowding and substandard living. In addition, the relatively large number of health needs (53/166 = 32%) is enhanced by our definition of needs. For example, in housing we were critical and included only emergency needs, while in health every need uncovered was included. It is also obvious that we are health oriented, and therefore are more keen to health needs. Thus we recognized and preserved each health need as a separate entity, while we consolidated many needs in other categories simply because we were not knowledgeable enough in the subject to appreciate differences. Finally, it must be recognized that many needs, especially in housing, that were known to be unsolvable were not included. Each team made decisions based on the reality of the situation. For example, most of the families contacted were entitled to better housing; however, it would be fanciful to believe that better housing could be obtained for all; therefore new housing was listed as a need only if the family was severely overcrowded or scheduled for relocation.

The twenty-two medical needs are a better yardstick of the newcomers' health in that they reflect the need for immediate medical care. We were somewhat disappointed that it was so high but certainly not surprised because of the popularly held opinion that "health is a low priority in the ghetto community."

Some individuals might be critical about the low number of employment needs, especially among a group heavily dependent on welfare. It was our feeling that the few requests for aid in securing jobs was due to the high percentage of families with only a female adult as the head. In those families that did have a male as head, most already were employed and requested help in obtaining more education.

Leading the list of needs for the senior citizens (Fig. 13.2) is the medical category with 64, followed by housing with 37, social 35, other health 33, welfare 17, food 12, job 9, and education 2. While it was expected that this population would have a higher number of medical than other health needs, due to the age of the members, it was again disturbing that the medical needs were so high. Part of this is due, no doubt, to the greater emphasis that the medical student-health guide teams placed on health-related needs. However, ignorance and neglect on the part of the population must figure to be the most important contributing factors. Which of the two, ignorance or neglect, played the dominant role, becomes an important question when designing a program to meet the medical needs of the community. We did not

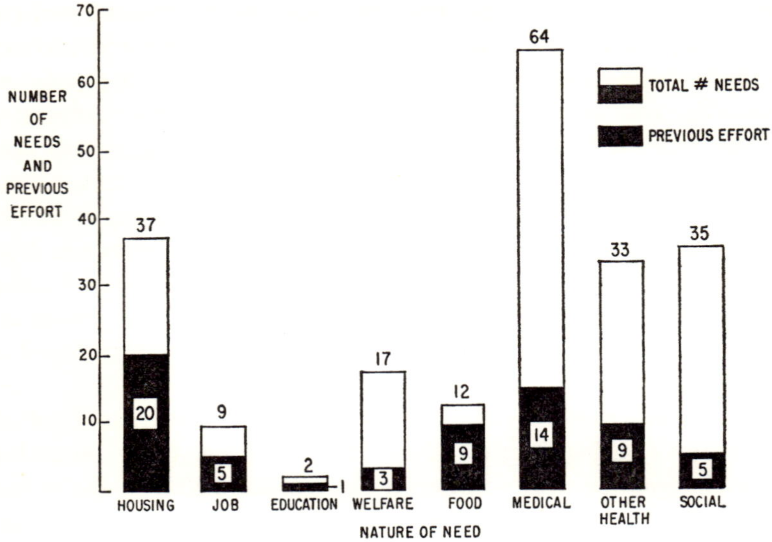

Figure 13.2. Number of needs by nature of need and family's previous effort to meet need for eighty-seven senior citizen families.

attempt to answer that question in the study, but it is our feeling that ignorance, rather than neglect, was the major cause of this population's apathy. A little support for this can be obtained indirectly from the data we gathered.

A point which we felt supported our subjective impression that the population is more ignorant than neglectful was that 57 of the 114 needs in the combined health and medical categories that had shown some progress (i.e. met, partially met, and in progress), obtained such status solely through education.* This, in addition, suggests that health is not as low a concern of the poverty population as generally believed.

Housing for the senior citizens, for the same reasons stated earlier, does not dominate the needs as would be expected. In fact, it is even less important in this group than in the newcomers. This is probably because their housing is better than the newcomers. This is supported by a very subjective evaluation of each

*Accumulated from individual result sheets.

home visited. We assessed the condition of each house and recorded whether it was excellent, good, fair, or poor. Of the newcomers' living quarters, none were excellent, 18 percent were good, 45 percent fair, and 36 percent poor. In comparison, 15 percent of the senior citizens had excellent housing, 40 percent had good, 29 percent fair, and only 16 percent poor.*

The high number of social needs results from the desire for companionship in this age group. Likewise, the few requests for jobs might be due to wanting to be useful.

Status of Needs at the Study Termination

Table 13.2 summarizes the status of the needs for both groups at the end of the study. Those needs listed under "In Progress" are needs in which some action has been taken, regardless of how minor, but because of the brevity of the study, solution of the need was not fully realized. It can be expected that one-half to two-thirds of these will eventually turn out to be unmet needs. It is of interest that almost identical percentages were obtained in the two groups.

TABLE 13.2
STATUS OF NEED IMPLEMENTATION BY TOTAL NEEDS FOR NEWCOMER AND SENIOR CITIZEN FAMILIES

	Newcomers		Senior Citizens	
Need Status	Number	Percent	Number	Percent
Met	48	29	61	29
Partially Met	5	3	10	5
In Progress	50	30	61	29
Unmet	63	38	77	37
Total	166	100	209	100

The final result of each need is presented in Figure 13.3 for the newcomers and in Figure 13.4 for the senior citizens. The highest portion of met needs in both medical and other health can be attributed, in part, to the increased efficiency of the teams

*Figures 13.1 and 13.2 show the number of needs in which the family made a previous effort to solve problems. Housing, as expected, has the right percentage. This probably correlates well with the severity of these needs; however, no attempt to link the two will be made.

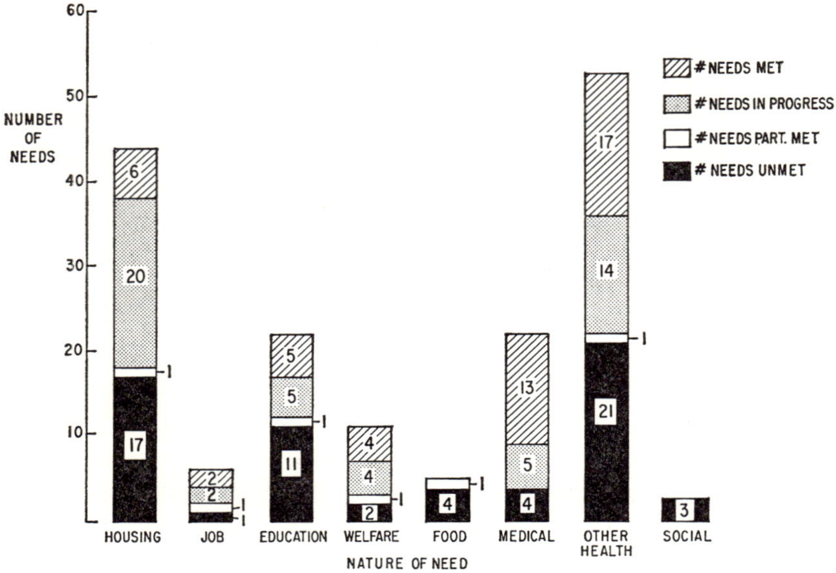

Figure 13.3. Status of need implementation by nature of need for firty-five newcomer families.

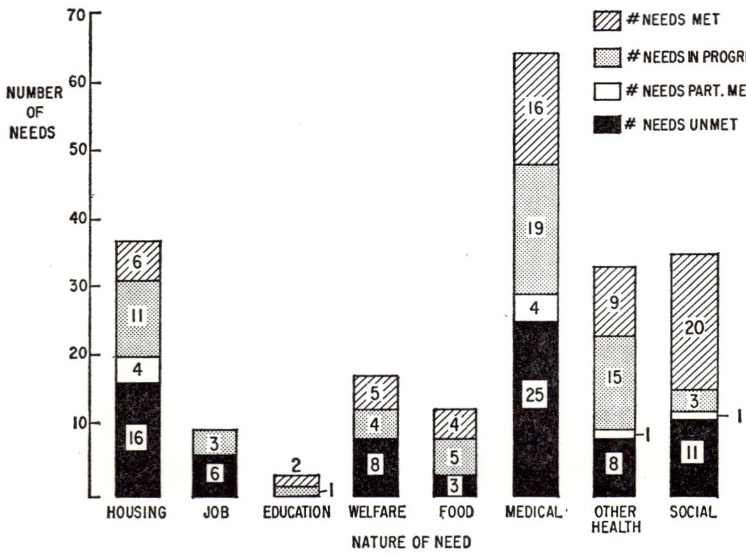

Figure 13.4. Status of need implementation by nature of need for eighty-seven senior citizen families.

in solving health-related problems. Most of the success in these areas is due, however, to the simplicity of the needs—if a person has an illness, treatment will usually be promptly given once requested.

Likewise, the high percentage of met needs in welfare for both groups, and social problems for the senior citizens, is due to the simplicity of the needs. That is, if someone is eligible for welfare he is not refused it. Housing, on the other hand, represents complex needs and the few needs that were met were minor ones; very few families were placed in better apartments or neighborhoods.

Table 13.3 shows the means by which the needs for each group were met, partially met, or in progress. It is from this table that the real importance of the study is evident. Of the ninety-two newcomer needs that showed progress toward solution, 79 percent was achieved through simple education of the family or through minimal assistance. The comparable figure for the senior citizen,

TABLE 13.3
MEANS OF IMPLEMENTATION FOR MET NEEDS AND REASONS FOR UNMET NEEDS FOR NEWCOMER AND SENIOR CITIZEN FAMILIES

	Newcomer	Senior Citizen
Total Number of Met, Partially Met, and In-Progress Needs	92*	129†
Means of Implementation:		
Education	54 (58%)	55 (43%)
Min. Assistance	19 (21%)	30 (23%)
Max. Assistance	19 (21%)	44 (34%)
Total Number of Unmet Needs	63	77
Reasons:		
Family Unmotivated	44 (70%)	43 (56%)
Agency Inefficient or Inaccessible	12 (17%)	20 (26%)
Financial Reason	4 (7%)	14 (18%)
No Solution	3 (6%)	0

*Eleven needs were excluded for the following reasons: 6 met through family's own initiative, 1 partially met with inefficient agency, and 4 in-progress with inefficient or inaccessible agency.

†Three needs were excluded as they were met through family's own initiative.

66 percent, while lower, is still impressive. Need implementation through maximal assistance was greater in the senior citizen group, 34 percent versus 21 percent in the newcomer group. This difference can, in part, be attributed to the decreased mobility of this older age group.

The reason accounting for the greatest number of failures was lack of motivation. This is not to imply negligence, because there is obviously a discrepancy between what we perceived as a need and what they did. In addition, we must consider our own deficiencies in not being able to convince them of the importance of solving all their needs. Worth noting is that agency inefficiency and inaccessibility plays a minor but substantial role.

Table 13.4 presents the frequency and time spent by medical student-health guide teams in working with study families. The total hours spent in contact with the families and agencies was 414 hours. From Table 13.3 it can be demonstrated that 221 needs had some progress. This represents then about two hours spent per "positive" action. More specifically, there were 109 met needs, meaning that about four hours were spent by medical student-health guide teams in solving each need. We considered such a small expenditure of time highly encouraging.

COMMENTS AND RECOMMENDATIONS

We applaud the Health Guides Project and believe that it is a valuable and important program to the Bedford-Stuyvesant community. Its strongest point is the utilization of people indigenous to the area in (a) evaluating the needs of the area and (b) relating to the community population. We see in this group the potential for an increasingly more active role, and thus propose an expansion of their activities, perhaps in providing additional social and health services.

A problem frequently encountered among senior citizens was that their chronic limitation of mobility prevented them from attending as many clinics or contacting as many agencies as they might otherwise have done. Similarly, lack of baby-sitters hampered newcomers' efforts. The remedy to this is by no means simple;

TABLE 13.4
FREQUENCY AND LENGTH OF CONTACTS FOR NEWCOMER AND SENIOR CITIZEN FAMILIES

	Family Type	Housing	Empl.	Educ.	Welfare	Food	Medic.	O. Health	Social	Sub-Total	Total
Number of Contacts with Family for Each Need	Newcomer	75	14	36	20	9	50	95	6	305	694
	Senior Citizen	60	16	7	33	24	117	64	68	389	
Time for Family Contacts (In Hours)	Newcomer	5+	3¼	6+	5⅓	1¼	7½	24+	4/5	53+	260
	Senior Citizen	19⅔	4½	1¼	13½	4½	126⅓	17½	19½	206+	
Number of Contacts With the Agency	Newcomer	30	5	15	10	1	15	18	0	94	206
	Senior Citizen	23	8	0	11	2	30	25	13	112	
Time for Agency Contacts (In Hours)	Newcomer	11¼	2⅔	6	7½	1¼	14¾	27¼	0	70½	153½
	Senior Citizen	12¼	4½	0	9	3½	28¾	20½	4½	83	

the answer may be an agency designed to cope with these problems.

It was found that 95 percent of the people in Bedford-Stuyvesant had at least one TV set or radio. Since there was a high percentage of needs met by virtue of education alone, we suggest that the use of these modes of communication, if feasible, would have positive effects.

We also would like to see established some type of agency to aid those who cannot speak English, acting specifically as interpreters and conducting classes in English at a very local level, i.e. within an apartment in a "Spanish-speaking" building if necessary. The manpower for such a program could come from college students, who could receive credit for their efforts, or by using bilingual welfare recipients.

APPENDIX 13A

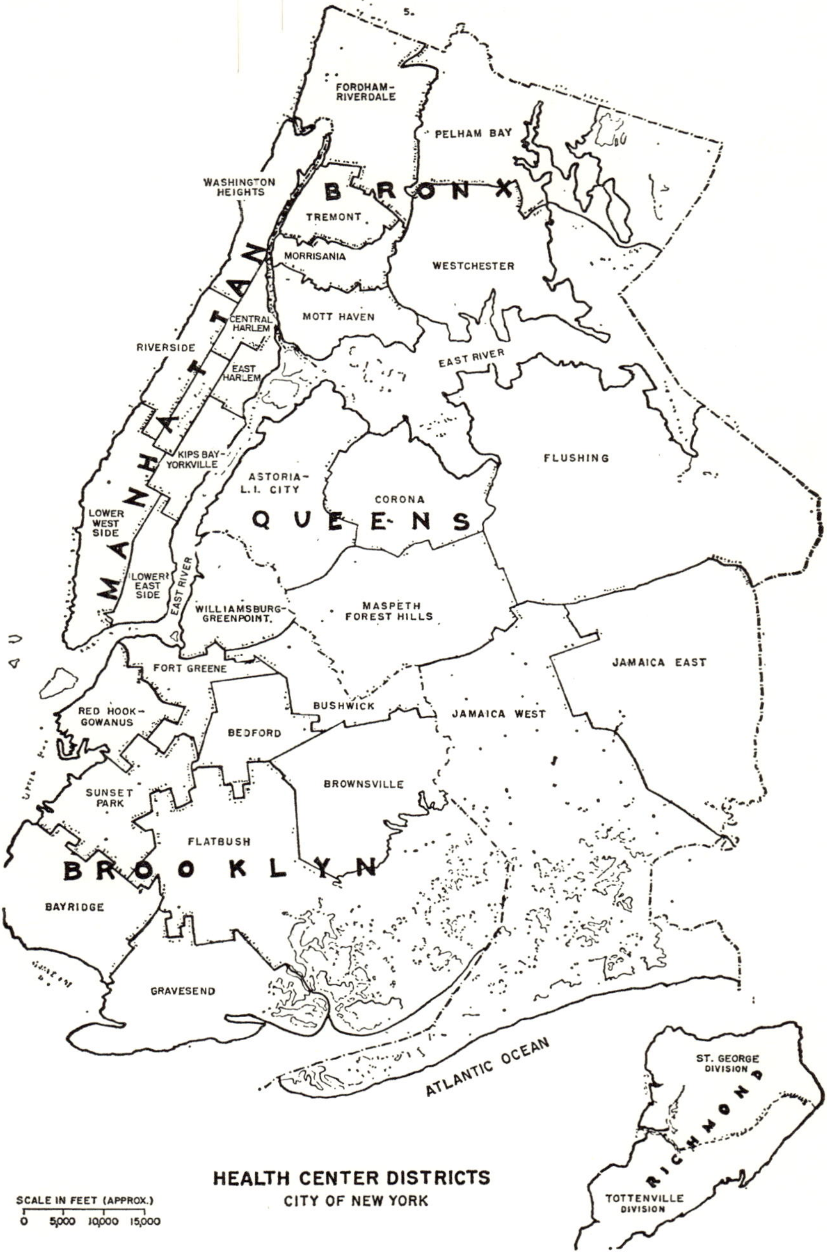

HEALTH CENTER DISTRICTS
CITY OF NEW YORK

APPENDIX 13B

CORNELL FAMILY STUDY
FORM 1—DEMOGRAPHIC INFORMATION

Date:
Name of Interviewer (Student): CFS #:
(Guide): HGP #:

I. *Head of Household:*
1. Name:
2. Marital status:
3. Telephone:
4. Address:
5. Race:

II. *Length of Residence:*
1. In New York City:
2. In Bedford-Stuyvesant:
3. In last home prior to N.Y.:

III. *Total Income:* $_____
Support Programs:
1. Welfare (Yes or No):
2. Medicare:
3. Medicaid:
4. Old Age Social Security:
5. Other Pensions:

IV. *Members in Household:*

	Sex	*Ed.*	*Age*	*Employed*	*Contribute to Support*
1. Head of household					
2. Spouse					
3. Children (list)					
4. Other (list)					

V. *Home Environment:*

1. Rent:
2. Flights of stairs:
3. Number of rooms:
4. Heat type:
5. Hot water?
6. Toilet (public or private) :
7. Cooking (public or private) :
8. Number of bedrooms:
9. Pests:
10. Peeling paint, cracked walls?

Overall Rating: E G F P

VI. *Medical History:*

	Date Last Physical Exam.	*Where Given*
1. Head of household		
2. Spouse		
3. Children (list)		
4. Other (list)		

Do you read the paper? (Yes or No) :
Which one?
Do you watch TV?
Do you listen to the radio?

Comments:

CORNELL FAMILY STUDY FORM 2—NEED SHEET

Name: *Date:* *Time Spent:*

Need:

Individual's Previous Efforts:

Suggested Approach:

I. *Results:* *Date:* *Time Spent:*

1. Did individual contact agency?
2. If "No," why not?
3. Did agency solve problem?
4. If "No," why not?

Suggested Approach:

II. *Results:* *Date:* *Time Spent:*

1. Did individual keep appointment?
2. If "No," why not?
3. Did agency solve problem?
4. If "No," why not?

Suggested Approach:

III. *Results:* *Date:* *Time Spent:*

1. Did individual keep appointment?
2. If "No," why not?
3. Did agency solve problem?
4. If "No," why not?

CORNELL FAMILY STUDY FORM 3
HEALTH CHECK-LIST FOR HOUSEHOLD MEMBERS

HGP #: *Sex:* *Age:*

CFS #:

Relationship to Household Head: Self Spouse Parent Child GP GC
Relative Other

General Health Status: Excellent Good Fair Poor Very poor

Chronic Mobility
Limitation: No limitation Has trouble getting around
Unable to get around Confined to house
Confined to bed

Presence of Specific Complaints and Medical Care for Them (Senior Citizens Only):

	Yes	*No*		*Yes*	*No*
Poor vision			Frequent headache		
Hearing difficulty			Frequent dizziness		
Loss of teeth			Speech difficulty		

Weakness of limbs
Chest pain or tightness
Shortness of breath
Chronic cough
Indigestion
Abdominal pain
Constipation
Back pain
Joint pain
Swelling of ankles
Feet troubles
Skin troubles
Urination troubles
Mental or emotional troubles
Has eye glasses
Has hearing aid
Has dentures
Seen by physician

Presence of Chronic Disease Told by Physician:
Hypertension Heart disease Stroke Diabetes
Asthma Peptic ulcer G-B disease Hernia Arthritis
Tuberculosis Mental disorders Other (specify)

Prenatal Care Received (Pregnant Women Only): Yes No

Well Baby Clinic Visit Done (Infants Under 1 Year Only): Yes No

Immunization Completed (Grade School and Pre-School-Age Children Only): Yes No

CORNELL FAMILY STUDY CARD 1
CORNELL UNIVERSITY MEDICAL COLLEGE–NEW YORK CITY HEALTH DEPARTMENT
DEMOGRAPHIC INFORMATION

CFS #: _____ Type Family: Senior Citizen _____ Newcomer _____

Number of People: _____ Weekly Income: _____ Home Size: _____

Rent: _____ Welfare: _____ Medicaid: _____ Medicare: _____

Soc. Sec.: _____ Other: _____

P.E. within Year: Father _____ Mother _____ Child (Fract) _____

Other _____

Child Age (<) : 1 2 3 4 5 6 7 8 9 10 11 12 13 14 15 16 17 18 19 20 21

H.H.: Male Female Other Adult	*Home Environment*
Age	Stairs: 1 2 3 4 5 6 7
Ethnic*	Heat Type: Oil Gas Steam Elect.
Employed	Hot Water: Yes No Sometimes
Education	Kitchen: Public Private
Res. in B-S	Bathroom: Public Private
Res. in N.Y.	Bedrooms: 1 2 3 4 5
Prior res.	Phys. Plant: E G F P
Read paper	Housekeeping: E G F P
Watch TV	
Listen radio	

*B—Black WI—West Indian W—White PR—Puerto Rican

CORNELL FAMILY STUDY CARD 2
CORNELL UNIVERSITY MEDICAL COLLEGE–
NEW YORK CITY HEALTH DEPARTMENT
FAMILY NEEDS

CFS #: ____

Nature of Need #: ____ None ____ Housing ____ Job ____ Welfare ____ Education ____ Food ____ Medical Care ____ Other Health ____ Social ____

Family Previous Efforts: Yes ____ No ____

Contacts (Family) ____ # Visits (Family ____
Time in Hrs (Family ____

Contacts (Agency ____ # Visits (Agency ____
Time in Hrs. (Agency) ____

Status at Study Term.: Need Met ____ Unmet ____ Part. Met ____
In Progress ____

If Unmet: Unmotivated ____ Agency Inacc. ____ Agency Ineff. ____
No Solution ____

If Met: Education ____ Min Assistance ____ Max Assistance ____

CORNELL FAMILY STUDY CARD 3
CORNELL UNIVERSITY MEDICAL COLLEGE–NEW YORK CITY HEALTH DEPARTMENT
TOTAL FAMILY NEEDS

CFS #	None	Hous.	Job	Educ.	Welf.	Food	Med. Care	Other Health	Social	Total
Family Previous Effort to Meet Need										
# of Needs										
# of Contacts (Fam)										
# of Contacts (Ag)										
# of Visits (Fam)										
# of Visits (Ag)										
Time in Hrs. (Fam)										
Time in Hrs. (Ag)										
# Unmet Needs										
# Met Needs										
# Part. Met Needs										
Average # Needs per Family										

APPENDIX 13C

COMMUNITY RESOURCES

I. If you see any evidence *of rats or mice, call*
Bedford-Stuyvesant Pest Control
Stuyvesant & Halsey Streets
Tel. 467-6464 . . . and tell your story.

II. If you have *any housing problem* (heat, hot water, peeling paint, garbage removal, etc.), *call*

a) Greater Crown Heights Community Development Council
1419 St. John's Place
Tel. 774-7322 . . . ask for Mr. Williams.

b) Mayor's Urban Task Force
1233 Fulton Street
Tel. 783-7767

For problems with the *landlord,* call

a) City Rent and Rehabilitation Administration
81 Willoughby Street
Tel. 643-7570

b) New York City Housing Authority
250 Broadway
Tel. 964-3000 . . . ask for Mr. Washington.

III. *Any health problems*

1. If you don't have Medicaid and your family makes more than $5000 per year, call
Bedford Health Center
485 Throop Avenue
Tel. IL 2-7880
2. If you have Medicaid or your family makes less than $5000 per year, call
Neighborhood Health Clinic
476 Nostrand Avenue
Tel 638-8575

IV. If you have a *welfare* problem or think you are eligible for it, call 344-8700 to find out which center will take you. Then call local center or visit in person early 8:00-10:00 A.M. or late 3:00-5:00 P.M.

For additional Assistance, call Welfare Rights Movement
(Mrs. Weens)
348 Tompkins Ave., Tel. 622-5187

FOR ANY PROBLEM, CALL . . .
HEALTH GUIDES PROJECT
6 BROOKLYN AVE., 638-9842, 9843, 9844

BEDFORD-STUYVESANT RESOURCE LIST
HOUSING

I. *Pest Control*

a) For Bedford-Stuyvesant area, use
Bedford-Stuyvesant Pest Control
Stuyvesant and Halsey Streets
Tel. 467-6464 . . . ask for Mr. Cryden or Mr. Gibbs.
Call this agency if there is any evidence of rats or mice but *not roaches.* They will inspect, do their work, and sue the landlord for costs.

b) For Brownsville, use
Brownsville Pest Control
Tel. 342-6517 . . . ask for Stan Brothway.

II. *Physical Plant*

a) Greater Crown Heights Community Development Council
1419 St. John's Place

Tel. 774-7322 . . . ask for Director Cleveland Williams.
They are efficient, and deal with problems of heat, hot water, plaster, garbage removal, etc.

b) Mayor's Urban Task Force
1233 Fulton Street
Tel. 783-7767
Hours: 9-5 P.M. They contact the agencies for you as sort of a middle-man referral agency.

c) New York City Housing and Redevelopment
597 Gates Avenue
They send inspectors but do not always produce good results.

d) New York City Housing Authority
250 Broadway
Tel. 964-3000 . . . ask for Mr. Washington.
They are the main branch of the city Housing Authority—they deal with all complaints

e) Emergency Repair Service (in Bedford-Stuyvesant)
Tel. 453-6035

f) Emergency Water Repair
Tel. 227-1400

g) Gas Emergency
Tel. 643-4050

h) Potholes in the street
Tel. WO 4-2110

i) Tow-aways
Tel. 757-1533

j) Street Lights
Tel. AS 4-4200

III. *Problems with landlord*

a) Mayor's Urban Task Force
1233 Fulton Street
Tel. 783-7767

b) Tenant Aid Division of Relocation Department
2 Lafayette Street
Tel. 565-6478

c) City Rent and Rehabilitation Administration
81 Willoughby Street
Tel. 643-7570
This agency enforces Rent Control, will cut rents if proper services are not administered by the landlord.

IV. *Relocation*

a) Urban Renewal—Building Management and Relocation Office 1600 Fulton Street

Services: "Landlord" for all buildings taken over by city, relocation of tenants, financial aid—moving expenses (depends on number of rooms vacated and bonus expenses (depends on number of rooms moved into).

b) City Housing Projects

Find out which housing project is desired, then contact that development (they are all listed in the phone book under New York City Department of Housing).

At this time, there seems to be more space available for senior citizens. Call

Carter G. Woodson Housing
New York City Housing Authority
Powell Street & Livonia Avenue
Tel. 949-1130

V. *Sanitation*

Mayor's Urban Task Force
1233 Fulton Street
Tel. 783-7767

VI. *Urban Renewal*

a) Model Cities
1563 Fulton Street
Hours: 9-5 P.M. . . . contact Mr. Knight.

b) Application for half-fare cards
Tel. 345-6363

c) Job training programs
Maintenance Crew Team for Senior Citizens—retired craftsmen skilled in carpentry, painting, electrical and mechanical repairs, concrete work, welding, pavement repairs, gardening.
Steady, part-time employment . . . call,
Tel. 467-1351 . . . ask for Mr. Ballantine.

d) Central Brooklyn Model Cities Housing, Management & Relocation
654 Gates Avenue
Tel. 491-7200
Register for Model Cities Program and obtain City Housing Applications.

This is a private organization that modernizes apartments and paints building facades. They are very good. They will paint an entire block if you have approval of two-thirds of the people on that block.

EDUCATION

I. a) Headstart
480 Tompkins Avenue
Tel. 789-6161 . . . ask for Mrs. Holmes, Mr. Burroughs, or Mrs. Haywood.
Children must be between 3 and 5 years of age. Program hours 9-3 P.M. Free lunches and instruction in basic subjects. (All branches have the same program.)

b) Day Camp—summer school for kids who have completed one year or more of school. Crafts, sports, trips, etc.

II. *High School Diploma*

a) State University Urban Center (Family Education Program)
470 Vanderbilt Avenue
Tel. 638-0308
Available only to parents with children in Headstart. Parents get courses on *any* educational level. Program begins in September, lasts one year. Family activities and field trips. Equivalency or college entrance diploma.

b) OIC
1024 Fulton Street
Tel. 857-3100
Applicant must be 17-55 years of age, must be a citizen, (if naturalized bring papers to register).
Average length of time spent in school: Basic education—6 months, Vocational education—6 months (one year total). Half- and full-day sessions available. No fees, no stipend given. September is earliest starting date. All graduates placed in jobs. *Must be in-person application.*

III. *Vocational Training*

a) OIC
1024 Fulton Street
Tel. 857-3100
(see above)

b) Urban Center

470 Vanderbilt Avenue
Tel. 638-0308
(see above)

c) Brooklyn Adult Training Center
475 Nostrand Avenue
Manpower training

IV. *Tutoring*

a) Contact local school or YIA, 1173 Fulton Street, Tel. 789-6161
b) For disabled children, contact Board of Education.
(M.D. certification necessary)

V. *Handicapped Education*

a) Brooklyn Social Service
285 Schermerhorn Street
Tel. TR 5-0710

EMPLOYMENT

I. *General*

a) Manpower
1249 Fulton Street
Tel. 789-4411
Hours: 8:30 A.M.-8:00 P.M. (Monday-Thursday)
For senior citizens—ask about PATH program: Personal Aid to the Homebound.

b) YIA—Neighborhood Youth Corps
6 Brooklyn Avenue
Tel. 789-6161, Ext. 285, 288

II. *Daycare Center*

a) New York City Department of Welfare
Division of Daycare Information and Counselling Service
601 East 9th Street
Tel. OR 3-4500, Ext. 19

b) 348 Tompkins Avenue
Social Service pays the $10 per week fee.

III. *Housekeepers*

a) Clinton Welfare Center
103 Clinton Street
Tel. 237-5370 (for location of local center)
Make the needs known to the welfare caseworker and get an M.D.'s certification of need.

b) DAB—for senior citizens—see handicapped.
c) American Cancer Society
1 DeKalb Avenue
Tel. UL 8-8200
Only for people disabled by cancer.

IV. *Social Security*
a) Social Security Administration
345 Adams Street
Tel. 596-4100 . . . call this number for all problems.
b) Chance—Social Service—will baby-sit and pay $10 to educate mothers on how to houseclean

HEALTH

I. *Narcotics Addiction*
a) SHUN
1854 Fulton Street
Tel. 756-5940 . . . ask for Miss King.
Hours: 9:30-12 A.M. for interview or first visit.
10:30-5:30 therapy sessions (group and work).
7:30 P.M. Wednesday—Community awareness sessions, counseling for parents of addicts.
b) 24-hour Addiction Information
Tel. 226-6900
c) Methadone Clinic
Brooklyn Hospital
DeKalb Avenue & Ashland Place
Tel. 270-4281
d) Addiction Research and Treatment Corp.
937 Fulton Street
Tel. 636-1000
Long waiting list. Applicant must be over 21 years of age. Complete physical given, counseling therapy and group therapy, recreation room. No referral from M.D. needed, just appear in person.

II. *Family Planning*
a) Planned Parenthood
Tel. 421-2290

III. *Abortion*

a) Information
Tel. 777-2015

IV. *Medicaid*

a) If people want information on whether they have it, call 790-3645 . . . or as a last resort 790-3652,3,4 (central index).

b) If a family earns less than $5000 but more than $3000, they may apply for Medicaid without welfare. This is done through
Medicaid Center
340 West 34th Street
Tel. 594-3050
However, the best way to register them for Medicaid is to bring them down to the Neighborhood Health Center of the Provident Society
476 Nostrand Avenue
Tel. 638-8575
They will register patient in addition to supplying medical care.

c) If a patient's family earns less than $3000, they may apply for welfare and Medicaid automatically comes with it.

V. *Medicare* (file through Social Security)

a) Social Security Administration
345 Adams Street
Tel. 596-4100

VI. *Child Abuse*

a) 67 Schermerhorn Street
An investigator will visit the family, the child will be placed in a home or institution, and legal action may be taken against the parents.

VII. *Clinics*

a) Bedford Health Center
485 Throop Avenue
Tel. GL 2-7880
Patients may be registered for all clinics without having to go in person; simply fill out one of the application forms that have been distributed.

Well baby clinic
Sick baby clinic
Prenatal care
Chest clinic (TB)
Immunizations
Dental clinic (for children less than 14 years old, recruitment through school program)
Social hygiene clinic
Mental health clinic
Nutrition counselling
Eye clinic and corrective lenses—not open during summer
General medical clinic (including health check-up)

b) Bedford Car Service
Tel. GL 2-7881, Ext. 41 . . . ask for Mrs. Turner.
For Medicaid eligible patients they will provide transportation.

c) Charles Drew Neighborhood Health Center
St. Mary's Hospital
Dental Clinic—Daily 1-5 P.M., M,W,F, 5-8 P.M.
Tel. 345-4000, 4001 . . . ask for Mr. David Rogers for information.

d) Brooklyn Eye and Ear Hospital
29 Greene Avenue
Tel. 852-5200

e) Neighborhood Health Center of the Provident Clinical Society
476 Nostrand Avenue
Tel. 638-8575
They give *complete* medical care with each patient having a private physician. Will take only patients eligible for Medicaid and will register them for it. They also provide free bus service for all those who need it.
All weekdays 9-5 P.M., Tuseday & Thursday 9-9 P.M.

VIII. *Emergency Rooms*

a) Bedford Health Center
Tel. GL 2-7880
Ambulance service to the local hospitals is provided.

b) Kings County Hospital
451 Clarkson Avenue
Tel. IN 2-4000

c) St. John's Hospital
480 Herkimer Street
Tel. 467-7000

IX. *Lead Poisoning*

a) Community Health Guide Project
6 Brooklyn Avenue
Tel. 638-9842

X. *Psychiatry*

a) King's County Hospital
Psychiatric Evaluation Department
Building "G"

XI. *Multiphasic Health Screening*

a) Brookdale Hospital Center
Linden Boulevard at Brookdale Plaza
Tel. HY 5-6900, Ext. 341 . . . ask for Mr. Glouer.
The patient gets a full physical examination and several laboratory examinations free of charge. The results are sent either to the patient's private physician or to a clinic (register the patient first).
Wednesday, no appointment needed. Other weekdays, appointment is needed. Takes about 2½ hours, only one visit.

XII. *Handicapped*

a) DAB (Housekeepers)
103 Clinton Street
Tel. 237-4090, 4337, 4338 . . . ask for Mr. Elkin or Mr. Patton.
General (for Senior Citizens only)
Transportation to clinics
Home management
Recreation
Living arrangements (homes, etc.) on M.D.'s recommendation Self care services, housekeeper (they supply funds—guides must find someone to do the work)

XIII. *Alcoholism*

a) King's County Hospital
451 Clarkson Avenue
Tel. IN 2-4000

WELFARE

I. General Social Service
250 Church Street
Tel. 344-8700 . . . call this number to find out to which welfare office the person belongs.
- a) For all social needs, contact local social worker.
- b) Some services: Bureau of Child Welfare
  Office of Community Relations
  Bureau of Fiscal Administration
  Bureau of Public Assistance—aid to dependent children, disabled, blind, old age, etc.
  Bureau of Resources
  Bureau of Shelter Services for Adults
  Day care centers for older persons
  Home maker services
  Chance—training for welfare mothers in many fields

II. Fulton Action Center
1574 Fulton Street
Tel. 778-1250 . . . ask for Mrs. Johnson.

III. Welfare Rights Movement
348 Tompkin Avenue (between Madison & Monroe)
Tel. 622-5187 . . . ask for Mrs. Weens.
These two agencies are comprised of eager ladies who work best as escorts to welfare centers and not advisors.
To obtain welfare:
1. Visit center, pick up application, and make appointment to see interviewer next morning.
2. After interview, investigator will visit applicant at home, accept or reject application.

COMMUNITY ORGANIZATIONS

I. *Legal Aid Society*
293 Adams Street
Tel. UL 5-8473
- a) Local: Bedford-Stuyvesant Legal Service
  1103 Fulton Street
  Tel. 638-9324

Free; open 9-5 P.M. weekdays. Must appear in person, but call about local information first.

II. *Block Associations*

III. *YIA (Youth-in-Action)*
1178 Fulton Street
Tel. 789-6161
Job training, family counseling, etc.

IV. *Recreation*
a) Breevort Houses Community Center
280 Ralph Avenue
Tel. 467-6350
Provides recreational services for boys and girls (5-13 years) Monday-Friday 3-5:15 P.M.
For boys and girls 14-18 yrs. Monday-Friday 7-10 P.M.
Vocational and college guidance, community improvement classes, for adults; *no fee*
b) Bedford Boys Club
Boys 7-17 years of age
c) YMCA
139 Monroe Street
Tel. 622-1100
d) St. John's Recreation Center
Prospect Place
All ages
e) Senior Citizens
Kingsboro Heights
f) Church Programs for Senior Citizens
g) PAL—Ages 7-17
185 Chancey Street
Brooklyn Borough Office
31 Snyder Avenue
Tel. 462-8639
PAL Youth Centers
110 West 9th Street
Tel. 875-6749
h) Boy Scouts (Girl Scouts) —Mrs. Williams
1400 Bureau Street
Brooklyn Borough Office

147 Remsen Street
Tel. TR 5-4900

i) Libraries
1. St. Marle's Avenue
2. Grand Army Plaza
3. Eastern Parkway and Albany Avenue
4. Macon & Lewis Streets
5. Franklin Street

j) William Reid Senior Citizen Center
447 King's Fourth Walk
Tel. 756-8400
Hours: 9-5 P.M. weekdays; 12-5 P.M. weekends and holidays. Offer counseling on health or social problems, 25¢ lunch, recreation room, group work projects, and assorted field trips.

k) Concord Church (Senior Citizens)
Marcy & Putnam Streets
Hours: 9-2 P.M. weekdays. No card playing; any denomination. Trips, etc. Very sincere small group.

l) For men:
Eleanor Roosevelt Housing Center
Maria Lawton Day Care Center for Senior Citizens
Hart & Stuyvesant Streets

APPENDIX 13D

SELECTED FAMILY STUDIES

CORNELL FAMILY STUDY NO. 1

FAMILY: S.
FAMILY TYPE: Senior Citizen
AGE OF SENIOR CITIZEN: 74
NUMBER OF PERSONS IN HOME: 1

Family History

Mrs. S., 74, was first seen on July 14, 1970, in her owned brownstone. A highly emotional and nervous individual, Mrs. S. was immediately seen to be suffering from a senile or mentally ill condition. She was found alone in the unkept basement rooms of the home, cooking a nearly empty pot of beans on the gas stove. She was receptive and capable of momentary rational conversation, but repeatedly related the events of an automobile accident that left her with a concussion and a memory "not what it used to be, don't you know." It was eventually learned that this accident occurred in the early 1930's. Her living conditions were unhealthy and the housekeeping poor. The upstairs bedroom area was practically abandoned and spider infested.

Attempts to question Mrs. S. as to family history (age, relatives, means of support, etc.) were to no avail due to her "loss of memory." She volunteered a stack of collected papers and bills but nothing was found dating after 1953. Evidence was found that she was a member of the Amalgamated Cleaners and Dyers Union in New York City and was a member of the Siloam Church. Neighbors had related that a husband, Mr. S., was presently in a city TB hospital and that a woman occasionally visited Mrs. S. Mrs. S. was not able to tell us whether her husband was in New York or even whether he was alive or not. Neighborhood children also told of helping Mrs. S. with food supplies on occasion. She maintained that there were no tenants living on the first or second floor, which seemed to be the case. She also felt that her grandson stayed with her at times but could give us no further information on this.

Mrs. S. gave the impression of a small and haggard, but strong and very active woman existing from day to day in her private world with little financial or social contact with the outside.

Family Needs
Mrs. S. could supply us with nothing helpful except a belief that her union paid for her automobile injuries and hospitalization. It would be necessary to determine through the agencies themselves whether Mrs. S. was receiving Social Security, Welfare, Medicaid, etc. and would require our investigation as to the whereabouts of her husband. Maximum assistance was necessary immediately to provide her with a means of support.

Implementation
St. John's Hospital was visited on July 21 to determine whether either Mr. or Mrs. S. had ever been a patient there. No record was found of them. Calls were made the following day, first to the Amalgamated Cleaners and Dyers Union. The Medical History Department searched its files and reported two days later that there was never any coverage for Mrs. S. involving an auto accident or otherwise. The Beneficiary Department had Mrs. S. listed as a "retired

worker" drawing $65 per month under claim number CLMA 168. Her benefits had begun following her "stop-work date" of June 20, 1963. She had failed to return the monthly required notice in June 1970 to receive her July 1970 benefits. She had signed all notices prior to that time.

They provided us with her Social Security number. We notified that office, which, after a search of records, could not locate any information on either her or her husband. They placed a request with the central Baltimore office and would call us in two weeks. On August 10, we were notified that she was receiving Social Security benefits. Contact was made with Mr. L., an administrative assistant for Social Service's D.A.B. unit. They had a record of requests in the winter of 1969 for aid in paying fuel oil bills by Mr. S.. Aid was discontinued when it was learned that his requests were not made as a tenant, but as a home owner. The unit had never visited his home and he was not heard from again.

When visiting the home on July 27, her brother, F.W., was found there. He was attempting to take her to Kings County Hospital Building "G" for psychiatric evaluation. Mr. W. lived further out on Long Island and, as a truck driver, had little free time in the past to see his sister. Yet, while driving his route late one evening he had run across his sister, wandering alone in the street, with only a coat on. His visit now was on a special day off, in order to help her. We encouraged her to take the ride with us in her brother's car.

The psychiatric unit spent two hours for evaluation, physical, and Medicaid application on Mrs. S.. She was seen to have a senile condition dangerous to her health and safety and was recommended for referral to the Brooklyn State Mental Hospital three blocks down the street. We spoke to Dr. M. at the hospital and she was admitted for an indefinite period. Immediately following this, a visit to Building "E," the chest wards, revealed that Mr. S. had been a patient there from June 11, 1970, to July 23, 1970. Mrs. S. had no recollection of Mr. S. having been home after that time. The brother, F.W., undertook to lock up the home and follow up in the financial affairs of Mrs. S..

A visit to the home on August 4 failed to find Mr. S. home. Then a chance visit on August 6 found Mr. S., 70 years old, sitting on his front steps. He refused to identify himself at first but we proceeded to talk to him. He was a very suspicious man who would tell us little about himself. He stated that he was going to have his wife committed when he got out of the hospital anyhow. Mr. S. had no plans to rent the apartment, which would have meant repairs. He was content to live on his Social Security. He refused any help other than a half-fare card, which he examined ten minutes before signing. He had been informed of the previous events by Mr. W. and had seen his wife twice and stated that she was doing well.

Comments

It was never discerned to what extent Mrs. S. was subsisting alone preceding our case involvement. The information shows that many "neighbors" knew of her condition, but none felt the need to bring it to the attention of welfare or the police. Our own visits found Mrs. S. at times rummaging through the trash barrels on the street and chasing children away from her stoop, while others looked on in amusement.

It is to the credit of the Kings County Psychiatric Evaluation Unit and Brooklyn State that Mrs. S. could be evaluated and admitted in one afternoon. Though the health guide team did not initiate the trip there, Mr. W. felt that we had helped in the admission process. The unit personnel recalled Mrs. S. from a previous visit one month before, though it is unclear as to who brought her then. She was not admitted at that time.

I believe Mrs. S. would have been happier at home, though her safety and care would have been tenuous. Her personality was one formed from a history of hard work handling heavy laundry machinery and it is disheartening to see this end in a life cultured under her particular living conditions.

CORNELL FAMILY STUDY NO. 3

FAMILY: D.
FAMILY TYPE: Senior Citizen
AGE OF SENIOR CITIZEN: 72
NUMBER OF PERSONS IN HOME: 2

Family History

Mrs. D., long divorced from her husband, lives with her daughter in a third-floor apartment. Mrs. D. appears slightly senile but is very

kind and helpful. She has lived in the Bedford-Stuyvesant area for thirty years now, much of that time with her daughter, Mrs. W. . She occupies two rooms of a six-room home and contributes toward the rent ($20 per month) . She currently draws only Social Security ($106 per month) .
Mrs. D.'s medical history is sporadic. She last saw a doctor three years ago at a King's County clinic. She was diagnosed as a diabetic but was taking no medicine.

The daughter, Mrs. W., has one son, now a paraplegic as a result of a house fall three years ago, who is a permanent patient at the Brooklyn Jewish Hospital. Mrs. W. spends nearly eight hours per day caring for her son at the hospital and is rarely free during the day. Her commitment prevents her from holding a job. She is separated from her husband.

Mrs. D. fell down a flight of stairs in her apartment house and was bedridden at home for several months without any medical care. There were apparently no broken bones or serious internal injuries, as she is now capable of walking the stairs and traveling several blocks on foot.

Mrs. D. candidly admitted that her daughter "wants her back home in North Carolina." Consequently the daughter takes little care of her as Mrs. W.'s hospitalized son occupies much of her time.

Nature of Family Needs and Development of Plan for Meeting Needs
An immediate problem concerned hot water which they have lacked for two months now. Previous efforts to notify the landlord had resulted in "someone" examining and patching the pipes and declaring that extensive replacement work would eventually be necessary. The apartment had been visited three times by inspectors from the real estate company. Believing that the landlord had had time to correct the problem, Mrs. D. was asked to contact the Crown Heights Community Council to acquire a petition and further help. Crown Heights had been successful when dealing with the city in earlier matters concerning housing in Brooklyn.

Mrs. D. claimed she was not covered by Medicare. Since she was eligible, we referred her to Social Security to request an application form be sent her. Mrs. D. further stated that she had at one time been covered by Medicaid, but had sent the card in for renewal one year ago and had heard nothing from them. She did follow with one phone attempt but called Social Security instead, obviously confused by the agencies. We asked her to call the Medicaid number we provided and inquire.

Mrs. D.'s physical condition warranted action. She felt generally ill, which she ascribed to her diabetes, was unable to use either of two sets of dentures acquired under her old Medicare coverage. She needed glasses, had infected fingers, scraped sore by fish scaling, arthritis in her right leg, and periodic dizziness. She was currently taking three aspirins a day. She professed to be planning to visit King's County at the time we first saw her.

Following our methodology outline, we recommended that she visit the Provident Society Neighborhood Health Center immediately. If she could not clear up her Medicaid problem with the office, the Provident would determine her eligibility. The Health Center also would provide dental and eye service for Mrs. D. the clinic's location nearby was a strong point.

Mrs. D. was also eligible for a half-fare subway-bus ticket. Her daughter, having complained of "nerves" resulting from her son's condition, was given a referral to the Bedford Health Center (where she was registered) . She had not seen a doctor in over a year either.

Implementation of the Plan
Our follow-up visit showed that Mrs. D. had not accomplished any of our requested contacts in that two-week period.

For the water problem, she claimed that the landlord was again contacted and had promised to send a plumber out. To give minimum assistance, we called Crown Heights at that time but were asked to call back that afternoon, which we then instructed Mrs. D. to do. A return visit showed that she had not called. Her daughter then called and was told to visit their office to pick up necessary petitions and obtain counselling; Mrs. W. promised to do that. Our limited study time has not allowed us to follow up.

Mrs. D., due partially to her senile state and partially to the lack of cooperation by her relatives, failed to contact any of the other agencies. Our health guide team personally called the Medicare

Records Office and learned that Mrs. D. was, indeed, enrolled in Medicare on a "Buy-in" list. The state paid her premiums as it was originally judged that she needed all her social security check monthly. The office promised a mailing of her new card in three weeks.

Our health guide team, having contacted Model Cities, was supplied with half-fare applications and cards. We were then able to give them the card in the home, and mail in the registered form. This we did for Mrs. D..

Mrs. D. had not visited the Provident Clinic or sought Medicaid coverage. The health guide, Mrs. B., called Provident Health Center for an appointment and, as was our policy, accompanied her on the initial visit on July 31, 1970. Mrs. D. was interviewed and application was made for Medicaid coverage by the clinic. She was seen by a doctor, and medicine prescribed for her infections. Blood tests and chest x-rays were scheduled and she was to return to the clinic, transportation provided by Provident, on August 3, 1970. This took approximately four hours.

A follow-up on August 4, 1970, indicated that Mrs. D. was not picked up on August 3, 1970, and a call to the clinic confirmed that an oversight had occured and notice of pick-up had not been attached to her file. We were given an August 5, 1970, appointment for her which was kept. Mrs. D. took her dentures to the clinic and was seen by the dentist. New plates are being made after correction of the old ones was ruled out. Mrs. D. thought the transportation service was excellent and eagerly awaited its arrival. She was treated very courteously at the clinic.

Our investigation into the Concord Church Golden Age Recreation Program convinced us that Mrs. D. could benefit from its socializing. As study time was short we immediately offered to accompany her there and did so on August 6, 1970. She was well received by the members there (only four) and will be participating in manual projects and fund-raising sales, etc.. She was very appreciative as we left her. A worker of the church routinely provides help in returning home.

Several observations can be made:

1. In dealing with the hot water problem, the inconvenience of heating the water was not enough to encourage persistent action on the part of the tenants. They were apparently quieted by a show of

interest by the landlord in sending someone out. The lack of precise knowledge of whom to call to complain contributed some to the inaction. But the telling explanation was offered by Mrs. W.: "People would rather have the same conditions and lower rent, than improvements and higher rent." It was unclear to us what changes had occurred in the rent during the two months of no hot water.

2. A family structure cannot always be relied upon to assume care for its members. Mrs. D. lived but two blocks from the Provident Clinic yet no one saw to it that she attended there or the more established Bedford Health Center. The lack of care after the stairs accident attests to this attitude.

3. The Provident Clinic deserves special recognition. Their attributes of comprehensive medical and dental care provided in an assessible manner through an invaluable transportation service and location has assured continuing care for Mrs. D., independent of her apathetic family. In all fairness, the D.-W. family represents a series of hardships uncommon in most situations. The devotion of Mrs. W. to her son is commendable except for her neglect of those in her family who were receiving no care at all.

4. Mrs. D. illustrates that a substantial change in the physical and social conditions of a person can be accomplished by a health guide team given the existing agencies (although Provident Clinic is new in its conception and operation).

CORNELL FAMILY STUDY NO. 6

FAMILY: E.
FAMILY TYPE: Senior Citizen
AGE OF SENIOR CITIZEN: 73
NUMBER OF PERSONS IN HOME: 1

Family History

Mr. E., a 73-year-old widower, lives a simple and unsophisticated life in a one-room apartment that is only in fair condition, but is clean.

A former truck driver, Mr. E. asks very little of friends who do most of his required errands. He has limited mobility due to chronic and fairly severe arthritis in his left knee. His eyes are bad, though he has an old pair of glasses to use. Mr. E.'s medical history indicates that he has not seen a doctor in over three years, when he was seeing a private practitioner. A continuing prescription dating from that time has been lost for months, and his condition of frequent boils, for which the medication was intended, bothers him occasionally.

Mr. E. receives about $134 monthly from Social Security and a union pension, $65 of which must go for rent. Mr. E. does have Medicare.

Mr. E. is quite friendly and well-liked in his neighborhood and passes many days sitting out in front of his apartment on the store stoop.

Family Needs

Mr. E. had been contacted by the Health Guide Donated Foods Program in January. He subsequently visited the agency and enrolled. He has not heard anything from them as of our first visit on July 8. Judging that Mr. E. already was educated to the agency, we provided minimum assistance by calling the Donated Foods office. A search of their files indicated that he was on the mailing list and would receive a card by July 25. He had applied in May, not in January.

Mr. E. had also lost his Medicare card. He had not seen any need to use it, so had not felt its loss. We referred him to the local Social Security office (to be reached by phone) to request a new card.

Mr. E.'s need for glasses and prescription medicine suggested that, if eligible, Medicaid could be a great benefit. Our initial suggestion was to phone the Medicaid office to request forms through the mail. He had heard of the program but did not understand its coverage.

Mr. E.'s lack of medical care and limitation of mobility suggested that a registration at the Bedford Health Center, and use of their ambulatory service, would be necessary. But Medicaid coverage was assumed necessary for this service and an effort here was delayed until he received a Medicaid card. During the following week this plan of implementation was found necessary.

Implementation

Mr. E. received his Donated Foods card on July 27 and on July 30 had a friend pick up the food at the Throop Station. This required 2½ hours via cab and the food received was mostly leftovers from previous handouts. The officials promised them better selections next month.

A revisit to Mr. E. on July 20 found him sitting out front of his apartment. He had entrusted his various referrals to a friend who had not reported back any results. Feeling that adequate time had passed for phone contacts with agencies, we provided the minimum assistance task of calling for him.

Three phone calls were required before an agency official would take time to search the files to locate Mr. E.'s Social Security number and determine if he did have Medicare coverage. He did and was promised a replacement card in two to three weeks. He received that card on July 26, only a week later.

Following our initial talks with Mr. E., the Provident Clinical Society's Neighborhood Health Center was located and it became evident that their concern with patients as indicated by transportation service and practice of determining Medicaid eligibility for prospective patients (this coverage being required for service) made this a practical solution to his medical needs.

The health guide team had been given the privilege of making appointments for prospective patients at the center and did this for Mr. E. on July 31. We were scheduled to accompany Mr. E. to the clinic but a visit to his home before his scheduled visit found him gone. A search at the clinic found him waiting—brought down on his own initiative by a friend who drove. He remained with him and took him home in a cab after the first visit.

In his $2\frac{3}{4}$ hours at the clinic Mr. E. was questioned and application filled out and sent in by the clinic for Medicaid coverage. In addition, he was seen by a doctor, diagnosed as hypertensive, 200/120, given a prescription and an EKG. He was also scheduled for blood tests and a chest x-ray on August 4, and later to be seen for eye and tooth care on August 12. The subsequent appointment would be handled by the clinic's own transportation.

Mr. E.'s drugs would have to be paid for with cash until his Medicaid was approved, still a six- to eight-week process by mail. This was not deemed an undue hardship for that period.

A revisit on August 5 found Mr. E. in good spirits. His trip to St. John's Hospital (back-up and laboratory care for Provident) the day before was quick and courteous; it took only two hours. The mini-bus transportation made the appointment convenient and even anticipated.

Comments

Mr. E. found health care inconvenient due to his arthritic condition and crisis-oriented outlook. He still had an underlying feeling that general checkups were needed, and when "confronted" with a concerned health team, was more than willing to attend a clinic (even to the point of arriving before the guide team could meet him at home). Help with overcoming the initial and perhaps general barrier to participation with service-oriented agencies has now allowed Mr. E. the prospects of continuing preventive health care. The operations of the Provident Health Center contributed in no small way to this accommodation.

CORNELL FAMILY STUDY NO. 16

FAMILY: G.
FAMILY TYPE: Senior Citizen
AGE OF SENIOR CITIZEN: 69
NUMBER OF PERSONS IN HOME: 1

Family History

Mrs. G., a widow of fourteen years, lives a comfortable and content life in her own brownstone apartments. She has three families as tennants. Mrs. G., a West Indian from Trinidad, represents the classic case of the prevalence of West Indian home owners in the Bedford-Stuyvesant area. She has a strong sense of community spirit and conscience, and is chaplain of her local block association. She is interested in restoration possibilities, and keeps up her home well. Her attitude toward the city is negative when she talks about the "hard burden" the city places on landlords.

Her medical history is uneventful, with no present illness. Her attitudes on health care are typically crisis oriented. Her last private doctor's visit was in 1968.

Mrs. G. was most impressed by our health team's interest in her. Questions concerning her home in Trinidad brought an exclamation of surprise. She was much more friendly on subsequent visits.

Family Needs

Mrs. G. expressed much frustration at having to pay monthly for Medicare coverage and then not being covered for glasses and dentures. She had an incomplete knowledge of what services were covered by this service. A previous experience with purchasing glasses resulted in her being referred to three different agencies (undetermined) in quest of Medicaid coverage which she did not even understand. She was now discouraged and mad about her lack of success with agencies (the run-around) and failure to have programs explained.

We explained Medicaid to her and asked her to send for an application. She did not disclose her income, and some question of her eligibility arose. We felt she should have an application, though.

Mrs. G. was scheduled to attend the Brookdale multiphasic screening clinic on the following Monday, July 13. This was at her own initiative. The results would be sent to her private doctor and a visit to him would follow.

Implementation
Mrs. G. did not contact Medicaid for an application as she expressed a deeper fear of discussing her income or revealing it on an application. Her initial explanation had been, "I did not have time to call" (two-week interval).

Her interest in acquiring an application was renewed due to our revisit and we supplied minimal assistance by addressing an envelope for her. The time limit of the study did not permit us to follow up here.

Mrs. G.'s multiphasic screening clinic visit was met with extreme enthusiasm. A two-hour visit encompassing a comprehensive and courteous series of tests given with respect for the patient impressed her most. She feels the program is a blessing and that all should have access to it. She will now see her doctor for the results.

Comments
Mrs. G. is a proud and energetic woman who was a victim of inadequate education by agencies of their services. Once she is motivated by clarification, Mrs. G. is capable of using agencies for her benefit.

CORNELL FAMILY STUDY NO. 32

FAMILY: T.
FAMILY TYPE: Senior Citizen
AGE OF SENIOR CITIZEN: 70
NUMBER OF PERSONS IN HOME: 1

Family History
Mrs. T. is a 70-year-old black woman who has been living by herself now for the two years since her husband died. In that time her health has deteriorated rapidly and she claims to have lost over one hundred pounds. When we saw her she could only walk about with great difficulty; the mere excitement of our visit caused her to become sufficiently agitated to have to lie down on the bed. Her pulse was weak and her heart beat rapidly. She would close her eyes and enter a faint, being unable to answer questions or be aware of anything at all.

Upon seeing the building where she lived for the first time, I was really taken aback. The entire six-story apartment was in utter shambles. The lobby had peeling paint, there was garbage strewn about, the stairs had several slats missing, and, since someone had removed a mail chute, there remained holes on each floor landing. Most amazing was that, despite the height of the building, the elevator was locked and inoperative.

In addition to all this, Mrs. T. informed us that the building had had heat for only one week during the previous three years, no hot water, and often no cold water. The elevator had not worked in *six years.* I could hardly believe that Mrs. T. lived on the sixth floor in a building with no elevator when she could hardly walk, let alone climb stairs. She told me that two days before she had collapsed while walking up them and had been taken to St. John's Hospital and was released. Several other times she had fainted while climbing the stairs and had been carried up to the top by neighbors.

Needs and Suggested Implementation
Mrs. T.'s needs were obviously many. First was medical attention, with possible hospitalization. I believed if she could be hospitalized and then sent to a nursing home. I could have avoided the difficulties surrounding Urban Relocation. But my disgust at the sight of this place prompted me to explore the problems of the building further. We left references for pest control, relocation, and emergency repair, but I did not expect her to be able to handle any of this by herself. She wasn't.

The next time, I returned and Mrs. T. looked so bad that I decided to take her down to the Neighborhood Health Clinic that very day. She already had a Medicaid card, through her monthly welfare payment of thirty-two dollars. Upon arriving at the clinic, Mrs. T. was again in a faint and the doctors made room in their busy schedule for her. She was given a complete examination and afterwards she seemed much better, both in health and in spirits. The doctors recommended placing her in St. John's Hospital for further tests and observation. However, when the nurse tried to secure a bed, there was none, so Mrs. T. had to return home. I called and visited her all that week to find out if she had gotten in and finally, five days after the visit to the clinic, she was admitted to St. John's. She was subsequently found to have severe heart damage and is currently in St. John's Hospital.

As for the building, results were not so direct and forthcoming. As there was no immediate need for relocation for Mrs. T., I investigated how things had gotten so bad at the apartment. When I asked Mrs. T. who the landlord was, she said Mr. S. but she had not seen him in months. She said she paid rent to a Mrs. B. on the first floor. Mrs. T. seemed to be of the opinion that Mr. S. no longer owned the building. When I went to see Mrs. B. I found out she was the treasurer of a tenant's association of which a Mrs. G. was the vice president and leader.

I contacted Mrs. G. and she told me this story. Last fall, since the tenants faced the prospects of another winter without heat or hot water, they contacted their city councilman, a Mr. T., who helped them organize a rent strike. They then had all rents cut in half. By this time, however, the building had come to the attention of the City Housing Department. They had inspected the building several times and found over two hundred and forty health violations at one time or another. I understood that Mr. S. was merely paying the summonses he received and not making any repairs. Finally, when Urban Renewal and a program called Restore came into the picture, Mr. S. vacated the building entirely. That seemed to leave the tenant committee in control of the rent collection, they were now a sort of de facto owner. But as Mrs. G. had neither the will power nor time to evict people for failure to pay rent, about one half of the tenants were either not paying or were far behind in the payments. I found it amazing that one half of the tenants were paying at all under these circumstances.

As my next step, I went to see a Mr. K. of the Fulton Park Urban Renewal and asked him what plans they had for the building and the entire block. He informed me that plans were under way for the Fulton Park Urban Renewal to purchase the building from Mr. S. (still uncertain at this point). They had acquired the rights to several other buildings on the block as well and plans had been drawn up for all of them. He promised me that at least there would be a boiler installed before winter to insure heat and hot water.

With this long-range promise in hand from a man who seemed to know what he was doing I tried to get something done immediately for the building and thus encountered an entire agency which did not know what it was doing. The Department of Housing referred me to the Department of Rent and Rehabilitation, who referred me to the Department for Emergency Repairs, who did not answer. I finally was told by the Department of Housing to come in person. The next day I did manage to contact the Emergency Repair Service, who promised to send out an investigator.

Despite several attempts I was never able to contact the landlord, Mr. S.. I had to abandon my work through city agencies at this point because I had other families to contend with. If I had had more time I would have liked to have had a general meeting of all tenants in the building to explain the situation more fully and convince them to pay rent to the tenants association, which would use the money only for repairs. I would have liked to establish some priorities based on the tenants in most need, and those who had kept up in their payments. Unfortunately, Mr. T., the city councilman involved, was on vacation for the three weeks but otherwise I would have liked to see what he could have contributed, short of putting the building to the torch.

As for Mrs. T., I spoke with Mrs. G. and she assured me that she would help Mrs. T. move into a vacant second-floor apartment if she returned to the apartment from the hospital. She also had available thirty-five dollars that Mrs. T. had laid out for repairs for a window and wall that collapsed.

In the interim I also contacted a Mr. P. from DAB who said he would provide funds for a housekeeper for Mrs. T., but that he had no manpower available to do the actual work. At this time Mrs. D. and Mrs. B. had suggested people whom they thought might be interested. Ideally Mrs. T. should have been placed in a nursing home under close medical care.

Comments

This case seemed to be a microcosm of all that I encountered in Bedford-Stuyvesant this summer. First, with proper supervision and aid, Mrs. T. was able to get good medical care, whereas on her own she had not, except in crises. All that was really needed was the information on the best facility in the area and a few dollars for transportation and a little effort. However, housing was never that simple. The seeming interaction of private ownership, city control, the myriads of agencies and the buckpassing, all in the framework of a society which does not emphasize social service, all made it difficult, if not impossible, to solve the problems.

CORNELL FAMILY STUDY NO. 43

FAMILY: M.
FAMILY TYPE: Senior Citizen
AGE OF SENIOR CITIZEN: 62
NUMBER OF PERSONS IN HOME: 1

Family History

Mrs. M. resides in the first-floor apartment of a red-tiled building which she owns. She is a widow and has lived in New York City approximately forty years. Her birthplace and earlier home was in Marion, South Carolina, about which she recalls very little.

When we first contacted Mrs. M., she was confined to her apartment with an advanced case of arthritis, an unrepaired telephone, and almost no contact with the outside world. She has not been outside her home since June of 1969. A friend was visiting when we arrived, whom we saw again on our several revisits in her role of procuring food and other necessities for the disabled woman.

Mrs. M. entertains little contact with the world outside her apartment. All contact with her family has been terminated, with the exception of one grandson whom she reared and who pays her a sporadic visit. From a nearby church, Reverend H., now occupied with World Evangelism, visits her occasionally with a word of friendship and encouragement. Sister G., a resident of Reverend H.'s church, is of some assistance in times of need.

In the beginning, Mrs. M. was very suspicious of any of our questions and thus reluctant to give us honest answers. Combined with a genuine premature loss of memory, these suspicions made communications difficult during the first visits. But once she saw ways that we could help her, she became very frank and helpful. By the end of our time with her, she was looking forward to our visits with unusual excitement. From a state of mind where she had almost given up hope for any relief of her problems, her outlook changed to a hard determination and "I'll never give up" attitude at the close of our five weeks.

In regard to her health, Mrs. M. has a number of problems. She was under no care for her arthritis; she had no dentures and inadequate glasses; she had frequent lapses of memory; she was lacking adequate financial assistance for her medical problems; she had a hazy idea about her birthday and lacked proper proof of age.

Not long ago, she had a bad fall for which she had an operation to relieve pain in her left knee, leg, and ankle. Pins placed in her knee joint greatly relieved the pain but immobilized the joint. This was the last time she had contact with a physician, which was at least a year ago.

In regard to her home environment, it must be noted that the physical condition of her home has deteriorated mainly due to neglect. Weeds and debris pollute the small patch of grass in front of the building; dirt and grease on the floors attract mice and roaches; some peeling paint lines the walls. Several mousetraps were scattered throughout the room. Although the building is sturdy with adequate toilet, cooking, and plumbing facilities, the painting and appearance has greatly deteriorated because of neglect.

In her home, Mrs. M. has three roomers (one man and two women) who pay a minimum of rent. This income is barely sufficient to meet the increasingly higher property taxes she must pay. She receives no welfare, Social Security, or pension. She does have a small life insurance policy with Liberty Life Insurance Company in Greenville, South Carolina.

Nature of Need and Development of Plan to Meet Needs

The specific health needs of Mrs. M. may be enumerated as follows: arthritic treatment, uniform and concentrated medical care, Medicaid, dentures, and new glasses. For Medicaid, dentures, new glasses, and for Medicare, she needs the guidance of a trained representative for proof of age and assessment of her financial and health conditions. Although she received some arthritic treatment earlier, she was unable to recall anything about the medicine or treatment. In conjunction with her health needs, Mrs. M. would like a homemaker whose function would be housekeeping and nutritional and other health care. In addition, Mrs. M. needs to have her phone repaired to improve her meager contact with the outside world.

Our plan to meet these immediate needs involved first, contacting the telephone repair service to reestablish telephone communications. Then we made arrangements to get her to the Neighborhood Health Center for several purposes: for direct assistance from a Medicaid representative to obtain financial assistance for her medical needs, for initial registration at the clinic, for a screening examination for medication for her arthritis, for later eye and dental appointments, for arrangements for any future transportation between her home and the necessary clinics and hospitals, for a doctor's referral to DAB* or other agency to procure the aid of a homemaker, for any additional medical care and social services that she may need.

Our plan also included preparing and mailing a letter to her insurance company to obtain information about her previously named beneficiary, the means of changing her beneficiary, the cash value of the policy, how to obtain that cash value, and borrowing privileges on the policy.

Implementation of the Plan

The first step in our approach to satisfying the needs and problems of Mrs. M. was to call the New York Telephone Repair Service for emergency telephone repair. We phoned on July 24th. Two weeks later it was still out of order even after a second call to the repair service. A new switchboard was to be installed in mid-August to alleviate all phone problems in the area, but conditions were the same at the end of the summer. This and other problems we faced with telephone service proved the poor reputation of the telephone company to be a fact.

Regarding the plan to meet her immediate health needs, we first referred her to the Neighborhood Health Center to see if she had enough motivation and assistance to contact them on her own. At our

*Disabled, Aged, and Blind—New York City Department of Social Services.

first revisit we found her in the same condition. She did not contact the clinic because of a lack of communication through phone or close friends and a lack of sufficient hope that she could be helped if she struggled there by herself. Thereupon we commenced a program to personally escort her to the clinic. We procured the services of a gypsy cab this time which cost us $1.25 each way to travel five blocks. Four hours were spent at the clinic and the following was accomplished: initial registration at the clinic, interview with a Medicaid representative arranged, placement under regular surveillance by a local social case worker, a medical examination and medicine to ease her suffering from arthritis, an appointment for St. John's Arthritis Clinic, appointments for her teeth and eyes, and a revisit to Neighborhood Health Center. We were extremely pleased with what was accomplished, particularly that transportation would be provided for her for all subsequent visits to hospitals and clinics.

We revisited Mrs. M. a week later on the day of her appointment at St. John's (August 3rd), and we discovered she was unable to see the doctor. She was ready on time, but the limousine driver was not punctual and she thus missed the doctors, who remain only a short time at the hospital. Therefore, an appointment was rescheduled for the following week (August 10th), the same day as her revisit to the Neighborhood Health Center. We lacked sufficient time for follow-up on the results of these visits.

On August 4th we saw her again to see how she was getting along. We were informed that the social service agent had visited her, reminding her of her appointment and so forth. We found it necessary then to take a trip to the Neighborhood Health Clinic, planning to have her prescription filled, which she had been unable to do.

Our last visit on August 6th was heartwarming since she spoke about how she missed us each day and had continued to look forward to our coming. She signed a letter which I had prepared to mail to her insurance company to obtain information about her policy. A copy was to be sent to me so I could review it and assist her in any way possible.

Comments

At the end of our time with Mrs. M., we were encouraged by all that was accomplished to bring about the eventual satisfaction of her social and health needs. Although we met some barriers with the phone company and transportation oversights, we did see great progress made in the areas of present and future long-term medical attention. Truly the most rewarding thing was to see the change in Mrs. M.'s attitude from despair and disillusionment to hope and fortitude. This dynamic change of heart alone could be termed a success story.

CORNELL FAMILY STUDY NO. 81

FAMILY: R.
FAMILY TYPE: Senior Citizen
AGE OF SENIOR CITIZEN: 81
NUMBER OF PERSONS IN HOME: 1

Family History

Mrs. R. is the youngest-looking 81-year-old this interviewer has ever seen. She was born in South Carolina but has lived in New York City since the age of two. The past thirty-eight of these years she has lived in Bedford-Stuyvesant. A practical nurse at Kings County Hospital for twenty years, she is a spry, trim woman who has no limitation of mobility. The age of her son (present at the interview) is equally deceptive. He is a 63-year-old railroad worker who looks like 40. He visits his mother daily to see to her needs, and he supplements her public assistance allowance of $150 per month. Besides her son, Mrs. R. has two daughters, both of whom are married and have families of their own. This is apparently an extremely tightly knit family unit as evidenced by the plethora of family pictures and memorabilia displayed on the walls.

Mrs. R. lives alone in a spacious six-room apartment on the fourth floor of a four-story building, for which she pays $54 a month. She meticulously cleans the apartment herself, and it is immaculate. She has her own bathroom and cooking facilities, adequate heating and water, and a receptive landlord. Housing is not a problem.

Seated next to Mrs. R. on the couch was a large feminine doll. Upon questioning, she revealed that the doll is her "companion"—she buys stockings for it, sleeps with it, and talks with it. She also envinced some evidence of paranoia (hides things), but her son attributes all of this to senility. Mrs. R. spends her days looking out the window and watching TV.

Mrs. R. has a very fatalistic attitude about death, and is quite prepared to sit back and accept it as a natural occurrence. In addition, the concept of preventative medicine is alien to her. Further, she cannot stand crowds or waiting in lines, and for those reasons will not attend clinics. Consequently, she has not had a physical examination in about eight years. The occasion for that was a course of treatment for arthritis at Cumberland Hospital.

Nature of Needs and Development of Plan for Meeting Needs

Actually, Mrs. R. has remarkably few needs for a woman her age. Although visibly well she should have a complete physical. She has hearing difficulty and probably needs a hearing aid. Since she is on Medicaid, these problems could be quite easily solved if she were registered at the Provident Health Center, which is right around the corner. Her son should accompany her on this and future visits. Her mental status is somewhat in question, and perhaps the companionship to be found at a senior citizens' club might be helpful. Finally, her son should get her a half-fare card, which she did not know existed.

Implementation of Plan for Meeting Needs

Surprisingly (to me), Mrs. R. registered at the health center on our suggestion and had a physical. She is currently in the process of getting a hearing aid through them, and was given vitamins as well. Her son also procured a half-fare card for her. Thus, the needs we assessed for this woman were met after she became convinced they were actually needs and was educated as to how to deal with them.

Comments

Mrs. R. was ignorant of the health facilities in the Bedford-Stuyvesant area, but given her attitudinal predisposition, I was dubious if she would avail herself of them even if she did know. Further, her son seemed too indulgent of his mother's whims to be effective in getting her to the clinic. I was pleasantly surprised on all counts.

CORNELL FAMILY STUDY NO. 83

FAMILY: R.
FAMILY TYPE: Senior Citizen
AGE OF SENIOR CITIZEN: 69
NUMBER OF PERSONS IN HOME: 1

Family History

Miss R. is a 69-year-old woman who lives alone in a three-room apartment on the second floor of a four-story building, for which she pays

$75 monthly in rent. Her heat was out most of the winter, and as of late she has had no hot water. This may be due to the fact that the building is condemned and is scheduled to be torn down next year. Understandably, relocation is Miss R.'s number one concern. Originally from Virginia, she has lived in New York City for fifty years. The last thirty-eight of those years have been spent at the same residence. Miss R. receives public assistance and Old Age Social Security totaling $170 monthly. She is covered by both Medicare and Medicaid. Socially, she is isolated. She has no family or friends (they have already been relocated), and spends her days at home alone.

Miss R. is under the care of a private physician in the area, and she recently had a complete physical which did not turn up anything that was not already known: she has arthritis, terrible sinuses, and heart disease. She cannot walk more than two or three blocks without getting out of breath. She is in need of new glasses, dentures, and quite possibly a hearing aid.

Nature of Family Needs and Development of Plan for Meeting Needs
When we first rang her bell, Miss R. mistook us for someone coming to restore her hot water, which had been gone for two weeks. Apparently, she had tried to work through Urban Renewal but had gotten nowhere. We thereupon referred her to the Housing Authority and gave her the number, suggesting that they might be able to help her more satisfactorily. Although she has more pressing problems than this, it was important to solve this one first, for without hot water she cannot bathe, and if she cannot bathe she refuses to leave the apartment, and if she does not leave the apartment she cannot work at solving her other problems.

Given the length of her residence in the same apartment (38 years), Miss R. should have been given priority in the relocation process when the building was condemned, but such was not the case. She is one of the few people remaining in the building. She has been packed for four months and is living out of trunks awaiting placement from Urban Renewal while a court order hangs over her head. According to her, this unfortunate situation can be traced to bureaucratic incompetence on the part of Urban Renewal, resulting from rapid turnover of help and apathy. (Her application has been lost *three* times). Miss R. justifiably refers to these people as "third-raters," an epithet I have adopted. Since she has exhausted her resources and has been repeatedly thwarted, the plan is for me to personally contact the agency.

In the realm of health, Miss R.'s problem is that her doctor does not accept Medicaid payment. Ideally, she should become registered at a clinic offering continuing care, pick-up service, and one that accepts Medicaid. Such a clinic is the nearby Neighborhood Health Center of the Provident Clinical Society. This clinic could also see to her possible need of a hearing aid, dentures, and new glasses. Thus we informed her of the facility and referred her to them.

As was mentioned earlier, Miss R. is socially isolated. Thus, she should be referred to a senior citizen's club in the area (Concord Church is the closest one).

Finally, when Miss R. registered for donated foods, she was sent to the depot at Bushwick Avenue. This is ridiculous, since she lives two blocks away from the Albany Avenue depot, and has trouble getting even that far. We apprised her of this fact and instructed her in the rite of transfer.

Implementation of Plan for Meeting Needs

Miss R., as we expected, contacted all the agencies we told her about. During the initial interview she displayed righteous indignation with respect to her treatment at the hands of the bureaucrats, and seemed determined to act on her own behalf if she only knew what to do. She contacted the Housing Authority and they sent a man out to fix the water pipes. She registered at the health center. She obtained a donated food transfer to the nearer depot. She joined the Concord Church Senior Citizen Club.

The only problem left unsolved is the most serious one—relocation. Urban Renewal had a different version of the R. vs. New York case. They claim that she has already been offered space in two projects in Borwnsville, but that she has turned them both down, insisting that she will go nowhere but the Senior Citizen Project on Bergen Street. Urban Renewal disavowed any knowledge of lost applications, but said that at any rate her application was now complete and all she can do is wait. Thus, Miss R. continues to live out of a trunk in the hope that a vacancy will arise at Bergen Street before the wreckers come.

Comments

I am stymied.

CORNELL FAMILY STUDY NO. 201

FAMILY: E.
FAMILY TYPE: Newcomer
NUMBER OF PERSONS IN HOME: 9

Family History

Mrs. E. has been in New York for only two years and Bedford-Stuyvesant for one since leaving her native South Carolina. She is separated and has three boys, ages 4, 3, and 2. She is unemployed, her total income being the $218 per month she receives from Social Service. Also living with the E. family in their bare 3½-room apartment is Mrs. E.'s sister, Mrs. W., and her four children, ages 7, 3, 2, and 1.

The physical structure of the apartment was one of the worst visited by the team, and Mrs. E.'s housekeeping was equally bad. The place was extremely filthy and scantily furnished. The furnishings consisted of an old couch and chair, a table with a broken TV in the living room, and a table with chairs in the kitchen.

Although the interview was close to noon, Mrs. E. was still in her robe and was quite inattentive. Mrs. W. was also in her robe and remained silent, slumped in a chair, throughout the interview. The team felt that she was either on drugs or extremely bored with what we were saying. Both the health guide and the medical student felt that both women were apathetic and had very low potential to follow through.

Needs and Implementation

Mrs. E. informed us that she was visited by a relocation representative about a month ago and told to find a new apartment, if possible, because hers would be torn down eventually. He also gave her an application for the city projects to complete and mail at that time. She completed the form, but neglected to mail it. She was urged to mail, or better yet, to deliver the form in person and make an emergency plea for top priority because of the overcrowding of their apartment. She was also urged to find her own apartment, rather than letting Relocation find one for her, because of the greater financial return.

It was also learned that Mrs. E. was not receiving welfare for any of her children, and that Mrs. W. was not receiving any welfare at all. They thought if the city knew Mrs. W. was living with Mrs. E., Mrs.

E. would receive less money. They were told this was not the case, and were referred to the Welfare Rights Organization for help.

The children were currently receiving their immunizations at the Provident Clinic and Mrs. E. was urged to make sure the children completed the series. However, she did not keep the appointment for the children's lead screening test set up by the guides who first visited her. She was given a second appointment.

Headstart was also discussed, but not given much chance of success because the only argument for it that impressed Mrs. E. was that it would give her more time. It was suggested that she contact the local school, which was only two blocks away, and see if she could enroll her 3- and 4-year-olds.

Finally, as we were leaving, a cousin of Mrs. E., who was visiting her, mentioned that Mrs. W. was sick and had had "a bad stomach ache" for the last two days. Because she had no Medicaid she was referred to King's County Hospital, and because of the emergency of the situation transportation money was given to her by the health guide. The cousin, who seemed quite capable, said she would accompany her there and would call the health guide offices once there to let us know the status of Mrs. W.'s illness. It was learned later, when we returned to the offices, that Mrs. W. was admitted to the hospital with a diagnosis of appendicitis.

On our return visit, Mrs. E. reported that she received $280 from welfare for her youngest son, and will continue to receive a small amount each month for him. Likewise, Mrs. W. registered with the Welfare Department, and will be receiving aid in the future. Mrs. E. reported keeping the screening test appointment for her children, and had, amazingly, washed her floors in the interim. She also informed us that she was pregnant again, and was referred to Provident for prenatal care and family planning once the child was born.

She was unmotivated, however, to do anything about the housing or Headstart. Plans were made to meet with her next week and accompany her to the school and to the Brooklyn Public Improvement Association (housing). The week delay would enable Mrs. E. to obtain a record of her children's immunizations from Provident. Since the children were going there for a dental checkup in a few days anyway, this involved little extra effort on her part.

On the specified date, we accompanied her to P.S. #256 where her 4-year-old was enrolled in Headstart. The school was unable to take her 3-year-old, but referred us to the Salvation Army next door who also ran a Headstart program that would be able to accommodate the 3-year-old. We went there and applied, but being a 3-year-old, he had least priority and was put on a waiting list. Because of the time spent at the school and Salvation Army, Mrs. E. was not able to go to the housing agency. Therefore, we went there in her behalf. They accepted her application, but because of the shortage, could offer no additional help in spite of the fact that she was pregnant and that nine people were living in the 3½-room apartment.

Comments
At the first interview, we were quite sure that Mrs. E. would be unlikely to follow through on our suggestions. In fact we considered Headstart to be the most important need simply because it would provide an alternative influence on the children. It was a great satisfaction to have Mrs. E. solve most of her needs by herself. Her case exemplifies the importance of education.

CORNELL FAMILY STUDY NO. 216

FAMILY: A.
FAMILY TYPE: Newcomer
NUMBER OF PERSONS IN HOME: 7

Family History
Mrs. A. came to New York from her native Puerto Rico 2½ years ago, and has been living in Bedford-Stuyvesant for the last four months. She is 28 years old, speaks only Spanish, and has six children (ages 12, 9, 6, 5, 3, 1). Because she speaks only Spanish the health guide, who is bilingual, did all of the interviewing.

Mrs. A. is not employed, but receives $428 each month from the Social Services. Her 4½-room apartment rents for $70 per month and is in very poor condition. At the time of our first interview, she had no furniture other than beds and some kitchen chairs. Mrs. A. had traveled to Manhattan two weeks previously and bought furniture with her rent money, but it had not been delivered yet. She chose the store in Manhattan, rather than one in Brooklyn, because it was owned by Spanish-speaking people and she could communicate with them.

The cement floor in Mrs. A.'s apartment has no covering of any kind, there are numerous cracks in the wall, and the large window in her kitchen is broken out so that the children are able to climb over the window sill into the back yard. The back yard is full of trash and garbage, and is an ideal breeding ground for rats and disease. Mrs. A. has already registered with the city to enter a project when an opening becomes available.

Family Needs
Mrs. A. is not receiving any welfare for her three youngest children. She has not been able to keep her appointments at the welfare center because she has trouble getting a baby-sitter and certainly cannot take her children with her.

Of Mrs. A.'s six children, only the 12-year-old has had any formal education. He has completed one year at P.S. #309, and is able to speak a little English. The 9-year-old daughter, L., is mentally retarded, deaf, and reported to be an epileptic. She has spent some time at Brooklyn Hospital, but it was not clear exactly what was done for her there. None of the children have received much medical care, specifically immunizations or general physical examinations, with the exception of C., age 3, who Mrs. A. reported has an operation about every eight months to change her sex. C. and L. are not the only children of Mrs. Aa's that have congenital deformities. Another child has very small or absent toenails, and another has six fingers on each hand.

Mrs. A.'s former social worker had arranged for Mrs. A. to have an "operation" so she could not have any more children. She was unable to keep this appointment because, again, she had no one who would care for her children while she was in the hospital. She also has a general problem of communicating with her social worker because her social worker does not speak Spanish.

Implementation of Needs
In accordance with the first phase of the study, Mrs. A. was given suggestions and referrals to aid her in solving her problems. Since

she could speak only Spanish, only agencies that had Spanish-speaking workers were utilized.

During the first interview, a neighbor visited Mrs. A. and was approached as to the possibility of baby-sitting for Mrs. A. while she went to the welfare center to find out about receiving financial aid for her three youngest, about receiving donated foods or food stamps; about a second appointment for a tubal ligation or some form of birth control, and about what that office could do for her mentally ill child. She was referred to the Bedford Health Clinic and given instructions on how to get there, so that her children could receive their immunizations, lead poisoning tests, and a general physical and dental examination. While there she could also talk with someone concerning family planning and her mentally defective child.

Mrs. A. lived within two blocks of two different schools, and it was suggested that she visit one or both with her 12-year-old as an interpreter and inquire about enrolling her 5- and 6-year-olds in Headstart, and also find out what the school system could do to help her learn the English language.
To meet her home repair needs, it was suggested that Mrs. A. have her bilingual sister contact the New York City Housing and Redevelopment Board at 597 Gates Avenue. Finally, Mrs. A. was instructed to complain to the furniture store about the poor service she was getting.

Because Mrs. A. was not contacted until two weeks into the study and because she had several difficult needs to solve for a person who could not speak English, it was decided not to let the entire week and a half lapse before visiting her again. Therefore, we returned one week later. At that time, Mrs. A.'s needs were no closer to being solved than the previous week.

She visited the Social Service Center, where she was informed that she had been transferred to a new center and would receive the name of her new social worker and his location by mail. She did not go to the Bedford Health Clinic because she could not get a baby-sitter. She also failed to contact either the schools or the home repair agency. Mrs. A. still had no furniture, but did contact the distributor. He told her that her furniture had been damaged and was sent back to the factory, and that she would be getting a new set within a few days.

We decided to wait another week for the Social Service to contact Mrs. A.. Likewise the furniture company was given another week before any intervention by us on behalf of Mrs. A. was undertaken. Thus, we concentrated on solving the health and educational needs of the children. That same day, we visited P.S. #9. They had no room in their Headstart for either the 5- or 6-year-olds, but would see that the 6-year-old started school this fall. They also told us of their "day camp" for children who had been to school before and urged us to enroll Mrs. A.'s 12-year-old. We then visited P.S. #309, where we were able to enroll both the 5- and 6-year-olds. It was a bonus to learn that they also had one Spanish-speaking teacher who would help ease the children into the new environment. The children were unable to begin school, however, until they had been immunized. We contacted the Bedford Health Clinic, but their immunization clinic is only open on Thursday mornings and we had to wait until then. At the same time, we were referred to the Ralph Avenue Station for the 3-year-old's immunizations and family planning for Mrs. A.. The earliest appointment we could get at the Ralph Avenue Station for the 3-year-old was, unfortunately, three weeks away, and for Mrs. A. over two weeks away. Both of these dates would be after the study had terminated, and might be hard for her to keep without some help.

On the day we were to revisit Mrs. A., the health guide was late because of a bus accident. This turned out to be fortunate in that Mrs. A. found her own interpreter—a young woman from Flushing who was visiting her sister, a neighbor of Mrs. A.'s. She not only acted as an interpreter until the health guide arrived, but volunteered to baby-sit while we went to the clinic.

At the clinic, the 5- and 6-year-olds received their vaccinations. We also tried to get a lead screening test done, but that clinic was not open while we were there. We were told that if we arrived at 9:00 A.M. the next time we came for immunizations, we might catch the man who draws blood before he leaves on his daily appointments. If not, we would have to come when the clinic was open, which constituted a separate trip.

When we returned from the clinic, the health guide accompanied Mrs. A. and the two children to the school and I remained behind to baby-sit for the others (the lady from Flushing had to return home to pick her own child up from school at 11:00 A.M. She did promise to return the following week to baby-sit again).

Mrs. A. had received her furniture by this time, but had still not heard from the Social Service Department. I called her old center and was referred to her new one, where I talked with a Mr. S.. He is the supervisor of her unit and knew nothing about her because they had not received her file from the previous center. He was receptive and considered her case a challenge. He specifically stated that he would have her social worker address himself to adjusting her welfare, to getting her on the food stamps program, and to seeing that her mentally ill child received the proper tests. He also stated that they would visit her shortly regardless of whether her file came or not.

We also visited the Bedford office of the City Redevelopment and Housing Maintenance Agency. They could do nothing for Mrs. A. yet, because broken windows are not considered an emergency during the summer. They suggested we return in the fall and file a complaint then.

A letter was mailed to a Mrs. B. at St. John's Hospital's Psychiatric Division about the status of the mentally ill child. They will then inform Mrs. A. by mail when to bring the child to the hospital.

At the final visit, the children received DPT and polio shots. Since it was the last week of the study, we were unable to see that they received all of the shots. We left a map of how to get to both the Bedford and Ralph Avenue clinics. The lady from Flushing said she would help Mrs. A. keep the immunization and family planning appointments.

Comments

Mrs. A. is tremendously hampered in solving her problems because she does not speak English and because her family size makes her immobile. It seems cruel to make her come to the Welfare Center instead of the worker visiting her, and it seems insane to have a worker assigned to her who cannot speak Spanish. She is very appreciative of outside help and will solve her problems with a little support.

It was learned at the final visit that the father of her last child would like to marry her, but that her family objects. She says he treats her well, has a job and a car, is bilingual, and has offered to fix up her apartment. In light of this, and that her family gave her absolutely no help while we were with her, we strongly urged that she marry him.

REFERENCES

1. Sunley, R. Family advocacy: From case to cause. *Social Casework, 51:*347-357, June 1970.
2. Young, M.M. People workers: A local health department's experience with health education aids. *Amer. J. Public Health, 59:*1845-1850, Oct. 1969.
3. Blum, H.L. The multipurpose worker and the neighborhood multiservice center: Initial experiences and implications of the Rodeo Community Service Center. *Amer. J. Public Health, 58:*458-468, Mar. 1968.
4. Wise, H.B. The family health worker. *Amer. J. Public Health, 58:*1828-1838, Oct. 1968.
5. Kent, J.A., and Smith, C.H. Involving the urban poor in health services through accommodation: The employment of neighborhood representatives. *Amer. J. Public Health, 57:*997-1003, June 1967.
6. Brown, G.E. *The Multi-Problem Dilemma.* Metuchen, New Jersey, Scarecrow Press, 1968.
7. Geisnar, L.L., and Ayres, B. *Measuring Family Functioning.* St. Paul, Minn., Greater St. Paul Community Chest and Council, 1960.
8. Blumenthal, H.T. *Medical and Clinical Aspects of Aging.* New York and London, Columbia University Press, 1962.
9. Gibson, C.D. The neighborhood health center. *Amer. J. Public Health, 50:*1188-1191, July 1968.
10. Hazell, K. *Social and Medical Problems of the Elderly.* Springfield, Thomas, 1966.
11. Henley, B.M. Helping the elderly find community services. *Amer. J. Nurs. 63:*89-92, April 1963.
12. Homburger, F., and Bonner, C. *Medical Care and Rehabilitation of the Aged and Chronically Ill,* 2nd ed. Boston, Little, Brown and Co., 1964.
13. Vedder, C.B., and Lefkowitz, A. *Problems of the Aged.* Springfield, Thomas, 1965

Chapter 14

PRIORITIES IN COMMUNITY HEALTH: THE CHALLENGE TO EPIDEMIOLOGY

GORDON T. STEWART

"He that will not apply new remedies must expect new evils; for time is the greatest innovator."

Francis Bacon, Essays, 24, ("Of Innovations")

IN THE PRECEDING chapters, we have presented approaches and achievements in some of the chief avenues of epidemiology, looking at the needs as well as the states of health and disease of people in selected communities, people in special categories and people in general. This width of approach and accomplishment is the main trend today in epidemiology, which has diversified itself by borrowing the elegant techniques and theories of biostatistics and genetics to make more meaningful the facts of human health variously gathered: by elementary shoe-leather explorations in Bedford-Stuyvesant, by talking to kids in Haight-Ashbury, by prospective surveillance in Framingham, or by more sophisticated, remote analyses elsewhere. The results in the various chapters speak for themselves and exemplify the commitment of epidemiology to service no less than to education and research. There is no need for further generalization about trends and achievements, which are so obvious in their applications to immediate, pressing problems of human health, nor is there any need to apologize for some editorial eclecticism, without which the book would have been unmanageably long and slow in publication. There is a need, however, to examine the extent to which epidemiology is developing effective intellectual and technical approaches to a parallel problem, that of the general assessment of needs and priorities and of health care in a very charismatic health scene.

There are times when it is necessary to reconsider familiar concepts both rapidly and radically. The present time is, if ever there was one, a time of rapid change in practically every aspect of human life and endeavor. Insofar as health is a prime condition affecting both, it is time to reconsider health as a major—perhaps the major—item in the human inventory.

HEALTH AND MEDICAL CARE

Health is a simple word for a concept of enormous complexity. Like other primal words (life, bread, love, self), it has its origin deep in all languages. In English, health comes from the Old English word "hāl" (whole), which still finds use in phrases like "hale and hearty" to express its positive meaning. The French word "santé" has its etymologic origin in the Latin "sanitas," with bifurcation in English (and some other languages) into "sanitary," which is one aspect of health, and "sanity," which is another.

Because differences in opinion, interpretation, and action are often semantic, it is helpful before proceeding further to think about the possible importance of these differences in the basic meaning of the word. Health is regarded as an index of the quality of life in practically all cultures, primitive and modern, but there is a profound difference between the qualities conveyed by the words "sanitary" and "sanity," though both are indubitably relevant. Similarly, the word "hygiene" had a holistic meaning in classical Greek which is not fully conveyed by its usage in modern English.[1] Interpretive divergences based upon these semantic differences have found their way historically into various cultures and affected the style and quality of life in modern societies. For instance, in many countries today, statutory authorities and legislation dealing with health are preoccupied with sanitation rather than sanity; with absence of certain diseases rather than all-round fitness; with the quality of optionals, like branded products, rather than the quality of essentials, like air, soil, and water. Correspondingly, traditional medicine is geared to treatment much more than to prevention of disease, illness, or disability (Table 14.1). The reasons here are stronger because there is an emotional as well as a philosophic drive involved: illness and disability arouse compassion in humanitarian societies, which therefore orient their medical expectations and rewards toward re-

TABLE 14.1
CONTRASTING PARADIGMS OF ORGANIC DISORDER AND ILLNESS

	Organic Disorder (Disease)	Illness (Disability)
Definition	Organic or biochemical damage Coordinated symptoms Observable derangement	Personal awareness of discomfort
Recognition	Diagnosis	Problem-solving
Management	Symptomatic or specific therapy	Knowledgeable intervention
Place	Clinic, hospital	Home, half way house
Resource	Technology	Supportive measures
Training of attendants	Diploma, degree	Apprenticeship, experience

lief of suffering and cure of illness. Medicine men, as priests of the healing art, have enjoyed status and authority for thousands of years but they have seldom sought or acquired equal status as teachers of the gospel of health even when—as in most organic diseases, until recently—they had little else to offer. Maintenance of health is therefore rooted, historically and professionally, in medical care,[2] which in the positive sense means relief of suffering but in the negative sense means preoccupation with illness, disability, and disease. In some societies, this preoccupation amounts to an obsession with sickness and leads to elaborate provisions for semisickness as a way of life in nursing homes, spas, and other resorts. Linked to this outlook was payment for services rendered, which meant in practice that service followed money and the suffering poor continued to suffer either from neglect or from charity. Social reforms in Europe before World War I led many countries to provide insurance against illness[1] by state-subsidized prepayment. This was a historic departure from the two fiscal extremes of payment for service, on the one hand, and charitable asylum, on the other; but it maintained the orientation toward illness though social reformers and critics of the system, like George Bernard Shaw, began to voice the heterodoxy that doctors should be paid to keep people well. The need and demand for more extensive insurance against a wider range of illnesses and disabilities gained momentum during and after World War II, and several countries established national organizations for this purpose, still laying emphasis primarily upon treatment of the sick. The British National Health Service, founded in 1948, was originally a National Sickness Service, comparatively efficient and undoubtedly humane in its working, but essentially unconcerned until recently with prevention of disease or disability or with promotion of positive health except insofar as antenatal care, early diagnosis of illness, and treatment could contribute. Most other developed countries now have similar systems, benevolent in concept and successful in easing, if not removing, the financial burden of illness but, in many countries still, even this degree of protection is very limited.

Health Care in the United States

In the United States, where public opinion is thought to resist the invasion of private health sectors by federal or state programs, the bulk of expenditure (about $70 billion annually) on "health" is on curative medical care, while at least the same amount is expended on indirect care, including over-the-counter medicines, self-medication, and unorthodox systems, practices, and cults. Inherent in this system—or nonsystem[3]—is the belief that quality of service is still dependent upon a fee-for-service-rendered and upon private enterprise, which is a keystone of American economy and popular philosophy. Incentives and value scales of professional health workers and of the general public conform, by and large, to this pattern. Meanwhile, medicine has advanced and diversified, with the result that provision for the diagnosis and treatment of disease, even minor disease, has become very elaborate, raising costs to levels which are now much higher than most individuals or even group insurance policies can afford. In consequence, issues of health have become so urgent that, in the words of President Nixon,[4] the nation faces a "massive crisis in health care." His view echoes widespread public, political, and professional concern over what has been more strongly described[5] as a "national health disaster," thus:

If one thing is clear in the United States of 1971, it is that health

> care is the fastest-growing failing business in the Nation—a $70 billion industry that fails to meet the urgent needs of our people. Today, more than ever before, we are spending more on health care and enjoying it less.
>
> In spite of our vaunted research and technology, unequaled by any other nation in the history of the world, America is an also-ran in the delivery of health care to our people.
>
> Almost every family knows the cruel burden of worry, frustration, and disappointment that mark our search for better health care. The average American lives in dread of illness and disability. He lives with the uncertainty of not knowing whether to seek medical care, or when to seek it, or where to find it, or how to pay for it.

With both political parties and influential sections of labor, professions, and public opinion in agreement, there is little doubt that the 92nd Congress will have to deal with health as a national crisis as well as a controversial political issue. But the agreement signifies only the common opinion and experience that the existing system has failed, and a better expectation for the future.

There is much disagreement, politically and professionally, about how health care can be improved. All plans so far formulated—the A.M.A. Medicredit,[6] the Nixon plan,[4] the Griffiths-Kennedy plan,[5] and others[7]—lay chief emphasis on the provision of more comprehensive care; the only definite suggestions for more effective prevention are periodic health checks, antenatal care, improved diagnostic facilities, and disease-oriented research, e.g. on cancer. Primary prevention is de-emphasized except insofar as existing organizations like the National Center for Disease Control and the National Institutes of Health will be maintained; there are no specific provisions for multifactor control of venereal disease, drug abuse, accidents, disorders of infants, mental disorders, environmental hazards, chemical poisoning, or dental disorders; nor is there any indication, except from unofficial groups,[8,9] about how urban planning, environmental improvement, transportation, manpower, health education, relief of poverty, and numerous other overlapping facets of the health problem are going to be incorporated in the plan at local, state, and federal levels or, in general, about how primary preventive care is going to be extended.

STRATEGY FOR HEALTH CARE

It is difficult to escape the view that the oversights in past and present planning, as well as the failure of the existing system, are due to one simple historical fact:[1] effort, initiative, and expenditure are overwhelmingly preoccupied with the provision of episodic medical care and with attention to disease, disability, or accidents *after* the event; logistically, this converts every person into a potential patient, a consumer of services related to his or her health. Inevitably, the techniques of consumer-based economy are therefore employed to make him expect and consume more of the available service, with the difference, as compared with other aspects of consumer economics, that techniques such as cost-benefit analysis, value for money, consumer protection, profit restriction, and corporate responsibility are seldom applied. The ultimate expression of this sickness orientation is declared in an increasing range of cliff-edge practices in which, at enormous cost, a few persons might receive temporary alleviation of symptoms or brief postponement of death. The relentless laws of sentimental supply and morbid demand are beginning to operate in this hitherto exclusive sector, raising the specter of more highly organized resuscitation, transplant surgery, and banks of spare organs for the hundreds of thousands of old people who at present die each year from cardiac, pulmonary, and renal insufficiency or who are rescued from terminal pneumonia to die of senility.

The question to be examined here is not that medical care even in its more esoteric forms is bad, but that there are limits in all fields of human endeavor; extension of medical care on contemporary lines could quickly exhaust available resources of energy, funds, and professional expertise, imperiling the maintenance of existing services and inhibiting the development of effective preventive services aimed at the alleviation of more extensive and socially more serious problems like retardation in childhood, poverty, ignorance, population-growth, malnutrition, mental illness, alienation, and drug dependence, none of which is effectively covered by standard health services or by any of the new plans.

Assessment of this wider meaning of health means consideration of the determinants of health not only biologically, demographically, and socially, but of the health of the body politic, for there can be no health if basic human needs are neglected or thwarted. A way must be found to describe and assess cultural, administrative, and political considerations as realistically as technical considerations in health programs.[10] Technical skill is nowadays adequate to control tuberculosis, venereal disease, and malnutrition; but administrative and political skills are not adequate, and the problems remain or even increase, as do pollution, crime, alienation, drug abuse, and numerous other pervasive threats to the health of all streams of any society, even among the "unyoung, the unpoor and the unblack,"[11] in the privileged as in the underprivileged. Realization of these wider aspects of health maintenance is boosting human ecology as a descriptive discipline; but for exact assessment of determinants, we still have to rely upon the epidemiological approach, which must, in turn, adapt itself to the new demands by redefining health in terms of the quality of life and by developing methods for assessing fitness as a congenial as well as a physical or disease-free adjustment to a given setting.[12] This is the new frontier for a discipline which has always been the basic science of public health and preventive medicine but which has been preoccupied, until now, with specific diseases of high prevalence: firstly with herd infections and epidemics, more recently with gross chronic afflictions[13,14] like heart disease, cancer, and stroke, but only occasionally with social or behavioral disorders. When serious attention has been paid, even retrospectively, to cultural and behavioral parameters like smoking[15] or dietary habits (Chaps. 2, 4, 5, and 7), the results have been highly informative and no less practical; it could well be said that the biggest practical contribution from any quarter to the prevention of chronic disease is the demonstration epidemiologically of the simple, quantitative relationship between smoking and heart disease, lung cancer, and brochitis.[16,17] The epidemiological approach to such problems usually has the added advantage that, though impersonal, it is humane, relying upon questions, observations, and limited experiments, with a minimum of interference with people's activities and comfort and with preservation of personal responsibility for personal health. It could fairly be said, also, that the dividends in relief of suffering and expenditure also are impressive: the most striking achievements in preventing cancer, namely of the cervix uteri and lung, have been accomplished by surveillance[18] at a fraction of the cost of experimental cancer research.

MULTIFACTORIAL ETIOLOGY OF DISEASE AND DISABILITY

In asserting the axiomatic quality of this concept, epidemiology stands in opposition to the Doctrine of Specific Etiology elaborated by Bretonneau,[19] which holds that for every disease there is a single, ascertainable cause. Fortified by the success of the Germ Theory between 1870 and 1900, Bretonneau's doctrine has been assimilated into medical reasoning to an extraordinary extent, with the result that immense efforts are still directed towards discovering single causes of every main threat to health—heart disease, metabolic disease, stroke, cancer, drug addiction, accidents, malnutrition—even when it is self-evident, as in the conditions mentioned, that multiple influences are operating. Politically, this mentality prevails in quest of the vain hope that identification of a single cause will always lead to a simple answer or technique, like vaccination against poliomyelitis or discovery of an ideal drug.

It is, in fact, questionable if the Doctrine of Specific Etiology has any logical place in medical science except indirectly by serving as a spur in the hunt for principal factors or agents[20] and for grading them in order of importance. The weakness of the doctrine is best illustrated by those very diseases in which, because chief agents are identifiable, it still finds its strongest applicability, e.g. in syphilis, diabetes, and chemical poisoning. Syphilis can be completely controlled prophylactically or therapeutically by an almost ideal drug, penicillin; yet its incidence is rising due to uncontrollable behavioral and societal factors which are equally germane to the disease (p. 370). Diabetes mellitus can be symptomatically controlled by insulin replacement—but without touching the cause. Chemical poisoning clearly results from chemicals, but elimination of hazards resulting from environmental chemicals is proving to be almost insurmountable because our way of life requires or tolerates them: lead poisoning is a clear example of this, especially among children.[25] It obviously cannot occur unless lead is inhaled or ingested, but environmental contamination makes involuntary ingestion inevitable. Lead in gasoline is inhaled by everyone in congested cities[22] and, while there is a continuing debate between governments, industries, and health scientists about the danger to health therefrom,[21-24] the elimination of this poison from the atmosphere is clearly desirable but difficult to enforce because of industrial practice and attitudes.[22-25] The use of lead in certain industries (car batteries, paint, plumbing) is a traditional occupational hazard.[26] Ingestion of lead by children is a certainty[21,27,28] in old, dilapidated dwellings and leads to serious, irreparable disease, including encephalopathy and mental retardation,[21,28] which may be epidemic in scale in some cities[26] and increasing.[29,30] Reports from Japan[31] confirming earlier reports from Sweden[32] and elsewhere strongly suggest that contamination of river water by cadmium causes osteomalacia, glycosuria, and aminoaciduria ("itai-itai" or "ouch-ouch" disease). Mercury,[33] other metals,[26] and numerous other named and unnamed chemicals add to the environmental hazard, though precise information about their effect on health seems always to be obtained after, rather than before, contamination is permitted.[30]

The prime cause of environmental pollution and poisoning is human behavior and industrial economy, which must therefore be assessed and included in multifactor control. In such situations, facts and figures speak for themselves if objectively presented. There is no need to await the demonstration of a trace metal or questionable carcinogen before controlling pollution, for complaints and mortality records[34-36] are equally valid as indicators of discomfort or hazard and much easier to obtain. It is beyond doubt that social and environmental inferiority, especially in urban districts, have a profound influence upon health from infancy onward.[10,37-41] The relatively high infant mortality rate in the United States is due, not to unknown diseases or to low socioeconomic levels per se,[38] but to disproportionately high rates in certain numerically large, underprivileged groups—40 per 1000 live births in Harlem compared with 13 per 1000 in Maspeth-Forest Hills, N.Y.[42] We stand in need of epidemiological investigation of these problems, not to see why they exist but why they continue to exist.

The epidemiological method requires detailed examination of as many variables as can be practicably handled whenever a disease or change in the health of a community is being investigated. Some variables such as age, sex, and occupation are included routinely, but in selecting others out of the many which might be relevant, great care and judgment are required to accord same priority to those which are most relevant.[13] This process necessarily lessens objectivity but has the compensating advantages of minimizing complexity and retaining common sense. The biggest advances have often resulted from testing limited hypotheses rather than by conducting elaborate surveys: it is questionable, for instance, if the "green finger" successes of Lind, Jenner, Snow, Semmelweis, Goldberger, or Doll would have been achieved by wide surveillances or multivariate analyses of any number of factors in the populations which they studied. This limitation of our methodology is well described by Sartwell in Chapter 1, for at the other extreme, critical evaluation of overlapping risk factors in chronic disease obviously requires elaborate planning of a prospective or retrospective surveillance, as in the Framingham Study (Chap. 6). To include the less tangible administrative, political, and behavioral factors, new techniques are required. But whatever the problem, the approach used for factor evaluation differs according to whether or not a chief cause or agent has been identified. If the former, then the search is for accessory factors like overcrowding, environmental pressure, malnutrition, or anxiety, which can precipitate or aggravate diseases without causing them. If no agent has been identified, the search first resembles a reconnaissance of an uncertain area and it is appropriate to consider, in such situations, how we proceed from uncertainty towards certainty.

Investigative Mentality and the Learning Process

The importance of observation, experiment, analysis, and inference in epidemiology is described in Chapter 2 and illustrated in all the chapters of this book. These are the formal processes in epidemiological disciplines[13,35] which, like all other Western sciences, rely upon formal logic for exposition on Hegelian lines, thus

Thesis ⟶ Antithesis ⟶ Synthesis.

The process of reasoning here depends upon conscious verbal thinking within an existing matrix or frame of reference. But there are situations in which the mechanism of learning may be less precise, especially when completely unfamiliar, innovative, or superficially illogical concepts arise. Whitehead[43] suggests that

Romance ⟶ Precision ⟶ Generalization,

culminating in a process whereby

Emotion ⟶ Logic ⟶ Philosophy.

Within these two contrasting concepts, there is room for more detail. Whitehead believes that new ideas develop ". . . predominantly through informal and unpremeditated talk." He believes in "the interspersed explanation" and distrusts formal approaches to teaching, learning, and above all to problematic questions. The investigation of a disease of unknown etiology falls squarely into this category, for it is a matter of historical record that discoveries leading to major advances in knowledge come less by orderly steps than by jumps or by thinking laterally[44] along previously separate frames of reference.[45] But this does not mean that we can leave our epidemiological explorations to initiation by chance or to bright ideas emerging from unstructured discussions, wonderful as these are when they happen. We have to look for new frames of reference sufficiently wide to accommodate salient input from the periphery and yet sufficiently small to keep the problem area demarcated.

To do this we might define Whitehead's interspersed, unpremeditated, or romantic idea simply as an imaginative observation, like Archimedes' bath water, Newton's apple, or Fleming's mold, wherein the essential quality is not chance alone but a chance occurrence presenting itself to a receptive and prepared mind.

The occurrence, the observation, and even the idea which follows are not, in themselves, enough to advance knowledge. In Whitehead's words,[43] "Ideas which are not utilized are positively harmful." What counts, as in other walks of life, is not the lucky strike but the follow-through.

Alternatively, the primer can be an abstract notion or empirical judgment—that the heart pumps blood, that cowpox might protect against smallpox, that inherited disorders differ from congenital ones, that germs might cause disease, that cigarette smoking might lead to cancer, that RNA might be the messenger carrying the code for protein synthesis. Again, the notion by itself is sterile unless it is followed up, and this is where the outcome depends almost entirely upon the diligence with which the systematic, structured surveillance, Hegelian dialectic, or experimental plan supersedes, yet accommodates, the unstructured primer and Socratic discussion—or, in other words, upon the transition from the romantic to the logical mechanism. Genius, to paraphrase Thomas Carlyle, is "10 percent inspiration and 90 percent perspiration," and this applies to all levels of ingenuity: "To innovate is not to reform," said Burke (1796) in a letter to a would-be reformer. We also in any experimental science have to register feedback, reevaluate our logic, and modify our plan accordingly, even if this means altering our hypothesis or, in Wertheimer's words,[46] approaching creativity by the "process of destroying one *gestalt* in favor of another."

We might therefore restate the stages of deliberate advance in knowledge on cybernetic lines (Fig. 14.1) so that the process be-

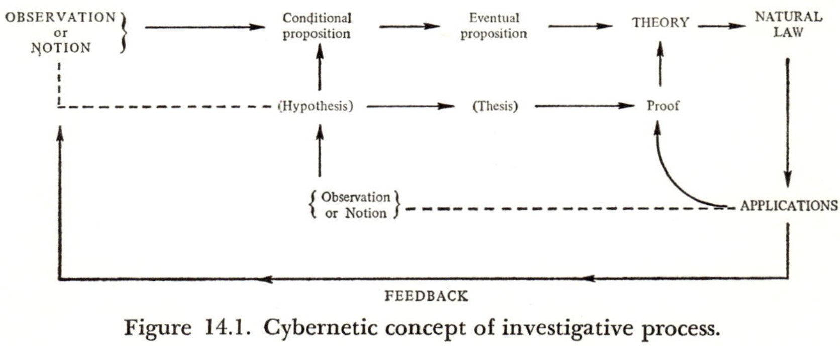

Figure 14.1. Cybernetic concept of investigative process.

comes cumulative and open-ended, unlike Hegelian learning and hypothesis testing. It then begins to harness the energy of personal experience, belief, and motivation. The romantic observation or notion is an instant cognizance of fact or possibility endowed with the dynamism of a first apprehension and with the vividness of novelty. Because it is unfettered by protocol or systematic procedure, it can be handled in various ways while plans for follow-up are developed. Then begins the systematic stage, in which speculation gives way to formal logic. Ideally, even the formal process preserves some of the initial thrill of exploration or "ideational excitement"[47] by setting its sights on the goal, whatever it is, before the field becomes filled with detail and procedure, i.e. with formulation, step-wise progression, and a limited capacity for admitting new notions. Success in surveillance and experiment depends not only upon achievement but also upon elaboration of a thesis which offers an intellectually satisfying explanation of the facts or, alternatively, upon rejection of a reasonable hypothesis. A good survey or a good experiment is one which is important even if the results are negative, as in the search for carcinogenicity of birth-control pills.

In epidemiological learning and research, the end is often unspectacular in that, one way or another, it was foreseen from the start: a given agent or factor is or is not concerned with a disease; health does or does not change as a result of some intervention, deliberate or accidental. Novelty usually comes at the beginning, with the notion or observation, not at the end as in synthetic chemistry and experimental physics. This makes epidemiology a hard discipline, for the sense of adventure, innovation, and creative outcome, which is an important part of investigative mentality, may be dispelled by the mechanism and prosaic outcome of the research itself. It has to be remembered, also, that most forms of secondary (i.e. systematic) learning are enormously inferior in tempo to natural (i.e. inquisitive, cognitive) learning: a child learns naturally to speak lucidly and effectively in five years or less but then takes ten years or more to learn grammar, composition, or another language much less effectively. This exemplifies the prime importance of the romantic and emotional components of learning, emphasized above, and makes the novitiate in epidemiology an important contributor to research, which can often be effectively included in the primary learning process (see Chaps. 2, 9, and 13). Expertise is needed in epidemiology less in the conduct than in the planning and analysis of research, which can proceed on disciplined lines which are laid down in standard works[13,14,34,35] but which must also allow for innovation in the scope no less than in the methods of the science.

Relevance of Data

There was a time when the collection of data or even of elementary facts was extremely difficult, and there are many domains, even in matters as critical as birth and death,[48] where the same is true today (p. 366). The census in the Domesday Book (1086) was unique, for nearly eight hundred years passed before Farr (1856) introduced vital statistics and a few denominators into health affairs. We are now in an age when mechanical methods make the compilation and processing of data and inventories on a large scale easy; hence the need for design, selection, and cerebration is greater.[49] There are few futilities more vulgar than the senseless compilation of data, yet because of the availability and lure of facilities this is increasingly a threat to the quality of epidemiological research because of its special dependence upon bulky data: the presentation of data untouched by human thought, the elaborate proof of the obvious, and the reiteration of knowledge already available are now as commonplace as they are wasteful.

In general, it may be said that knowledge is directional when it leads from uncertainty to a degree of certainty; information is the input relevant to the reduction of uncertainty in the given frame of reference. All other information, however interesting in itself, is redundant. In epidemiology, unlike the exact sciences, input is heterogeneous and evaluation therefore interdisciplinary. The task of defining relevance is correspondingly difficult: everything which a community does or possesses is conceivably relevant on the time axis to their health. As knowledge expands, it becomes necessary to look closely at interrelationships—for instance, between genetics and epidemiology, as in Chapter 3, or between behavior and disease or disability, as in Chapters 2 and 4. Knowledge is often restricted into artificial compartments by what Felix Frankfurter has called "the curse of departmentalization" and by the cultural irresponsibility inherent in excessive specialization,[50] but there is currently an equal danger of its being dispersed by excessive generalism and interdepartmentalization. Academic institutions usually draw a distinction between a department, which is an administrative entity, and a discipline, which has a scholastic meaning and demarcates convenient limits for the planning of investigative activities, including teaching, in interdisciplinary subjects like epidemiology. The task of correlating biological with behavioral, social, and environmental data is the unique but formidable challenge in epidemiology, demanding constant innovation in parametric and nonparametric methods so that, almost literally, chalk may be compared with cheese, hard water with atherosclerosis, occupational activity with peptic ulceration, lethargy with cardiac dysfunction, sexual behavior with precancerous change in the cervix uteri—all of these, and many others, with intermediate and additional variables, like genetic constitution, diet, hours of rest, occupation, and environment.

The lesson in these achievements and aims of epidemiology is not new, for it is historically a fact though still not widely realized that most of the major improvements in community health result from social rather than medical progress.[1] There are some notable exceptions to this rule, such as the introduction of specific therapeutic and prophylactic agents, like vitamins, antibiotics, hormones, and vaccines, and of improved diagnostic methods; but the fact remains. Opportunities for more extensive practical applications of new work, for example, in environmental improvement, genetic counseling, family planning, population study, child development, dental fitness, and physical fitness generally, are now present; diseases like the venereal infections and trachoma could be abolished: the necessary knowledge and technical resources are available, though techniques of application are still sadly underdeveloped. We know, for instance, that blindness due to trachoma is completely preventable if tetracycline eye ointment and elementary precautions against dust are made available to children in endemic zones; yet trachoma remains the commonest cause of blindness in many populous parts of the world. The answer here is simple epidemiologically but apparently difficult economically. In many other threats to health, none of the answers are simple: to control the new epidemic of venereal disease and drug abuse (Chaps. 9 and 12) in children and adolescents, we need to deal with a much wider range of factors in homes, news media, schools, and streets and somehow to include as potent determinants, also, factors beyond the normal competence of the health professional, such as bribery, intimidation, prostitution, gang influence, pushing, and organized crime. Point-by-point assessment of these imponderables is impossible, for the situation changes monthly. The only solution is to seek cooperation where it can be found and apply our elementary knowledge to multi-factor control: these epidemics in our cities today will be contained, not by other drugs or by group therapy, but by planned cooperation among parents, children, schoolteachers, police, interested citizens, and legislators to increase awareness and to arouse the emotional drives of compassion and concern which originate discovery (p. 573) and never fail to move society. In recognizing this opportunity, we have to recognize also some contemporary gaps, gaps which can be filled only if administrative, political, and economic impediments are pulled—or dragged—into the arena of health affairs and out again to clear the ground for more urgent and purposeful action.

The other gap—though in many ways it is an extension of the same gap—is the void of knowledge about and professional commitment to health as a quality of life. Despite great and growing public and political concern for welfare and civil rights of all communities, there is a pathetic, sometimes tragic indifference to realistic parameters and logistics. Longevity has become not an extension of life but a postponement of death; fecundity has become a menace; over-the-counter abortion is the latest medical response to consumer demand; freedom has become a license to destroy, a threat to itself and an ally of anarchy; while, at the other extreme, rigid attitudes and bureaucracy are strangling the causes which they are trying to champion in the delivery of health care. The real maladies of the age—morbid aggression, alienation, self-destruction, environmental squalor, educational deprivation —are largely ignored, while the end results pile up to consume health and welfare services. These and many other inconsistencies in health-related activities are often regarded as political and, therefore, outside the province of the health professional; but they are, in reality, inseparable from what is, or should be, the common goal: improved health in the community and the adequate provision of preventive care for all whose health is indifferent or threatened.

Lastly, if quality of life be the essential character of the common goal, there are questions of values, of morals, of beliefs which cannot be considered except philosophically. There is danger in the health professional's assuming that he has any rights or superior knowledge in this part of the frontier, but he has immense responsibilities,[50-52] the main one being to ensure that such questions are not ignored and that the health, whether of an individual or a community, will never become a matter for mechanistic, impersonal, and therefore inhuman debate or decision.

In this book, trends in epidemiology are presented as contributions to human culture no less than to technical progress in the assessment of health problems and delivery of health care, which are the ultimate responsibilities of all health professionals. Disease and illness are part of human history but they are not otherwise interesting except insofar as they can be prevented, ameliorated, or cured.

REFERENCES

1. Sigerist, H.J. *On the Sociology of Medicine*. New York, MD Publications, 1960.
2. Levi-Strauss, C. *Structural Anthropology*. New York, Doubleday Anchor, 1967.
3. Huntley, R.R. *Inquiry, 7*:15, 1970.
4. Nixon, Richard M. As reported in the *New York Times,* Feb. 19, 1971.
5. Kennedy, E.M. Health security for America. In *Proceedings and Debates of the 92d Congress,* first session, Jan. 25, 1971.
6. *Amer. Med. Ass. News,* Mar. 1, 1971.
7. *New Eng. J. Med., 284*:241, 1971.

8. Health is a community affair. In *Report of the National Committee on Community Health Services*. Cambridge, Mass., Harvard University Press, 1967.
9. Kass, E.H. (Ed.) *Preventive Approaches to Chronic Diseases. Millbank Mem. Fund Quart. 47,* (No. 3) 1969.
10. Susser, M.W., and Watson, W. *Sociology in Medicine*. London, New York, and Toronto, Oxford University Press, 1962.
11. *The Manchester Guardian Weekly,* Dec. 17, 1970.
12. Stewart, G.T. *Lancet, 2:*115, 1970.
13. MacMahon, B., Pugh, T. F., and Ipsen, J. *Epidemiologic Methods*. Boston and Toronto, Little, Brown & Co., 1960.
14. Lillienfeld, A.M., Peterson, E., and Dowd, J. E. *Cancer Epidemiology: Methods of Study*. Baltimore, Johns Hopkins Press, 1967.
15. Stocks, P. *Brit. J. Cancer, 6:*99, 1952.
16. Doll, R., and Hill, A.B. *Brit. Med. J., 1:*1399, 1964.
17. Washington, D. C., Public Health Service Publication No. 1103, 1964.
18. Wilson, J.M.G., and Jungner, G. *Principles and Practices of Screening for Disease*. Geneva, World Health Organization, 1968.
19. Bretonneau, P. *Des Inflammations Speciales*. Paris, 1826.
20. Stewart, G.T. *Lancet, 1:*1077, 1968.
21. *Control of Lead Poisoning in Children*. Washington, D.C. U.S. Dep't of Health, Education, and Welfare, Dec. 1970.
22. *Sci. Amer., 224:*15, 1971.
23. *Wall Street Journal,* Mar. 26, 1970.
24. Mackintosh, D.R. *J. Environ. Health, 32:*292, 1969.
25. *Wall Street Journal,* Mar. 17 and Sept. 30, 1970.
26. *Scientist and Citizen*. St. Louis, Mo., Committee for Environmental Information, 1968, vol. 10.
27. *Facts about Lead and Pediatrics*. New York, Lead Industries Assoc., Inc., 1969.
28. Jacobziner, H. *Clin. Pediat. (Phila.), 5:*277, 1966.
29. *New York Times,* May 12, 1970.
30. *The Nation's Health*. New York, American Public Health Ass'n., 1971.
31. Tsuchiya, K. *Keio J. Med., 18:*181, 1969.
32. Friberg, L. *Arch. Ind. Health, 20:*401, 1959.
33. *Morbidity and Mortality, 19,* 26. Atlanta, Nat'l. Comm. Dis. Center, 1970.
34. Morris, J.N. *Uses of Epidemiology,* 2nd ed. Baltimore, Williams & Wilkins Co., 1964.
35. Fox, J.P., Hall, Carrie E., and Elveback, Lila R. *Epidemiology: Man and Disease*. London, Macmillan, 1970.
36. Hodgson, T.A. *Environ. Sci. Technol., 4:*589, 1970.
37. Martin, A.E. *Urban Studies, 4:*1, 1967.
38. Mechanic, D. *Medical Sociology*. New York, Free Press, 1968.

39. Stockwell, E.G. *Amer. J. Public Health, 53*:956, 1960.
40. Gardner, M.J., Crawford, M.D., and Morris, J.N. *Brit. J. Prev. Soc. Med., 23*:133, 1969.
41. Holland, W.W., Halil, T., and Bennet, A.E. *Brit. Med. J., 2*:205, 1969.
42. Erhardt, C.L., Abramson, H., Pakter, J., and Nelson, F. *Arch. Environ. Health, 20*:743, 1970.
43. Whitehead, A.N. *The Aims of Education*. New York, Macmillan, 1959.
44. De Bono, E. *New Think: The Use of Lateral Thinking in the Generation of New Ideas*. New York, Basic Books, 1968.
45. Koestler, A. *The Ghost in the Machine*. New York, Macmillan, 1967.
46. Wertheimer, A. Quoted by Gerard, R.W. In Ghiseln, G. (Ed.) *The Creative Process*. New York and Toronto, New American Library, 1952, p. 231.
47. James, W. *Textbook of Psychology*. London, Macmillan, 1930.
48. Heasman, M.A., and Lipworth, L. *Studies on Medical and Population Subjects, No. 20: Accuracy of Certification of Cause of Death*. London, H.M., Stationery Office, 1966.
49. *Inquiry, 7*:3-50, 1970.
50. Bruher, J.G. *J. Med. Educ., 46*:166, 1971.
51. Tabershaw, I. *Arch. Environ. Health, 18*:811, 1969.
52. Gardner, J.W. *No Easy Victories*. New York, Harper & Row, 1968.

INDEX

D

N

O

P